Hyperactivity and attention disorders of childhood

Second edition

Edited by

Seija Sandberg

Royal Free and University College Medical School, London

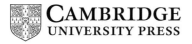

CAMBRIDGE
UNIVERSITY PRESS

PUBLISHED BY THE PRESS SYNDICATE OF THE UNIVERSITY OF CAMBRIDGE
The Pitt Building, Trumpington Street, Cambridge, United Kingdom

CAMBRIDGE UNIVERSITY PRESS
The Edinburgh Building, Cambridge CB2 2RU, UK
40 West 20th Street, New York, NY 10011-4211, USA
477 Williamstown Road, Port Melbourne, VIC 3207, Australia
Ruiz de Alarcón 13, 28014 Madrid, Spain
Dock House, The Waterfront, Cape Town 8001, South Africa

http://www.cambridge.org

First published 1996
Second edition 2002

Printed in the United Kingdom at the University Press, Cambridge

Typeface Dante MT 11/14pt   *System* Poltype® [V N]

A catalogue record for this book is available from the British Library

Library of Congress Cataloguing in Publication data

Hyperactivity and attention disorders of childhood / edited by Seija Sandberg. – 2nd ed.
      p.   cm. – (Cambridge child and adolescent psychiatry)
Rev. ed. of: Hyperactivity disorders of childhood / edited by Seija Sandberg. 1996.
Includes bibliographical references and index.
ISBN 0 521 78961 3 (PB)
1. Attention-deficit hyperactivity disorder.   I. Sandberg, Seija.   II. Hyperactivity disorders of
childhood.   III. Cambridge child and adolescent psychiatry series.
[DNLM: 1. Attention Deficit Disorder with Hyperactivity – Child. WS 350.8.A8 H998 2002]
RJ506.H9 H97 2002
618.92'8589 – dc21   2001043388

ISBN 0 521 78961 3 paperback

Every effort has been made in preparing this book to provide accurate and up-to-date information which is
in accord with accepted standards and practice at the time of publication. Nevertheless, the authors, editors
and publisher can make no warranties that the information contained herein is totally free from error, not
least because clinical standards are constantly changing through research and regulation. The authors,
editors and publisher therefore disclaim all liability for direct or consequential damages resulting from the
use of material contained in this book. Readers are strongly advised to pay careful attention to information
provided by the manufacturer of any drugs or equipment that they plan to use.

Hyperactivity and attention disorders of childhood

Building on the success of the first edition and addressing the advances in the field since its publication, Seija Sandberg has brought together a distinguished international team to review the area of attention deficit and hyperactivity disorders (ADHD) in children and young adults.

This new edition is thoroughly revised and updated. Some chapters, such as those dealing with the genetic background and the adult form of the disorder, are completely new. And some of the areas dealt with in the first edition are being covered by new authors in the second. The writers are among the world's leading experts, both researchers and clinicians, in the area. This will be essential reading for all professionals involved in the management and care of people with ADHD.

From reviews of the first edition:

'Presents an extremely informative and readable discussion of hyperactivity and the critical facets of the disparity between Europe and North America in the approach to attention-deficit-hyperactivity disorder . . . It should be particularly valuable for trainees in pediatrics, psychiatry, and neurology who treat attention deficits in children.'
New England Journal of Medicine

'It would be a good one to keep in a department, as a source of information for practice and teaching. Trying to understand the underlying mechanisms is engrossing and Sandberg's book contributes to our attempts to unravel fundamental aspects of human behaviour.'
Journal of the Royal Society of Medicine

Cambridge Child and Adolescent Psychiatry

Child and adolescent psychiatry is an important and growing area of clinical psychiatry. The last decade has seen a rapid expansion of scientific knowledge in this field and has provided a new understanding of the underlying pathology of mental disorders in these age groups. This series is aimed at practitioners and researchers both in child and adolescent mental health services and developmental and clinical neuroscience. Focusing on psychopathology, it highlights those topics where the growth of knowledge has had the greatest impact on clinical practice and on the treatment and understanding of mental illness. Individual volumes benefit both from the international expertise of their contributors and a coherence generated through a uniform style and structure for the series. Each volume provides firstly an historical overview and a clear descriptive account of the psychopathology of a specific disorder or group of related disorders. These features then form the basis for a thorough critical review of the etiology, natural history, management, prevention and impact on later adult adjustment. Whilst each volume is therefore complete in its own right, volumes also relate to each other to create a flexible and collectable series that should appeal to students as well as experienced scientists and practitioners.

Editorial board

Series editor   Professor Ian M. Goodyer   *University of Cambridge*

Associate editors

Professor Donald J. Cohen
Yale Child Study Center

Dr Robert N. Goodman
Institute of Psychiatry, London

Professor Barry Nurcombe
The University of Queensland

Professor Dr Helmut Remschmidt
Klinikum der Philipps-Universität, Germany

Professor Dr Herman van Engeland
Academisch Ziekenhuis Utrecht

Dr Fred R. Volkmar
Yale Child Study Center

Already published in this series:

Outcomes in Neurodevelopmental and Genetic Disorders edited by Patricia Howlin 0 521 79721 7 PB

Practical Child and Adolescent Psychopharmacology edited by Stan Kutcher 0 521 65542 0 PB

Specific Learning Disabilities and Difficulties in Children and Adolescents: Psychological Assessment and Evaluation edited by Alan and Nadeen Kaufman 0 521 65840 3 PB

Psychotherapy with Children and Adolescents edited by Helmut Remschmidt 0 521 77558 2 PB

The Depressed Child and Adolescent second edition edited by Ian M. Goodyer 0 521 79426 9 PB

Schizophrenia in Children and Adolescents edited by Helmut Remschmidt 0 521 79428 5 PB

Anxiety Disorders in Children and Adolescents: Research, Assessment and Intervention edited by Wendy Silverman and Philip Treffers 0 521 78966 4 PB

Conduct Disorders in Childhood and Adolescence edited by Jonathan Hill and Barbara Maughan 0 521 78639 8 PB

Autism and Pervasive Developmental Disorders edited by Fred R. Volkmar 0 521 55386 5 HB

Cognitive Behaviour Therapy for Children and Families edited by Philip Graham 0 521 57252 5 HB 0 521 57626 1 PB

Hyperactivity Disorders of Childhood edited by Seija Sandberg 0 521 43250 2 HB

Contents

Contributors

Joanne Barton
Department of Child and Adolescent
Psychiatry
University of Glasgow
Caledonia House
Royal Hospital for Sick Children
Yorkhill
Glasgow G3 8SJ, UK

Jan K. Buitelaar
Division of Child and Adolescent Psychiatry
University Medical Center Utrecht, B.01.324
PO Box 85500
3508 GA Utrecht
The Netherlands

F. Xavier Castellanos
ADHD Research Unit
Child Psychiatry Branch
National Institute of Mental Health
10 Center Drive (Building 10), Room 3B-19
Bethesda, MD 20892-1251
USA

Erika Hagemann
School of Psychology
Curtin University of Technology
GPO Box U 1987
Perth
Western Australia

David A. Hay
School of Psychology
Curtin University of Technology
GPO Box U 1987
Perth 6845
Western Australia

Ellen Heptinstall
Department of Child and Adolescent
Psychiatry
Institute of Psychiatry
De Crespigny Park
London SE5 8AF, UK

Ting-Pong Ho
Department of Psychiatry
University of Hong Kong
Queen Mary Hospital
Pokfulam
Hong Kong

Peter S. Jensen
and the MTA Group
Columbia and New York City University
1051 Riverside Drive, no. 78
New York, NY 10032
USA

Jana Kreppner
Institute of Psychiatry
De Crespigny Park
Denmark Hill
London SE5 8AF, UK

Patrick W. L. Leung
Department of Psychology
The Chinese University of Hong Kong
Shatin, New Territories
Hong Kong

Florence Levy
School of Psychiatry
University of New South Wales
Sydney, NSW
Australia

Ernest S. L. Luk
Maroondah Hospital
Child and Adolescent Mental Health Service
Wundeela Centre
21 Ware Crescent
Ringwood East
Victoria 3135
Australia

Sheryl Olson
Department of Psychology
The University of Michigan
525 E. University
Ann Arbor, MI 48109-1109
USA

Soo Hyun Rhee
Department of Psychology
Emory University
532 N. Kilgo Circle
Atlanta, GA 30322
USA

Penny Roy
Social, Genetic and Developmental
Psychiatry Research Centre
Institute of Psychiatry
De Crespigny Park
Denmark Hill
London SE5 8AF, UK

Michael Rutter
Social, Genetic and Developmental
Psychiatry Research Centre
Institute of Psychiatry
De Crespigny Park
Denmark Hill
London SE5 8AF, UK

Seija Sandberg
Department of Psychiatry and Behavioural
Sciences
Royal Free and University College Medical
School
Wolfson Building
48 Riding House Street
London W1N 8AA, UK

Russell Schachar
Department of Child Psychiatry
University of Toronto
The Hospital for Sick Children
555 University Avenue
Toronto
Canada M5G 1X8

Joseph A. Segeant
Klinische Neuropsychologie
De Boelelaan 1109
1081 HV Amsterdam
The Netherlands

James Swanson
UCI Child Develoment Center
University of California, Irvine
19262 Jamboree
Irvine, CA 92715
USA

Eric Taylor
Department of Child and Adolescent
Psychiatry
Institute of Psychiatry
De Crespigny Park
London SE5 8AF, UK

Brian Toone
Department of Psychological Medicine
King's College Hospital
Denmark Hill
London SE5 9RS, UK

Jaap J. Van der Meere
Laboratory of Experimental Clinical
Psychology
University of Groningen
Grote Kruisstraat 2/1
9712 TS Groningen
The Netherlands

Irwin D. Waldman
Department of Psychology
Emory University
532 N. Kilgo Circle
Atlanta, GA 30322
USA

Preface

Hyperactivity is still sometimes portrayed as an arbitrary, unreliable and even invalid diagnostic entity that adds nothing to, or even obscures, our understanding of disruptive behaviour disorders in children. The evidence, however, supports a different view. The diagnosis, based as it has been largely on clinical observation and consensus, has proven useful for clinical practice and science. The studies performed in the past decade indicate a prevalence of between 5 and 10%, with the higher rate mostly found among primary school-age boys. Lower figures have been reported for girls, preschoolers and adolescents. The disorder shows a high degree of persistence over time, and a substantial comorbidity with learning problems, oppositional/conduct disorders, depression and anxiety disorders.

This second edition not only presents thoroughly updated reviews of the topics covered in the first edition, but also ventures into new fields such as genetics, the effects of early institutional rearing and the adult form of the disorder. As was the case first time round, a group of internationally renowned experts and leading researchers in the fields of psychology, psychiatry and brain sciences have been brought together to present a multifaceted but interlocking account of the condition.

Despite recent attempts at harmonization, differences in diagnostic practice continue to influence the prevalence of the disorder, resulting in 10- or even 100-fold differences being quoted between the USA and the UK, for example. Including or excluding coexisting disorders and preference for a categorical over a quantitative approach are some of the reasons for this. However, as the criteria in both were developed with school-age boys in mind, they share a continuing ambiguity as to whether and how they should be adjusted when applied to very young children, girls, adolescents and adults.

Indeed, until quite recently, the literature may have given the impression that hyperactivity was solely a problem of male children, as study after study concentrated on boys only. The strategy was justified to a point. Male predominance is a consistent finding, with girls appearing to be protected against the development of hyperactivity. However, it is now acknowledged that, once their symptoms reach the threshold of caseness, girls exhibit behaviour that is similar to that of boys, while clear differences exist regarding the forms of social maladjustment in teenage years, for example.

The study of cultural influences on the expression of childhood psychiatric disorders is another relatively recent development. The studies that have so far been carried out have shown that, even in disorders with a strong biological basis such as hyperactivity, cultural influences nevertheless exert an impact on how individuals and their families experience, interpret and respond to the disorder, and on how society responds to the individual's behaviour.

Many attempts have been made to validate the clinical concept of hyperactivity in the laboratory. Given that the manifestation of its primary symptoms largely depends on the type of environment in which the child is observed, the laboratory approach also has its limitations. The somewhat unexpected finding from laboratory studies has been that children with attention deficit, as defined by behavioural descriptions by parents, teachers and clinicians, are not deficient in their basic attentional abilities, but that their task efficiency is highly sensitive to state manipulations. Clinicians may therefore be presenting parents and teachers with the wrong questions, and the parents may be accurate when they report that the child's symptoms show themselves especially in boring conditions, but practically disappear when the child is truly interested in what he or she is doing, or is motivated by the task.

The situation regarding cognition and learning is more complex than at the time of the first edition. This is partly due to the introduction of subtypes of the disorder, and to the increasing rate of diagnosis of attention problems in children who in the past might have ended up as 'controls'. Hence, the questions have changed from which cognitive problems occur in children with attention disorders to which problems occur in which particular attention disorders. The question of the heterogeneity of attention problems has become a key issue. There is also new evidence suggesting that hyperactivity, language learning disability and reading disorder share a common inherited aetiological component.

Family, adoption and twin studies allow several general conclusions to be drawn about the aetiology of hyperactivity and attention disorders. The most important of these is that the symptoms are highly heritable. Molecular genetic studies have to date concentrated mainly on the candidate genes in the dopamine system. Recent studies also provide converging evidence that the phenotype of hyperactivity/inattention is characterized by neuropsychological deficits in executive functions and reduced size of neuroanatomical regions in the frontal lobes, basal ganglia and cerebellum. Primary genetic factors are proposed to have their strongest direct effects on the development and function of the cerebellum, thus leading to dysregulated neurotransmission in childhood and adolescence, and to deficient neuronal networks in adulthood. The fact that medications, such as stimulants, temporarily improve the dysregulated systems is consistent with the model of the underlying deficit.

The role of early caregiving in the development of hyperactivity is likely to be more significant than was previously assumed. Evidence for this comes from recent attachment research, and from studies incorporating attachment constructs with wider socioecological influences, broader patterns of family relationships, biological influences on parent–child relationships and psychosocial contributions to brain biology. Thus, there clearly seem to be multiple pathways to hyperactivity, and to its later outcomes. Furthermore, risk factors associated with negative outcomes appear to be additive within developmental periods and cumulative across time.

Psychosocial factors likely to have causal importance for hyperactivity and attention disorders include maternal depression and negative parent–child interaction. As these factors often occur together with other psychosocial adversity, the mechanisms by which they lead to hyperactivity may vary from case to case. New in this area of research are studies showing that experiences can determine brain growth, or cause organic brain pathology, especially when impacting on very young immature brains. Furthermore, important interconnections appear to exist between genetic and environmental influences on behaviour and cognition. Studies of Romanian child adoptees also suggest that an institutional rearing in early years predisposes to a pattern of inattention and hyperactivity, often associated with a lack of specificity in selective attachments and a lack of social boundaries, as reflected in an undue friendliness with strangers.

Despite decades of research on treatment, few controlled studies have examined the effectiveness of long-term treatments. The reported (MTA) study exceeds other studies of child treatment in size, scope and length. The findings indicate that long-term treatments involving systematic frequent medication management with parent guidance greatly reduce children's symptoms of hyperactivity, oppositional-aggressive behaviours and anxiety, while also enhancing other areas of functioning. In certain circumstances, however, psychosocial treatments offer a definite advantage over medication.

The recognition that hyperactivity and inattention symptoms may persist into adulthood is a recent development. Many authorities, however, continue to question the very existence of the disorder in adults, and there are keen debates about its prevalence and indications for pharmacological treatment. Future studies need to address these issues using population-based samples, preferably taking as their starting point the longitudinal studies of childhood cohorts, and employing uniform standardized diagnostic procedures. More also needs to be known about the consequences of the remitted syndrome for subsequent personality and cognitive development, and for social and occupational adjustment.

Seija Sandberg

1

Historical development

Seija Sandberg[1] and Joanne Barton[2]

[1]Department of Psychiatry and Behavioural Sciences, Royal Free and University College Medical School, London, UK
[2]Department of Child and Adolescent Psychiatry, University of Glasgow, Glasgow, Scotland, UK

Introduction

The constellation of overactivity, poor impulse control and inattention has been given a variety of diagnostic labels over the years. Although at present attention deficit hyperactivity disorder and hyperkinetic disorder are popular diagnoses, they are relative newcomers in the diagnostic classification of child psychiatry. For example, even the latest (1957) edition of the child psychiatry textbook by Kanner contained no reference to hyperactivity as a diagnostic entity. The same applied to the 1969 edition of a widely used text on child psychology by Johnson and Medinnus (1969), with even the term 'attention span' only mentioned on two of the total of 657 pages. A well-regarded textbook on experimental child psychology (Reese and Lipsitt, 1970) did include a section on attention processes, but without any reference to attention deficit hyperactivity disorder. Yet evidence of attention psychology going back at least to the latter half of the nineteenth century has been well documented (James, 1890; Spearman, 1937). On the European continent, however, the condition was recognized and referred to as 'hyperkinetic disorder' in Hoff's (1956) major textbook of general psychiatry. So, whilst hyperactivity tends to be thought of as a particularly American phenomenon, the history of the use of the term tells us otherwise. Though new as a diagnostic entity, hyperactive behaviour in children has been detected and treated for much longer. Indeed, the diagnosis of 'dextro-amphetamine response disorder' was in common use in the former German Democratic Republic (DDR: Göllnitz, 1981).

The current conceptualization of the disorder represents a stage in a complex and varying developmental history, and therefore in order to appreciate our present perspective it is important to consider the chronological course in the unfolding of the concept itself. In this chapter, an overview of the history of hyperactivity and attention disorders will be presented, especially as they have appeared in the western texts. Relatively more attention will also be given to publications up to the 1960s, after which time studies on the condition began to mushroom. This revised version contains some modifications and additions to the text of the first edition.

References to behavioural disturbance in childhood of a similar nature to that seen in hyperactivity disorders can be found in the writings of Hoffmann (1845), Maudsley (1867), Clouston (1899), Ireland (1877) and others from the middle of the 1800s. However, the earliest clear descriptions of the disorder are those by Still and Tredgold in the early 1900s. Their work will be discussed and examined in the context of the prevailing social and scientific climate. Both authors presented their analysis of the behavioural characteristics of a relatively small group of children, some of whom bear close resemblance to the hyperactive children of today. Still (1902) attributed such behaviour to a 'defect of moral control', believing it to be a biological defect, which was inherited or resulted from some pre- or postnatal injury. His ideas about causation are best understood in the context of the widespread support given at that time to social Darwinism.

The theory of damage occurring in the early stages of the individual's development, though often mild and undetected, was adopted by Tredgold (1908); and at a later stage by others, such as Pasamanick et al. (1956a), as an attempt to explain the behavioural problems seen in hyperkinetic children. The encephalitis epidemic in 1917–18 played a significant part in the history of hyperactivity. Following the epidemic, clinicians were confronted with children suffering from behavioural and cognitive sequelae, many presenting with the core features of what would today be termed hyperactivity.

For the first half of the twentieth century, the predominant view regarding the causation of hyperactivity was that of an association with brain damage. A plethora of terms such as 'organic drivenness' and 'minimal brain damage' were used to describe the disorder. During this period, the similarity between the behaviour of hyperactive children and that of primates subjected to frontal lobe lesions was noted. This was used by several investigators to support the idea that hyperkinetic disorders were due to defects in forebrain structures, despite the lack of evidence of such lesions in many children.

During the fourth and the fifth decades of the last century, a series of papers were published which marked the beginnings of child psychopharmacology in general, and the pharmacotherapy of behaviourally disturbed children in particular. By the end of the 1950s, the concept that brain damage was the single important factor in the development of hyperkinesis was challenged. 'Minimal brain dysfunction' was substituted for 'minimal brain damage'. At the time, a variety of hypotheses were put forward regarding the causation of hyperactivity, including the psychoanalytic theory of poor parenting. With the decline of the concept of 'minimal brain dysfunction', the idea of the 'hyperactive child syndrome' was being developed, with Stella Chess (Chess, 1960) as one of its chief proponents. Chess differed from her predecessors in that she viewed the prognosis of hyperactive children as reasonably good, with the condition having resolved by puberty in most cases. By the end of the 1960s the prevailing view was that hyperkinesis represented a form of brain dysfunction, and presented with a variety of symptoms, of which motor overactivity was the most predominant.

It was during the 1960s that the split developed between Europe and North America over the conceptualization of hyperkinesis. Clinicians in Europe maintained a narrower view of the disorder, seeing it as a rare syndrome of excessive motor activity, usually occurring in conjunction with some signs of brain damage. In North America, on the other hand, hyperactivity was seen as being relatively common, and in most cases not necessarily associated with overt signs of brain damage. The differences became highlighted in the diagnostic classificatory systems used (*International Classification of Disease* (ICD); World Health Organization, 1992 and *Diagnostic and Statistical Manual of Mental Disorders* (DSM: American Psychiatric Association, 1980), respectively).

In the 1970s, the emphasis moved away from motor overactivity and began to focus on the attentional aspects of the disorder. A number of authors demonstrated that hyperactive children had great difficulty with tasks involving sustained attention. At the same time, there was also a growing belief that hyperkinetic behaviour was due to environmental causes. This coincided with a move towards a healthier lifestyle and disquiet about the 'drugging' of schoolchildren. The idea that hyperactivity was, at least in every other case, due to an allergic reaction to food substances, particularly food additives, became popular at this time. Technological advance and other cultural influences were also put forward as causative factors. An additional development of the decade was the increase in the number of studies investigating the psychophysiology of hyperactivity.

During the 1980s the explosion of research in the field continued. With this came the development of research criteria and standardized assessment procedures. Advancements were also made in the area of treatment, with new methods involving cognitive-behavioural therapies. Hyperactivity came to be seen as a condition with a strong hereditary component, chronic in nature and causing significant handicap in the areas of academic achievement and socialization; treatment required the complementary skills of a variety of professionals.

Throughout the 1990s hyperactivity and attention disorders continued to generate more research literature than any other child psychiatric disorder. The breadth and range of the subject matter of this literature are enormous and encompass research into the genetics and neurobiological bases of hyperactivity, together with studies examining the relative efficacy of different treatment methods. The 1990s also saw the development of management guidelines, including the European Society for Child and Adolescent Psychiatry guidelines (Taylor et al., 1998), and the American Academy of Child and Adolescent Psychiatry practice parameters (Dulcan, 1997), in an attempt to facilitate standardization in practice. These guidelines emphasize the importance of individualized, multimodal, multidisciplinary assessment and treatment of hyperactivity and attention disorders by practitioners experienced in the field. Increasingly, it is also recognized that these disorders can and do persist through adolescence and into adulthood. Hence, the past decade has also seen a surge of interest in their presentation and treatment in adults.

Early medical explanations

The modern history of hyperactivity disorders is traditionally seen to begin with the writings of Sir George Frederick Still (1902) and Alfred F. Tredgold (1908), with many authors acknowledging that our present concept of hyperactivity has its foundation in their work (Ross and Ross, 1982). Preceding the studies by Still and Tredgold, extensive descriptions of hyperkinetic children, mostly in the form of individual case studies, had already appeared in the psychiatric literature of the nineteenth century (Hoffmann, 1845; Maudsley, 1867; Ireland, 1877; Bourneville, 1897; Clouston, 1899) and continued to be published in the early decades of the twentieth century (Pick, 1904; Boncour and Boncour, 1905; Scholz, 1911; Heuyer, 1914).

Overexcitability and mental explosiveness: forerunners of hyperactivity?

Clouston (1899) described a series of very difficult morbid conditions that 'occur in neurotic children, but lie on the borderland of psychiatry'. He hypothesized that the disorders were all due to some dysfunction in the 'brain cortex', and were pathogenically 'states of deranged reactiveness of the neurones of the higher regions of the brain'. The derangement had arisen because the higher centres of the brain, responsible for inhibiting activity, had in some way been weakened and therefore become unable to cope with the amount of 'energising they have to control'.

Clouston, however, emphasized that such disorders should not be classified as 'out and out mental disorders'. He believed that the conditions were ultimately caused by 'hereditary and congenital peculiarities', with defects in the 'subtle and obscure process of central nerve development in childhood' acting as predisposing agents. He further postulated that certain areas of the brain 'running ahead' in their development, compared to others, were causing the derangement of its function. This in turn caused 'explosions which spread into other centres'.

A series of morbidities was outlined which, as Clouston proposed, all resulted from the same pathology; one of these resembles the attention deficit hyperactivity disorder of today. He called it 'simple hyperexcitability', arguing that the disorder resulted from 'undue brain reactiveness to mental and emotional stimuli'. It affected children from the age of 3 years until puberty, with overactivity and restlessness being the main symptoms. The disorder came in bursts and lasted from a few months to years. During the bursts the child would grow thin, not sleep and deteriorate in educational performance. Such clinical signs were ascribed to the children showing a 'delirium of pleasure in response to nice things', and interpreted as an exaggeration of the response one would expect from a child of nervous temperament.

The common feature of such disorders, according to Clouston, was the 'explosive condition of the nerve cells in the higher cortex'. In his view this was comparable to the overactivity of the motor cortex seen in persons suffering from epilepsy. Referring to the by then well-established findings that the process of brain development in childhood comprises rapid cell multiplication accompanied by the cells gradually becoming more stable, he argued that in the children suffering from 'hyperexcitability' this process of nerve stability does not occur, resulting in the children growing up with 'irregular explosive tendencies'.

The recommended treatment for such conditions was the use of bromides, 'fearlessly in large doses up to the point when symptoms of bromism are beginning to show themselves'. Clouston did, however, emphasize that the drugs should not be used in isolation. Instead, the children should at the same time be given a good diet, plenty of fresh air, 'suitable amusement, companionship and employment'. The aim of the treatment was to 'reduce the cell catabolism and the reactiveness of the cerebral cortex whilst not interfering with brain anabolism'. The treatment had to be carefully monitored in order to ensure that it did not 'go too far'.

Still and the defect of moral control

The first clear, systematic accounts of hyperactivity are attributed to Sir George Frederick Still (1868–1941), a paediatrician and the first professor of children's diseases at King's College Hospital, London. Professor Still is, however, most notable for his description of chronic rheumatoid arthritis in children, commonly known as Still's disease. In 1902, Still presented the Cloustonian lectures to the Royal College of Physicians describing the case histories of 20 children, whose presentation was similar to what we at present would call hyperactivity. In his descriptions, features such as extreme restlessness and 'almost choreiform' movements were frequently mentioned. Another common characteristic was that of 'an abnormal incapacity for sustained attention', causing school failure even despite normal intellect. In their behaviour, many of the children were mischievous, destructive and violent, and appeared not to respond to punishment.

According to Still, this pattern occurred more often in boys than in girls, became frequently apparent by early school years, was sometimes accompanied by peculiarities of physical appearance (e.g. epicanthic folds and high-arched palate), seemed often to be a function of temperament, generally showed little relationship to the child's training and home environment, and commonly shared a poor prognosis. Thus, Still described many of the characteristics and associations we recognize today. Still suggested that the children he was describing suffered from a 'defect of moral control', whereby they demonstrated 'the reckless disregard for command and authority in spite of such training and discipline as experience shows will render a healthy child law-abiding'. Instead, such children displayed 'immediate gratification of self without regard either to the good of others or to the larger and more remote good of self'. Still also noted that, although many of the children with this condition came from chaotic families, a substantial proportion of them lived in homes where they appeared to receive an adequate upbringing. In fact, when refining his criteria for children with the disease, Still decided to exclude those who had been exposed to poor child-rearing. This led him to hypothesize that the 'defect of moral control' was due to some 'morbid physical condition', which was either inherited or resulted from a perinatal or postnatal injury.

The degree of uncertainty about the causation of the condition provided a logical basis for separating the children with such problems into subgroups. Still proposed a distinction between children with demonstrable gross lesions of the brain; those with a variety of acute diseases, conditions and injuries that would be expected to result in brain damage, although none could be demonstrated; and those with hyperactive behaviours that could not be attributed to any known cause. Thereby, Still laid the groundwork for the historical equivalents of three major diagnostic categories of brain damage, minimal brain dysfunction and hyperactivity. In doing this, he also sowed the seeds for a terminological confusion so prevalent in the literature of hyperactivity over decades to come, but confusion that also gave the impetus for much excellent research on the nature of hyperactivity and its treatment.

Still's theories about his patients are best understood in the context of the prevailing socioeconomic and scientific climate. During the nineteenth century the UK underwent significant economic, political and social change. The economy became increasingly centred on factories in small towns, moving away from farming and the land. Unemployment was common and those in employment often worked long hours and were poorly paid. A distinct class hierarchy dominated society, with the lower classes being perceived as immoral and inferior (Rowntree, 1901). Considerable adversity afflicted the lower classes as a result of the socioeconomic changes and this was reflected in rising infant mortality, poor physical health in general, and learning difficulties and delinquency in children. However, the intellectual and moral deficiencies of the lower classes tended to be identified as the cause, rather than the consequence, of their circumstances.

Concurrent with these developments was the rise of positivism in contemporary science, with beliefs that the progress of society could be achieved through the development of objective science. It was especially the theories of Darwin that provided a scientific rationale for various kinds of social deviance, with hypotheses suggesting that the environment conferred a selective advantage to some types of biological variation (Darwin, 1859). Deduced from his theories, the notion for the 'survival of the fittest' became elevated to the status of a 'law', in an attempt to explain social phenomena. Likewise, poor health could easily be viewed as a form of inherited weakness and inferiority. This social Darwinism soon found wide support among intellectuals and social reformers.

In keeping with the prevailing trend of his day, Still was keen to adopt the principles of social Darwinism and set out to explain the 'defects of moral control' of the children he was asked to treat. He claimed that moral consciousness and moral control were essentially innate characteristics. They were also 'the highest and latest product of mental evolution'. However, because they constituted a relatively recent evolutionary advance, they were also fragile and showed 'a special liability to loss and failure in development'.

Hyperactivity due to neuropathic diathesis

To support Still's reports of hyperactive behaviour pattern occurring when brain damage was suspected, but could not be substantiated, Tredgold (1908) presented further evidence in children. He proposed that some forms of brain damage, such as birth injury or relatively mild anoxia, though undetected at the time, could express themselves as behaviour problems or learning difficulties when the child is faced with the demands of early school years. Alfred F. Tredgold was a member of the English Royal Commission on Mental Deficiency. His book, *Mental Deficiency (Amentia)*, was published in 1908, updated in 1914, and remained in publication until 1952. In the book, Tredgold described many children who exhibited features of hyperactivity, and he is attributed by a number of authors (Ross and Ross, 1982) as being the first to provide an account of 'minimal brain damage'.

Tredgold's descriptions of hyperactivity derived from his observations of a group of child patients whom he labelled as 'high-grade feeble minded'. Although incapable of making use of education as provided in school, such children would in his judgement nevertheless benefit from individual attention and instruction. He also noted that a number of the children exhibited a variety of physical anomalies, including abnormalities of the palate, soft neurological signs, abnormal head shape and size and poor coordination.

Apart from being educationally inferior, the children were also prone to criminal behaviour, despite having been raised in an adequate environment. Tredgold shared Still's belief that moral deficiency resulted from the effect of some 'organic abnormality on the higher levels of the brain', and argued that the areas of the brain where the 'sense of morality' was located were the product of the more recent development in the course of human evolution, and were therefore more susceptible to damage. Tredgold believed that such moral deficiency was caused by the inheritance of some brain defect that was being passed on from generation to generation: being able to take various forms, it resulted in hyperactivity, migraine, mild forms of epilepsy, hysteria and neurasthenia. He called the defect by various names, such as 'neuropathic diathesis', 'psychopathic diathesis', 'blastophoria' or 'germ corruption'. In his view, environmental circumstances played no significant role in the causation of such mental or moral deficiency.

With regard to the influence of slum life and all its associated conditions in producing amentia, it is necessary to sound a note of warning. It does happen sometimes that the real mental defectives of our large towns hail from the slums, although I do not think such is disproportionately the case. Still, a sufficient number of defective children come from such areas to make the superficial enquirer content with that which is apparent, jump on the conclusion that the pernicious environment is therefore the cause of their defect. My own enquiries have convinced me that in the great majority of these slums cases, there is pronounced morbid inheritance, and that their environment is not the cause, but the result, of that heredity (Schachar, 1986, p. 23).

In the decades that followed, a wide range of deviance was attributed to the interaction of brain disorder and constitutional predisposition by leading medical authorities on both sides of the Atlantic. Such biological variation could in turn have several different outcomes, ranging from school failure (Cornell, 1912), to criminality (Healy, 1915). In contrast, psychological and social explanations for cognitive and behavioural deviations were explicitly rejected. The core debate revolved around the relative contributions of inheritance and birth injury as factors of prime importance in leading to disturbed adaptability towards one's surroundings (Henderson, 1913).

Sequelae of the encephalitis epidemic

The link between hyperactive behaviour and demonstrable brain damage was strengthened by the epidemic of encephalitis spreading across Europe and the USA in 1917–18. In its aftermath, many clinicians encountered children who, though having survived the infection, subsequently presented with behaviour problems and cognitive deficits. Hyperactivity, catastrophic changes in personality and learning difficulties were among the predictable sequelae of the disease (Hohman, 1922; Ebaugh, 1923). The term 'postencephalitic behaviour disorder' was adopted to encompass the various consequences. Observations of the child victims of subsequent outbreaks of encephalitis confirmed the same pattern of symptoms (Bender, 1943; Gibbs et al., 1964). Cantwell (1975) and many others date the development of North America's interest in hyperactivity to the encephalitis epidemic.

Hohman (1922), Ebaugh (1923) and Strecker and Ebaugh (1924) argued that the children who showed persisting problems with behaviour following the epidemic were also the ones who had been most severely affected by the disease, and in most cases were left with severe brain dysfunction. As such, however, only the problems of few of the children described would fit the present-day criteria for attention deficit hyperactivity disorder. It is also to be acknowledged that the available evidence was for an association between severe damage and severe behavioural disturbance. For some reason, this was subsequently extrapolated to claim that a similar connection existed between minimal brain damage and lesser degrees of disordered conduct.

As was the case with Still's disease, the influences of social Darwinism were also brought to bear on the sequelae of encephalitis, with the assumption that there was some inherited predisposition to developing the disease. People who contracted illnesses, such as encephalitis, were believed to be in some way constitutionally inferior (Bassoe, 1922; Bond and Appel, 1931).

Hyperkinetic disease

In the early 1930s, Kramer-Pollnow described a syndrome characterized by extreme restlessness, distractibility and speech disorder. He called it 'hyper-kinetische Erkrankung' (hyperkinetic disease) and classified it as a form of childhood psychosis, usually of unknown origin (reported by Hoff, 1956, pp. 537–53). The extreme restlessness, commencing in the third or fourth year of life, often came on suddenly, 'after a period of quiet', and was frequently followed by an epileptic seizure. The restlessness reached its most severe form at the age of 6, and then gradually decreased, with most cases achieving almost complete recovery. Disturbances of speech and general mental development were often noted before the onset of restlessness.

The children were also described as being easily distracted. Their excessive motor activity, chaotic and aimless in nature, appeared to occur as a succession of uncorrelated impulses with no aim other than to respond to a stimulus. Their play also seemed to lack purpose, with toys tending to be broken rather than played with. The 'lack of discrimination', as noted, bears a resemblance to the 'impulsivity' described in children suffering from hyperkinetic disorders of today. The paucity of the children's interpersonal relationships was likewise remarked upon. They were also more often aggressive towards other children rather than playing with them. Any attempts to restrain the child would be met with opposition and struggling.

The speech disorders, as recorded, consisted of poor articulation and 'inarticulate labelling'; the children's vocabulary was thought not to increase until their recovery from the condition. However, their intelligence, when observed daily at home, appeared to be higher than that detected on formal cognitive testing. It was also argued that the disorder could be differentiated from others such as schizophrenia, dementia infantilism, encephalitis and schizophrenia-like psychoses.

In total, 15 children presenting with 'hyperkinetic disease' were described. Of these one died, three suffered from definite mental defect, three recovered from the restlessness but were left with permanently impaired intelligence, four recovered partially, whilst another two recovered completely. The remaining two children were less than 7 years old and were therefore felt still to be within the 'hyperactive stage'.

A small compilation of cases with similar presentation had also been published in Italy a few years previously (de Sanctis, 1925). Indeed, after having examined the evidence collected by both Kramer-Pollnow and de Sanctis, Hoff concluded the topic of 'Hyperkinetische Erkrankung', as part of his three-lecture series on child psychiatry to his Viennese medical students, by adopting a revised view. He stated clearly that, rather than a form of psychosis, the hyperkinetic disease was due to some kind of endogenous disturbance of brain metabolism – and quite possibly had a hereditary basis (Hoff, 1956, p. 544).

In the Soviet Union, on the other hand, hyperactivity appears to have been a well-acknowledged condition almost from the inception of the new federal state. According to Isaev and Kagan (1981), as early as the 1920s Soviet child psychiatrists Gurevich, Kashchenko (1919), Simson (1929) and Jogikhes (1929) are recorded as having emphasized that hyperactivity was a combination of a medical and a pedagogical problem. In addition, Gurevich (1925) had described in some detail the work done at a 'psychoneurological sanatorium' school, established in 1919. The school was meant for 'near-normal children with minor aberrations', such as nervousness and general neurological imbalance. It also seems that the view of hyperactivity as a condition closely akin to 'hypersthenic form of neurasthenia' guided Soviet child psychiatrists' approach to the diagnosis, aetiological explanations and treatment of the disorder for decades to come. The medication aspect of the treatment often consisted of a mixture of stimulants and tranquillizers, the relative proportions of which were determined by the assumed ratios of excitatory and inhibitory processes operating in the child's nervous system (Isaev and Kagan, 1978, 1981). Likewise, in the former DDR, where terms such as 'an erethic child' were used to describe hyperkinesis, the nature of medication treatment depended on whether or not the restlessness was accompanied by rapid tiring. In the former instance, stimulants were the choice, and in the latter it was tranquillizers (Göllnitz, 1981).

Organic drivenness

In 1934, Kahn and Cohen described three patients whose clinical condition was marked by hyperkinesis, an inability to remain quiet, abruptness, clumsiness and explosiveness of voluntary activity. The authors argued that all the symptoms were secondary to a central behaviour abnormality – hyperactivity. This, in turn, was a result of 'organic drivenness, or a surplus of inner impulsion', originating from an abnormality in the organization of the brain stem, often caused by trauma, or 'prenatal encephalopathy or birth injury'. Acknowledging that in a number of such hyperactive children no history of trauma could be confirmed, Kahn and Cohen postulated that a congenital defect in the activity-modulating system of the brain stem was the cause of the condition. In their view, both the over- as well as the underdevelopment of certain areas of the brain were capable of leading to the same endresult. They also added that features such as soft neurological signs, e.g. twitching, and minor congenital dysmorphisms were evidence of the constitutional nature of these deficits.

Further evidence of a causative link between brain damage and hyperactivity was provided by studies of epilepsy and other brain disorders (Clark, 1926; Lord, 1937; Preston, 1945). Also, children with confirmed lead poisoning were often found to sustain severe neurological and psychological sequelae, one of the latter being a behavioural expression of hyperkinesis, short attention span and impulsivity (Byers and Lord, 1943). The characteristics of the children suffering from 'motor restlessness syndrome', as it appeared in the early recorded descriptions in Soviet child psychiatry (Sukhareva, 1940), are strikingly similar.

Associations with primate research

Studies carried out in the latter half of the nineteenth century (Fernier, 1876) had shown that frontal lobe ablation in monkeys produced excessive restlessness and poor concentration. During the 1930s, several researchers noted that there was a similarity between the behaviour shown by primates who had undergone frontal lobe ablation and that of hyperactive children (Blau, 1936; Levin, 1938). This was taken as evidence in support of hyperkinetic behaviour in children as the result of some defect in forebrain structures, even though signs of such lesions could not always be demonstrated in all affected individuals.

Psychostimulant treatments and their effect on theory of hyperkinesis

The efficacy of amphetamines in the treatment of hyperkinesis was discovered purely by accident by Charles Bradley, working at the Emma Pendleton Bradley Home in Providence, Rhode Island, USA. The details of the discovery are described in a letter from Mortimer D. Gross to the editor of the *American Journal of Psychiatry* in 1995 (Gross, 1995). In this letter, Gross recalls the story of the breakthrough as recounted to him by M.W. Laufer. Bradley and his colleagues, having been impressed by the ideas of Kahn and Cohen (1934), also working at the centre, decided to join in the efforts to demonstrate the nature of structural abnormalities in the brain which they believed were the cause of disruptive behaviour in children. For this purpose, pneumoencephalograms were widely employed, with the consequence that many of the children were left with severe headaches. The headaches were thought to be due to the loss of spinal fluid and Bradley believed that if he could stimulate the choroid plexus to produce spinal fluid more rapidly, the headaches would be alleviated. He chose benzedrine as the most potent stimulant available at that time.

Most of the children given benzedrine (amphetamine derivative) for their headaches also showed a clear improvement in their behaviour and school performance (Bradley, 1937); in some there was also a rise in intelligence test scores (Bradley and Green, 1940), which was attributed to the drug's favourable effect on the child's emotional attitude towards the test. Furthermore, it was noted that a wide range of children benefited from the medication, and that the therapeutic effect was not specific to any particular behaviour, although the children who improved least turned out to have a demonstrable structural neurological deficit (Bradley and Bowen, 1940, 1941).

The mechanism of the drug's action was at first attributed to its effect of stimulating higher inhibitory centres, thereby producing increased voluntary control. In addition, Bradley (1957) commented on the importance of the euphoriant effect of amphetamines. He believed that children with behaviour problems, many of whom showed marked overactivity and restlessness, were unhappy, and that their deviant behaviour was their way of conveying this. Therefore, giving them amphetamines made them less unhappy, and took away some of their need to behave badly.

Laufer (1975) later suggested that the reason the drug was not widely used until the mid 1950s was because of the prevailing psychoanalytic climate, which resisted the idea that hyperactive behaviour had an organic basis. Laufer and his colleagues took up the cause of amphetamines and set out to investigate the neurological mechanism underlying the 'hyperkinetic impulse disorder', and the action of amphetamines (Laufer and Denhoff, 1957; Laufer et al., 1957). Attempting to secure some sound evidence for the drug's effectiveness, in the face of strong competition from those who promoted the role of poor parenting as the cause for hyperactive-type behaviour problems, was an uphill struggle.

Laufer's research was heavily built on the work of two of his contemporaries, Gastaut (1950) and Magoun (1952). Gastaut had developed a photometrozol stimulation test, which involved administering the drug metrozol whilst lights were flashed at the child. The resulting myoclonic jerks of the forearm and spike-wave patterns on the EEG were then carefully monitored. Magoun's work centred on the importance of the ascending reticular activating system in preserving alertness.

Hypothesizing that abnormalities of the reticular activating system led children to be overalert and overactive, Laufer et al. (1957) embarked on a study of children with 'emotional disturbance', dividing them into those who showed evidence of 'hyperkinetic impulse disorder' and those who did not. They found that the hyperkinetic group required less metrozol to induce myoclonic jerks in response to the stroboscope compared with the nonhyperkinetic group. However, when the hyperkinetic children were given amphetamines, the amount of metrozol required increased to the same level as in the nonhyperkinetic children. The authors postulated that the central nervous system deficit of overactive children was located in the area of the thalamus. As a result of this, excess stimulation was not filtered out, but instead passed through to the brain, causing the child to behave in an overactive manner.

It has later been pointed out that Laufer's research did suffer from certain methodological flaws; for example, there had been a failure to record the photo-metrozol levels of the nonhyperkinetic children. However, even though the original study has never been replicated, Laufer's early work has definitely fuelled much interest in the study of biological treatments in childhood hyperactivity.

From minimal brain damage to minimal brain dysfunction
Minimal brain damage/minimal damage to the brain
The belief that brain damage could be inferred laid the foundation for the concept of minimal brain damage (Ehrenfest, 1926; Smith, 1926; Doll et al., 1932; Ingalls and Gordon, 1947). The publications and 'minimal stimulation' classroom programmes by Strauss and his associates (Strauss and Werner, 1942, 1943; Strauss and Lehtinen, 1947; Lehtinen, 1955) further helped to promote the idea that hyperactive behaviour was caused by minimal brain damage. The group studied the psychopathology and educational needs of children residing in the Wayne County Training School, Michigan, USA. The school provided rehabilitation for children considered to be of borderline intelligence, or 'higher grade morons'. Strauss and Kephart (1955) suggested that the borderline children should be divided into two distinct groups, which they called 'exogenous' and 'endogenous'. The 'exogenous' children had histories of physical damage to the central nervous system, either due to trauma or inflammatory process, but no family history of mental retardation. The medical histories of the 'endogenous' children did not contain any evidence of physical damage to the brain, but the children came from families with a history of mental retardation. The two groups also differed with regard to their behaviour and current functioning: the 'exogenous' children responded poorly to teaching, and appeared to be overactive and easily distracted. Prompted by their observations, the group set out to determine the nature of the brain-injured child's deficit, and to develop appropriate educational programmes for such children.

As a result of their observations, Strauss and Werner (1943) concluded that the behaviour of the brain-injured children closely resembled that of brain-injured adults. This led them to postulate species-specific innate patterns of behaviour. When a child suffers a brain injury these particular behavioural patterns are triggered by less intense stimuli, but produce more intense responses than is the case with adults. Although their initial studies were based on intellectually impaired children, the authors argued that there was no reason why these same behaviour patterns should not indicate brain damage in children of normal intelligence.

Research findings like these were appealing at the time, because they provided a biological explanation for children's behaviour problems and educational failure. They also excited paediatricians and child psychiatrists who, when trying to help such children, had grown disillusioned and dissatisfied with the lack of success of treatments based largely on psychoanalytic theories. Although welcomed by many, the conclusions by Strauss and his colleagues were also met with scepticism by a number of people. The main criticisms related to the lack of clarity of the criteria by which organic brain disorder was defined. Also, the educational programmes that had been guided by the research frequently turned out to be ineffective (Cruickshank et al., 1961), and the attempts to replicate the psychometric results proved unsuccessful in most instances (Weatherwax and Benoit, 1962).

At the same time as the theories put forward by Strauss and his coworkers were struggling to gain wider acceptance, the validity of the concept of minimal brain damage was strengthened by a substantial body of fetal and animal research. Epidemiological studies demonstrated a strong association between maternal and fetal factors and subsequent behaviour problems in children (Lilienfeld et al., 1955; Pasamanick et al., 1956b), and results of animal studies supported a relationship between disordered behaviour and minor degrees of brain damage (Cromwell et al., 1963). Empirical evidence for a significant link between histories of anoxia at birth and later disorders of development appeared particularly suggestive (Graham et al., 1957), as did the systematic clinical observations of the behaviour of children suffering from epilepsy (Ounsted, 1955), and of other forms of organic brain disorder (Ingram, 1956).

The term 'minimal brain damage syndrome' was a diagnosis also widely used by Soviet and east European clinicians and researchers from the 1950s, at least until the end of the 1970s. Particularly, a constellation of several (even dozens of) symptoms, such as dyslexia, dysgraphia, dyscalculia, attention problems, overall cognitive difficulties and aggression, in addition to motor restlessness, merited the diagnosis in the Soviet practice (Badalyan et al., 1978;

Isaev and Kagan, 1978; Kovalev, 1979). In the former DDR, hyperkinesis was viewed as one aspect of encephalopathy (organic brain syndrome), not indicating any specific illness (Göllnitz, 1981). Rather, a combination of biologically and neurologically tangible symptoms, together with the child's interactions with his or her environment, formed the syndrome (Laehr, 1975). Also, the term 'uninhibited child with choreatic symptoms' was used (Lemke, 1953).

The continuum of reproductive casualty

The introduction of the concept of a continuum of damage, with a corresponding continuum of medical, behavioural and educational consequences, by Pasamanick and his colleagues presented a theoretical step forward (Knobloch et al., 1956; Pasamanick et al., 1956a,b). The argument was based on the observation that the cause of perinatal death in babies whose mothers had had severe complications of pregnancy, and/or where the pregnancy ended prematurely, was usually due to brain injury. Therefore, amongst the group of infants who did not die, some would be severely injured and develop a variety of disorders. Depending on the severity and location of the injury, the disorders ranged from cerebral palsy through conduct disorders and learning difficulties to mild behaviour problems (Pasamanick and Knobloch, 1961). These findings stemmed from a study of children referred to the Division of Special Services of the Baltimore Department of Education, with nonreferred children from the same classrooms being used as controls. The referred children were found to be three times more likely than the controls to have a history of perinatal complications such as anoxia or premature birth. This was particularly true of those children who presented with hyperactive-type behaviours. In a subsequent prospective study, involving 500 children who had been born prematurely, the incidence of such developmental abnormalities was found to increase with decreasing birth weight (Knobloch and Pasamanick, 1966). Although the findings were mainly interpreted as lending support for the role of gestational and perinatal factors in the later development of hyperactivity, an association between socioeconomic status, race and complications of pregnancy was also recorded. There was a higher incidence of perinatal events in lower socioeconomic and nonwhite populations. This led the authors to conclude that the perinatal complications and adverse environmental factors most likely stemmed from the same social disadvantage.

Minimal dysfunction replaces minimal damage

While Pasamanick and his colleagues were promoting their research as providing evidence for a link between minimal brain damage and hyperactivity, several authors criticized the idea, increasingly doubting the concept of brain damage as the sole cause of children's hyperactive behaviour. Birch (1964), Rapin (1964) and Herbert (1964) all questioned the assumption that, if brain damage caused behaviour problems, then all children with behaviour problems must have brain damage – even though there might be no physical evidence to support the presence of damage.

Coinciding with this, the Oxford International Study Group of Child Neurology (MacKeith and Bax, 1963) also contended that brain damage should not be inferred from behaviour alone, and recommended that the term 'minimal brain damage' be replaced by 'minimal brain dysfunction' (MBD). It also advocated attempts to reclassify the heterogeneous group of children, subsumed under this label, into a number of more homogeneous subgroups. In one of the longest-established London medical schools, the professor of psychiatry (Pond, 1967, p. 127), specializing in problems of behavioural disturbance and brain damage, also adopted a very sceptical view, and stated: 'There are . . . no absolutely unequivocal clinical signs, physiological tests or psychological tests, that prove a relationship between brain damage and any particular aspect of disturbed behaviour'.

In the USA, a national task force formulated an official definition of the disorder (Clements, 1966):

The term minimal brain dysfunction syndrome refers . . . to children of near average, average, or above average general intelligence with certain learning or behavioral disabilities ranging from mild to severe, which are associated with deviations of function of the central nervous system. These deviations may manifest themselves by various combinations of impairment in perception, conceptualisation, language, memory, and control of attention, impulse, or motor function . . . during the school years, a variety of learning disabilities is the most prominent manifestation (quotation by Ross and Ross, 1982).

The definition was welcomed by those who believed hyperactivity to be an unequivocal diagnostic sign of brain damage (Wender, 1971), but criticized by many (Routh and Roberts, 1972; Rutter, 1977). Gomez (1967), the head of child neurology at the Mayo Clinic, expressed his views on the topic without undue reservation: To him the term 'minimal brain dysfunction' stood for 'maximal neurologic confusion'. Although the term 'MBD' was useful in emphasizing the role of organic factors in the causation of hyperactivity, and thus providing something of a challenge to the psychoanalytic views of the time, proposing that the disorder was due to poor parenting, it was eventually recognized as being overinclusive. 'MBD' was subsequently replaced by more specific terms relating to particular behavioural and developmental disorders, such as dyslexia, learning disabilities and language disorders. These terms were based on observed disabilities rather than hypothesized underlying mechanisms.

Emergence of behavioural definitions

Three decades elapsed between Still's (1902) description of children with hyperactive behaviour unrelated to either demonstrable brain damage or a history of suggestive damage and the first comprehensive discussion of hyperactive children. In 1935, Childers noted that only a small proportion of cases with hyperactivity seemed aetiologically related to substantiated or inferred brain damage. His deliberation on children with no evidence of brain damage is notable for the differentiation made between the hyperactive child and the brain-damaged child.

Hyperkinetic behaviour syndrome

During the late 1950s and early 1960s, dissatisfaction with the term 'MBD' was growing. The influential publications by Laufer and his associates (Laufer and Denhoff, 1957; Laufer et al., 1957), which introduced the concepts and terms of 'hyperkinetic behaviour syndrome' and 'hyperkinetic impulse disorder', signalled the onset of final acceptance of the construct of hyperactivity as we know it now.

Chess (1960) also emphasized the importance of excessive motor activity as a defining feature of the disorder, and that this should be observed rather than taken on as an anecdotal account from the parents. In addition, she moved away from attributing the disorder to poor parenting or brain damage. Her findings were based on a group of 36 children, termed hyperactive, in a whole sample of 881 children attending a private practice. The features, documented in detail, resemble the present criteria of attention deficit hyperactivity disorder, including sex ratio and age of onset. Aggression and impulsivity were seen as associated characteristics. Chess (1960) proposed that in most cases the disorder was due to 'physiologic hyperactivity', but also noted that hyperactivity could be associated with mental retardation, schizophrenia or organic brain damage. A treatment approach incorporating behaviour modification, medication, special educational provision and psychotherapy was recommended.

The changes in the concept and terminology served as a stimulus for a series of important empirical investigations (Smith, 1962; Werry et al., 1964; Huessy, 1967) and descriptive clinical studies (Bakwin and Bakwin, 1966; Stewart et al., 1966; Werry, 1968). By the late 1960s, the concept of hyperactivity was firmly established in the literature.

First systematic tools for assessment

In the late 1960s, Conners and his team developed parent and teacher rating scales for the assessment of symptoms of hyperactivity (Conners, 1969, 1970). At that time, these questionnaire-based instruments presented an invaluable step forward in allowing for a standardized measurement of children's behaviour with a particular emphasis on hyperactivity. Although initially devised for the measurement of change in behaviour during drug treatment, the scales have also been successfully employed in epidemiological research.

Psychophysiology and the importance of arousal level

Several psychological models have attributed hyperactive behaviour to an abnormality in the level of arousal in the central nervous system. However, the direction of postulated abnormality has been a matter of considerable dispute. The models viewing the deficit as one of overarousal have interpreted hyperactivity as a behavioural manifestation of an overaroused, or highly aroused central nervous system (Kahn and Cohen, 1934; Strauss and Lehtinen, 1947; Laufer et al., 1957; Freibergs and Douglas, 1969). The underarousal models, on the other hand, have conceptualized the condition as a compensatory response by a suboptimally aroused individual through increased sensory input (Bradley, 1937; Werry and Sprague, 1970).

The psychophysiology of hyperactivity was extensively investigated during the 1970s. Several studies were published during this time examining a variety of physiological aspects, such as EEG, galvanic skin response, averaged evoked responses, etc. (Satterfield and Dawson, 1971; Satterfield et al., 1972, 1974; Satterfield, 1973). Many of these also had considerable methodological problems and were highly criticized (Hastings and Barkley, 1978). One of the weaknesses of the psychophysiological research was that the studies were often based on outdated theories of the 1950s suggesting, for example, that hyperactivity was due to cortical overarousal. If anything, the evidence generated suggested that hyperactive children had a slower than normal response to stimulation, thus detracting from theories of overstimulated cortices in these children.

Deficits of attention and motivation

The 1970s saw a proliferation of research into hyperactivity and a fast-growing volume of literature on various aspects of the disorder. Particularly in the USA, features such as short attention span, impulsivity and distractibility, previously considered to be associated characteristics, were now included in the defining symptoms. At the same time, the popularity of the concept of MBD was declining due to the lack of scientific evidence in its favour.

One of the turning points in the history of hyperactivity was when, in the early 1970s, Douglas and her team at McGill University suggested that motor overactivity was not the core symptom in the syndrome of hyperkinesis, but rather deficits in the ability to sustain attention and control impulsive responding were more important. Douglas also argued that these were the areas in which stimulant medication was most effective (Douglas, 1972).

Employing a series of measures to assess the behavioural and cognitive aspects of the disorder, the McGill team demonstrated that hyperactive children experienced more problems with sustained attention, particularly in situations where there were distractions, but that they were not generally more learning- or reading-impaired, or more distractible than normal children. However, in situations where the children were given continuous and immediate reinforcement, the hyperactive ones could perform at near normal and even normal levels of attention (Freibergs and Douglas, 1969). Another important observation was that, while the excessive motor restlessness usually declined by the early teens, the difficulties in sustained attention and impulse control often persisted into adolescence.

One of the doubtless merits of the systematic and detailed work of Douglas and her colleagues was that it helped to establish a tradition of high-quality research in the study of cognitive aspects of hyperactivity. Another notable feature of her contribution has been the way it was guided by theory, which can be tested and revised when necessary; these are characteristics so often found wanting in the mushrooming hyperactivity research.

The work of Douglas and her team has definitely been influential in shaping the study of hyperactivity. It was probably the main reason for the American Psychiatric Association (1980) altering the diagnostic terminology in DSM-III to attention deficit disorder ± hyperactivity, thus focusing on the attentional aspects of the disorder, rather than on the motor overactivity. Although the theory of Douglas has subsequently been questioned in part, it nevertheless provided the impetus for a new generation of high-quality research in the various aspects of hyperactivity, including the individual processes of attention, motivation and inhibitory control. It has undoubtedly facilitated the development of links between the study of attention as a behavioural manifestation of central processing of information and the neuroanatomical and neurotransmitter processes, providing the focus for the more recent research in the field of hyperactivity and attention problems.

The role of the environment

In the 1970s the trend against drugging children with behaviour disorders was accompanied by a number of alternative theories explaining the causation of hyperactivity. One such explanation, gaining longlasting popularity, was that of food allergy. Feingold (1975) suggested that children demonstrated hyperactive behaviour as a result of an allergic or toxic reaction to food substances, especially food additives. This theory caught the imagination of both professionals and lay people. Several studies were set up to investigate the concept; the more rigorous of these have found no or minimal effect of food substances on the behaviour of children.

Poor parenting as a causative factor in hyperactivity was put forward by both psychoanalysts (Bettelheim, 1973) and behaviourists (Willis and Lovaas, 1977). Psychoanalysts suggested that an excessively negative reaction from an intolerant mother to a child who demonstrates a negative or hyperactive temperament would lead to the clinical presentation of hyperactivity. According to behaviourists, noncompliant and hyperactive behaviour developed as a result of poor conditioning to stimulus control by parental commands and instructions. However, in the search for psychosocial causes, the finding which was of possibly greatest potential importance was that by Tizard and Hodges (1978), demonstrating an association between institutional upbringing and hyperactive behaviour. It suggested that a lack of continuity in parenting may impair the development of the normal modulation of activity and attention. The importance of disrupted core relationships for the development of hyperactive behaviour pattern was also highlighted by the observational study of Routh (1980), and the theoretical model of 'learned ineffectiveness' by Glow and Glow (1979). Other attempts by researchers and clinicians to come to terms with the new, rapidly spreading childhood disease were to seek explanations in wider social ecology (Gadow and Loney, 1981; Gittelman, 1981; Whalen and Henker, 1980a). Thus, causes were looked for in the various social problems of urban living, deteriorating schools and ever-expanding traffic, disposing to lead poisoning.

The 1970s also saw the beginning of a vigorous sociological and medicolegal debate about the implications of the increasingly popular diagnosis of hyperactivity. Block (1977), for example, suggested that technological development, leading to rapid cultural change, was responsible for children becoming hyperactive. The resulting increased excitation and environmental stimulation could in 'pre-disposed' children cause hyperactive behaviour of clinical severity. Conrad (1976), on the other hand, argued that the expansion of the clinical diagnosis stemmed at least partly from the existence of powerful drug treatments for children's disruptive behaviours. The drugs, of course, had existed long before then, but their availability was convenient when physicians became increasingly confronted with referrals of children with puzzling troublesome behaviours, especially from schools. The issue was also seized by authors of more popular texts. In the USA, for example, journalists Schrag and Divoky (1975) published a book about the 'myth' of childhood hyperactivity and in the UK Steven Box (1977), in a widely read sociological journal, referred to the 'scandalous silence' surrounding the mass labelling and drugging of schoolchildren who failed to conform. Whalen and Henker (1980b) also drew attention to the apparent increased tolerance for diagnostic ambiguity and for a greater tendency to make the diagnosis of hyperactivity once there was evidence of the child's behaviour having improved by the drug treatment. Messinger (1975) went even further by arguing that pure profit-making motives were a major force. As drug companies were benefiting greatly from the sale of stimulants, they were also keen to promote any research likely to increase the detection of hyperactivity.

The issue of a syndrome

The question of whether hyperactivity constitutes a syndrome (O'Malley and Eisenberg, 1973), in the sense of sharing a unitary cluster of symptoms, a common cause in terms of major aetiological factors, a consistent response to treatment, a predictable natural course, and whether or not it differs from other disorders, especially conduct disorder, in terms of these factors, has been a difficult one to settle. At times, the argument has led to considerable polarization of views, with some seeing the whole issue as more of a hindrance to the progress of research (Ross and Ross, 1982), while others have regarded it as an invaluable stimulus for good study (Rutter, 1982).

The interest generated by the syndrome issue has led a small but determined group of investigators to search for empirical support for the disorder. This process has helped to sharpen both the theoretical reasoning behind it (Quay, 1979; Shaffer and Greenhill, 1979; Rie and Rie, 1980; Sandberg, 1981; Rutter, 1982) and, most notably, to improve the search for aetiological processes (Shaffer et al., 1974; Loney et al., 1978, 1981; Sandberg et al., 1978; Schachar et al., 1981; Taylor, 1983). The net result has been an appreciable scientific advancement starting from the early 1970s and which is likely to continue for some time. The scientific and clinical developments of the 1980s and 1990s are the subjects of the individual contributions to both editions of this book, and, therefore, outside the remit of this chapter.

REFERENCES

American Psychiatric Association (1980). *Diagnostic and Statistical Manual of Mental Disorders*, 3rd edn. Washington, DC: American Psychiatric Association.

Badalyan, L.O., Zhurba, L.T. and Mastyukova, E.M. (1978). Minimalnaya mozgovaya disfunktsiya u detei: Nevrologichesky aspekt. *Zurnal Nevropatologii i Psikhiatrii*, **78**, 1441–6.

Bakwin, H. and Bakwin, R.M. (1966). *Clinical Management of Behavior Disorders in Children*. Philadelphia: Saunders.

Bassoe, P. (1922). Diagnosis of encephalitis. *Journal of the American Medical Association*, **79**, 223–5.

Bender, L. (1943). Postencephalitic behavior disorders in children. In *Encephalitis: A Clinical Study*, ed. J.B. Neal, pp. 361–85. New York: Grune and Stratton.

Bettelheim, B. (1973). Bringing up children. *Ladies Home Journal*, **90**, 28.

Birch, H.G. (1964). *Brain Damage in Children. The Biological and Social Aspects*. Baltimore: Williams and Wilkins.

Blau, A. (1936). Mental changes following head trauma in children. *Archives of Neurology and Psychiatry*, **35**, 722–69.

Block, G.H. (1977). Hyperactivity: a cultural perspective. *Journal of Learning Disabilities*, **110**, 236–40.

Boncour, P. and Boncour, G. (1905). *Les Anomalies Mentales chez les Ecoliers, Etude Medicopédagogique*. Paris: Alcan.

Bond, E.D. and Appel, K.E. (1931). Treatment of post encephalitic children in hospital school. *American Journal of Psychiatry*, **10**, 815–28.

Bourneville, E. (1897). *Le Traitement Médico-Pédagogique des Différentes Formes de l'Idiotie*. Paris: Alcan.

Box, S. (1977). Hyperactivity: the scandalous silence. *New Society*, **42**, 458–60.

Bradley, C. (1937). The behavior of children receiving Benzedrine. *American Journal of Psychiatry*, **94**, 577–85.

Bradley, C. (1957). Characteristics and management of children with behavior problems associated with organic brain damage. *Pediatric Clinics of North America*, **4**, 1049–60.

Bradley, C. and Bowen M. (1940). School performance of children receiving amphetamine (Benzedrine) sulfate. *American Journal of Orthopsychiatry*, **10**, 782–8.

Bradley, C. and Bowen, M. (1941). Amphetamine (Benzedrine) therapy of children's behavior disorders. *American Journal of Orthopsychiatry*, **11**, 91–103.

Bradley, C. and Green, R. (1940). Psychometric performance of children receiving amphetamine (benzedrine) sulfate. *American Journal of Psychiatry*, **97**, 388–94.

Byers, R.K. and Lord, E.E. (1943). Late effects of lead poisoning on mental development. *American Journal of Diseases of Children*, **66**, 471–94.

Cantwell, D.P. (1975). *The Hyperactive Child*. New York: Spectrum.

Chess, S. (1960). Diagnosis and treatment of the hyperactive child. *New York State Journal of Medicine*, **60**, 2379–85.

Childers, A.T. (1935). Hyperactivity in children having behavior disorders. *American Journal of Orthopsychiatry*, **5**, 227–43.

Clark, L.P. (1926). Psychology of essential epilepsy. *Journal of Nervous and Mental Disease*, **63**, 575–85.

Clements, S.D. (1966). *Task Force One: Minimal Brain Dysfunction in Children*. National Institute of Neurological Diseases and Blindness, monograph no. 3. Washington, DC: US Department of Health Education and Welfare.

Clouston, T.S. (1899). Stages of over-excitability, hypersensitiveness, and mental explosiveness in children and their treatment by the bromides. *Scottish Medical and Surgical Journal*, **IV**, 481–90.

Conners, C.K. (1969). A teacher rating scale for use in doing studies with children. *American Journal of Psychiatry*, **126**, 884–8.

Conners, C.K. (1970). Symptom patterns in hyperkinetic, neurotic and normal children. *Child Development*, **41**, 667–82.

Conrad, P. (1976). *Identifying Hyperactive Children*. Massachusetts: Lexington Books.

Cornell, W.S. (1912). *Health and Medical Inspection of School Children*. Philadelphia: F.A. Davis.

Cromwell, R.L., Baumeister, A. and Hawkins, W.F. (1963). Research in activity level. In *Handbook of Mental Deficiency*, ed. N.R. Ellis, pp. 632–63. New York: McGraw-Hill.

Cruickshank, W.M., Bentzen, F.A., Ratzeburgy, F.H. and Tannhauser, M.T. (1961). *A Teaching Method for Brain Injured and Hyperactive Children: A Demonstration Pilot Study*. Syracuse, New York: Syracuse University Press.

Darwin, C.R. (1859). *On the Origin of Species by Means of Natural Selection or the Preservation of the Favoured Races in the Struggles for Life*. London: John Murray.

de Sanctis, S. (1925). *Neuropsichiatria Infantile*. Stockholm: Rome.

Doll, E.A, Phelps, W.M. and Melcher, R.T. (1932). *Mental Deficiency due to Birth Injuries*. New York: Macmillan.

Douglas, V. I. (1972). Stop, look and listen: the problem of sustained attention and impulse control in hyperactive and normal children. *Canadian Journal of Behavioral Science*, **4**, 259–82.

Dulcan, M. (1997). Practice parameters for the assessment and treatment of children, adolescents and adults with attention-deficit hyperactivity disorder. *Journal of the American Academy of Child and Adolescent Psychiatry*, **36** (suppl. 10), 85s–121s.

Ebaugh, F.G. (1923). Neuropsychiatric sequelae of acute epidemic encephalitis in children. *American Journal of Diseases of Children*, **25**, 89–97.

Ehrenfest, H. (1926). *Birth Injuries of the Child. Gynecological and Obstetrical Monographs*. New York: Appleton.

Feingold, B. (1975). *Why Your Child is Hyperactive*. New York: Random House.

Fernier, D. (1876). *The Functions of the Brain*. New York: Putnam.

Freibergs, V. and Douglas, V.I. (1969). Concept learning in hyperactive and normal children. *Journal of Abnormal Psychology*, **74**, 388–95.

Gadow, K. D. and Loney, J. (1981). *Psychosocial Aspects of Drug Treatment for Hyperactivity*. Boulder, CO: Westview.

Gastaut, H. (1950). Combined photic and Metrazol activation of the brain. *Electroencephalography and Clinical Neurophysiology*, **2**, 249–61.

Gibbs, F., Gibbs, E., Spies, H. and Carpenter, P. (1964). Common types of childhood encephalitis. *Archives of Neurology*, **10**, 1–11.

Gittelman, M. (1981). *Strategic Interventions for Hyperactive Children.* Armonk, NY: Sharpe.

Glow, P.H. and Glow, R.A. (1979). Hyperkinetic impulse disorder: a developmental defect of motivation. *Genetic Psychology Monographs,* **100**, 159–231.

Göllnitz, G. (1981). The hyperkinetic child. In *Strategic Interventions for Hyperactive Children,* ed. M. Gittelman, pp. 80–96. Armonk, NY: Sharpe.

Gomez, M.R. (1967). Minimal cerebral dysfunction (maximal neurologic confusion). *Clinical Pediatrics,* **10**, 589–91.

Graham, F.K., Caldwell, B.M., Ernhart, C.B., Pennoyer, M.M. and Hartmann, A.F., Sr. (1957). Anoxia as a significant perinatal experience: a critique. *Journal of Pediatrics,* **50**, 556–69.

Gross, M.D. (1995). Origin of stimulant use for treatment of attention deficit disorder. *American Journal of Psychiatry,* **152**, 298–9.

Hastings, J.E. and Barkley, R.A. (1978). A review of psychophysiological research with hyperactive children. *Journal of Abnormal Child Psychology,* **7**, 413–47.

Healy, W. (1915). *The Individual Delinquent.* Boston: Little Brown.

Henderson, L.J. (1913). *The Fitness of the Environment.* New York: Macmillan.

Herbert, M. (1964). The concept and testing of brain damage in children – a review. *Journal of Child Psychology and Psychiatry,* **5**, 197–217.

Heuyer, G. (1914). *Enfants anormaux et délinquants juveniles.* Paris: Thèse de médécin.

Hoff, H. (1956). *Lehrbuch der Psychiatrie,* vol. II. Basel: Benno Schwabe.

Hoffmann, H. (1845). *Der Struwwelpeter.* Frankfurt: Literarische Anstalt.

Hohman, L.B. (1922). Post encephalitic behavior disorders in children. *Johns Hopkins Hospital Bulletin,* **33**, 372–5.

Huessy, H.R. (1967). Study of the prevalence and therapy of the choreatiform syndrome or hyperkinesis in rural Vermont. *Acta Paedopsychiatrica,* **34**, 130–5.

Ingalls, T.H. and Gordon, J.E. (1947). Epidemiologic implications of developmental arrests. *American Journal of Medical Science,* **241**, 322–8.

Ingram, T.T.S. (1956). A characteristic form of overactive behaviour in brain-damaged children. *Journal of Mental Science,* **102**, 550–8.

Ireland, W.E. (1877). *On Idiocy and Imbecility.* London: Churchill.

Isaev, D.N. and Kagan, V.S. (1978). Sostoyanie giperaktivnosti u detei: Klinika, terapiya, reabilitatsiya. *Zurnal Nevropatologii i Psikhiatrii,* **78**, 1544–9.

Isaev, D.N. and Kagan, V.E. (1981). A system of treatment and rehabilitation of hyperactive children. In *Strategic Interventions for Hyperactive Children,* ed. M. Gittelman, pp. 97–111. Armonk, NY: Sharpe.

James, W. (1890). *The Principles of Psychology.* New York: Holt.

Johnson, R.C. and Medinnus, G.R. (1969). *Child Psychology: Behavior and Development,* 2nd edn. New York: Wiley.

Kahn, E. and Cohen, L.H. (1934). Organic drivenness. A brain stem syndrome and an experience with case reports. *New England Journal of Medicine,* **210**, 748–56.

Kanner, L. (1957). *Child Psychiatry,* 3rd edn. Springfield, IL: Charles C. Thomas.

Knobel, M., Wolman, M.B. and Mason, E. (1959). Hyperkinesis and organicity in children. *Archives of General Psychiatry,* **1**, 310–21.

Knobloch, H. and Pasamanick, B. (1966). Prospective studies on the epidemiology of reproductive casualty. Methods, findings, and some implications. *Merrill-Palmer Quarterly*, **12**, 27–43.

Knobloch, H., Rider, R., Harper, P. and Pasamanick, B. (1956). Neuropsychiatric sequelae of prematurity: a longitudinal study. *Journal of the American Medical Association*, **161**, 581–5.

Kovalev, V.V. (1979). *Psikhiariya Detskogo Vozrasta (Psychiatry of Childhood)*, pp. 41–3. Moscow: Medicina.

Laehr, H. (1975). Über den Einfluß der Schule auf die Verhinderung von Geistesstörungen. *Allgemeine Zeitschrift der Psychiatrie*, **32**, 216.

Laufer, M.N. (1975). In Osler's day it was syphilis. In *Explorations in Child Psychiatry*, ed. E.J. Anthony, pp. 105–24. New York: Plenum Press.

Laufer, M. and Denhoff, E. (1957). Hyperkinetic behavior syndrome in children. *Journal of Pediatrics*, **50**, 463–74.

Laufer, M.W., Denhoff, E. and Solomons, G. (1957). Hyperkinetic impulse disorder in children's behavior problems. *Psychosomatic Medicine*, **19**, 38–49.

Lehtinen, L.E. (1955). Preliminary conclusions affecting education of brain-injured children. In *Psychopathology and Education of the Brain-injured Child. Progress in Theory and Clinic*, eds. A.A. Strauss and N.C. Kephart, pp. 165–91. New York: Grune & Stratton.

Lemke, R. (1953). Das enthemmte Kind mit choreiformer Symptomatik. *Psychiatrie, Neurologie und Medizinische Psychologie*, **5**, 290–4.

Levin, P.M. (1938). Restlessness in children. *Archives of Neurology and Psychiatry*, **39**, 764–70.

Lilienfeld, A.M., Pasamanick, B. and Rogers, M. (1955). Relationship between pregnancy experience and the development of certain neuropsychiatric disorders in childhood. *American Journal of Public Health*, **45**, 637–43.

Loney, J., Langhorne, J.E. and Paternite, C.E. (1978). An empirical basis for subgrouping the hyperkinetic/minimal brain syndrome. *Journal of Abnormal Psychology*, **87**, 431–41.

Loney, J., Kramer, J. and Milich, R. (1981). The hyperkinetic child grows up: predictors of symptoms, delinquency and achievement at follow-up. In *Psychosocial Aspects of Drug Treatment for Hyperactivity*, eds. K.D. Gadow and J. Loney, pp. 381–415. Colorado: Westview Press.

Lord, E.E. (1937). *Children Handicapped by Cerebral Palsy*. New York: Commonwealth Fund.

MacKeith, R.C. and Bax, M.C.O. (1963). *Minimal Cerebral Dysfunction: Papers from the International Study Group held at Oxford, September 1962*. Little Club Clinics in Development Medicine, No. 10. London: Heinemann.

Magoun, H.W. (1952). An ascending reticular activating system in the brain stem. *Archives of Neurology and Psychiatry*, **67**, 145–54.

Maudsley, H. (1867). *The Physiology and Pathology of the Mind*. London: Macmillan.

Messinger, E. (1975). Ritalin and MBD: a cure in search of a disease. *Health/PAC Bulletin*, **12**, 1–17.

O'Malley, J.E. and Eisenberg, L. (1973). The hyperkinetic syndrome. *Seminars in Psychiatry*, **5**, 95.

Ounsted, C. (1955). The hyperkinetic syndrome in epileptic children. *Lancet*, ii, 303–11.

Pasamanick, B. and Knobloch, H. (1961). Epidemiological studies on the complications of pregnancy and the birth process. In *Prevention of Mental Disorders in Children. Initial Explorations*, ed. A. Caplan, pp. 74–94. New York: Basic Books.

Pasamanick, B., Knobloch. H. and Lilienfeld, A.M. (1956a). Socio-economic status and some precursors of neuropsychiatric disorder. *American Journal of Orthopsychiatry*, **26**, 594–601.

Pasamanick, B., Rogers, M.E. and Lilienfeld, A.M. (1956b). Pregnancy experience and the development of behavior disorder in children. *American Journal of Psychiatry*, **112**, 613–18.

Pick, A. (1904). Uber einige bedeutsame Psycho-Neurosen des Kindesalters. *Sammlung zwangsloser Abhandlungen aus dem Gebiete der Nerven- und der Geisteskrankheiten*, **5**, 1–28.

Pond, D.A. (1967). Behavior disorders in brain-damaged children. In *Modern Trends in Neurology*, ed. D. Williams, pp. 125–34. London: Butterworth.

Preston, M.I. (1945). Late behavioural aspects found in cases of prenatal, natal, and postnatal anoxia. *Journal of Pediatrics*, **26**, 353–66.

Quay, H.C. (1979). Classification. In *Psychopathological Disorders of Childhood*, 2nd edn, eds. H.C. Quay and J.S. Werry, pp. 1–42. New York: Wiley.

Rapin, I. (1964). Brain damage in children. In *Practice of Pediatrics*, vol. 4, ed. J. Brennemann. Hagerstown: M.D. Prior.

Reese, H.W. and Lipsitt, L.P. (1970). *Experimental Child Psychology*. London: Academic Press.

Rie, H.E. and Rie, E.D. (1980). *Handbook of Minimal Brain Dysfunctions: A Critical Review*. New York: Wiley.

Ross, D.M. and Ross, S.A. (1982). *Hyperactivity: Current Issues, Research and Theory*, 2nd edn. New York: Wiley.

Routh, D.K. (1980). Developmental and social aspects of hyperactivity. In *Hyperactive Children: The Social Ecology of Identification and Treatment*, eds. C.K. Whalen and B. Henker, pp. 55–73. New York: Academic Press.

Routh, D.K. and Roberts, R.D. (1972). Minimal brain dysfunction in children: failure to find evidence for a behavioral syndrome. *Psychological Reports*, **31**, 307–14.

Rowntree, B.S. (1901). *Poverty: A Study of Town Life*. London: Macmillan.

Rutter, M. (1977). Brain damage syndromes in childhood: concepts and findings. *Journal of Child Psychology and Psychiatry*, **18**, 1–21.

Rutter, M. (1982). Syndromes attributed to 'minimal brain dysfunction' in childhood. *American Journal of Psychiatry*, **139**, 21–33.

Sandberg, S.T. (1981). The overinclusiveness of the diagnosis of hyperkinetic syndrome. In *Strategic Interventions for Hyperactive Children*, ed. M. Gittelman, pp. 8–38. New York: Sharpe.

Sandberg, S.T., Rutter, M. and Taylor, E. (1978). Hyperkinetic disorder in clinic attenders. *Developmental Medicine and Child Neurology*, **20**, 279–99.

Satterfield. J.H. (1973). EEG issues in children with minimal brain dysfunction. *Seminars in Psychiatry*, **5**, 35–46.

Satterfield, J.H. and Dawson. M.E. (1971). Electrodermal correlates of hyperactivity in children. *Psychophysiology*, **8**, 191–7.

Satterfield, J.H., Cantwell, D.P., Lesser, L.I. and Podosin, R.L. (1972). Physiological studies of the hyperkinetic child. *American Journal of Psychiatry*, **128**, 1418–24.

Satterfield, J.H., Cantwell, D.P. and Satterfield, B.T. (1974). Pathophysiology of the hyperactive child syndrome. *Archives of General Psychiatry*, **31**, 839–44.

Schachar, R.J. (1986). Hyperkinetic syndrome: historical development of the concept. In *The*

Overactive Child, ed. E.A. Taylor, pp. 19–40. Clinics in Developmental Medicine, no. 97, Spastics International Publications. Oxford: Blackwell.

Schachar, R., Rutter, M. and Smith, A. (1981). The characteristics of situationally and pervasively hyperactive children: implications for syndrome definition. *Journal of Child Psychology and Psychiatry*, **22**, 375–92.

Scholz, F. (1911). *Die Charakterfehler des Kindes*. Leipzig: E.H. Mayer.

Schrag, P. and Divoky, D. (1975). *The Myth of the Hyperactive Child*. New York: Pantheon.

Shaffer, D. and Greenhill, L. (1979). A critical note on the predictive validity of 'the hyperkinetic syndrome'. *Journal of Child Psychology and Psychiatry*, **20**, 61–72.

Shaffer, D., McNamara, N. and Pincus, J. (1974). Controlled observation on patterns of activity, attention, and impulsivity in brain-damage and psychiatrically disturbed boys. *Psychological Medicine*, **4**, 4–18.

Smith, G.B. (1926). Cerebral accidents of childhood and their relationships to mental deficiency. *Welfare Magazine*, **17**, 18–33.

Smith, A. (1962). Ambiguities in concepts and studies of 'brain-damaged' 'organicity'. *Journal of Nervous and Mental Disease*, **135**, 311–26.

Spearman, C. (1937). *Psychology down the Ages*, vol. 1. London: Macmillan.

Stewart, M.A., Pitts, F.N., Craig, A.G. and Dieruf, W. (1966). The hyperactive child syndrome. *American Journal of Orthopsychiatry*, **36**, 861–7.

Still, G.F. (1902). The Coulstonian lectures on some abnormal physical conditions in children. *Lancet*, **1**, 1008–12; 1077–82; 1163–8.

Strauss, A.A.and Kephart, N.C. (1955). *Psychopathology and Education of the Brain Injured Child*, vol. 2. *Progress in Theory and Clinic*. New York: Grune and Stratton.

Strauss, A.A. and Lehtinen, L.E. (1947). *Psychopathology and Education of the Brain-Injured Child*. New York: Grune and Stratton.

Strauss, A.A. and Werner, H. (1942). Disorders of conceptual thinking in the brain-injured child. *Journal of Nervous and Mental Disease*, **96**, 153–72.

Strauss, A.A. and Werner, H. (1943). Comparative psychopathology of the brain injured child and the traumatic brain injured adult. *American Journal of Psychiatry*, **99**, 835–8.

Strecker, E.A. and Ebaugh, F.G. (1924). Neuropsychiatric sequelae of cerebral trauma in children. *Archives of Neurology and Psychiatry*, **12**, 443–53.

Sukhareva, G.E. (1940). Neskolko polozhenyo printsipakh psikhiatricheskoi diagnostiki. *Voprossy Detskoi Psikhiatrii*, pp. 1–38. Moscow: Medicina.

Taylor, E.A. (1983). Drug response and diagnostic variation. In *Developmental Neuropsychiatry*, ed. M. Rutter, pp. 348–68. New York: Guilford Press.

Taylor, E.A., Sergeant J., Doepfner M. et al. (1998). Clinical guidelines for hyperkinetic disorder. European Society for Child and Adolescent Psychiatry. *European Journal of Child and Adolescent Psychiatry*, **7**, 184–200.

Tizard, B. and Hodges, J. (1978). The effect of early institutional rearing in the development of eight-year-old children. *Journal of Child Psychology and Psychiatry*, **19**, 99–118.

Tredgold, A.F. (1908). *Mental Deficiency (Amentia)*. New York: W. Wood.

Weatherwax, J. and Benoit, E.P. (1962). Concrete and abstract thinking in organic and nonorganic mentally retarded children. In *Readings on the Exceptional Child: Research and Theory*, eds. E.P. Trapp and P. Himmelstein, pp. 500–8. New York: Appleton-Century-Crofts.

Wender, P.H. (1971). *Minimal Brain Dysfunction in Children*. New York: Wiley.

Werry, J.S. (1968). Developmental hyperactivity. *Pediatric Clinics of North America*, **15**, 581–99.

Werry, J.S. and Sprague, R.C. (1970). Hyperactivity. In *Symptoms of Psychopathology*, ed. C.G. Costello, pp. 397–417. New York: Wiley.

Werry, J.S., Weiss, G. and Douglas, V. (1964). Studies on the hyperactive child: I. Some preliminary findings. *Canadian Psychiatric Association Journal*, **9**, 120–30.

Whalen, C.K. and Henker, B. (1980a). *Hyperactive Children: The Social Ecology of Identification and Treatment*. New York: Academic Press.

Whalen, C.K. and Henker, B. (1980b). The social ecology of psychostimulant treatment: a model for conceptual and empirical analysis. In *Hyperactive Children: The Social Ecology of Identification and Treatment*, eds. C.K. Whalen and B. Henker, pp. 3–54. New York: Academic Press.

Willis, T.J. and Lovaas, I. (1977). A behavioral approach to treating hyperactive children: the parent's role. In *Learning Disabilities and Related Disorders*, ed. J.B. Millichap, pp. 119–40. Chicago: Year Book Medical.

World Health Organization (1992). *ICD-10. Classification of Mental and Behavioural Disorders. Clinical Description and Diagnostic Guidelines*. Geneva: World Health Organization.

2

Epidemiological aspects: what have we learned over the last decade?

Jan K. Buitelaar

Division of Child and Adolescent Psychiatry, University Medical Centre Utrecht, Utrecht, Netherlands

Introduction

By the study of a disorder in the general population, epidemiology attempts to accomplish a number of goals. The first one is to determine the prevalence rate and the distribution of a disorder. This implies the answering of questions such as what is the proportion of the population at risk that develops the disorder within a given time period? And also, who has the disorder, where and when? Epidemiology may further be very useful in looking at the boundaries of a disorder. Where does a disorder shade off into normality, and at which level of symptom severity, or of functional impairment, does an individual become a case? A third goal of epidemiology is to examine the mechanisms that explain how a particular individual got the disorder. What are the risk and protective factors that influence the presence of the disorder, and how do these factors interact and evolve over time? Finally, epidemiology is concerned with the need for and the use of services, including the assessment of the determinants of help-seeking behaviour, and the investigation of referral pathways. Up-to-date epidemiological data are therefore an essential prerequisite for rational mental health policies and appropriate planning of services. They will also provide necessary background information to clinicians and researchers in the design of preventive interventions and treatment programmes (Verhulst and Koot, 1992, 1995).

In the previous edition (Buitelaar and van Engeland, 1996), epidemiological contributions on hyperactivity disorders published between 1981 and 1991 were discussed. The focus of the present version is on epidemiological work that has been published from 1991 onward. In addition to summarizing findings on prevalence and distribution, special consideration will be given to issues that have attracted interest over the last years. These include the boundaries of hyperactivity disorders and the establishment of diagnostic thresholds, the measurement of functional impairment, long-term stability and course of hyperactivity disorders in community-based samples, and the adequacy of standard rating scales.

Defining caseness

Unlike diseases that can be identified from physical signs and symptoms, or from laboratory parameters, the classification of caseness for psychiatric disorders relies primarily on a description of behaviour. Information on behaviour may be derived from observations by parents, teachers and professionals as well as from self-report, and this information may extend from readily overt behaviour units to more covert emotions and cognitions. The absence of a definite diagnostic test for any psychiatric disorder at the current state of knowledge implies diagnostic uncertainty (Zarin and Earls, 1993). Among clinically referred children the judgement of an expert will resolve this uncertainty and serve as a gold standard. In epidemiology, however, this is of little use, for obvious practical and budgetary reasons. Hence, it is of crucial importance for epidemiologists to make explicit how diagnostic information is to be organized in order to arrive at a definition of caseness and a classification of individual cases.

Classification of hyperactivity disorders

Both classification systems for psychopathology that are widely used, the *Diagnostic Statistical Manual* (DSM) of the American Psychiatric Association (APA), and the *International Classification of Disease* (ICD) of the World Health Organization (WHO), include definitions of hyperactivity disorders. In 1994, the DSM nomenclature witnessed the transition from DSM-III-R to DSM-IV (Chapter 5). DSM-III-R included a diagnostic category of attention deficit hyperactivity disorder (ADHD) that was defined by a single list of 14 symptoms, covering inattention, impulsivity and hyperactivity (APA, 1987). The diagnostic threshold was set at the presence of any eight symptoms. DSM-III-R also included a category called undifferentiated attention deficit disorder (UADD) that was believed to be comparable to attention deficit disorder without hyperactivity (ADD) in DSM-III (APA, 1980). No clear criteria for the diagnosis of UADD were provided, however. As a consequence, DSM-III-R-defined ADHD was viewed as a single disorder that included individuals with varying combinations of symptoms of inattention, hyperactivity and impulsiveness. Clinically, thus, ADHD was found to represent an extremely heterogeneous group. DSM-III-R, in addition, provided the following criteria for the clinical severity of ADHD: 'mild' was noted for cases with few, if any, symptoms in excess of the diagnostic threshold and minimal or no functional impairment in school and in social relationships; 'moderate' referred to symptom and impairment levels intermediate between 'mild' and 'severe'; and 'severe' was associated with cases demonstrating many symptoms in excess of the threshold, and significant impairment in functioning at home and school, and with peers.

DSM-IV retained the same diagnostic label as DSM-III-R (attention deficit hyperactivity disorder, ADHD), but provided a modified and extended list of diagnostic criteria (APA, 1994). The DSM-IV definition of ADHD contains a list of 18 symptoms spread over three separate dimensions: inattention (IA, nine symptoms), hyperactivity (H, six symptoms) and impulsivity (I, three symptoms). Furthermore, DSM-IV recognizes three subtypes of ADHD: combined type (at least six IA symptoms and six H and/or I symptoms), inattentive type (at least six IA symptoms), and hyperactive/impulsive type (at least six H and/or I symptoms). In contrast to previous DSM editions, DSM-IV further stipulates that the ADHD symptoms must be present in two or more settings (e.g. at school and at home). The revised definition of ADHD in DSM-IV is based on a number of factor analytic studies of ADHD symptoms in individuals from both clinic-referred and community samples (Lahey et al., 1988; DuPaul, 1991; Bauermeister et al., 1992; Pelham et al., 1992). These analyses have provided consistent support that two separate dimensions underlie ADHD: the first one consists of inattention symptoms, and the second one of hyperactivity and impulsivity symptoms. The validity of this distinction was further bolstered by evidence that these two dimensions differ in course and correlates. Inattention appears to be more stable over time than hyperactivity or impulsivity, which show a greater relative decline with increasing age. Hyperactivity-impulsivity symptoms are more strongly correlated with oppositional and antisocial behaviours than is inattention (Frick et al., 1994; Lahey et al., 1994). The way in which the diagnostic threshold of six symptoms for DSM-IV was finally derived reflects a growing appreciation of the importance of measuring functional impairment in addition to counting symptoms, which was a common practice earlier. Functional impairment will be discussed in more detail later in this chapter.

The latest version of ICD describes a category of hyperkinetic disorder (HKD) based on an almost identical list of 18 symptoms as in DSM-IV (WHO, 1992). However, there are differences between ICD-10 and DSM-IV in the way these symptoms serve as a basis for classification. A diagnosis of HKD requires the presence of each three – inattention (at least six out of nine symptoms), hyperactivity (at least three out of five symptoms) and impulsivity (at least one out of four symptoms). Furthermore, a major subdivision is made between HKD and hyperkinetic conduct disorder, a category reserved for the combination of HKD and conduct disorder. The presence of other comorbid conditions such as depressive or anxiety disorders, however, excludes the diagnosis of HKD. Finally, the criteria for cross-situational pervasiveness are more rigorous in ICD-10 than in DSM-IV. As a result, HKD is a more strictly defined subset of ADHD combined type (Chapter 5).

Categories versus dimensions

The approach to classification, in which a number of symptoms from a list constitutes a threshold that has to be met or passed, explicitly acknowledges that disorders are dimensional phenomena (Boyle et al., 1996) – symptoms can be substituted for one another to achieve a threshold. In this way, ADHD may be conceived of as the extreme end of a complex trait that is continuously distributed in the general population and includes inattention, hyperactivity and impulsivity as its subdimensions. This is in line with evidence from rating-scale data obtained from large populations of children (Rowe and Rowe, 1997). These data show a continuous distribution of scores, with progressively smaller number of subjects having scores at the extreme end. Analyses of large sets of parent and teacher ratings of primary schoolchildren on a scale that comprised the 18 DSM-IV ADHD symptoms provided further support for this dimensional view (Gomez et al., 1999). Confirmatory factor analyses on parent and teacher ratings favoured the two-factor (inattention vs. hyperactivity/impulsivity) and three-factor (inattention vs. hyperactivity vs. impulsivity) models of AD/HD symptoms at the population level, though the differences in fit between the two- and three-factor models were relatively minor (Gomez et al., 1999).

Important questions then are whether the category at the extreme end differs only by degree, or also by kind, and whether there are nonarbitrary and valid ways to establish a cutoff between a disorder as present or absent. The answer certainly depends on how and where we look, i.e. which dependent variables are chosen. In the DSM-IV field trial for ADHD among a clinic-referred sample of children aged 4–17 years, the diagnostic threshold of six symptoms was derived by calibrating the number of symptoms against measures of general and specific functional impairment (Lahey et al., 1994). This information, taken from a clinic population, may not be applicable to general population samples, as clinic referral in itself is already a sign of functional impairment, and the underlying response patterns of the two groups may differ (Boyle et al., 1996). The results of a study that systematically evaluated the implications of choosing different thresholds to classify DSM-III-R ADHD by using data from the Ontario Child Health Study (Boyle et al., 1996) are informative. Three methods are of particular interest here:

(1) using an extreme score of one standard deviation above the mean on parent and teacher scales, plus the perception that the child needed professional help

(2) using an extreme score of one standard deviation above the mean on parent and teacher scales, plus the perception of the informant that the child exhibited impairment in school (teacher), or in social relationships (parents)

(3) establishing a threshold on a rating scale by using the weighted information of a structured interview with parents and a child psychiatric interview with teachers

These methods resulted in roughly similar relative odds between the cases classified as ADHD and two associated correlates, parental arrest and developmental problems of the child. However, the results also showed considerable variation in prevalence estimates and in the patterns of comorbidity with conduct disorder. Moreover, when the overlap within informants was examined regarding children classified as ADHD, disagreements were far more frequent than agreements. One may therefore conclude that the use of different approaches to establish thresholds strongly affects what the findings will be. And further, that there is no generally agreed-upon approach that is superior on conceptual or empirical grounds. More empirical work should be done to develop measures of functional impairment and distress, as well as to derive rational decision rules to classify subjects.

A different and so far hardly explored perspective is that of aetiology. Are similar causal factors involved along the entire range of the dimension? Or alternatively, do cases at the extreme end of the dimension involve qualitatively different aetiological factors? A recent twin study provided evidence that ADHD reflects a highly heritable trait with about similar amounts of genetic loading across the range of phenotypic expression (Levy et al., 1997). This does not necessarily mean, however, that similar genes are involved at various cutoffs across the dimension; molecular genetic data are needed to clarify this. Looking at environmental risk factors, obstetric adversity and abnormalities at neurological examination were found in significantly higher percentages of children with severe ICD-10-defined HKD compared to children with ADHD according to DSM-III-R (Taylor et al., 1991). The suggestion clearly is that these early influences have an impact on brain development and determine the severity of the phenotypic expression.

Structured interviews vs. checklists

Information about psychiatric disorders in the general population is usually gathered by problem checklists that are self-rated or completed by important informants, and by structured interviews. Each approach has its merits and demerits. Checklists can be sent and returned by mail, and therefore are of relatively little expense. They can be completed at a time most convenient to the respondent, and allow information to be obtained from large populations. Structured interviews on the other hand enable more detailed information to be collected, for example, about symptom onset and duration. They also offer opportunities for resolving resistances, providing extra information and over-coming literacy problems. Compared to checklists, however, interview procedures are more time-consuming and expensive. Along with these practical contrasts between checklists and interviews, over the last years there has been increasing convergence regarding the descriptive content. Frequently, check-lists are now used that comprise items derived from the DSM schemes and have been subjected to factor analytic procedures to test the validity of syndromal structures, as detailed above concerning ADHD (DuPaul, 1991). At the same time, respondent-based structured interviews have been developed that involve strictly predefined questions and limited response options, thus leaving minimal room for interpretation by the interviewer (Shaffer et al., 2000). In epidemiological studies, these interviews are typically administered by trained nonprofessionals.

In a comparison of checklists vs. interviews for classifying DSM-III-R ADHD in an epidemiological data set, the differences in test–retest reliability and validity of the two methods were small (Boyle et al., 1997). No matter whether cases were classified by checklist or by interview as having ADHD, strong and significant associations were found with impaired social functioning and poor school performance (Boyle et al., 1997). This means that information about symptom onset and duration, as obtained by interview, does not offer surplus value when examining the association with external validators. Since there was little agreement about which individuals met the criteria for caseness, both methods are likely to involve considerable measurement error. Ultimately there does not appear to be much to choose between the two methods, aside from economic savings and reduction in time for respondents when using checklists.

Epidemiological surveys of ADHD in the period 1990–2000

Methodology

Table 2.1 summarizes the design and main findings of 11 questionnaire-based studies on the epidemiology of ADHD that were published between 1990 and 2000. The methodological diversity was less than in studies of earlier times, since the majority (7/11) of studies both used questionnaires based on DSM-III-R or DSM-IV items for ADHD, and spanned a rather similar age range, from 5 to about 14 years. The data of two reports were based on Conners' questionnaires. Two studies focused on the epidemiology of ADHD in adults and covered an age range of 17–84 years. Teacher information was mostly used for the studies in children and adolescents. One study utilized both parent and teacher reports, and therefore allows a comparison of the information from the two sources (Gomez et al., 1999). The studies in adults were based on self-report data.

The design and findings of 19 studies that used a diagnostic interview approach to case definition have been outlined in Tables 2.2 and 2.3. As is apparent, these studies present considerable variations in design and methodology. One study is limited to preschoolers (Lavigne et al., 1996), five studies focus on children aged 6 and 10 years, five others only include children from 10 to 15 years of age, and the remaining eight projects study a broader age range somewhere between 6 and 17 years. Twelve studies used a two-stage design in which the community sample was first screened with a questionnaire such as the Child Behavior Checklist (CBCL), sometimes with the related Teacher Report Form (TRF) and Youth Self-report Form (YSF) added, the Rutter scales, or the Conners scales. The children who had scores above a predetermined cutoff point (screen-positives), and a subsample of screen-negative children, were invited for detailed evaluations in the second stage. The remaining studies (7/19) employed a one-stage design in which as many parents and/or children of the initial sample as possible were interviewed (Cohen et al., 1993b; Fergusson et al., 1993; Schaughency et al., 1994; Shaffer et al., 1996; Costello et al., 1997; Simonoff et al., 1997; Breton et al., 1999). In most cases the preferred structured diagnostic interview was the Diagnostic Interview Schedule for Children (DISC: 9/19 studies); other interview schemes used were the Child and Adolescent Psychiatric Assessment (CAPA: 3/19), the Diagnostic Interview for Children and Adolescents (DICA) and the Schedule for Affective Disorders and Schizophrenia for School-Age Children (K-SADS: each 1/19). All studies but three were designed to establish the prevalence of any psychiatric disorder, and were able to provide data on ADHD as a component of this more general enterprise. Three projects had a more restricted focus, specifically aiming to identify cases with ADHD, and to investigate the cognitive and psychosocial correlates of these (Taylor et al., 1991; Landgren et al., 1996; Leung and Connolly, 1996; Leung et al., 1996).

Prevalence of ADHD in children and adolescents

Because of important differences in the choice of informant (parent vs. teacher), and in the statistical procedures to define a cutoff, the findings on prevalence of the two studies (Wang et al., 1993; Rowe and Rowe, 1997) that incorporated Conners' questionnaires cannot be appropriately compared, in spite of including children of a similar age range. For children between 5 and 14 years of age, the prevalence of DSM-III-R-defined ADHD on the basis of teacher report varied from 6.5% to 10.9% (Pelham et al., 1992; Baumgaertel et al., 1995; Wolraich et al., 1996). The six studies that provided information on ADHD according to the DSM-IV scheme found a prevalence in this age range between 8.1% and 17.8% (Baumgaertel et al., 1995; Wolraich et al., 1996, 1998; Gaub and Carlson, 1997; Gomez et al., 1999; Pineda et al., 1999). The likely explanations for these discrepant findings are differences in case definition, and particularly whether functional impairment was taken into consideration. For example, when measures of impairment of peer relationships and academic achievement were added to the count of symptoms, the total prevalence of ADHD dropped from 16.1% to 6.8% in one study (Wolraich et al., 1998). Another study only took symptoms into account if endorsed as 'very much' (Gaub and Carlson, 1997), which is discrepant from the approach adopted in other studies on DSM-IV items that aggregated symptoms endorsed as 'much' and 'very much' (or as 'often' and 'very often'). Wolraich et al. (1998) showed that changing the cutoff point from 'often' and 'very often' to only 'very often' resulted in a reduction of identified cases by about 36%. Two studies applied both DSM-III-R and DSM-IV criteria, and thus allow a direct comparison between these classification systems (Baumgaertel et al., 1995; Wolraich et al., 1996). The results converge, in that DSM-IV criteria systematically increase the prevalence of ADHD by a factor of 1.6. This is not surprising given the introduction of the hyperactive-impulsive type and the reentry of the inattentive type of ADHD in DSM-IV.

As shown in Table 2.3, the studies using psychiatric interviews are reporting a prevalence of any psychiatric disorder between 14.2% (Simonoff et al., 1997) and 35.5% (Verhulst et al., 1997), with nine studies being remarkably consistent in finding a prevalence of any disorder within a close range between 19.9% and 26.3%. These estimates are based on the application of the so-called 'or' rule, in

Table 2.1. Studies using questionnaires on the epidemiology of attention deficit hyperactivity disorder (ADHD) in the period 1990–2000

Study	Size	Age (years)	Frame	Assessment	Prevalence (%)	Other findings
Pelham et al., 1992	931	5–14	National sample in the USA	Teacher questionnaire (Disruptive Behavior Disorders Rating Scale – DSM-III-R items)	DSM-III-R 6.5	
Wang et al., 1993	4290	5–13	Public schools in Taiwan	Conners' Teacher Questionnaire	9.9 (optimal cutoff determined using receiver operator characteristics analysis)	M/F 3.3 : 1 (prevalence in boys 14.9, in girls 4.5)
Baumgaertel et al., 1995	1077	5–12	10 public schools in Regensburg, Germany	Teacher questionnaire (all DSM-IV and DSM-III-R items for ADHD)	DSM-III-R 10.9 DSM-IV: IA 9.0 HI 3.9, C 4.8 Total 17.8	M/F 5 : 1 for HI and 2 : 1 for IA Comorbidity: ODD 23.9% Age: not reported
Wolraich et al., 1996	8258	5–11	All schools in middle Tennessee county, USA	Teacher questionnaire (all DSM-IV and DSM-III-R items for ADHD)	DSM-III-R 7.3 DSM-IV: IA 5.4 HI 2.4, C 3.6 Total 11.4	M/F 4 : 1 for HI and 2 : 1 for IA Age: not reported Comorbidity: ODD 30.2%, CD 15.6%, ANX/DEP 21.6%
Murphy and Barkley, 1996	720	17–84	Convenient sample of individuals that applied for a first licence or renewed their driver's licence	Self-report questionnaire (all DSM-IV items for ADHD) for current symptoms and symptoms in childhood	DSM-IV IA 1.3 HI 2.5, C 0.8 Total 4.7 (cutoff 6/9 criteria)	M/F no significant differences Significant decline with age for all symptoms
Rowe and Rowe, 1997	6841	5–14	Cluster-designed representative sampling of school-age children in Victoria, Australia	Parent ratings on Conners' Abbreviated 10-item Parent–Teacher Questionnaire Confirmatory factor analysis revealed a five-item subscale inattentive/overactive	3.4–4.0 (using as cutoff a total weighted score of 2 on the inattentive/overactive scale)	M/F: 1.8 at 5–6 years till 5.8 at 12–14 years Increase of prevalence from 4–5 years to 12–14 years in boys, and decrease over these ages in girls

Study	N	Age	Method	Prevalence	Comments
Gaub and Carlson, 1997	2744	5–10	Teacher questionnaires (SNAP-IV, DSM-IV-based items of ADHD and ODD)	DSM-IV: IA 4.5 HI 1.7, C 1.9 Total 8.1	No effect of age
Wolraich et al., 1998	4323	5–12	Teacher questionnaire (all DSM-IV items for ADHD)	DSM-IV IA 8.8 HI 2.6, C 4.7 Total 16.1 DSM-IV plus impairment IA 3.2 HI 0.6, C 2.9 Total 6.8	M/F 3:1 for HI and 2:1 for IA Age: not reported Comorbidity: ODD 36.5%, CD 9.6%, ANX/DEP 20.8%, LD 11.3%, LI 4.4%
Pineda et al., 1999	540	4–17	Parent questionnaire (DSM-IV ADHD rating scale)	DSM-IV: IA 4.2 HI 8.5, C 3.3 Total 16.0	M/F 1.5:1 (not significant) Higher total prevalence at 6–11 years (18.2%) and in low SES (22.5%)
Gomez et al., 1999	1275	5–11	Parent and teacher questionnaire (DSM-IV ADHD rating scale)	Parent ratings: DSM-IV IA 4.2 HI 2.7, C 2.9 Total 9.9 Teacher ratings: IA 5.8 HI 0.9, C 2.1 Total 8.8 Parent and teacher: IA 1.6 HI 0.2, 0.6, 2.4	M/F 2.5:1 for parent ratings, 3.3:1 for teacher ratings and 5.3:1 for ratings of parents and teachers. Age effect on the HI scale completed by parents (younger higher scores) but not on the IA scale and not on teacher ratings
Kooij et al., unpublished work	1780	18–74	Self-report questionnaire (all DSM-IV ADHD items for current symptoms, and three questions about hyperactivity, impulsivity and inattention in childhood)	DSM-IV: IA 0.4 HI 0.5, C 0.4 Total 1.3 (cutoff for current symptoms 6/9 criteria) IA 0.5 HI 1.6 C 1.1 Total 3.2 (cutoff for current symptoms 4/9 criteria)	M/F no significant differences No significant age effects

M/F, male/female ratio; IA, ADHD inattentive type; HI, ADHD hyperactive/impulsive type; C, ADHD combined type; total sum of inattentive, hyperactive/impulsive and combined type of ADHD; SNAP-IV, Swanson Nolen and Pelham scale for DSM-IV; ODD, Oppositional defiant disorder; CD, conduct disorder; ANX, anxiety disorder; DEP, depressive disorder; LD, learning disorder; LI, language impairment; SES, socioeconomic status.

Table 2.2. Studies in the period 1990–2000 on the epidemiology of attention deficit hyperactivity disorder (ADHD) using structured interviews: design

Study	Location	Size	Age (years)	Frame	Case definition
Taylor et al., 1991	Newham, East London, UK	2462 (194)[a]	6–7	All boys at school in Newham	DSM-III-R, ICD-10
Fergusson et al., 1993	Christchurch, New Zealand	961–986[b]	15	Birth cohort of 1265 children born in Christchurch area in 1977	DSM-III-R
Cohen et al., 1993a,b	New York, USA	975 (776)	10–13	Second follow-up of multistage random community sample	DSM-III-R
Schaughency et al., 1994	Dunedin, New Zealand	943 (943)	15	Follow-up of Dunedin birth cohort	DSM-III (adapted by using cutoff 1 SD above mean for symptom count)
Gomez-Beneyto et al., 1994	Valencia, Spain	1200 (320)	8, 11 and 15 (each 400)	Multistage random community sampling	DSM-III-R
Jensen et al., 1995	Washington DC, USA	482 (126)	6–17	Military post	DSM-III-R and impairment
Lavigne et al., 1996	Chicago, USA	3860 (510)	2–5	Children visiting paediatricians in the Chicago area	DSM-III-R
August et al., 1996	Minnesota, USA	7231 (318)	6–10	Sample of all children of 22 elementary schools	DSM-III-R
Leung et al., 1996	Hong Kong	3069 (611)	6–10, boys only	Random sample of primary schools in Hong Kong	DSM-III, DSM-III-R and ICD-10
Costello et al., 1996a,b	Great Smoky Mountains Study, North Carolina, USA	4500 (1015)	9, 11, and 13 (first wave of overlapping cohort design)	Screening-stratified sampling from general population	DSM-III-R and various measures of impairment
		(970)	10–14 Second wave		DSM-IV and impairment
		(928)	11–15 Third wave		DSM-IV and impairment
		(820)	12–16 Fourth wave		DSM-IV and impairment

Reference	Location	Age and design	N (n)	Sample	Diagnostic criteria
Costello et al., 1997	Qualla Boundary, North Carolina, USA	9, 11 and 13 (overlapping cohort design with four annual waves)	450 (450)	All American Indian children	As in Costello et al., 1996a,b
Landgren et al., 1996	Mariestad, Sweden	6	589 (95)	Birth cohort of 2 years	DSM-III-R
Shaffer et al., 1996	Four sites (Connecticut, Georgia, New York and Puerto Rico), USA	9–17	1285 (1285)	Random community (multisite)	DSM-III-R and impairment
Verhulst et al., 1997	Netherlands	13–18	853 (272–4)	Stratified multistage cluster and random sampling from general population	DSM-III-R and impairment (CGAS)
Simonoff et al., 1997	Virginia, USA	8–16, longitudinal cohort study	2824 (1412 families)	Sample of twins born between 1974 and 1983 in Virginia	DSM-III-R
Steinhausen et al., 1998	Canton of Zurich, Switzerland	7–16	1964 (399)	Stratified random sample	DSM-III-R
Rohde et al., 1999	Porto Allegro, Brazil	12–14	1013 (191)	Cluster random sample of school	DSM-IV and impairment (CGAS)
Breton et al., 1999	Quebec, Canada	6–14	2400[b]	Stratified random sample	DSM-III-R and impairment
Almqvist et al., 1999	Finland	8–9	5813 (435)	Multistage stratified random sample	DSM-III-R

[a]Numbers in brackets refer to the number of participants interviewed in a two-stage design.

[b]All participants were interviewed.

CGAS, Children's Global Assessment Scale.

Table 2.3. Studies in the period 1990–2000 on the epidemiology of attention deficit hyperactivity disorder (ADHD) that used structured interviews: assessment and findings

Study	Assessment	Prevalence	Other findings concerning ADHD
Taylor et al., 1991	First stage: Rutter scale A (parents), Rutter scale B, supplemented with items from the Conners Teacher Questionnaire (teachers) Second stage: battery of attentional performance tests, behaviour observation and neurological examination (child), PACS (parents), standardized interview (teachers)	Any psychiatric disorder: not assessed ADHD (DSM-III-R) 17% ADD 1.5% PH 9% HKD (ICD-10) 1.7%	Comorbidity: CD 46%, ED 14% SES − (ADD +) Cognitive impairments: lower IQ and attention deficits in ADD and HKD Adverse family factors correlated with persistence of disorder Perinatal adversity and neurological abnormalities in HKD
Fergusson et al., 1993	DISC (child) and Revised Behavior Problems Checklist (parents) for ADHD and ODD diagnoses	Any psychiatric disorder 22.1% (self-report), 13.0% (parent) ADHD (DSM-III-R) 2.8% (self-report), 3.0% (parent), 4.8% ('or' rule)	Males 5.7%, Females 2.7% Comorbidity: ODD/CD (OR 23.6) Depression (OR 4.5) Substance abuse (OR 7.0)
Cohen et al., 1993a,b	DISC (child and parent) interview	Any psychiatric disorder: not reported ADHD (DSM-III-R) 9.3%	Age: ADHD at 10–13 years 12.8%, 14–16 years 9.0%, 17–20 years 6.0% Male/female 1.90
Schaughency et al., 1994	DISC (child) and Revised Behavior Problems Checklist (parents) for ADHD diagnoses	Any psychiatric disorder 22.0% (severe disorder 10.0%) ADHD (DSM-III) 4.9% (child)	Males 6%, females 3.6% Comorbidity ODD/CD 30% Anxiety/depression 23%
Gomez-Beneyto et al., 1994	First stage: CBCL Second stage: K-SADS (parent and child) interview	Any psychiatric disorder 21.7 % (severe disorder 4.4%) ADHD (DSM-III-R) 7.6%	Age: ADHD at 8 years 14.4%, 11 years 5.3%, 15 years 3.0%
Jensen et al., 1995	First stage: CBCL Second stage: DISC (parent, child) interview	Any psychiatric disorder 18.6% (parent), 8.8% (child), 26.3% ('or' rule) ADHD (DSM-III-R) 11.9% (parent), 0.8% (child), 15.1% ('or' rule)	Prevalence of ADHD when the diagnosis is accompanied by service need/use: 2.4% (parent), 0.7% (child), 2.7% ('or' rule)
Lavigne et al., 1996	First stage: CBCL Second stage: play observation, developmental evaluation, Rochester Adaptive Behavior Inventory	Any psychiatric disorder 21.1% (severe disorder 8.3%) ADHD (DSM-III-R) 2% (severe ADHD 1.5%)	Males 2.4%, Females 1.3% Comorbidity 20/23 (87%) of ADHD cases had comorbid disorders

Study	Method	Prevalence	Comorbidity/Correlates
August et al., 1996	First stage: screen of 10-item Conners' Questionnaire (teachers, then parents) Second stage: DICA (parent) interview	ADHD (DSM-III-R) 5.6% (unweighted since only screen-positives were interviewed)	Comorbidity ODD 32% CD 12% Depression 30% Anxiety 34%
Leung et al., 1996	First stage: screen of Rutter questionnaire (parents, teachers) Second stage: parent interview (PACS), teacher interview, battery of cognitive tests, neurological examination	ADDH (DSM-III) 6.1% ADHD (DSM-III-R) 8.9% HKD (ICD-10) 0.8%	Attentional problems in pervasive hyperactive children, but not in children with mixed hyperactive/conduct problems Different correlates for pervasive hyperactive and situational hyperactive children
Costello et al., 1996a,b	First stage: screen of externalizing items of CBCL. Second stage: CAPA interview (parent, child); ADHD diagnosis only based on parent interview	Any psychiatric disorder 20.3% ADHD (DSM-III-R) 1.9%	Males 2.9%, females 0.95% Comorbidity: ODD/CD 33.3% (OR 10.2) Depression 12.8% (OR 11.1) Anxiety 12.8% (OR 2.6)
	CAPA interview (parent, child)	ADHD (DSM-IV) 1.0%	Comorbidity: ODD/CD 35.5% (OR 11.7) Depression 7.2% (OR NS) Anxiety 17.2% (OR 5.6)
	CAPA interview (parent, child)	ADHD (DSM-IV) 0.9%	Comorbidity: ODD/CD 22.1% (OR 8.7) Depression 17.2% (OR NS) Anxiety 17.2% (OR 7.4)
	CAPA interview (parent, child)	ADHD (DSM-IV) 1.0%	Comorbidity ODD/CD 13.9% (OR NS) Depression 0 %, anxiety 0%
Costello et al., 1997	CAPA interview (parent, child)	First wave: ADHD (DSM-III-R) 1.3% Second wave: ADHD (DSM-IV) 1.3% Third wave: ADHD (DSM-IV) 1.0% Fourth wave: ADHD (DSM-IV) 0.4%	Comorbidity: ODD/CD 25% (OR NS) Depression 0%, anxiety 0% Comorbidity: ODD/CD 50% (OR 11.9) Depression 50%, anxiety 0% Comorbidity: ODD/CD 67% (OR 43) Depression 33%, anxiety 33% Comorbidity: ODD/CD 100% Depression 0%, anxiety 0%

Table 2.3. (cont.)

Study	Assessment	Prevalence	Other findings concerning ADHD
Landgren et al., 1996	First stage: parent questionnaires (10-item Conners; psychomotor items), teacher questionnaire (attention, language) and screen by doctor for motor problems Second stage: neurodevelopmental, neuropsychiatric and psychological examinations (child), interview on DSM-III-R ADHD items (parents)	ADHD (DSM-III-R) 4.0% DAMP 6.9%	Male/female 5.7:1 Comorbidity: 8/14 (57%) of ADHD cases also met criteria for DAMP; 8/27 (30%) of DAMP cases met criteria for ADHD
Shaffer et al., 1996	DISC (child and parent) interview	Any psychiatric disorder 10.2% (parent), 12.3% (child), 20.9% ('or' rule) (CGAS <70 and specific impairment) ADHD (DSM-III-R) 2.8% (parent), 1.1% (child), 4.1% ('or' rule) (CGAS <70 and specific impairment)	
Verhulst et al., 1997	First stage: CBCL, TRF and YSF Second stage: DISC (child and parent) interview	Any disorder 21.5% (self-report), 21.8% (parent), 2.6%, (child) 35.5% ('or' rule), 4.0% (both) ADHD 1.3% (self-report), 1.8% (parent), 2.6% ('or' rule), 0.4% (both)	No significant sex differences Comorbidity 8/12 (75%) of ADHD cases had comorbid disorders
Simonoff et al., 1997	CAPA (parent and child) interview	Any psychiatric disorder with impairment 14.2% ADHD (DSM-III-R) 1.4%	Males 2.4%, female 0.8% No significant age effect Comorbidity ODD/CD 40% (OR NS)
Steinhausen et al., 1998	First stage: CBCL and YSF (11–17 years) Second stage: DISC (child and parent) interview	Any psychiatric disorder 22.5% ADHD (DSM-III-R) 5.3%	Males 6.1%, female 3.3%

Study	Method	Results	Demographics
Rohde et al., 1999	First stage: ADHD DSM-IV rating scale (teacher) Second stage: clinical interview with parent and child (applying DSM-IV criteria for ADHD and other disruptive disorders)	ADHD (DSM-IV) IA 2.0% HI 0.8% C 3.0% Total 5.8% (child and parent information, using 'or' rule)	Male/female 1:1 Comorbidity ODD 21.7%, CD 26.1%
Breton et al., 1999	DISC (child 12–14 years, parent, teacher interview; cartoon-based notebook (child 6–11 years)	Any psychiatric disorder 19.9% (parent), 15.8% (child) ADHD (DSM-III-R) 4% (parent), 3.3% (child), 8.9% (teacher)	Male/female 2.9:1 (parent) to 5.1:1 (teacher) Age: 6–8/12–14 years OR ~2.2 (sign)
Almqvist et al., 1999	First stage: Rutter Parent Scale, Rutter Teacher Scale, Children Depression Inventory Second stage: interview with parents (semistructured, according to Rutter–Graham)	Any psychiatric disorder 21.8% ADHD (DSM-III-R) 7.1%	Males 11.3%, females 2.9%

OR, odds ratio; HKD, hyperkinetic disorder; ADD, attention deficit disorder; ADDH, attention deficit disorder with hyperactivity (DSM-III); ADDH, attention deficit disorder without hyperactivity (DSM-III); ED, emotional disorder; DISC, Diagnostic Interview Schedule for Children; DICA, Diagnostic Interview for Children and Adolescents; CAPA, Child and Adolescent Psychiatric Assessment; PACS, Parental Account of Childhood Symptoms; PH, pervasive hyperactivity; CBCL, Child Behavior Checklist; K-SADS, Schedule for Affective Disorders and Schizophrenia for School-Age Children; TRF, Teacher Report Form; YSF, Youth Self-report Form; DAMP, disorders of attention, motor deficits and perception; CGAS, Children's Global Assessment Scale; NS, not significant.

Other abbreviations: see footnotes to Table 2.1.

which a disorder is considered to be present when endorsed by information from either the parent or the child. This consistency is even more remarkable given that these studies covered an age range from preschool (Lavigne et al., 1996) to late adolescence (Fergusson et al., 1993; Schaughency et al., 1994), and used various methodologies. There is much greater variance in the reported prevalence of DSM-III-R ADHD. The highest rate comes from Jensen et al. (1995) who report an overall prevalence of 15.1% of ADHD among children aged between 6 and 17 years. These data are based on a rather small community sample, and consequently the confidence intervals are wide. All three studies that used the CAPA interview came up with the lowest prevalence rates in the range of 1.4–1.9% (Costello et al., 1996b, 1997; Simonoff et al., 1997). The CAPA interview retrieves information from the parent covering only the past 3 months for conferring a diagnosis of ADHD, whereas the DISC interview collects information from the parent over the past 6 months. Furthermore, the CAPA interview does not incorporate information from the child, while the DISC is usually applied to children aged 9 or older. However, these differences in procedures can hardly explain the variation in prevalence estimates. For example, in the study by Shaffer et al. (1996), parent information would only amount to a prevalence of 2.4%, but in the Jensen et al. (1995) study it amounts to up to 11.9%. The other nine studies provide estimates of DSM-III-R-based ADHD between 2.0% and 9.3%. Excluding the study in preschoolers (Lavigne et al., 1996), the prevalences between 5.3% and 9.3% seem reasonably comparable with the estimates obtained in questionnaire-based studies. Not one of the interview-based studies applied both DSM-III-R and DSM-IV criteria, which precludes a comparison of the prevalences obtained by both systems.

The studies primarily designed to examine the prevalence of ADHD have produced widely divergent estimates (4.0%, 8.9% and 17%; Taylor et al., 1991; Landgren et al., 1996; Leung et al., 1996). This may be explained by the fact that the London and Hong Kong studies only included boys, and that the Swedish study had a rather small sample size with large confidence intervals. This range of estimates seems to be less, if at all, a result of age differences since the ages in the London and Swedish studies were similar. The prevalence of the more strictly defined ICD-10-based hyperkinetic disorder in boys was between 0.8% and 1.7% (Taylor et al., 1991; Leung et al., 1996).

Influence of gender

All questionnaire studies report an excess of boys with ADHD over girls, with ratios of total ADHD between 1.5 and 5.8, though the lowest ratio of 1.5 in one study is not significant (Pineda et al., 1999). The interview studies found gender ratios between 1.8:1 and 4:1, with the exception of that by Verhulst et al. (1997) in which no significant gender difference in prevalence could be observed. Gender differences may be partly a function of informant use, since teacher reports have led to greater gender-related differences in prevalence than parent reports (Breton et al., 1999). For a more extensive discussion on gender influences, see Chapter 4.

Influence of age

The data about the effect of age in the range between 5 and 17 years on the frequency of ADHD symptoms, and on the prevalence of ADHD types, have, however, been far less consistent. Pineda et al. (1999) found that the prevalence of total ADHD based on parent ratings was higher in children between 6 and 11 years of age than in the 4–5-year-olds, or in the 12–18-year-olds. Furthermore, in the 4–11-year-olds the hyperactive-impulsive type predominated, whereas in the oldest group the inattentive type was most frequent. In contrast, children with any of the three subtypes of ADHD had a rather similar mean age in Gaub and Carlson's (1997) study. Gomez et al. (1999), on the other hand, documented a significant age effect on hyperactivity-impulsivity symptoms for parent, but not for teacher ratings, with higher scores at a younger age, but failed to find an age effect on inattentive symptoms. On Conners' Abbreviated Scale completed by parents, a significant age effect was found for boys, but not for girls, with higher scores at age 12–14 years than at age 4–5 years (Rowe and Rowe, 1997). Such a gender by age interaction effect was absent in other studies. Three studies that used questionnaires did not provide a breakdown of the data according to age (Baumgaertel et al., 1995; Wolraich et al., 1996, 1998). Overall, parent information provides stronger support than teacher information for age differences, particularly concerning hyperactivity-impulsivity symptoms.

Age seems to be one of the major modifying variables of prevalence among interview-based studies. Children at preschool age have not yet gone through the entire risk period to develop ADHD. Not surprisingly, then, Lavigne et al. (1996) found a prevalence of 2.0% DSM-III-R ADHD at age 2–5 years. On the other hand, studies including adolescents between 13 and 18 years of age have reported prevalences between 2.6% and 4.9% (Fergusson et al., 1993; Schaughency et al., 1994; Verhulst et al., 1997). Higher prevalences between 5.3% and 9.6% were reported in studies that included children between 6 and 13 years of age (August et al., 1996; Steinhausen et al., 1998; Almqvist et al., 1999; Rohde et al., 1999). The important influence of age is further confirmed by studies that systematically examined age effects on prevalence. In the

Canadian study by Breton et al. (1999), the prevalence was 5.8% at age 6–8, 4% at age 9–11 and 2.5% at age 12–14 years. In Valencia, Spain, the prevalence among 8-year-old children was 14.4%, among the 11-year-olds 5.3%, and among the 15-year-olds 3% (Gomez-Beneyto et al., 1994). Finally, in a longitudinal cohort study, the prevalence was 12.9% at age 10–13 years, 9% in the 14-year-olds, and 6% in the 16-year-old children (Cohen et al., 1993b). In summary, the epidemiological data from interview studies clearly indicate that prevalence declines with age.

Informant perspective

Parent ratings on inattentive and hyperactivity-impulsivity symptoms were higher than teacher ratings for both boys and girls in a DSM-IV rating-scale study (Gomez et al., 1999). This suggests that parent ratings are less likely to be confirmed by teachers than vice versa. In this particular study, teacher ratings also showed higher test–retest reliabilities and higher internal consistencies than parent ratings (Gomez et al., 1999). The results are in contrast to those of Breton et al. (1999) who found much higher prevalences of ADHD as reported by teachers. This latter result is, however, more in line with the experience of many clinicians who believe that the structured classroom situation makes higher demands on the ability to sustain attention and to control behaviour than the situation at home. As a consequence, children are more likely to be considered inattentive, hyperactive or impulsive at school than at home. Earlier epidemiological work had also pointed to a greater contribution to the diagnosis by teachers than by parents (Szatmari et al., 1989).

Further data that are relevant to the issue of informant perspective are provided by a community study from Hong Kong (Ho et al., 1996; Leung et al., 1996). This study compared the behavioural, developmental and cognitive correlates of pervasively hyperactive children (i.e. meeting threshold criteria on a rating scale both at home and at school) with the ones of children who were only hyperactive at home (situational home hyperactive), or who were only hyperactive at school (situational school hyperactive), and with the ones of nonhyperactive controls. The pervasively hyperactive children differed systematically from normal controls on actometer measures of motor activity. By contrast, the situationally hyperactive groups could not be discerned from the normal children by their motor activity. Home hyperactivity was associated with poor family relationships, whereas school hyperactivity was linked to low intelligence, clumsiness, reading problems and other difficulties in scholastic achievements. A unique characteristic of the pervasively hyperactive children, compared to the other groups of children, was the high percentage of language delay (Ho et al., 1996). Overall, these results cast serious doubt on the validity of home hyperactivity as a clinical syndrome. Furthermore, the findings urge caution against lumping together school hyperactivity and pervasive hyperactivity, given their rather different correlates. In any case, this study lends support to the importance of the school situation in diagnosing ADHD.

Subtypes of ADHD

Among clinically referred children the combined type of ADHD is diagnosed much more often than the inattentive or hyperactive-impulsive types (Lahey et al., 1994). At the population level, however, five out of six studies report that the inattentive type of ADHD is the most common one, and occurs in about 50% of the ADHD cases defined on the basis of teacher information (Baumgaertel et al., 1995; Wolraich et al., 1996, 1998; Gaub and Carlson, 1997; Gomez et al., 1999) or parent information (Gomez et al., 1999). Apart from the data of the second to the fourth waves in the studies using the CAPA interview (Costello et al., 1996b, 1997), only one reported on the prevalence of DSM-IV subtypes of ADHD (Rohde et al., 1999). The results confirmed the findings of questionnaire studies in that the inattentive type constituted a substantial component (about 35%) of total ADHD.

Clinical studies had previously indicated that the three types of ADHD exhibited different patterns of associated characteristics. The combined type of ADHD was diagnosed more often among boys of a younger age, whereas children with the inattentive type were somewhat older and mostly girls (Lahey et al., 1994). Furthermore, the combined type was associated with greater severity of general impairment and high rates of comorbid externalizing disorders. In contrast, the ADHD inattentive type showed stronger links with specific impairments of cognitive and learning functions, and with comorbid internalizing disorders (Lahey et al., 1994). It was expected that replication of these findings in population-based samples would provide further support for the validity of the DSM-IV ADHD subtypes. This was indeed what the data generally showed. The inattentive type was identified relatively more often in girls, with boy:girl ratios from 2:1 to 3:1 for inattentive ADHD, and from 3:1 to 7:1 for hyperactive-impulsive ADHD (Baumgaertel et al., 1995; Wolraich et al., 1996, 1998; Gaub and Carlson, 1997; Gomez et al., 1999). Furthermore, inattentive symptoms were correlated with low rates of associated oppositional and conduct problems, high rates of poor academic performance (Baumgaertel et al., 1995; Wolraich et al., 1996; Gaub and Carlson, 1997) and high rates of comorbid internalizing problems and language impairments (Wolraich et al., 1998) when compared to the symptoms of hyperactivity-impulsivity.

Comorbidity

The rates of comorbid disorders are rather high in both questionnaire and interview studies, and include oppositional defiant disorder (22–35%), conduct disorder (15%) and affective disorders (anxiety and/or depression, 25%). A recent review and metaanalysis of comorbidity in community-based samples that included a number of studies described in Tables 2.2 and 2.3, as well as some studies published earlier than 1990, concluded that there is a statistically significant association between ADHD and conduct disorder (median odds ratio (OR) 10.7), ADHD and depressive disorders (OR 5.5) and ADHD and anxiety disorders (OR 3.0; Angold et al., 1999a). The interested reader may consult this thoughtful review for further considerations of theoretical models, causes and interpretations of these comorbidities.

Prevalence and distribution of ADHD in adults

Two reports are available on the epidemiology of ADHD in adults based on self-report data. The first used a convenience sample of individuals who applied for their first driving licence or wished to renew one. The total prevalence of ADHD was 4.7% when using the cutoff of 6/9 criteria as defined in DSM-IV for both current and childhood functioning (Murphy and Barkley, 1996). The second study administered the ADHD DSM-IV rating scale for current symptoms and three key questions on childhood symptoms to a sample of adult primary-care patients (Kooij et al., unpublished work). The conventional cutoff of 6/9 current symptoms and at least two symptoms in childhood produced a total prevalence of 1.3%. When measures of functional impairment were incorporated in the analyses, a cutoff of 4/9 current symptoms proved to offer the best balance in differentiating cases from noncases (Kooij et al., unpublished work). This would result in a prevalence of total ADHD of 3.2%. With the cutoff of 6/9 current symptoms, about one third of the ADHD cases in both studies were of the inattentive type. A lowering of the cutoff to 4/9 current symptoms, however, gave evidence of a clear shift from the inattentive type towards the hyperactive-impulsive and the combined types of ADHD at adult age. Obviously, this reflects the fact that the majority of adults with four or more inattentive symptoms also have four or more hyperactive-impulsive symptoms, and thus qualify for the ADHD combined type. The reverse, however, for adults with four or more hyperactive-impulsive symptoms, is not true. These results are unexpected, given the preponderance of the inattentive type of ADHD in children in population-based samples, and the stronger decline of hyperactive-impulsive than of inattentive symptoms at older age (Biederman et al., 2000). The relatively strong representation of hyperactive-impulsive ADHD at adult age is also not in line with the view that this subtype is particularly present among preschoolers who have not been challenged enough by task-related demands in school, and have not yet developed clinically significant inattentive symptoms (Lahey et al., 1994).

The caveat to be made, of course, is that the adult studies rely on self-report data. Two-stage designs that have utilized structured psychiatric interviews to establish ADHD symptoms in adults have not yet been performed. This means that our knowledge about the validity and reliability of self-report data on ADHD symptoms remains limited. A recent report provided evidence for a strong correlation between adult self-report data and reports by partners of current ADHD symptoms, and between adult self-reports and their parents' ratings of childhood symptoms (Murphy and Schachar, 2000). In a follow-up study of adolescents, who in childhood had been identified as having ADHD, self-report information was found to underestimate the severity of ADHD symptoms (Danckaerts et al., 1999). On the other hand, self-report data were a good predictor of general outcome. In a similar way, self-report data about ADHD symptoms at age 15 in the Dunedin birth cohort study showed little overlap with information by the parents, but did correlate rather well with a number of external validators such as measures of functional impairment (Schaughency et al., 1994).

Both adult studies failed to establish significant gender differences. This is in accordance with clinical experience in adult ADHD clinics where about equal numbers of men and women are seen on the basis of self-referral or referral by primary-care professionals. The two adult studies have opposite findings regarding age influences above 18 years. While using the same age blocks of 17–29 years, 30–49 years and above 50 years, Murphy and Barkley (1996) reported a significant decline of all symptom dimensions with age, whereas Kooij et al. (unpublished work) did not. Sample variation (car drivers vs. primary-care patients) may be relevant here to explain this discrepancy.

For a fuller discussion on the adult form of the disorder, see Chapter 14.

Cognitive correlates

The study with the most extensive data set on cognitive and attentional correlates of hyperactivity is reported by Taylor and colleagues (1991). In the second stage of the London survey, cognitive performance was examined in five carefully defined contrast groups of children, namely a pure hyperactive group (defined as pervasively hyperactive on both parent and teacher questionnaires), a pure conduct disorder group, a mixed hyperactive-conduct disorder group, a group of children with attentional problems without hyperactivity

(ADD acording to DSM-III) and a normal control group. The battery of psychological tests administered included five subtests from the Wechsler Intelligence Scale for Children – Revised (WISC-R: similarities, vocabulary, block design, object assembly and digit span), reading tests, a Continuous Performance Task (CPT), a central-incidental learning test, a Matching Familiar Figures (MFF) test and the Paired Associate Learning (PAL) test. As a result, the ADD group proved to be clearly different from the normal group in revealing a lower IQ, more speech problems and in having poorer reading skills. The mixed hyperactive-conduct group was also delayed in reading abilities, but not lower in IQ. The hyperactive and conduct groups were neither different from one another, nor different from the normal group in IQ, speech or reading skills. On a composite score of attention performance the ADD and the mixed groups were found to be significantly impaired by comparison with the normal children. Also, the hyperactive group were behind in attention performance compared to the conduct group. All the same differences reported in speech and reading skills and in attention performance were found even with covarying IQ. The authors concluded that the ADD children were characterized by marked general cognitive impairments, including deviations in IQ, speech and reading skills and attention performance. The pervasively hyperactive children manifested more subtle attention deficits compared to the conduct-disordered children, but not such a general cognitive deficit.

When shifting the analysis to the still more restrictive definition of hyperkinetic disorder, hyperkinetic boys revealed more general cognitive deficits compared both with the conduct disorder and pervasive attention deficit disorder with hyperactivity (ADDH) boys. Deficits included lower IQ scores, reading delay and deviations on digit span, MFF and PAL tests. In summary, both the ADD and hyperkinetic children were characterized by general cognitive and attentional problems, while pervasive ADDH was associated with more subtle attention impairments which were not severe enough to be manifest in IQ tests. The overall position of pervasively hyperactive boys on cognitive tests was intermediate between that of the hyperkinetic syndrome and normal boys.

In a rather similar design, pervasively hyperactive Chinese boys recruited from a community sample (Leung et al., 1996) were markedly more distractable on the Stroop test when compared to normally developing children (Leung and Connolly, 1996). Such an attentional deficit, however, was not found in the mixed group of children with pervasive hyperactivity and conduct problems. The most likely explanation for this unexpected finding is the greater clinical, and probably also aetiological, heterogeneity of this mixed group

(Leung and Connolly, 1996). In this context, it is worth noting that in studies involving clinically referred patients with ADHD, contradictory findings concerning cognitive deficits have been reported (Schachar and Tannock, 1995). For a more extensive consideration of the cognitive aspects, see Chapter 7.

Psychosocial correlates

A number of earlier community studies had shown that ADHD was more prevalent in populations with lower socioeconomic status, but that this similarly applied to other psychiatric disorders as well, making it a nonspecific finding (Buitelaar and van Engeland, 1996). The most informative data on psychosocial correlates of hyperactivity disorders were collected by Taylor et al. (1991). In the London survey the ADD group appeared to be associated with low occupational status of the parents and lower social class. Further, measures of family relationships did differ for the mixed hyperactive-conduct group, and for the hyperkinetic disorder group, compared to the other groups. It turned out that persistence of disorder at follow-up 9 months later was significantly associated with the presence of intrafamilial problems and maternal depression. For a further discussion on psychosocial aspects, see Chapter 11.

Further issues

Subthreshold cases and boundaries of ADHD

So far, few attempts have been made to exploit the potential of epidemiology in answering questions about the boundaries of disorders and in establishing meaningful diagnostic thresholds. What is the stability of a subthreshold classification? To what extent is the classification of subjects just falling below the threshold due to measurement error, or to temporal fluctuations in symptom severity, or because of both of these possibilities? Are subjects with subthreshold ADHD at high risk of developing ADHD or other forms of psychopathology later in life? Or, alternatively, is subthreshold AD/HD a result of the presence of other primary psychiatric disorders such as affective conditions? To take the example of oppositional defiant disorder (ODD), Angold and Costello (1996) were able to demonstrate that the large majority of children who had two or three symptoms – a number just below the threshold of four symptoms of ODD in DSM-IV – and had functional impairment were clearly disturbed and met validity markers such as perceived need for treatment, service use or parental burden. At follow-up 1 year later, approximately half of the subthreshold group of ODD were still impaired and about 10% had developed conduct disorder, an outcome not significantly different from that of children who had earlier met the full requirements for ODD.

Returning now to ADHD, children with subthreshold ADHD symptoms were significantly more impaired on the Children's Global Assessment Scale (CGAS) than non-ADHD children in a community study (Scahill et al., 1999). Children with clinical DSM-III-R-defined ADHD, by contrast, were more impaired in psychosocial adaptation than subthreshold children, and had in addition stronger signs of family dysfunctioning and higher rates of comorbid disorders. At the very least, these findings suggest that subthreshold ADHD may be a clinically meaningful condition that requires more study.

Measurement of impairment

It is increasingly recognized that the measurement of functional impairment is important in ascertaining psychopathology. Merely to count the number of symptoms is no longer felt adequate for case detection in epidemiology, nor in clinical practice (Bird, 1999). For example, children with subthreshold disorders and impaired functioning were at equally high risk for later psychopathology as children with threshold diagnoses but without impairment (Angold et al., 1999b; Costello et al., 1999). The presence of a clinical diagnosis on its own did not carry a poor prognosis, unless in conjunction with serious functional impairment. Much work is still to be done in improving ways of measuring impairment. In the ADHD DSM-IV field trial, the number of hyperactivity and impulsivity symptoms was related to general impairment as measured by the CGAS. By contrast, the number of inattention symptoms was unrelated to the CGAS, but associated with specific impairments such as problems in completing homework, accuracy and quantity of academic work completed in the classroom, and with peer sociometric status (Lahey et al., 1994). However, these analyses left unanswered the question to what extent impairment was due to the presence of comorbid disorders rather than to ADHD symptoms. Furthermore, by calibrating the diagnostic threshold to the mean level of impairment of clinically referred cases, an element of circularity is introduced. Structured interview schemes such as the DISC (Shaffer et al., 2000) and the CAPA (Angold and Costello, 2000), therefore, now intend to measure the degree of impairment associated with a particular diagnosis. Each module includes a series of questions to probe whether specific symptoms lead to parental concern and parental burden, interference with family activities or with the participation in social relationships with peers, obstacles in performing academic work, signs of subjective distress or seeking help. We need to learn more about how impairment is related to, but is also different from, symptom severity and symptom count, and to pervasiveness and persistence of symptoms.

Stability of classification and natural history

A series of studies have examined the diagnostic stability of ADHD in clinic-referred samples (Barkley et al., 1990; Hart et al., 1995; Biederman et al., 1996). These studies included a 4–8-year prospective follow-up from childhood into adolescence. The reported diagnostic persistence of DSM-III-R-defined ADHD appeared to be between 75% and 85%. Predictors of persistence were young age, severity of hyperactivity and impulsivity symptoms, initial presence of comorbid conduct disorder (Hart et al., 1995), positive family history for ADHD, high levels of psychosocial adversity, greater functional impairment, comorbid bipolar disorder and multiple anxiety disorders (Biederman et al., 1996). In addition, symptoms of hyperactivity and impulsivity showed a greater decline with increasing age than was the case with symptoms of inattention (Hart et al., 1995; Biederman et al., 2000). The interpretation of the results obtained from clinic samples, however, is complicated by referral bias, treatment bias and labelling bias. Follow-up studies of children with ADHD identified in the general population are in principle able to overcome these limitations. In a 9-month follow-up assessment of a school-based sample of childen rated as pervasively hyperactive, a 64% persistence rate was reported (Taylor et al., 1991). This suggests that a substantial minority of ADHD cases remit within 1 year of receiving the diagnosis. Persistence was associated with higher initial rates of conduct disorder on both parent and teacher questionnaires, and with family problems in the form of maternal mental illness, previous divorce of the parents and high levels of critically expressed emotion (Taylor et al., 1991). In a somewhat similar study with a follow-up 3 and 4 years after the initial diagnosis of DSM-III-R-defined ADHD, 38% of cases were found to have a fully persistent disorder that was present at all assessments (August et al., 1998). Another 31% were classified as moderately persistent by having the diagnosis at one but not at both of the follow-up assessments, and 31% qualified as desisters. Again, persistence was associated with higher levels of comorbid oppositional defiant and conduct disorder at baseline, higher levels of ineffective child management practices and more concerns related to coping, parental control and marital satisfaction (August et al., 1998). It is important to appreciate that the designs of these studies do not allow to differentiate whether these family correlates are the result of parenting, reflect a more severely disturbed child with a persistent disorder, or are in themselves the cause of persistence (Taylor et al., 1991; August et al., 1998). The greater decline over time of hyperactivity and impulsivity symptoms compared with inattention, as inferred from clinic-based studies, could be further confirmed in this community sample (August et al., 1998).

Data on persistence of ADHD in children from the general population are also provided by Cohen et al. (1993a). Cases with ADHD identified in the first wave of this longitudinal project (Cohen et al., 1987) were split into three levels of severity: mild ADHD just met the DSM-III criteria of ADHD on the basis of either parent or child responses to the diagnostic interview; moderate and severe ADHD met the DSM-III criteria and in addition had scores on a scale that included all relevant items for ADHD of more than one and more than two standard deviations above the population mean, respectively. At follow-up $2\frac{1}{2}$ years later, the conditional probability of those initially diagnosed with ADHD at any level of severity to be rediagnosed as ADHD was 42%. The odds of the diagnosis at follow-up for those who were diagnosed in the original assessment were nearly 16 times as high as the odds of the diagnosis for those not previously diagnosed. Split into the three levels of severity of ADHD at the original assessment, the OR was nearly 60 for severe ADHD, and about 10 for both mild and moderate ADHD. Finally, only 32% of cases diagnosed at follow-up were new cases with ADHD. Age and gender did not significantly affect the persistence of ADHD (Cohen et al., 1993a).

Interesting findings about the natural history of ADHD are further provided by 9-year follow-up of children identified with pervasive hyperactivity at age 6–7 years in the London community study (Taylor et al., 1996). The threshold for hyperactivity as defined by the parent and teacher questionnaires in this study was considerably lower than that for a clinical diagnosis of ADHD. This is illustrated by the fact that only 37/84 (44%) and 16/84 (19%) pervasively hyperactive cases met DSM-III criteria for ADHD and ICD-10 criteria for hyperkinetic disorder, respectively (Taylor et al., 1991). The results of the follow-up, therefore, are also informative about the long-term risks of subclinical levels of hyperactivity. At follow-up, 12/51 (24%) children with initial pervasive hyperactivity met the full criteria for DSM-III-R ADHD. The corresponding numbers for those meeting criteria for hyperkinetic disorder at follow-up were 6/51 (12%). Initial pervasive hyperactivity was further associated with an increased prevalence of any psychiatric disorder, compared with that found among the initially nonhyperactive children (45% vs. 15%). Initial hyperactivity as a continuous measure strongly predicted both later hyperactivity and later conduct problems, and this was independent from the level of early conduct problems (Taylor et al., 1996). Later antisocial behaviour and violence, poor peer relations and academic problems in school were all long-term correlates of initial hyperactivity, but not of initial conduct problems. Self-reported smoking habits, alcohol or drug use, instead, were not linked to early hyperactivity (Danckaerts et al., 2000). All in all, this study demonstrates that pervasive hyperactivity in childhood is an important risk factor for developmental outcome in late adolescence in various domains of functioning, and that this risk extends to children at subthreshold levels of hyperactivity.

Adequacy of standard rating scales

Attention has been drawn to a number of methodological issues endemic to the designs of questionnaire-based studies on psychopathology, including ADHD (Rowe and Rowe, 1997). One of these relates to the fact that all commonly applied questionnaires like the CBCL, Conners' scales, Rutter scales and scales using DSM-based items only include negatively worded items. The emphasis on negative items is at the expense of a more balanced assessment and easily induces rater bias. From a statistical point of view, the result is a strongly skewed distribution of scores at the population level (Rowe and Rowe, 1997). A study of more than 800 school-age children rated by their teachers on the ADHD DSM-IV rating scale illustrates how this practice leads to overidentification of children with extremely abnormal scores. Using a statistical cutoff of 1.65 standard deviations above the mean, 8.4% of the population were identified, instead of the expected 5% (Swanson et al., unpublished work). The authors were also able to show that the use of both negative and positive assessments could remedy this problem. For example, in the Strengths and Weaknesses of ADHD-symptoms and Normal-behaviors (SWAN) rating scale, items were rephrased. Instead of phrasing the first DSM-IV symptom as 'often fails to give close attention to details and makes careless mistake', the item was worded as 'how does this child pay attention to details?'. The use of a seven-point rating system ranging from 'far below average' ($+3$) to 'far above average' (-3), and anchored in the middle to average behaviour scored as zero (0), resulted in strongly improved distributional properties of the scale. Such instruments will allow researchers to define individuals within the normal and supernormal range of a trait without too much measurement error. This is of great importance for all kinds of high-risk studies, including those investigating molecular genetics.

Concluding remarks

The studies that were informative about ADHD in the general population, and performed over the past 10 years, provide evidence, though not equivocally, for a prevalence of DSM-III-R-defined ADHD between 5% and 10%. The higher prevalence, close to 10%, is mostly found in the age range between 6 and 11 years. The prevalence is relatively lower among preschoolers and among adolescents. Boys outnumber girls 2–4 times. Though few studies to date have incorporated the DSM-IV nomenclature, the findings suggest that the DSM-IV definition of ADHD is overinclusive compared to DSM-III-R, and seems to raise the prevalence by a factor of 1.6. In particular the inattentive subtype of ADHD appears to be responsible for this increased prevalence, and constitutes between 35% and 50% of all ADHD cases identified in the community. The correlates, as predicted for the subtypes of ADHD, regarding associations between the inattentive type and learning problems and affective comorbidity, and between the hyperactive-impulsive and combined type and generally impaired psychosocial adaptation and comorbid oppositional and conduct disorders, were confirmed in community studies. Also, ADHD identified in the community is far from a transient disorder. Exactly the opposite is found, with high rates of persistence of disorder over time. The first data of ADHD in nonreferred samples of adults indicate a prevalence between 1.3% and 4.7%. The adult studies further suggest that the cutoff of six out of nine criteria is too stringent for adult cases. Instead, a cutoff of five, or even four, criteria would be more appropriate, as cases with four or more criteria exhibit serious impairment in psychosocial adaptation (Kooij et al., unpublished work). The male/female ratio among adults with ADHD is fairly equal. Since there is no evidence that symptoms of ADHD show a faster decline over age in boys than in girls, support is lent to the view that ADHD in girls remains undetected in earlier childhood and adolescence, and is generally underdiagnosed. Finally, comorbidity of ADHD with oppositional and conduct disorder, depressive disorders and anxiety disorders is substantial in the general population, and a true finding that cannot be explained away by methodological artefacts (Angold et al., 1999a).

The progress in our understanding of the epidemiology of ADHD, however, has been slow, and less than one may have wished. Few studies have incorporated information from both parents and teachers to create the opportunity to examine the differential characteristics of home situational ADHD, school situational ADHD and pervasive ADHD. In spite of the fact that all studies including structured psychiatric interviews with the parents have also collected information from the parent about the school situation, the question to what extent parents are reliable informants about the presence of ADHD in school, and if so, which parents, remains unclear. Furthermore, the information provided by the parent is typically aggregated over both the home and school situations, and is therefore not amenable to further differentiation. Also, few studies have been able to examine carefully selected subgroups of children with regard to the associated cognitive and neurobiological characteristics. Likewise, the important social problems of children with ADHD, and the overlap with pervasive developmental disorders, have been incompletely covered by the published studies. Finally, in the study of developmental pathways of ADHD, and of its causal mechanisms, much remains to be desired. Hopefully, ongoing and future studies will try to meet these research challenges.

REFERENCES

Almqvist, F., Puura, K., Kumpulainen, K. et al. (1999). Psychiatric disorders in 8–9-year-old children based on a diagnostic interview with parents. *European Child and Adolescent Psychiatry*, **8** (suppl. 4), 17–28.

American Psychiatric Association (APA) (1980). *Diagnostic and Statistical Manual of Mental Disorders*, 3rd edn (DSM-III). Washington, DC: APA.

American Psychiatric Association (APA). (1987). *Diagnostic and Statistical Manual of Mental Disorders*, 3rd edn revised (DSM-III-R). Washington, DC: APA.

American Psychiatric Association (APA). (1994). *Diagnostic and Statistical Manual of Mental Disorders*, 4th edn (DSM-IV). Washington, DC: APA.

Angold, A. and Costello, E.J. (1996). Toward establishing an empirical basis for the diagnosis of oppositional defiant disorder. *Journal of the American Academy of Child and Adolescent Psychiatry*, **35**, 1205–12.

Angold, A. and Costello, E.J. (2000). The Child and Adolescent Psychiatric Assessment (CAPA). *Journal of the American Academy of Child and Adolescent Psychiatry*, **39**, 39–48.

Angold, A., Costello, E.J. and Erkanli, A. (1999a). Comorbidity. *Journal of Child Psychology and Psychiatry*, **40**, 57–88.

Angold, A., Costello, E.J., Farmer, E.M., Burns, B.J. and Erkanli, A. (1999b). Impaired but undiagnosed. *Journal of the American Academy of Child and Adolescent Psychiatry*, **38**, 129–37.

August, G.J., Realmuto, G.M., MacDonald, III, A.W., Nugent, S.M. and Crosby, R. (1996). Prevalence of ADHD and comorbid disorders among elementary school children screened for disruptive behavior. *Journal of Abnormal Child Psychology*, **24**, 571–95.

August, G.J., Braswell, L. and Thuras, P. (1998). Diagnostic stability of ADHD in a community sample of school-aged children screened for disruptive behavior. *Journal of Abnormal Child Psychology*, **26**, 345–56.

Barkley, R.A., Fischer, M., Edelbrock, C.S. and Smallish, L. (1990). The adolescent outcome of hyperactive children diagnosed by research criteria: I. An 8-year prospective follow-up study. *Journal of the American Academy of Child and Adolescent Psychiatry*, **29**, 546–57.

Bauermeister, J.J., Alegria, M., Bird, H., Rubio-Stipec, M. and Canino, G. (1992). Are attentional-hyperactivity deficits unidimensional or multidimensinal syndromes? Empirical findings from a community survey. *Journal of the American Academy of Child and Adolescent Psychiatry*, **31**, 423–31.

Baumgaertel, A., Wolraich, M.L. and Dietrich, M. (1995). Comparison of diagnostic criteria for attention deficit disorders in a German elementary school sample. *Journal of the American Academy of Child and Adolescent Psychiatry*, **34**, 629–38.

Biederman, J., Faraone, S., Milberger, S. et al. (1996). Predictors of persistence and remission of ADHD into adolescence: results from a four-year prospective follow-up study. *Journal of the American Academy of Child and Adolescent Psychiatry*, **35**, 343–51.

Biederman, J., Mick, E. and Faraone, S.V. (2000). Age-dependent decline of symptoms of attention-deficit hyperactivity disorder: impact of remission definition and symptom type. *American Journal of Psychiatry*, **157**, 816–18.

Bird, H.R. (1999). The assessment of functional impairment. In *Diagnostic Assessment in Child and Adolescent Psychopathology*, eds D. Shaffer, C.P. Lucas and J.E. Richters, pp. 209–29. New York: Guilford Press.

Boyle, M.H., Offord, D.R., Racine, Y. et al. (1996). Identifying thresholds for classifying childhood psychiatric disorder: issues and prospects. *Journal of the American Academy of Child and Adolescent Psychiatry*, **35**, 1440–8.

Boyle, M.H., Offord, D.R., Racine, Y.A. et al. (1997). Adequacy of interviews vs checklists for classifying childhood psychiatric disorder based on parent reports. *Archives of General Psychiatry*, **54**, 793–9.

Breton, J.J., Bergeron, L., Valla, J.P. et al. (1999). Quebec child mental health survey: prevalence of DSM-III-R mental health disorders. *Journal of Child Psychology and Psychiatry*, **40**, 375–84.

Buitelaar, J.K. and van Engeland, H. (1996). Epidemiological approaches to hyperactivity. In *Hyperactivity Disorders*, S. Sandberg, ed., pp. 26–68. Cambridge: Cambridge University Press.

Cohen, P., Velez, N., Kohn, M., Schwab-Stone, M. and Johnson, J. (1987). Child psychiatric diagnosis by computer algorithm: theoretical issues and empirical tests. *Journal of the American Academy of Child and Adolescent Psychiatry*, **26**, 631–8.

Cohen, P., Cohen, J. and Brook, J. (1993a). An epidemiological study of disorders in late childhood and adolescence – II. Persistence of disorders. *Journal of Child Psychology and Psychiatry*, **34**, 869–77.

Cohen, P., Cohen, J., Kasen, S. et al. (1993b). An epidemiological study of disorders in late childhood and adolescence – I. Age- and gender-specific prevalence. *Journal of Child Psychology and Psychiatry*, **34**, 851–67.

Costello, E.J., Angold, A., Burns, B.J. et al. (1996a). The Great Smoky Mountains study of youth. Functional impairment and serious emotional disturbance. *Archives of General Psychiatry*, **53**, 1137–43.

Costello, E.J., Angold, A., Burns, B.J. et al. (1996b). The Great Smoky Mountains study of youth. Goals, design, methods, and the prevalence of DSM-III-R disorders. *Archives of General Psychiatry*, **53**, 1129–36.

Costello, E.J., Farmer, E.M., Angold, A., Burns, B.J. and Erkanli, A. (1997). Psychiatric disorders among American Indian and white youth in Appalachia: the Great Smoky Mountains study. *American Journal of Public Health*, **87**, 827–32.

Costello, E.J., Angold, A. and Keeler, G.P. (1999). Adolescent outcome of childhood disorders: the consequences of severity and impairment. *Journal of the American Academy of Child and Adolescent Psychiatry*, **38**, 121–8.

Danckaerts, M., Heptinstall, E., Chadwick, O. and Taylor, E. (1999). Self-report of attention deficit and hyperactivity disorder in adolescents. *Psychopathology*, **32**, 81–92.

Danckaerts, M., Heptinstall, E., Chadwick, O. and Taylor, E. (2000). A natural history of hyperactivity and conduct problems: self-reported outcome. *European Child and Adolescent Psychiatry*, **9**, 26–38.

DuPaul, G.J. (1991). Parent and teacher ratings of ADHD symptoms: psychometric properties in a community-based sample. *Journal of Clinical Child Psychology*, **20**, 245–53.

Fergusson, D.M., Horwood, L.J. and Lynskey, M.T. (1993). Prevalence and comorbidity of DSM-III-R diagnoses in a birth cohort of 15-year olds. *Journal of the American Academy of Child and Adolescent Psychiatry*, **32**, 1127–34.

Frick, P.J., Lahey, B.B., Applegate, B. et al. (1994). DSM-IV field trials for the disruptive behavior disorders: symptom utility estimates. *Journal of the American Academy of Child and Adolescent Psychiatry*, **33**, 529–39.

Gaub, M. and Carlson, C.L. (1997). Behavioral characteristics of DSM-IV ADHD subtypes in a school-based population. *Journal of Abnormal Child Psychology*, **25**, 103–11.

Gomez, R., Harvey, J., Quick, C., Scharer, I. and Harris, G. (1999). DSM-IV AD/HD: confirmatory factor models, prevalence, and gender and age differences based on parent and teacher ratings of Australian primary school children. *Journal of Child Psychology and Psychiatry*, **40**, 265–74.

Gomez-Beneyto, M., Bonet, A., Catala, M.A., Puche, E. and Vila, E. (1994). Prevalence of mental disorders among children in Valencia, Spain. *Acta Psychiatrica Scandinavica*, **89**, 352–7.

Hart, E.L., Lahey, B.B., Loeber, R., Applegate, B. and Frick, P.J. (1995). Developmental change in attention-deficit hyperactivity disorder in boys: a four-year longitudinal study. *Journal of Abnormal Child Psychology*, **23**, 729–49.

Ho, T.P., Luk, E.S., Leung, P.W. et al. (1996). Situational versus pervasive hyperactivity in a community sample. *Psychological Medicine*, **26**, 309–21.

Jensen, P.S., Watanabe, H.K., Richters, J.E. et al. (1995). Prevalence of mental disorder in military children and adolescents: findings from a two-stage community survey. *Journal of the American Academy of Child and Adolescent Psychiatry*, **34**, 1514–24.

Lahey, B.B., Pelham, W.E., Schaughency, E.A. et al. (1988). Dimensions and types of attention deficit disorder. *Journal of the American Academy of Child and Adolescent Psychiatry*, **27**, 330–5.

Lahey, B.B., Applegate, B., McBurnett, K. et al. (1994). DSM-IV field trials for attention deficit hyperactivity disorder in children and adolescents. *American Journal of Psychiatry*, **151**, 1673–85.

Landgren, M., Pettersson, R., Kjellman, B. and Gillberg, C. (1996). ADHD, DAMP and other neurodevelopmental/psychiatric disorders in 6-year-old children: epidemiology and co-morbidity. *Developmental Medicine and Child Neurology*, **38**, 891–906.

Lavigne, J.V., Gibbons, R.D., Christoffel, K.K. et al. (1996). Prevalence rates and correlates of psychiatric disorders among preschool children. *Journal of the American Academy of Child and Adolescent Psychiatry*, **35**, 204–14.

Leung, P.W. and Connolly, K.J. (1996). Distractibility in hyperactive and conduct-disordered children. *Journal of Child Psychology and Psychiatry*, **37**, 305–12.

Leung, P.W., Luk, S.L., Ho, T.P. et al. (1996). The diagnosis and prevalence of hyperactivity in Chinese schoolboys. *British Journal of Psychiatry*, **168**, 486–96.

Levy, F., Hay, D.A., McStephen, M., Wood, C. and Waldman, I. (1997). Attention-deficit hyperactivity disorder: a category or a continuum? Genetic analysis of a large-scale twin study. *Journal of the American Academy of Child and Adolescent Psychiatry*, **36**, 737–44.

Murphy, K. and Barkley, R.A. (1996). Prevalence of DSM-IV symptoms of ADHD in adult licensed drivers: implications for clinical diagnosis. *Journal of Attention Disorders*, **3**, 147–61.

Murphy, P. and Schachar, R. (2000). Use of self-ratings in the assessment of symptoms of attention deficit hyperactivity disorder in adults. *American Journal of Psychiatry*, **157**, 1156–9.

Pelham, W.E.J., Gnagy, E.M., Greenslade, K.E. and Milich, R. (1992). Teacher ratings of DSM-III-R symptoms for the disruptive behavior disorders. *Journal of the American Academy of Child and Adolescent Psychiatry*, **31**, 210–18.

Pineda, D., Ardila, A., Rosselli, M. et al. (1999). Prevalence of attention-deficit/hyperactivity disorder symptoms in 4- to 17-year-old children in the general population. *Journal of Abnormal Child Psychology*, **27**, 455–62.

Rohde, L.A., Biederman, J., Busnello, E.A. et al. (1999). ADHD in a school sample of Brazilian adolescents: a study of prevalence, comorbid conditions, and impairments. *Journal of the American Academy of Child and Adolescent Psychiatry*, **38**, 716–22.

Rowe, K.S. and Rowe, K.J. (1997). Norms for parental ratings on Conners' abbreviated Parent-Teacher-Questionnaire: implications for the design of behavioral rating inventories and analyses of data derived from them. *Journal of Abnormal Child Psychology*, **25**, 425–51.

Scahill, L., Schwab-Stone, M.E., Merikangas, K.R. et al. (1999). Psychosocial and clinical correlates of ADHD in a community sample of school-age children. *Journal of the American Academy of Child and Adolescent Psychiatry*, **38**, 976–84.

Schachar, R. and Tannock, R. (1995). Test of four hypotheses for the comorbidity of attention-deficit hyperactivity disorder and conduct disorder. *Journal of the American Academy of Child and Adolescent Psychiatry*, **34**, 639–48.

Schaughency, E., McGee, R., Raja, S.N., Feehan, M. and Silva, P.A. (1994). Self-reported inattention, impulsivity, and hyperactivity at ages 15 and 18 years in the general population. *Journal of the American Academy of Child and Adolescent Psychiatry*, **33**, 173–84.

Shaffer, D., Fisher, P., Dulcan, M.K. et al. (1996). The NIMH Diagnostic Interview Schedule for Children Version 2.3 (DISC-2.3): description, acceptability, prevalence rates, and performance in the MECA study. Methods for the Epidemiology of Child and Adolescent Mental Disorders Study. *Journal of the American Academy of Child and Adolescent Psychiatry*, **35**, 865–77.

Shaffer, D., Fisher, P., Lucas, C.P., Dulcan, M.K. and Schwab-Stone, M.E. (2000). NIHM Diagnostic Interview Schedule for Children version IV (NIMH DISC-IV): description, differences from previous versions, and reliability of some common diagnoses. *Journal of the American Academy of Child and Adolescent Psychiatry*, **39**, 28–38.

Simonoff, E., Pickles, A., Meyer, J.M. et al. (1997). The Virginia Twin Study of adolescent behavioral development. Influences of age, sex, and impairment on rates of disorder. *Archives of General Psychiatry*, **54**, 801–8.

Steinhausen, H.C., Metzke, C.W., Meier, M. and Kannenberg, R. (1998). Prevalence of child and adolescent psychiatric disorders: the Zurich epidemiological study. *Acta Psychiatrica Scandinavica*, **98**, 262–71.

Szatmari, P., Offord, D.R. and Boyle, M.H. (1989). Ontario Child Health Study: prevalence of attention deficit disorder with hyperactivity. *Journal of Child Psychology and Psychiatry*, **30**, 219–30.

Taylor, E., Sandberg, S., Thorley, G. and Giles, S. (1991). *The Epidemiology of Hyperactivity*. Oxford: Oxford University Press.

Taylor, E., Chadwick, O., Heptinstall, E. and Danckaerts, M. (1996). Hyperactivity and conduct problems as risk factors for adolescent development. *Journal of the American Academy of Child and Adolescent Psychiatry*, **35**, 1213–26.

Verhulst, F.C. and Koot, H.M. (1992). *Child Psychiatric Epidemiology. Concepts, Methods, and Findings*. Newbury Park, CA: Sage Publications.

Verhulst, F.C. and Koot, H.M. (1995). *The Epidemiology of Child and Adolescent Psychopathology*. Oxford: Oxford University Press.

Verhulst, F.C., Van der Ende, J., Ferdinand, R.F. and Kasius, M.C. (1997). The prevalence of DSM-III-R diagnoses in a national sample of Dutch adolescents. *Archives of General Psychiatry*, **54**, 329–36.

Wang, Y.C., Chong, M.Y., Chou, W.J. and Yang, J.L. (1993). Prevalence of attention deficit hyperactivity disorder in primary school children in Taiwan. *Journal of the Formosan Medical Association*, **92**, 133–8.

Wolraich, M.L., Hannah, J.N. and Pinnock, T.Y. (1998). Examination of DSM-IV criteria for attention-deficit hyperactivity disorder in a county-wide sample. *Journal of Developmental and Behavioral Pediatrics*, **19**, 162–8.

Wolraich, M.L., Hannah, J.N., Pinnock, T.Y., Baumgaertel, A. and Brown, J. (1996). Comparison of diagnostic criteria for attention-deficit hyperactivity disorder in a county-wide sample. *Journal of the American Academy of Child and Adolescent Psychiatry*, **35**, 319–24.

World Health Organization (WHO) (1992). *ICD-10. Classification of Mental and Behavioural Disorders. Clinical Description and Diagnostic Guidelines*. Geneva: WHO.

Zarin, D.A. and Earls, F. (1993). Diagnostic decision making in psychiatry. *American Journal of Psychiatry*, **150**, 197–206.

3

Cross-cultural/ethnic aspects of childhood hyperactivity

Ernest S. L. Luk[1], Patrick W. L. Leung[2] and Ting-Pong Ho[3]

[1]Department of Psychological Medicine, Monash University, Victoria, Australia; [2]Department of Psychology, The Chinese University of Hong Kong, Hong Kong; [3]Queen Mary Hospital, Hong Kong

Cross-cultural study of childhood psychopathology is an exciting and rapidly developing field. Its primary concern is how cultural factors influence the aetiology, expression, course, outcome and epidemiology of childhood mental disorders. The magnitude of the cultural influences is presumably related to the nature of a disorder. If the disorder is a developmentally inappropriate increase of behaviour with no organic cause, then the variability displayed by this disorder across different cultures is expected to be high. However, even in neurological disorders with a strong biological component, cultural influences can still exert an impact on how the individual and family experience, interpret and respond to the disorder and how society responds to the individual's behaviour. This chapter reviews the cross-cultural aspects of a childhood disorder, hyperactivity, and discusses how cross-cultural data shed light on aiding our understanding the disorder.

Hyperactivity refers to an enduring style of behaving in an overactive, inattentive and impulsive fashion (Taylor, 1986). It is a broad behavioural description of children's behaviour and does not carry any aetiological implication. Currently, there are two official diagnostic systems which confer a diagnosis for the disorder – the DSM system (*Diagnostic and Statistical Manual of Mental Disorders*) of the American Psychiatric Association (APA) and the ICD system (*International Classification of Diseases*) of the World Health Organization (WHO). Previously the two systems differed in some important aspects, but in their current versions, the ICD-10 and DSM-IV, there is presently more convergence. The ICD-10 (World Health Organization, 1994) terms the disorder of hyperactivity as hyperkinetic disorder and emphasizes the cooccurrence of some features from all three main symptom groups, namely, inattention, overactivity and impulsivity. The DSM-IV (American Psychiatric Association, 1994) also recognizes these three symptom groups, but allows subdivision into two – an inattention subtype and a hyperactivity-impulsivity subtype. Both subtypes are considered separable, independent variants of the disorder of hyperactivity, officially termed as attention deficit hyperactivity disorder (ADHD). There is a third variant of the disorder, which is the combined type of both the former two subtypes. In the review that follows, we will use the generic term 'hyperactivity', and unless otherwise specified, this refers to a condition defined by all three symptom groups.

Though hyperactivity has been studied extensively, research has been largely limited to Caucasian males (Samuel et al., 1997). The important question is whether the results of the bulk of the research would apply to other ethnic or cultural groups. In addition, it is important to remember that hyperactivity is a concept developed in western culture and based on clinical observation. This concept may be entirely unheard of in other cultures. It may be a 'culture-bound' syndrome related to the 'cultural tempo' (Block, 1977) or 'permissiveness' (Ho, 1981) of the western culture. This question gives the initial impetus for the cross-cultural study of hyperactivity.

Is hyperactive behaviour reported in other ethnic or cultural groups?

Hyperactivity as a clinical condition worthy of attention was first reported at the turn of the twentieth century (Schachar, 1986). Since then, this phenomenon has been reported in various ethnic or cultural groups in different parts of the world. Apart from North America and Europe, it has also been reported in Africa, South America and Asia (Minde and Cohen, 1978; Shen et al., 1985; Brito, 1987).

In the initial cross-cultural studies, the most popular way of measuring hyperactive behaviour was by parent report or teacher report questionnaires. The Conners' Teacher Rating Scale (CTRS; Conners, 1969) was probably among the most commonly used questionnaires for the measurement of hyperactivity. Good psychometric properties have been demonstrated when it is used in different cultures. Table 3.1 reports the comparison of the various symptoms of hyperactivity across different cultures, namely overactivity, inattention and impulsivity.

Table 3.1 shows that the various symptoms of hyperactivity have been reported in different ethnic or cultural groups with a range of 2.1–7.9% for overactivity, from 3.8% to 13.4% for inattention, and from 2.1% to 7.7% for 'impulsivity'. Two points are worth noting. First, there appears to be a fair amount of variation in the percentages of hyperactive behaviour reported, even though the sources accounting for the variation are not immediately obvious. None the less, despite the variation, the various symptoms of hyperactivity are reported to be present across different ethnic or cultural groups.

Table 3.1. Cross-cultural comparison of overactive, inattentive and impulsive behaviour items in the Conners' Teacher Rating Scale[a]

Behaviour	Australia (Holborow et al., 1984)		New Zealand (Werry and Hawthorne, 1976)		Germany (Sprague et al., paper presented, 1977)		USA (Werry et al., 1975)		Hong Kong (Luk et al., 1988a)	
	(2)	(3)	(2)	(3)	(2)	(3)	(2)	(3)	(2)	(3)
Restless, overactive	13.0	5.0	12.0	7.9	14.3	3.2	4.8	2.1	15.3	7.1
Constantly fidgeting	13.6	4.8	21.8	7.4	9.9	2.9	11.3	2.1	20.2	9.6
Fails to finish, short attention span	10.5	7.0	16.0	9.6	17.2	5.5	8.3	2.8	19.4	6.4
Inattentive, distractible	13.6	7.2	21.8	13.4	19.9	6.9	11.4	3.8	27.5	11.9
Excitable, impulsive	13.9	5.5	16.0	7.7	12.4	3.1	6.2	2.1	16.0	5.6
Disturbing other children	12.0	5.4	16.3	8.9	11.3	3.2	6.9	2.1	11.3	5.0

[a]Numbers are percentages. (2), pretty much; (3), very much.

Factorial validity – factor analytic studies

Are the above findings sufficient to prove that hyperactivity is not a 'culture-bound' syndrome but exists across different cultures? A definitive answer is probably premature. The above does show that individual symptoms of hyperactivity are present across different cultures, but there are more criteria to be met before hyperactivity as a clinical syndrome can be established to be present in ethnic or cultural groups other than in Caucasian children. The individual symptoms must also demonstrate the same unique clustering when examined in a different culture. This is called factorial validity. The statistical procedure of factor analysis has been used to examine this issue (Conners, 1969; Werry and Hawthorne, 1976; Glow and Stevenson, 1981; Trites et al., 1982; Taylor and Sandberg, 1984; Luk et al., 1988a). Results of studies analysing the CTRS are summarized in Table 3.2.

The original Conners' factor structure comprised two separate factors for hyperactivity and inattention (Conners, 1969). This was supported in a later study by Werry et al. (1975). This is interesting, as this separation coincides with the current DSM-IV position. However, in the ICD-10 tradition, it is predicted that hyperactivity and inattention should covary. In subsequent studies with Caucasian children in different parts of the world, support has emerged for a combined hyperactivity-inattention factor (Glow and Stevenson, 1981; Trites et al., 1982; Taylor and Sandberg, 1984). However, the Hong Kong study with Chinese children raises another issue; there was a combined hyperactivity-conduct disorder factor within a community sample (Luk et al., 1988a). This casts doubt on the independence of the syndrome of hyperactivity in a Chinese culture. Subsequently, another study in Hong Kong with children having various problems such as physical disabilities, mental retardation and maladjustment found two separate hyperactivity and conduct disorder factors (Leung et al., 1989). None the less, there is always a strong overlap of items between the two factors, even when they are separable.

Schachar et al. (1981) reported the results of factor analysis of another set of popular questionnaires – Rutter teacher and parent rating scales. There was a separate factor of three items indicating behaviour commonly attributed to hyperactivity, apart from the two existing antisocial and neurotic factors. The two questionnaires have also been used with non-Caucasian samples in different Asian communities. There are mixed findings. Two studies, in Japan (Morita et al., 1990) and Hong Kong (Ho et al., 1996), supported the existence of an independent hyperactivity factor. However, two studies in mainland China produced discrepant results: one failed to find an independent

Table 3.2. Comparison of factor analyses in different studies

Item	Conners (1969)	Luk et al., (1988a)	Taylor et al., (1991)	Werry et al., (1975)	Glow and Stevenson (1981)	Trites et al. (1982)
12	C	/	C	C	C	C
15	C	C-H	C	C	C	C
17	C	C-H	C	H	C	H-I
21	C	C-H	C	C	C	C
25	C	/	/	C	C	C
31	C	C-H	C	C	C	C
32	C	C-H	C	C	C	C
36	C	C-H	C	C	C	C
38	C	C-H	C	C	C	C
18	C	C-H	A	C	A	C
19	C	/	A	C	A	C
20	C	C-H	A	C	A	C
1	H	C-H	H-I	H	H-I	H-I
2	H	C-H	H-I	H	H-I	H-I
5	H	C-H	H-I	H	H-I	H-I
6	H	C-H	C	H	H-I	H-I
14	H	C-H	H-I	H	H-I	H-I
29	H	C-H	C	/	C	H-I
4	I	/	H-I	/	/	H-I
7	I	I	H-I	H	H-I	H-I
8	I	I	H-I	I	H-I	H-I
11	I	I	/	I	/	/
24	I	/	/	I	/	/
26	I	/	/	/	/	/

C, conduct problem; H, hyperactivity; I, attentive-passive; A, antisocial; H-I, combined factor of hyperactivity and inattentiveness; C-H, combined factor of hyperactivity and conduct problem; /, items not loaded in factor of conduct problem or hyperactivity or inattention.

hyperactivity factor (Wang et al., 1989), while another showed a combined hyperactive-aggressive factor (Ekblad, 1990).

Parent and teacher rating scales are not meant to be an exact instrument. Items on them are written in simple but general statements that require a fair amount of personal judgement from the respondents to make a rating. This may account for some of the discrepant findings using questionnaires. Perhaps interview measures with more exact definitions of the behaviours under examination should instil more confidence in their findings. Taylor et al. (1986) devised such an interview measure and applied it to British children with disruptive disorder. Factor analysis produced a separate hyperactivity factor apart from conduct disorder factor. The same measure was subsequently used with a group of Hong Kong Chinese clinic children and the same factor structure emerged (Luk et al., 1991).

On balance, despite some inconsistency, there seem to be sufficient positive findings from the questionnaire and interview studies to suggest that hyperactive behaviours do indeed cluster in a similar way across different cultures. This supports the proposition that a behaviour pattern characterized by overactivity, inattention and impulsiveness does exist regardless of the nature of the society or the ethnicity of the children it is measured in. However, the findings also raised two further issues. First, even if separate factors for hyperactivity and conduct disorder emerge in factor analysis, they are found to be moderately correlated, leaving lingering questions about the usefulness of the concept of hyperactivity as distinct from conduct problems. Second, the emergence of two separate overactivity-impulsivity and inattention factors in some of the earlier studies by Conners (1969) and Werry et al. (1975) precede the current DSM-IV system of subtyping hyperactivity. Recently, Achenbach and McConaughy (1997) also reported in the USA such a subdivision in the attention problem subscale of their teacher rating scale – the Teacher Report Form. Cross-cultural support of this DSM-IV system of subtyping hyperactivity is currently lacking with respect to the above-cited studies using Conners' Teacher Rating Scale and Rutter's Parent and Teacher Scales. Perhaps there is a measurement problem; the Rutter scales have only three items for hyperactivity. It would be difficult to have further subdivisions among such a small number of items. This, however, does not explain the results with the Conners Scale.

External validity

Given that there is sufficient evidence to support a clustering of inattentive, impulsive and overactive behaviours to form a recognizable syndrome cross-culturally, one can still raise the query whether this behavioural pattern carries a similar clinical identity or meaning across cultures or ethnic groups. One way of examining this issue is to test whether this behavioural pattern exhibits the same kinds of external correlates (e.g. associated deficits or risk factors) across cultures or ethnic groups. These external correlates very often help to define a more comprehensive syndromal picture of a disorder, describing its various facets in addition to its symptomatology. In other words, we are testing whether hyperactivity displays the same external validity across cultures or ethnic groups.

In a large-scale epidemiological study on hyperactivity conducted in Hong Kong with community sample of Chinese schoolboys, hyperactivity was found to be associated with the following external correlates (Leung et al., 1996a,b):

(1)   more exposure to biological risks such as complications in the neonatal period, prematurity/postmaturity and low/high birth weight
(2)   more histories of motor and, particularly, language delays
(3)   neurological abnormality
(4)   cognitive impulsiveness (i.e. a faster reaction time but more errors in a visual matching task)
(5)   cognitive inattentiveness (i.e. fewer correct hits, more false positives and a longer reaction time in a vigilance task)
(6)   a lower IQ
(7)   a lower reading score
(8)   teacher-rated academic backwardness.

This pattern of external correlates replicates essentially what has been found in western communities (Taylor et al., 1991; Leung et al., 1996a; Barkley, 1998). In other words, the same diagnosis of hyperactivity carries a similar clinical identity or meaning across western and nonwestern (Chinese) cultures. This in turn supports the presence of the same disorder in Chinese children.

Separation of hyperactivity and conduct disorder

Some of the cross-cultural factor analytic studies reviewed above, including some with Chinese children, have cast doubt on the separability of hyperactivity and conduct disorder. This raises a fundamental query of whether hyperactivity can be regarded as an independent disorder, i.e. whether hyperactivity has discriminative validity as a disorder from another disorder such as conduct disorder. Some years ago this issue was the subject of controversy even within western communities (Schachar, 1991). One way of examining this issue is to test whether hyperactivity and conduct disorder have different patterns of external correlates. One good example of this effort is a study in the UK by Taylor and his colleagues (Taylor et al., 1986). Hyperactivity was associated with greater motor activity, younger age, poorer cognitive performance and more minor neurological deficits. Conduct disorder was associated with impairment of family relationships and adverse social factors. The findings suggest that the two disorders, though frequently comorbid with each other, can be distinguished by their differing patterns of external correlates, indicating that they may have different characteristics, risk factors or aetiologies. Schachar (1991) concluded in his review that there was sufficient accumulated evidence to support an independent syndrome apart from conduct disorder.

To test whether hyperactivity retains its discriminative validity against conduct disorder across cultures, a comparable study, cited above (Leung et al., 1996a,b) using the same instruments was carried out with Hong Kong Chinese schoolboys. The external correlates for hyperactivity in Chinese schoolboys have been listed above. With the exception of academic backwardness and IQ, conduct disorder in Hong Kong displayed none of the above associations. Instead, it was related to family disharmony involving excessive maternal criticism, lack of maternal warmth, ineffective parental coping with the child's problems and parental inconsistency in child management strategies. Furthermore, hyperactivity was found to be a risk factor in the development of conduct disorder, but the reverse was not true (Ho et al., 1996). In other words, hyperactivity and conduct disorder are distinguishable from each other by differing patterns of external correlates such as neurodevelopmental impairment, specific cognitive deficits of inattention and impulsivity, family disharmony and course of development. These findings match well with those reported in western countries (Taylor et al., 1991; Leung et al., 1996a). This is further proof of the cross-cultural validity of the disorder of hyperactivity, maintaining its separation from its closest associate, conduct disorder, in Chinese culture.

Cross-cultural comparison of hyperactivity using behaviour rating scales

So far, the data from cross-cultural studies, cited above, support the thesis that the disorder of hyperactivity maintains its factorial, external and discriminative validity across different cultures. In other words, a pattern of behaviour involving overactivity, inattention and impulsiveness, which is distinct from other behavioural problems, can be found cross-culturally and carries the same clinical identity or meaning. Given such an overall conclusion, it is meaningful to proceed to compare the prevalence of the disorder across cultures. One of the easiest ways to do so is to use behaviour rating scales, such as the CTRS.

Based on Conners' original factor structure, the factor scores of the CTRS as applied in different countries are compared and shown in Table 3.3.

As can be seen from Table 3.3, the Hong Kong Chinese children and the New Zealand children, mainly from European descent, received the highest ratings on the factor of overactivity/impulsiveness, inattention and conduct

Table 3.3. Cross-national findings on Conners' Teacher Rating Scale scores

	South London (Taylor and Sandberg, 1984) (n = 437)		Mid-west USA (Werry et al., 1975) (n = 291)		New Zealand (Werry and Hawthorne, 1976) (n = 418)		Hong Kong (Luk et al., 1988a) (n = 914)		Canada (Trites et al., 1979) (n = 14 083)	
	Mean	SD	Mean	SD	Mean	SD	Mean	SD	Mean	SD
Conduct problem										
Boys	0.39	/	0.21	0.93	0.60	0.53	0.42	0.47	0.25	0.44
Girls	0.20	/	0.08	0.30	0.42	0.47	0.18	0.30	0.15	0.31
Inattention-passive										
Boys	0.70	/	0.60	0.58	0.96	0.60	1.01	0.50	0.63	0.66
Girls	0.51	/	0.43	0.55	0.71	0.58	0.72	0.52	0.40	0.55
Tension/anxiety										
Boys	0.52	/	0.29	0.29	0.61	0.46	0.55	0.38	0.48	0.52
Girls	0.52	/	0.35	0.35	0.73	0.56	0.66	0.44	0.56	0.56
Hyperactivity										
Boys	0.84	/	0.56	0.56	1.07	0.73	1.03	0.78	0.65	0.76
Girls	0.46	/	0.25	0.25	0.58	0.65	0.40	0.51	0.30	0.53

/, no data.

Table 3.4. Percentage of children identified as 'hyperactive' in different countries according to cutoff selected on the abbreviated Conners' Teacher Rating Scale

	Boys (%)	Girls (%)
Cutoff >1.5		
USA ($n = 291$: Werry et al., 1975)	9	2
New Zealand ($n = 418$: Werry and Hawthorn, 1976)	22	9
Germany ($n = 5357$: Sprague et al., paper presented, 1977)	12	5
Canada ($n = 14\,083$: Trites et al., 1979)	21	8
Australia ($n = 1759$: Holborow et al., 1984)	18	5
Italy ($n = 344$: O'Leary et al., 1985)	19.9	2.6
Hong Kong ($n = 914$: Luk et al., 1988a)	17.7	5.6
Cutoff >2 sd		
USA (>1.5)	9	2
New Zealand (>2.1)	5	4
Germany (>1.8)	6	3
Canada (>2.1)	7	2
Australia (>1.9)	8.8	2.4
Italy (>2)[a]	7.5	1.3
Hong Kong (>1.95)	7.1	0.5

[a]The actual mean $+ 2$ sd was 1.87.

problems. In contrast, very little difference is seen in the tension/anxiety factor scores.

The prevalence of a disorder can be obtained by designating a cutoff point on a rating scale. If an absolute magnitude is used, the lowest cutoff score employed so far is that of 1.5 applied to the mean of the abbreviated version of the CTRS (ATRS: Goyette et al., 1978; Holborow and Berry, 1986). The score of 1.5 was deduced from the original study of Werry and his colleagues (1975), and it was equivalent to about 2 standard deviations (sd) above the mean. Studies carried out in other countries have different means and sd. Barkley (1982), for example, has recommended that the cutoff should be set at 2 sd above the mean. Table 3.4 summarizes the results of a number of epidemiological investigations and demonstrates the rates of 'hyperactivity' when based on cutoffs which are 1.5 and 2 sd above the mean on the ATRS in such cross-cultural comparisons.

Table 3.4 clearly indicates that if 2 sd above the mean is used as the cutoff, then the prevalence of the disorder of hyperactivity is fairly similar across cultures. However, the results also reveal other important issues. All the studies showed a skewing of the distribution curve to the right and therefore the percentages of children above 2 sd are more than that predicted by a normal distribution curve. In addition, there is a consistent sex difference, with boys having a higher rate than girls. Significant differences are also found when the children's socioeconomic backgrounds are considered. Some studies have found an increase in the rates of hyperactivity in urban areas as compared with rural areas (Schachar et al., 1981; Offord et al., 1987; Luk et al., 1988a; Goodman and Stevenson, 1989). However, when there is a marked difference in the degree of poverty between rural and urban areas, then the poor rural area will show a higher rate of hyperactivity (Glow and Stevenson, 1981; Shen et al., 1985; Weisz et al., 1987a). It is also of interest to note that the findings in Hong Kong and China have turned out to be contrary to those previously predicted. The earlier literature suggests that hyperactivity is uncommon in the Chinese population (Ho, 1981), but this clearly does not appear to be the case with the studies reviewed.

In a more recent study, Caucasian and African American boys aged from 5 to 18 years were again compared using a behaviour rating scale (Reid et al., 1998). Teachers completed an ADHD-IV Rating Scale–school version, which consisted of 18 items directly adapted from the ADHD symptom list as specified in the DSM-IV. A random sample of 381 African-American and 1359 Caucasian Americans from public schools were included. Teachers rated the African-American students higher on all the behaviour items across all age groups. The mean scores for the African-American group were significantly higher than the Caucasian American group for both the inattention factor and the hyperactivity-impulsiveness factor. Once again, this suggests that hyperactivity is not exclusive to Caucasian children and even that they do not have the highest rate.

Problems of using behaviour rating scales for cross-cultural comparison

Several studies have pointed out the inappropriateness of relying on behaviour rating scales for cross-cultural comparison. Even though similar factorial structures may emerge from a behaviour rating scale applied cross-culturally, they are unlikely to be identical in terms of exact items involved. Furthermore, Reid et al. (1998), for example, using statistical structural equation modelling analysis and multidimensional scaling analysis, showed that the behaviour rating scale did not perform identically across the African and Caucasian American groups and that there were different relations between items across groups.

Given such differences, the cross-cultural comparison can only be considered as a gross approximation.

There is another inherent problem with rating scales. They rely upon the perception and judgement of the respondents. Different cultural groups may have different systematic tendencies in the direction of rating, possibly due to some cultural traditions. Mann et al. (1992) asked 37 mental health professionals from China, Indonesia, Japan and the USA to rate hyperactive-disruptive behaviours in standardized videotape vignettes of four 8-year-old boys participating in individual and group activities. A behaviour rating scale was also provided. All of the mental health professionals were experienced in treating children and all but one had worked with children who were diagnosed as hyperactive. Results showed that Chinese and Indonesian clinicians gave significantly higher scores of hyperactive-disruptive behaviours than did their Japanese and American colleagues. This finding suggests that the thresholds for the judgement of hyperactivity vary significantly across cultures. The Chinese and Indonesian clinicians must have a lower threshold so that they judge the same behaviour as more hyperactive than their Japanese and American counterparts. This systematic shift occurs even among well-trained child mental health professionals. This phenomenon undermines our confidence in looking at the cross-cultural comparison by rating scales.

Differences in prevalence of hyperactivity across cultures by diagnosis

In the past, there was a huge difference in the frequency of the clinical diagnosis of hyperactivity between the UK and the USA. Taylor (1985) compared the diagnostic rates across the Atlantic by examining data from clinic records, including drug prescription records, case registries and epidemiological studies. He came up with an estimate of the diagnosis being about 20 times higher in the USA than in the UK.

Data from questionnaire studies (as shown in Tables 3.3 and 3.4) provide no support for such a huge difference between the two countries. It was later found in a joint UK–USA study that the difference was probably due to differences in diagnostic practices under the ICD and DSM traditions (Prendergast et al., 1988). Case histories of 6–11-year-old boys were evaluated by British and American researchers. There was very little difference in the diagnostic rate between the two specially trained researchers in terms of the diagnosis of hyperkinetic syndrome according to ICD-9 (World Health Organization, 1978) and attention deficit disorder according to DSM-III (American Psychiatric

Association, 1980). However, ICD-9 did generate much fewer diagnoses of the disorder than did DSM-III. So the ICD system probably commands a more stringent diagnosis than that of the DSM system. The latest versions, ICD-10 (World Health Organization, 1994) and DSM-IV (American Psychiatric Association, 1994), despite various changes, have not altered their fundamental differences in diagnostic stringency. In fact, some researchers would consider hyperkinetic syndrome as a subset of the American attention deficit hyperactivity disorder, possibly as a more refined phenotype (Swanson et al., 1998a). The lesson seems clear for cross-cultural comparison; the same diagnostic system or standardized measures must be used before cross-cultural differences can be meaningfully interpreted.

To date, there are only a handful of studies reporting the prevalence of hyperactivity by diagnosis in non-Caucasian children. Bhatia et al. (1991) reported in India a prevalence of 5.2% DSM-III diagnosis with children aged 3–4 and an amazing 29% with adolescents aged 11–12. However, this sample is not an epidemiological one, but instead a clinic sample of paediatric outpatients. It is unsure how this characteristic of the sample may account for the high prevalence rate of hyperactivity among the adolescent group. There are two epidemiological studies, both with Chinese children. A study in mainland China reported prevalence rates of 6% and 9% DSM-III diagnosis of hyperactivity in urban and rural areas respectively (Shen et al., 1985). Recently, another study in Hong Kong with Chinese schoolboys reported 0.8% for hyperkinetic disorder (ICD-10), 6.1% for attention deficit disorder with hyperactivity (ADDH: DSM-III), and 9.8% for ADHD (DSM-IIIR: Leung et al., 1996b). The ICD-10 diagnostic criteria are accepted as more stringent and thus the lower prevalence rate comes as no surprise. A recent authoritative review of hyperactivity when the Hong Kong figures were compared to those reported in other western countries showed that they were quite compatible (Swanson et al., 1998a). The prevalence was about 5–10% in the DSM tradition and 1–2% in the ICD tradition. This prompts the conclusion that hyperactivity is a worldwide phenomenon (Barkley, 1998) and is not 'culture-bound' so that changing the 'western permissiveness' will not make it go away (Anderson, 1996).

Direct comparison of two epidemiological studies of hyperactivity between Hong Kong and the UK

The Hong Kong study (Leung et al., 1996b), cited above, can be directly compared to a previous British study (Taylor et al., 1991). The comparison was made possible by adopting similar methodology and instruments – a two-stage epidemiological design using the same measures and similar cutoffs at both screening and diagnostic stages. The subjects in both studies were all boys, aged 5–7. The British sample, totalling 2433, was the total population sample of a London borough while the Chinese sample, totalling 3069, was a probabilistic sample based on a representative sampling of local schools. When data from the two groups of hyperactive children were jointly analysed and compared, there were systematic cross-cultural differences (Luk et al., 1993).

In general, objective measures of activity (by mechanical actometer and direct observation) and attention (by Continuous Performance test) suggested a three-tier situation. The British hyperactive children displayed the most overactivity and inattention. The British normal controls and the Chinese ADHD children were in the middle while the Chinese normal controls showed the least overactivity and inattention. In the assessment of impulsivity (by Matching Familiar Figures test), the British hyperactive children exhibited the expected impulsivity, i.e. quick responding but a lot of errors. On the other hand, the Chinese hyperactive children were both quick and accurate in their responding, which was similar once again to the performance of the British controls.

In sum, objective measures of the three main symptoms of hyperactivity, i.e. overactivity, inattention and impulsivity, in Chinese hyperactive children re-vealed that their magnitude was similar to that of the British normal controls. In other words, if the former were to be put into the British context, they would be regarded as normal. However, back in the Chinese context, the behaviours of the Chinese hyperactive children were excessive or defective by local standards. This was because the Chinese controls displayed an even lower activity level and better attention. In other words, the Chinese had a lower baseline which meant that behaviours which would be judged normal in the UK were excessive or defective in a Chinese population. None the less, the finding remained that Chinese hyperactive children, in an absolute term, displayed a much more subdued pattern of cognitive and behavioural deficits/ excesses than their British counterparts.

The above findings are preceded by a previous study between Asian and English boys in the UK (Sonuga-Barke et al., 1993). Asian children were observed to be much lower in objective measures of hyperactivity, although they had similar teacher ratings on hyperactivity in relation to the English group. The more recent comparative study, described above, has extended this finding to other core symptoms of hyperactivity, namely, attention deficit and impulsivity.

This review so far has traced how issues surrounding the cross-cultural aspects of childhood hyperactivity have been dealt with and researched on. In the early days, there was an open query that hyperactivity was a product of the western permissive, individualistic culture – a 'culture-bound' syndrome, predicted to be very rare or even nonexistent in the more restrictive and collectivist Asian culture. However, emerging cross-cultural studies in Asian populations begin to debate this proposition. There are studies which demonstrate that the construct of hyperactivity as a disorder retains its factorial, external and discriminative validity across cultures. Questionnaire and diagnostic studies have reported largely similar prevalence rates of hyperactivity in Asian populations as compared to Caucasian. It appears that the cross-cultural issue that starts off the series of research may have been resolved. Childhood hyperactivity is shown to be a worldwide phenomenon and not a 'culture-bound' syndrome.

The proclamation of the above conclusion in the 1990s (Anderson, 1996; Barkley, 1998) also coincides with a period of time during which there was a major shift of focus in research on hyperactivity in the western world. Tannock (1998) reviewed that there was a marked increase of studies looking at the biological basis of the disorder. Preliminary evidence points to a dysfunction of the frontal striatal networks in the brain (which control attention and response organization) that may be of genetic origin (Swanson et al., 1998a; Tannock, 1998). There is multiple evidence from family, adoption and twin studies. Stevenson (paper presented, 1994) summarized that the average estimated heritability of symptoms of hyperactivity was 0.80 (range = 0.50–0.98). Environmental factors, possibly influenced by cultural traditions, combined with all nongenetic sources of neurological impairments, account for about 10–15% of the variance in hyperactive symptoms (Goodman and Stevenson, 1989). The strong hereditary influence in hyperactivity may also contribute to an apparent link between poor child management and hyperactivity – a link that may be attributable to a parent's own hyperactivity (Frick and Jackson, 1993). Thus, even aspects of the home environment which were once thought to be nongenetic may have genetic elements involved (Plomin, 1995). The resolution of hyperactivity as a worldwide phenomenon and the discovery of a strong genetic component in its aetiology appear to confer a diminishing role to cross-cultural studies. However, the findings from the direct comparison of Chinese and British hyperactive and control children give rise to new and interesting cross-cultural or cross-ethnic questions. While the Chinese and British both have hyperactive children by comparison with their own controls, the findings that Chinese hyperactive children have more subdued excesses/deficits in all three major symptom domains and that Chinese normal children in fact have a lower baseline in all these areas demand explanations that can have wide-ranging implications for understanding various aspects of the disorder. As an extension of Plomin's (1995) suggestion on the genetic involvement in even some aspects of social (i.e. home) environment, it must be noted that some of the differences between cultural groups may not be cultural but may be genetic due to different ethnicity. Thus, in the following section, we propose a model on the cross-cultural and cross-ethnic aspects of childhood hyperactivity as a way of conceptualizing the potential impact of cultural and ethnic influences or perhaps their interaction with various aspects of the disorder. The Chinese/British differences will be used as an example in this model for illustration.

Cultural/ethnic influence on the genetic basis of childhood hyperactivity

One of the approaches to examine cross-ethnic differences in psychopathology is the study of gene polymorphism. While there are no published empirical data on cross-ethnic differences in the genetic basis of childhood hyperactivity, the cross-ethnic study of alcoholism can be an illustrating example. It has been found that the prevalence rate of alcoholism is lower in Chinese than in Caucasians. One possible explanation is the cross-ethnic differences in the rates of alcohol metabolism. Alcohol is first oxidized to acetaldehyde, then broken down to acetate by aldehyde dehydrogenase (ALDH). A variant of the ALDH2 allele is deficient in eliminating acetaldehyde, leading to the accumulation of acetaldehyde, and subjects experience flushing and tachycardia after ingestion of alcohol. These physiological changes would exert a prohibiting effect on further drinking and provide protection against developing alcoholism. It was found that this ALDH2 variant is more common among Chinese than Caucasian people, and it is more common among nonalcoholics than alcoholic subjects (Chen et al., 1996). In short, the cross-ethnic difference in the ALDH2 polymorphism provides an explanation for the cross-ethnic differences in the prevalence of alcoholism. Given the strong hereditary influence in hyperactivity as evinced in family, adoption and twin studies, it is natural that researchers have recently moved towards directly searching for a candidate gene for the disorder. Part of the cross-ethnic similarities/differences in hyperactivity could be related to gene polymorphism.

The focus of genetic research on childhood hyperactivity is on the dopamine system. This is because effective drugs for hyperactivity act primarily on the dopaminergic and noradrenergic systems. Furthermore, brain imaging studies with hyperactive children indicate abnormality in neurological structures with rich dopamine innervations such as the frontal striatal circuitry. Thus, an initial focus of research is on the dopamine type 2 gene, but findings have been inconsistent (Kelsoe et al., 1989; Comings et al., 1991; Gelernter et al., 1991; Blum et al., 1996). Another candidate gene explored is dopamine transporter gene because drugs for hyperactivity inhibit the dopamine transporter. Two publications confirmed an association between the one allele (480 bp) of the dopamine transporter locus (DAT1) and hyperactivity (Cook et al., 1995; Gill et al., 1997), but a recent report failed to replicate the finding (Swanson et al., 1998b).

The dopamine receptor D4 gene (*DRD4*), which encodes one of the five known protein receptors that mediate the postsynaptic action of dopamine, is another potential candidate gene. These receptors are located in the frontal and prefrontal cortical regions of the brain, suggesting that they may be involved in the executive control and regulation of attention. Swanson and his colleagues have published two studies reporting that the 7-repeat allele in *DRD4* is associated with hyperactivity (Lahoste et al., 1996; Swanson et al., 1998b). To date, there has been a series of subsequent studies confirming the association (Faraone et al., 1999).

The potential candidacy of 7-repeat allele in *DRD4* as the genetic linkage to hyperactivity is particularly interesting for cross-ethnic studies with the Chinese. In a recent worldwide survey of the *DRD4* gene in 36 different populations, the 7-repeat allele was found to be very rare among Asian populations. In fact, among the 182 Chinese tested, none had the 7-repeat allele (Chang et al., 1996). The above finding has made a compelling case for replicating a genetic study in Chinese hyperactive children. It poses a stringent test on the 7-repeat allele (*DRD4*) hypothesis, given that this allele is expected to be absent in Chinese people. In other words, if the 7-repeat allele is found to be present in Chinese hyperactive children, it will provide a very solid support for its association with hyperactivity. On the other hand, if the 7-repeat allele is absent in Chinese hyperactive children, this will prompt a serious rethink on the validity of this hypothesis for hyperactivity. First, this allele may not simply be the site of genetic variant accounting for hyperactivity. On the other hand, it may be close or associated with the real site, giving important clues for further exploration. Second, there may be ethnic differences which are hitherto unsuspected. The 7-repeat allele hypothesis is perhaps only valid with Caucasian but not with Chinese children. Third, however meticulously we may have matched the phenotype of Chinese hyperactive children to that of Caucasian children, there may be subtle subtypes within the disorder that arise from different genetic and nongenetic causes. There could be multiple genes and each gene may account for a facet of childhood hyperactivity. The possibilities are indeed many; and cross-ethnic data from the Chinese will be very useful here and guide future efforts in the pursuit of the genetic aetiology of hyperactivity as well as in the demarcation of potential subtypes among the disorder (Swanson et al., 1998b).

Cultural/ethnic influence on the presentation of symptoms of childhood hyperactivity

In adult psychiatry, cross-cultural comparisons of major psychiatric disorders have indicated differences in symptom presentation. Studies of depressive disorders have, for example, demonstrated that among nonwestern samples of depressed patients, there is an increase of somatization and a decrease in depressive affect and cognition compared with patients diagnosed in western countries (Jablensky et al., 1981; Kleinman, 1982). Likewise, a study by WHO of first-contact cases of schizophrenia found that the symptoms of patients from developing countries were more often characterized by voices speaking to subjects, and by visual hallucinations, while patients from developed countries more often suffered from systematized delusions, primary delusions, delusional mood and thought insertion (Sartorius et al., 1986). In the light of these observations, it would be surprising if there were no differences in the presentation of symptoms across cultures for childhood hyperactivity. And indeed there are; the Chinese hyperactive children display a more subdued symptomatology compared to their British counterparts. In fact, normal Chinese children have an even lower baseline in relevant hyperactive behaviours. There may be both biological and cultural explanations for this.

Several studies on infant temperament have suggested that there may indeed be some ethnic differences in the temperament of infants. Bronson (1972) noted less motor reactivity to novel stimuli among infants of Asian ancestry compared with those of Caucasian origin. Freedman and Freedman (1969) and Ko (paper presented, 1988) reported Chinese infants to be more easily habituated, calmed and consoled than infants of Caucasian origin. The link between these allegedly inborn constitutional characteristics and the later behavioural symptoms is yet to be explored, but the implication does point to a genetic difference due to ethnicity. Perhaps there are some protective genes which are responsible for the overall reduction of intensity of hyperactive behaviour in the Chinese population. Once again, this requires a cross-ethnic genetic study with Chinese and Caucasian children.

Cultural differences may also be in force. Two main factors should be considered: child-rearing practice and the school environment. The 'problem suppression-facilitation' model described by Weisz et al. (1987b) would appear to be relevant for this discussion. It suggests that cultural factors may specifically suppress the development of certain child problems and facilitate the development of certain other problems.

There exists a good deal of evidence to suggest that there are considerable differences in child-rearing practices between different societies. In order to illustrate some of the salient issues, the differences between western developed countries and Chinese cultures are compared. Several themes emerge which are likely to be relevant to hyperactivity. First, Chinese parents are concerned about the expression of physical aggression in their children (Ekblad, 1986; Ho, 1986). Second, Chinese parents tend to foster dependence, whereas assertiveness and independent behaviour are encouraged by western parents (Ho, 1986). Third, academic achievement is strongly emphasized by Chinese parents. To sit down and concentrate on academic work is a very important part of the training (Chen and Stevenson, 1989). If these child-rearing practices have an impact on the behaviour of children, then it would be reasonable to hypothesize that there would be a suppressing effect on hyperactive symptoms.

The school environment is also different. For example, in the primary schools of Hong Kong, the classes are generally more structured. Children are expected to sit still and concentrate on their assigned task. Also, they are usually forbidden to leave their seat. The classroom routines in the first few years of primary school in countries like the UK or New Zealand tend to be very different. For example, in most lessons children are allowed to move around in the classroom. They are encouraged to carry out tasks they are interested in at their own pace. Considering the problem suppression-facilitation model, it is reasonable to hypothesize that the classroom situation in Hong Kong is likely to suppress hyperactive behaviour whereas in the UK and New Zealand, hyperactive behaviour may in fact be facilitated.

The 'problem suppression-facilitation model' is supported by a series of studies carried out by Weisz and his colleagues in an Asian country, Thailand, examining two broad-band behaviour problem dimensions: overcontrolled behaviour (i.e. emotional problems such as fearfulness, worrying, somatizing) on the one hand and undercontrolled behaviour on the other (i.e. disruptive behaviours such as disobedience, fighting, arguing; Achenbach and Edelbrock,

1978). Thailand is a Buddhist country where children's undercontrolled behaviour (e.g. aggression) is disapproved of and discouraged, and their inhibition and other overcontrolled behaviour are likely to be condoned and even encouraged. Weisz and his colleagues compared the problem behaviour of Thai children with US children and hypothesized that Thai children would have more problems involving overcontrolled behaviour and fewer problems involving undercontrolled behaviour.

Three studies were conducted to test this prediction. The first study is most supportive (Weisz et al., 1987b). Based on a clinic sample of Thai and American children, overcontrolled problems were reported by parents as much more prevalent in Thailand than in the USA; undercontrolled problems, on the other hand, were reported to be much more prevalent in US children than in Thailand. In the second study (Weisz et al., 1987a), the Child Behavior Checklist (CBCL), a parental questionnaire, was used to examine a community sample of Thai and American children. It was found that the Thai children were rated much higher on items indicating overcontrolled behaviour compared with the US children. In contrast, no differences in rating were found for undercontrolled behaviour problems. In other words, there seems to be support for the facilitation and not the suppression hypothesis. In addition, the Thai children had significantly higher overall problem scores than the US children. In the third study (Weisz et al., 1989), the Teacher's Report Form was used. The Thai children had significantly higher scores on both overcontrolled and on undercontrolled behaviour compared with the US children. Furthermore, the scores for overcontrolled behaviour were significantly higher than the scores for undercontrolled behaviour among the Thai children, whereas within the US sample the reverse was true. The results pertaining to the cross-cultural comparison do not fit well with the facilitation-suppression hypothesis, even though it can be argued that the within-culture results do show some degree of support.

On balance, it is fair to say that there is at least some partial support for the facilitation-suppression hypothesis. On the other hand, the unpredicted cross-cultural findings, particularly from the third study using the teacher's rating, prompted Weisz and his colleagues to seek additional explanation. They proposed an 'adult distress threshold' hypothesis, suggesting that the Thai adults had a lower threshold for recognizing children's problem behaviour than their US counterparts (Weisz et al., 1988). This hypothesis has, in fact, far-reaching implications for the cross-cultural study of hyperactivity. Previous studies with Chinese children using teachers' or parents' rating scales have produced scores on hyperactive behaviours which are commensurate with, or even higher than, those reported on Caucasian children, including British children (Luk et al., 1988a; Ho et al., 1996). These give the impression that the Chinese children would exhibit at least the same magnitude or intensity of hyperactive behaviour, if not more. However, the Hong Kong–UK study, described above, indicated that when objective measures were used, the Chinese hyperactive children, in fact, displayed more subdued overactivity, inattention and impulsivity (Luk et al., 1993). The message is clear: in future research, rating scales cannot be solely relied upon for cross-cultural/ethnic comparison but objective measures, including direct observation of behaviour, activity measures, such as actigraph or cognitive tests of cognitive functioning, should also be used. The study of hyperactivity fortunately benefits from the increasing availability of these objective measures.

There may be some indirect, tentative evidence from the joint findings of the Hong Kong–UK study (Luk et al., 1993) to support Weisz's model of a suppression effect in Asian culture so that the magnitude or intensity of hyperactive behaviour in the Chinese is reduced as regarding the population. Chinese parents, by comparison to their British counterparts, were found to be less rejecting and critical towards their hyperactive and control children, while at the same time they seemed to have better management skills and interparental agreement. One can argue that positive parenting may be instrumental in reducing hyperactive behaviour. On the other hand, because of the cross-sectional design of the study, it is equally valid to construe that the less critical and more effective parenting is a response to children with milder symptomatology due to constitutional or genetic reasons. This may represent a phenomenon of gene–environment correlation in which genetic differences produce differences in exposure to certain adverse or protective environments (Plomin and Rutter, 1998). Chinese children with a genetically more placid temperament will elicit a more accepting family environment that in turn helps to reduce further the level of any disorderly, hyperactive behaviour. So it is too early to conclude with a purely cultural explanation.

Furthermore, the above is a broad generalization on Chinese child-rearing practices, serving as a post hoc explanation to cross-cultural differences in hyperactivity. It must be noted that there are significant variations in child-rearing practices in different Chinese communities (Lin and Fu, 1990; Cheng Lai et al., 2000). Given such heterogeneity, one cannot be sure how far these broad generalizations on child-rearing practices and their explanation for cross-cultural differences are applicable to all Chinese.

Cultural/ethnic influence on the recognition of, and help-seeking for, hyperactivity

The 'adult distress threshold model' suggests that culturally mediated adult attitudes may help to determine which particular child behaviours are considered to be problematic and which will go over the adult's threshold for distress, and therefore result in a referral for help. This model has far-reaching implications in accounting how culture may influence the recognition of, and help-seeking for, hyperactivity.

In a study with a community sample of Hong Kong Chinese children, teachers were asked to fill in the Conners' Teacher Rating Scale and subsequently they were asked to judge whether the students whom they had previously rated had displayed behavioural or emotional problems which required a referral to mental health professionals, provided that the resources were unlimited (Luk et al., 1988a,b). Several interesting results emerged. First, as shown in Table 3.3, teachers in Hong Kong rated the children higher on the subscales of conduct problems, hyperactivity and inattention, but not on tension/anxiety when compared with results from similar studies carried out in other countries. This would suggest that teachers in Hong Kong may have a lower threshold for the recognition of hyperactive or conduct problems.

Second, a total of 55 students were considered as requiring referral for help, giving a referral rate of 6.3%. The referred group and the nonreferred group were compared, as shown in Table 3.5. The referred group had significantly higher mean scores on conduct and hyperactivity problems, but not on anxiety/tension problems, compared with the children who were not referred. This suggests that teachers in Hong Kong are more likely to refer conduct problems or hyperactivity for help, as compared with children whose psychological problems are predominantly of the internalizing type.

The validity of the CTRS in Hong Kong children was examined in another study (Luk and Leung, 1989). The total scores which defined sensitivity and specificity of the CTRS for the detection of conduct disorder and hyperactivity were established. For 100% specificity and 100% sensitivity, the CTRS total scores are respectively 44 and 12. A score of 36 gave an optimal specificity of 88% and sensitivity of 83%. These CTRS scores were then used to study the validity of the referrals, 'hypothetically' made by the teachers. Table 3.6 summarizes the results.

There was a significant difference between the CTRS scores of the referred and nonreferred groups. This generally supports the validity of the teacher

Table 3.5. Comparison of referred and nonreferred students

	Referred (n = 55)		Nonreferred (n = 819)		
	Mean	SD	Mean	SD	P^a
CTRS scores					
Total score	0.80	0.42	0.56	0.38	0.000
CTRS factor scores					
Factor 1 (conduct)	0.59	0.56	0.29	0.40	0.000
Factor 2 (inattentive/passive)	1.23	0.56	0.86	0.56	0.000
Factor 3 (anxiety/tension)	0.60	0.36	0.59	0.42	0.94
Factor 4 (hyperactivity)	1.06	0.89	0.73	0.73	0.008

$^a P$ value according to t-test or χ^2-test.
CTRS, Conners' Teacher Rating Scale.

Table 3.6. Distribution according to different Conners' Teacher Rating Scale (CTRS) scores

CTRS total score	Referred (n = 50)	Nonreferred (n = 783)	P value χ^2-test
>36	20	147	
			0.01
<36	30	636	
>44	12	75	
			0.001
<44	38	710	

Note: CTRS total score >36 specificity = 88%, sensitivity = 82.9%; >44 specificity = 100%.

referrals. However, 75 cases whose scores were above the CTRS score of 44 (specificity 100%) were not referred. The probability that these 75 students would require professional help was very high. They represented 86.2% of the cases above the cutoff point of 44. These results suggest that, while teachers in Hong Kong may have a lower threshold for the recognition of hyperactivity or conduct problems, and they tend to refer children with problems of undercontrolled behaviour more readily than with overcontrolled behaviour, they tend to have a high threshold for making a referral for help. The study has not explored the reasons behind the disinclination for making referrals for help.

One possible reason is the lack of knowledge about the nature of the problems and the benefits of professional help (Pavuluri et al., 1996).

A recent study from Florida, USA, serves as a good example of cross-cultural differences in this important area (Bussing et al., 1998). A sample of African-American and Caucasian parents of children at high risk for hyperactivity was surveyed by telephone and subsequently participated in face-to-face interviews addressing their explanatory models of hyperactivity. Results indicated significant cultural/ethnic differences in knowledge and sources of information about hyperactivity. Fewer African-American parents reported that they had ever heard of hyperactivity, or that they knew some or a lot about it. They were more likely to attribute hyperactivity to excessive sugar in the diet. They also reported that they obtained less information regarding hyperactivity from physicians as well as less use of and less preference for written information materials (newspapers, journals, library).

For the time being, the adult distress threshold model is proposed as a post hoc explanation to account for higher teachers' or parents' ratings in some nonwestern cultures. Research has not gone far enough to explore the cultural/ethnic factors behind the development of such a lower threshold for hyperactivity, the reluctance in making a referral, and the lack of knowledge about the disorder.

Cultural/ethnic influence on the comorbidity of childhood hyperactivity

Childhood hyperactivity is frequently associated with comorbid conditions. Among the commonest is conduct disorder (Biederman et al., 1991). Children in whom hyperactivity and conduct disorder occur together tend as a group to have more severe symptoms and worse prognosis (Szatmari et al., 1989; Barkley et al., 1990). Research on Chinese hyperactive children with comorbid conduct problems reported similar results, further underlining the diagnostic significance of comorbid conduct disorder across cultures or ethnic groups (Leung et al., 1996a).

A previous study, cited above, using the CTRS with Chinese children in mainstream schools found a combined hyperactivity-conduct problem factor (Luk et al., 1988b). This was in contrast to the other studies based on Caucasian children, which reported separate factors (Table 3.2). These factor analytical results suggest that hyperactivity in Chinese children may have a higher frequency of comorbid conduct problems. However, subsequent studies, using either CTRS or Rutter Parent and Teacher Questionnaires, found separate factors for hyperactivity and conduct problems (Ho et al., 1996; Leung et al.,

1989). Thus, on balance, there is insufficient evidence for a combined factor in Chinese children. This in turn weakens the support for conjecture on a higher rate of comorbid conduct problems in Chinese hyperactive children.

Affective disorders, including anxiety and depression, are also known to be frequently associated with hyperactivity (Biederman et al., 1991). A recent study on African-American children confirmed the same tendency across cultures or ethnicity (Samuel et al., 1998). Nineteen African-American children with DSM-III-R ADHD and 24 African-American children without ADHD were compared. Children with ADHD had a much higher lifetime rate of mood disorders.

It appears that the high frequency of hyperactivity comorbid with other disorders such as conduct disorder or affective disorders is confirmed across cultures or ethnicity. The follow-up question is to explore whether different cultures or ethnicity have an impact on the exact rates of comorbidity with different disorders. Comorbidity by itself is a very complex phenomenon, but it also provides a fertile ground for researching into the aetiology of psychiatric disorders (Angold et al., 1999). Cross-cultural/ethnic data would obviously help.

Cultural/ethnic influence on the management of childhood hyperactivity

Cultural factors are also likely to influence how mental health problems are to be managed in a society. They may, for example, help to protect or aggravate the problems, and they may interact differently with different characteristics of the problems.

The first issue is the availability of services for child mental health problems. In the developing countries, child psychiatry as a discipline still remains relatively underdeveloped. This is likely to contribute to hyperactivity being underreferred and underdiagnosed. Hyperactive children are probably considered as simply naughty, and managed accordingly. Second, behavioural management of hyperactivity and its comorbid oppositional defiant disorder/conduct disorder is a popular approach in western countries. However, it has been warned that this approach must take into consideration the child-rearing practices of the society (Forehand and Kotchick, 1996). Third, the acceptance of drug treatment may vary. In some places, a diagnosis of hyperactivity is often followed by drug treatment, whereas in other places, there may be a general ethos against using psychotropic medication for behaviour problems in children. In fact, even within the same service setting and when health care utilization was controlled, it has been documented that Afro-Americans were 2.5 times less likely to receive methylphenidate than Caucasians in a statewide survey of prescription patterns in the USA (Zito et al., 1997). Fourth, the school environment makes a lot of difference. In the developing countries, schools often have a high student/staff ratio with usually more than 40 students per class. The teachers usually adopt a more structured teaching approach. Students are expected to follow the pace of the teacher and to fit in with the school system instead of the school working out a more individualized programme for them. This makes management in the school situation more difficult. There has been little systematic cross-cultural study of the impact of these cultural factors with respect to the overall efficacy of the management of hyperactive children across different cultures.

Ethnic differences in drug response and biotransformation could be another important aspect of cultural/ethnic influences on the management of childhood hyperactivity. A recent study examined the association of alleles of candidate genes for ADHD and the response to stimulant medication among a group of African-American children (Winsberg and Comings, 1999). Homozygosity of the 10-repeat allele of the dopamine transporter gene (*DAT1*) was found to be significantly associated with a poor response to methylphenidate therapy. Though ethnic differences in biotransformation of methylphenidate have not been studied, the CYP2D6 (a type of cytochrome P450 isoenzyme that metabolizes tricyclic antidepressants, selective serotonin reuptake inhibitors and antipsychotics) has received some attention. About 1% of Asians are poor metabolizers for this enzyme compared to 3–10% of Caucasians. However, about one-third of extensive metabolizers in Asians have a mutation that decreases the activity of the enzyme (Lin et al., 1995). The net effect suggested that Asians might require a lower dosage of these psychotropic medications to achieve the same drug level or therapeutic response. The genetic effect on child psychopharmacology is a very complex issue (Cook, 1999). Much more work will need to be done before it can lead to an improvement in our current clinical practice.

Cultural/ethnic influence on the outcome of childhood hyperactivity

Several long-term follow-up studies have been carried out in western countries showing that childhood hyperactivity is a chronic disorder and leads to a poor prognosis (Barkley et al., 1990; Klein and Mannuzza, 1991; McGee et al., 1991; Taylor et al., 1996). In adult psychiatry, it has been shown that schizophrenia, especially in the females, has a better prognosis in the developing countries compared with the developed ones (Leff, 1988). The findings have also suggested that, for a schizophrenic patient, finding a role in the family and the community that is optimal for his or her functioning is very important in determining the prognosis of the illness. In the developing countries, there is a higher chance of this happening. It is an open question whether anything comparable might apply to the long-term outcome of childhood hyperactivity. To date, there are few published reports on outcome studies conducted in developing or nonwestern countries.

A model for the cross-cultural/ethnic aspects of childhood hyperactivity

Figure 3.1 summarizes the points raised above. The Chinese population in Hong Kong will be used here as the basis for discussion and illustration. There is some evidence that, constitutionally, Chinese children have a more placid innate temperament. Culturally, the Chinese child-rearing practice, school environment and social expectation may also tend to suppress activity level and facilitate inhibition. On the one hand, these ethnic and cultural factors combine to imply a lower vulnerability to hyperactivity and thus may lead to a lower prevalence rate. However, on the other hand, while Chinese hyperactive children may display a more subdued pattern of behavioural and cognitive deficits, their behaviour is still considered to be diagnosable as a disorder in view of the societal norm of a lower baseline with respect to hyperactive behaviour in the general Chinese population. Therefore, given the emphasis in Chinese culture on order and discipline, Chinese parents and teachers tend to have a lower tolerance of hyperactivity and report high ratings of hyperactivity. The prevalence of the diagnosis of hyperactivity is also found to be within the range of those reported in western countries. The concept of hyperactivity is unfamiliar to Chinese adults.

In parental ratings, hyperactivity symptoms tend to be mixed up with conduct problems. The threshold for referring children for help is generally high among the Chinese population. Thus, only severe cases may be referred. Chinese adults tend to accept medical practitioners' opinion, including pre-scriptions of medication for treatment of hyperactivity. However, there are considerable difficulties in helping children to adjust to the more structured and demanding Chinese school system. At present there are no data on the long-term outcome of hyperactivity in Chinese children.

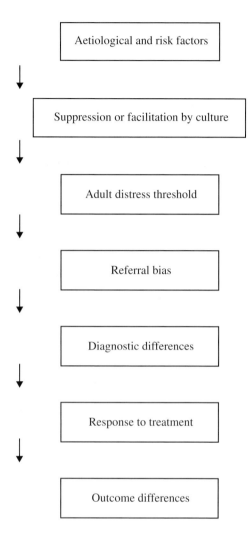

Figure 3.1   A model for the cross-cultural aspects of childhood hyperactivity.

Conclusions

In an insightful review of the relationship between molecular genetics and child developmental research by Plomin and Rutter (1998), it is noted that in complex disorders such as hyperactivity, there is likely to be more than one gene involved and their influences are likely to be probabilistic rather than deterministic; the exact outcome will also be shaped by environmental (including cultural) factors. This is the reason why the authors conclude: 'far from genetics leading to a mechanistic biological determinism, the finding of genes will provide the opportunity to unravel the complicated causal processes involved in the interplay between nature and nurture over the lifespan' (Plomin and Rutter, 1998, p. 1238). This is where studies involving different cultural/ethnic groups can play an important role in the future. The orientation of previous cross-cultural studies has tended to focus mainly on the impact of cultural influences on behaviour. Given the recent advances in genetics, there is a growing awareness of the genetic basis of many behavioural disorders – hyperactivity being one example. Cross-cultural studies should take on an expanded role by examining not only the cultural traditions but also the genetics of the different ethnic groups. Such cross-cultural/ethnic studies provide a powerful vehicle for scientific investigation as they can extend the range of variation or diversity in variables that a single culture or ethnicity cannot provide, e.g. the rarity of 7-repeat allele in *DRD4* in the Chinese or the suppression effects of a more restrictive, collectivist Asian culture. Such a variation or diversity is invaluable in human research since researchers cannot ethically subject human subjects to experimental manipulation. Cross-cultural/ ethnic studies thus provide the required natural laboratory for quasiexperimentation. The involvement of both cultural/social and biological/genetic factors in these studies also prevents the unnecessary and artificial division of nature and nurture in the study of human behaviour. Each piece of behaviour, including those referred to as hyperactive, is ultimately a product of both nature and nurture.

REFERENCES

Achenbach, T.M. and Edelbrock, E.S. (1978). The classification of child psychopathology: a review and analysis of empirical efforts. *Psychological Bulletin*, **85**, 1275–1301.

Achenbach, T. and McConaughy, S. (1997). *Empirically Based Assessment of Child and Adolescent Psychopathology: Practical Applications*, 2nd edn. Thousand Oaks, CA: Sage.

American Psychiatric Association. (1980). *DSM-III: Diagnostic and Statistical Manual of Mental Disorders*, 2nd edn. Washington, DC: American Psychiatric Association.

American Psychiatric Association. (1994). *Diagnostic and Statistical Manual of Mental Disorders (DSM-IV)*. Washington, DC: American Psychiatric Association.

Anderson, J.C. (1996). Is childhood hyperactivity the product of western culture? *Lancet*, **348**, 73–4.

Angold, A., Costello, E. and Erkanli, A. (1999). Comorbidity. *Journal of Child Psychology and Psychiatry*, **40**, 57–87.

Barkley, R.A. (1982). Defining hyperactivity/ADD: a working set of references. *Advances in Clinical Child Psychology*, **5**, 153–80.

Barkley, R. (1998). *Attention Deficit Hyperactivity Disorder*, 2nd edn. New York: Guilford Press.

Barkley, R.A., Fischer, M., Edelbrock, C.S. and Smallish, L. (1990). The adolescent outcome of hyperactive children diagnosed by research criteria: I. An 8-year prospective follow-up study. *Journal of American Academy of Child and Adolescent Psychiatry*, **29**, 546–57.

Bhatia, M.S., Nigam, V.R., Bohra, N. and Malik, S.C. (1991). Attention deficit disorder with hyperactivity among paedriatic outpatients. *Journal of Child Psychology and Psychiatry*, **32**, 297–306.

Biederman, J., Newcorn, J. and Sprich, S. (1991). Comorbidity of attention deficit hyperactivity among paediatric outpatients. *American Journal of Psychiatry*, **148**, 564–77.

Block, G. (1977). Hyperactivity: a cultural perspective. *Journal of Learning Disabilities*, **110**, 236–40.

Blum, K., Cull, J.G., Braverman, E.R. and Comings, D.E. (1996). Reward deficiency syndrome. *American Scientist*, **84**, 132–45.

Brito, G. (1987). The Conners Abbreviated Teacher Rating Scale: Development of norms in Brazil. *Journal of Abnormal Child Psychology*, **15**, 511–18.

Bronson, G.W. (1972). Infants' reactions to unfamiliar persons and novel objects. *Monographs of the Society for Research in Child Development*, **37** (3. Serial No. 148).

Bussing, R., Schoenberg, N.E. and Perwien, A.R. (1998). Knowledge and information about ADHD: evidence of cultural differences among African-American and white parents. *Social Science Medicine*, **46**, 919–28.

Chang, F.M., Kidd, J.R., Livak, K.J., Pakstis, A.J. and Kidd, K.K. (1996). The world-wide distribution of allele frequencies at the human dopamine D4 receptor locus. *Human Genetics*, **98**, 91–101.

Chen, C.S. and Stevenson, H.W. (1989). Housework: a cross-cultural examination. *Child Development*, **60**, 551–61.

Chen, W., Loh, E., Hsu, Y. et al. (1996). Alcohol metabolising genes and alcoholism among Taiwanese Han men: independent effect of ADH2, ADH3 and ALDH2. *British Journal of Psychiatry*, **168**, 762–7.

Cheng Lai, A., Zhang, Z. and Wang, W. (2000). Maternal child-rearing practices in Hong Kong and Beijing Chinese families: a comparative study. *International Journal of Psychology*, **35**, 60–6.

Comings, D.E., Comings, B.G., Muhleman, D. et al. (1991). The dopamine D2 receptor locus as a modifying gene in neuropsychiatric disorders. *Journal of the American Medical Association*, **266**, 1793–800.

Conners, C.K. (1969). A teachers rating scale for use in drug studies with children. *American Journal of Psychiatry*, **126**, 884–8.

Cook, E. (1999). The early development of child psychopharmacogenetics. *Journal of the American Academy of Child and Adolescent Psychiatry*, **38**, 1478–81.

Cook, E.H., Stein, M.A., Krasowski, M.D. et al. (1995). Association of attention deficit disorder and the dopamine transporter gene. *American Journal of Human Genetics*, **56**, 993–8.

Ekblad, S. (1986). Social determinants of aggression in a sample of Chinese primary school children. *Acta Psychiatrica Scandinavica*, **73**, 515–23.

Ekblad, S. (1990). The children's behaviour questionnaire for completion by parents and teachers in a Chinese sample. *Journal of Child Psychology and Psychiatry*, **31**, 775–91.

Faraone, S.V., Biederman, J., Weiffenbach, B. et al. (1999). Dopamine D-sub-4 gene 7-repeat allele and attention deficit hyperactivity disorder. *American Journal of Psychiatry*, **156**, 768–70.

Forehand, R. and Kotchick, B. (1996). Cultural diversity: a wake-up call for parent training. *Behaviour Therapy*, **27**, 187–206.

Freedman, D.G. and Freedman, N.C. (1969). Behavioural differences between Chinese American and European-American newborns. *Nature*, **224**, 1227.

Frick, P.J. and Jackson, Y.K. (1993). Family functioning and childhood antisocial behaviour: yet another reinterpretation. *Journal of Clinical Child Psychology*, **22**, 410–19.

Gelernter, J.O., O'Malley, S., Risch, N. et al. (1991). No association between an allele at the D2 dopamine receptor gene (DRD1) and alcoholism. *Journal of the American Medication Association*, **266**, 1801–7.

Gill, M., Daly, G., Heron, S., Hawi, Z. and Fitzgerald, M. (1997). Confirmation of association between attention deficit hyperactivity disorder and a dopamine transporter polymorphism. *Molecular Psychiatry*, **2**, 311–13.

Glow, R. and Stevenson, J. (1981). Cross-validity and normative data on the Conner's Parent and Teacher rating scales. In *The Psychosocial Aspects of Drug Treatment for Hyperactivity*, K.D. Gadow and J. Loney, eds, pp. 107–50. Colorado: Westview Press.

Goodman, R. and Stevenson, J. (1989). A twin-study of hyperactivity – I. An examination of hyperactivity scores and categories derived from Rutter Teacher and Parent questionnaires. *Journal of Child Psychology and Psychiatry*, **30**, 671–89.

Goyette, C., Conners, C.K. and Ulrich, R.F. (1978). Normative data on revised Conners Parent and Teacher rating scales. *Journal of Abnormal Child Psychology*, **6**, 221–36.

Ho, Y.F. (1981). Childhood psychopathology: a dialogue with special reference to Chinese and American cultures. In *Normal and Abnormal Behaviour in Chinese Culture*, A. Kleinman and T. Lin, eds, pp. 137–56. Dordrecht, Holland: D. Reidel.

Ho, Y.F. (1986). Chinese patterns of socialisation: a critical review. In *The Psychology of the Chinese People*, M.H. Bond, ed. pp. 1–15. Hong Kong: Oxford University Press.

Ho, T.P., Leung, P.W.L., Luk, S.L. et al. (1996). Establishing the constructs of childhood behavioural disturbances in a Chinese population: a questionnaire study. *Journal of Abnormal Child Psychology*, **24**, 417–31.

Holborow, P. and Berry, P. (1986). A multinational, cross-cultural perspective on hyperactivity. *American Journal of Orthopsychiatry*, **56**, 320–2.

Holborow, P., Berry, P. and Elkins, J. (1984). Prevalence of hyperkinesis: a comparison of three rating scales. *Journal of Learning Disabilities*, **17**, 411–15.

Jablensky, A., Sartorius, N., Giulbinat, W. and Ernberg, G. (1981). Characteristics of depressive patients contacting psychiatric services in four cultures. *Acta Psychiatrica Scandinavica*, **63**, 308–18.

Kelsoe, J.R., Ginns, E.I., Egeland, J.A. et al. (1989). Re-evaluation of the linkage relationship between chromosome 11p loci and the gene for bipolar affective disorder in the Old Order Amish. *Nature*, **342**, 238–43.

Klein, R.G. and Mannuzza, S. (1991). Long-term outcome of hyperactive children: a review. *Journal of the American Academy of Child and Adolescent Psychiatry*, **30**, 383–7.

Kleinman, A. (1982). Depression and neurasthenia in the People's Republic of China. *Culture, Medicine and Psychiatry*, **6**, 1–80.

Lahoste, G.J., Swanson, J.M., Wigal, S.B. et al. (1996). Dopamine D4 receptor gene polymorphism is associated with attention deficit hyperactivity disorder. *Molecular Psychiatry*, **1**, 121–4.

Leff, J. (1988). *Psychiatry around the Globe, A Transcultural View*, 2nd edn. London: Gaskell.

Leung, P., Luk, S. and Lee, P. (1989). Problem behaviour among handicapped children in Hong Kong: a factor-analytic study with Conners' Teacher's Rating Scale. *Psychologia*, **32**, 120–8.

Leung, P.W.L., Ho, T.P., Luk, S.L. et al. (1996a). Separation and comorbidity of hyperactivity and conduct disturbance in Chinese school boys. *Journal of Child Psychology and Psychiatry*, **37**, 841–53.

Leung, P.W.L., Luk, S.L., Ho, T.P. et al. (1996b). The diagnosis and prevalence of hyperactivity in Chinese school boys. *British Journal of Psychiatry*, **168**, 486–96.

Lin, C. and Fu, V. (1990). A comparison of child-rearing practices among Chinese, immigrant Chinese and Caucasian-American parents. *Child Development*, **61**, 429–33.

Lin, K. Anderson, D. and Poland, R. (1995). Ethnicity and psychopharmacology: bridging the gap. *Psychiatric Clinics of North America*, **18**, 635–47.

Luk, S.L. and Leung, P.W.L. (1989). Conner's Teachers' Rating Scale – a validity study in Hong Kong. *Journal of Child Psychology and Psychiatry*, **30**, 785–93.

Luk, S.L., Leung, P.W.L. and Lee, P. (1988a). Conner's Teacher Rating Scale in Chinese Children in Hong Kong. *Journal of Child Psychology and Psychiatry*, **29**, 165–74.

Luk, S.L., Leung, P.W.L., Lee, P. and Lieh-Mak, F. (1988b). Teachers' referral of children with mental health problems – a study of primary schools in Hong Kong. *Psychology in Schools*, **25**, 121–9.

Luk, S.L., Leung, P.W.L. and Yuen, J. (1991). Clinic observations in the assessment of pervasiveness of childhood hyperactivity. *Journal of Child Psychology and Psychiatry*, **32**, 833–50.

Luk, S.L., Lieh Mak, F., Leung, P.W.L. et al. (1993). *A Hong Kong–United Kingdom Cross-cultural Study of Childhood Hyperactivity: A Research Report to Croucher Foundation*. Hong Kong: Department of Psychiatry, University of Hong Kong.

Mann, E.M., Yoshiko, I., Mueller, C.W. and Akihisa, T. (1992). Cross-cultural differences in rating hyperactive-disruptive behaviors in children. *American Journal of Psychiatry*, **149**, 1539–42.

McGee, R., Partridge, F., Williams, S. and Silva, P. (1991). A twelve-year follow-up of preschool hyperactive children. *Journal of American Academy of Child and Adolescent Psychiatry*, **30**, 224–32.

Minde, K.K. and Cohen, N.J. (1978). Hyperactive children in Canada and Uganda: a comparative evaluation. *Journal of the American Academy of Child Psychiatry*, **17**, 476–87.

Morita, H., Suzuke, M. and Kamoshita, S. (1990). Screening measures for detecting psychiatric disorders in Japanese secondary school children. *Journal of Child Psychology and Psychiatry*, **31**, 603–71.

Offord, D.R., Boyle, M.H., Szatmani, P. et al. (1987). Ontario Child Health Study: II. Six-months prevalence of disorder and rates of service utilization. *Archives of General Psychiatry*, **44**, 832–6.

O'Leary, K.D., Vivian, D. and Nisi, A. (1985). Hyperactivity in Italy. *Journal of Abnormal Child Psychology*, **13**, 485–500.

Pavuluri, M., Luk, S.L. and McGee, R. (1996). Help-seeking for behaviour problems by parents of preschool children: a community study. *Journal of the American Academy of Child and Adolescent Psychiatry*, **35**, 215–22.

Plomin, R. (1995). Genetics and children's experiences in the family. *Journal of Child Psychology and Psychiatry*, **36**, 33–68.

Plomin, R. and Rutter, M. (1998). Child development, molecular genetics and what to do with genes once they are found. *Child Development*, **69**, 1223–42.

Prendergast, M., Taylor, E., Rapoport, J.L. et al. (1988). The diagnosis of childhood hyperactivity: a U.S.–U.K. cross-national study of DSM-III and ICD-9. *Journal of Child Psychology and Psychiatry*, **29**, 289–300.

Reid, R., DuPaul, G., Power, T. et al. (1998). Assessing culturally different students for attention deficit hyperactivity disorder using behaviour rating scales. *Journal of Abnormal Child Psychology*, **3**, 187–98.

Samuel, V., Curtis, S., Thornell, A. et al. (1997). The unexplored void of ADHD and African-American research: a review of the literature. *Journal of Attention Disorders*, **1**, 197–207.

Samuel, V.J., Biederman, J., Faraone, S.V. et al. (1998). Clinical characteristics of attention deficit hyperactivity disorder in African American children. *American Journal of Psychiatry*, **155**, 696–8.

Sartorius, N., Jablensky, A., Korten, A. et al. (1986). Early manifestations and first contact incidence of schizophrenia in different cultures. *Psychological Medicine*, **16**, 909–28.

Schachar, R.J. (1986). Hyperkinetic syndrome: historical development of the concept. In *The Overactive Child*, E. Taylor, ed., pp. 19–40. Oxford: Blackwell.

Schachar, R. (1991). Childhood hyperactivity. *Journal of Child Psychology and Psychiatry*, **32**, 155–91.

Schachar, R., Rutter, M. and Smith, A. (1981). The characteristics of situationally and pervasively hyperactive children: implications for syndrome definition. *Journal of Child Psychology and Psychiatry*, **22**, 373–92.

Shen, Y.C., Wang, Y.F. and Yang, X.L. (1985). An epidemiological investigation of minimal brain dysfunction in six elementary schools in Beijing. *Journal of Child Psychology and Psychiatry*, **26**, 777–88.

Sonuga-Barke, E.J.S., Minocha, K., Taylor, E. and Sandberg, S. (1993). Inter-ethnic bias in teachers' ratings of childhood hyperactivity. *British Journal of Developmental Psychology*, **11**, 187–200.

Swanson, J., Sergeant, J., Taylor, E. et al. (1998a). Attention-deficit hyperactivity disorder and hyperkinetic disorder. *The Lancet*, **351**, 429–33.

Swanson, J.M., Sunohara, G.A., Kennedy, J.L. et al. (1998b). Association of dopamine receptor (DRD4) gene with a refined phenotype of attention deficit hyperactivity disorder (ADHD): a family-based approach. *Molecular Psychiatry*, **3**, 38–41.

Szatmari, P., Boyle, M. and Offord, D.R. (1989). ADHD and conduct disorder: degree of diagnostic overlap and differences among correlates. *Journal of the American Academy of Child and Adolescent Psychiatry*, **28**, 865–72.

Tannock, R. (1998). Attention deficit hyperactivity disorder: advances in cognitive, neurobiological and genetic research. *Journal of Child Psychology and Psychiatry*, **39**, 65–100.

Taylor, E. (1985). Syndrome of overactivity and attention deficit. In *Child and Adolescent*

Psychiatry, Modern Approaches, M. Rutter and L. Hersov, eds., 2nd edn, pp. 424–43. Oxford: Blackwell.

Taylor, E. (1986). Childhood hyperactivity. *British Journal of Psychiatry*, **149**, 562–73.

Taylor, E. and Sandberg, S. (1984). Hyperactive behaviour in English school children: a questionnaire survey. *Journal of Abnormal Child Psychology*, **12**, 143–56.

Taylor, E., Schachar, R., Thorley, G. and Wieselberg, M. (1986). Conduct disorder and hyperactivity I: Separation and hyperactivity of antisocial conduct in British child psychiatric patients. *British Journal of Psychiatry*, **149**, 760–7.

Taylor, E., Sandberg, S., Thorley, G. and Giles, S. (1991). *The Epidemiology of Childhood Hyperactivity*. New York: Oxford University Press.

Taylor, E., Chadwick, O., Heptinstall, E. and Danckaerts, M. (1996). Hyperactivity and conduct problems as risk factors for adolescent development. *Journal of the American Academy of Child and Adolescent Psychiatry*, **35**, 1213–26.

Trites, R.L., Dugas, E., Lynch, G. and Ferguson, H.B. (1979). Prevalence of hyperactivity. *Journal of Paediatric Psychology*, **4**, 179–88.

Trites, R.L., Blouin, A.G.A. and Laprade, K. (1982). Factor analysis of the Conner's Teacher rating scale. Based on a normative sample. *Journal of Consulting and Clinical Psychology*, **50**, 615–23.

Wang, Y.F., Shen, Y.C., Gu, B.M., Jia, M.X. and Zhang, A.L. (1989). An epidemiological study of behaviour problems in school children in urban areas of Beijing. *Journal of Child Psychology and Psychiatry*, **30**, 907–12.

Weisz, J.R., Suwanlert, S., Chaiyasit, W. et al. (1987a). Epidemiology of behavioural and emotional problems among Thai and American children: parent repots for ages 6 to 11. *Journal of the American Academy of Child and Adolescent Psychiatry*, **26**, 890–7.

Weisz, J.R., Suwanlert, S., Chaiyasit, W. and Walter, B.R. (1987b). Over and under controlled referral problems among children and adolescents from Thailand and the United States: the Wat and Wai of cultural differences. *Journal of Consulting and Clinical Pscyhology*, **55**, 719–26.

Weisz, J.R., Suwanlert, S., Chaiyasit, W. et al. (1988). Thai and American perspectives on over and under controlled child behaviour problems: exploring the threshold model among parents, teachers and psychologists. *Journal of Consulting and Clinical Psychology*, **56**, 601–9.

Weisz, J.R., Suwanlert, S., Chaiyasit, W. et al. (1989). Epidemiology of behavioural and emotional problems among Thai and American children: teacher reports for ages 6–11. *Journal of Child Psychology and Psychiatry*, **30**, 471–84.

Werry, J.S. and Hawthorne, D. (1976). Conner's teacher questionnaire – norms and validity. *Australian and New Zealand Journal of Psychiatry*, **10**, 257–62.

Werry, J.S., Sprague, R.L. and Cohen, M.N. (1975). Conner's teacher rating scale for use in drug studies with children – an empirical study. *Journal of Abnormal Child Psychology*, **3**, 217–29.

Winsberg, B. and Comings, D. (1999). Association of the dopamine transporter gene (DAT1) with poor methylphenidate response. *Journal of the American Academy of Child and Adolescent Psychiatry*, **38**, 1474–7.

World Health Organization. (1978). *International Classification of Diseases*, 9th edn. Geneva: World Health Organization.

World Health Organization. (1994). *ICD-10: International Classification of Mental and Behavioural Disorders*. Geneva: World Health Organization.

Zito, J., Safer, D., dosReis, S., Magder, L. and Riddle, M. (1997). Methylphenidate patterns among Medicaid youths. *Psychopharmacology Bulletin*, **33**, 143–7.

4

Sex differences and their significance

Ellen Heptinstall and Eric Taylor

Department of Child and Adolescent Psychiatry, Institute of Psychiatry, London

Until quite recently, the literature on attention deficit hyperactivity disorder (ADHD) and hyperkinetic disorder (HKD) may have given the impression that they were solely problems of males, since study after study concentrated on boys only. Such a strategy may well be justified. There is little doubt that a male predominance is one of the consistent findings about ADHD and HKD and this must raise the possibility that affected females are in some ways different. The research approach of studying the sexes separately has much to be said for, but for a long time, the process tended to stop with the investigation of boys. However, in recent years there has been a considerable increase of interest in the question of sex differences in ADHD and HKD, both in terms of the practical concerns of clinicians treating girls and in terms of finding answers to questions about the aetiology of the disorder which could account for the sex differences. In particular, recent research has aimed at describing differences between affected males and affected females.

In recent years a major advance in ADHD research has been the use of genetically informative strategies to illuminate the question of how psychopathology develops. It seems probable that this approach will in future provide more satisfactory answers to this question. However, at the moment different studies contradict each other on key questions and the reasons for these contradictions are not obvious.

One particular problem in the methodology needs to be highlighted from the very beginning. Two of the key issues on the development of psychopathology are highly interdependent; these are the size of gender differences in prevalence of ADHD and HKD and the similarities and differences between the sexes. This interdependence arises because it is not clear how far different studies compare like with like. In many clinic-referred samples the sex differences are extreme (nine boys to one girl). If, as has been suggested, these differences are due to the identification of ADHD cases and a higher level of severity of the disorder in girls, it may well be that girls are found to have worse problems than boys. Compared with clinic-referred samples, gender differences in the population are typically much smaller (two boys to one girl). This situation may represent 'true' differences in prevalence because girls might be recognized as ADHD on milder grounds than boys. If this is the case, ADHD girls could be expected to be less severely affected than ADHD boys. The possibility that ADHD boys and girls are compared on different levels of severity is not completely avoided by the systematic use of the same interviews and rating scales for both sexes. It is not at all certain that a rating for hyperactive behaviour, for example, would be made in the same way by a person rating a boy as a person rating a girl.

What anchor points might be chosen to determine whether the same level of severity is present in male and female ADHD cases? Objective measures of activity and cognition, heritability estimates and molecular genetic variations might all be chosen. However, if ADHD in girls is defined at a level that generates equal heritability, it will no longer be possible to examine whether the sexes differ in their pattern of inheritance. From a psychiatric perspective, the most relevant choice would be impact; that is, whether the adverse outcome is comparable between the sexes, but insufficient knowledge from longitudinal studies is available. A lack of certainty in case definition is consequently a major problem for researchers seeking to draw conclusions from the rather contradictory literature.

We shall describe the empirical findings that are available so far, before going on to consider issues about the nature and possible aetiology of the sex differences. Above all, we hope to contribute to the clinical debate about sex differences in ADHD and HKD, both in terms of symptoms and aetiology.

Empirical studies of sex differences

Sex differences in prevalence

The most consistent finding in studies of ADHD and HKD has been the unequal representation of the sexes. Still (1902) first noted that in clinic-referred children problem behaviour or 'moral deficiency' or 'defects of moral control', as it was then termed, was more common in boys than in girls. Since then, many studies have reported an overrepresentation of boys in both ADHD and HKD.

However, there have been considerable variations in the reported boy/girl ratios. In the USA, clinic-referred children with ADHD were found to have a ratio varying from five boys to one girl to nine boys to one girl (Goodyear and Hynd, 1992; Lahey et al., 1994). In the UK, Thorley (1984) and James and

Taylor (1990) found a ratio of three boys to one girl in samples of clinically diagnosed HKD children. There is little doubt that referral criteria contribute to the overrepresentation of boys in clinic-referred samples. Several studies have argued that ADHD boys have higher rates of conduct disorder (CD) and other externalizing problems compared with ADHD girls. This pattern is likely to result in ADHD boys displaying more disruptive behaviour than ADHD girls, which in turn results in boys being more frequently referred than girls (Gaub and Carlson 1997; Jensen et al., 1997; Biederman et al., 1999).

Reporting the conclusions of a conference on sex differences in ADHD convened by the National Institute of Mental Health (NIMH) in the USA, Arnold (1996) has stated that it is not clear whether the sex differences in clinic referral indicate that girls are preferentially treated in different settings (e.g. home and school); whether their needs are simply overlooked; whether girls have less need than boys or whether it is in fact the result of a combination of these probabilities. The conference also agreed that the 'true' sex ratio is likely to be lower than in clinic-referred samples, but will probably never approach 1 : 1 as long as the same diagnostic criteria are used for both sexes.

Population-based studies of ADHD and HKD have generally reported less pronounced sex differences than clinic-based studies. Using both the Rutter A and B scales (for parents and teachers respectively), Taylor et al. (paper presented, 1998) reported a ratio of fewer than three boys to one girl. Studies relying on the Achenbach Child Behavior Checklist found an overall sex ratio of three boys to one girl (Szatmari, 1992; Gaub and Carlson, 1997). The variations in sex ratios in these studies are likely to be influenced by differences in measurements and sampling characteristics. Raters' bias is also considered to contribute significantly to differences in sex ratios. Studies using teacher questionnaire ratings only (McGee et al., 1987) reported a higher proportion of ADHD boys compared to ADHD girls than studies using both parent and teacher ratings (Szatmari et al., 1989b; McGee and Feehan, 1991). Gaub and Carlson (1997) have speculated that these variations may reflect a different basis for ratings by parents and teachers. They argue that parents are more likely to recognize ADHD symptoms in girls because they compare their daughters with other girls, many of whom are likely not to have ADHD symptoms. Teachers, on the other hand, may compare ADHD girls with ADHD boys to a norm influenced by the boys since they display more overt behaviour problems. McGee and Feehan (1991) have suggested that teachers tend to underrecognize ADHD symptoms in girls because girls are less likely than ADHD boys to exhibit behaviour management problems.

Variations in age may also have contributed to higher or lower sex ratios.

Brown et al. (1991) have reported that as ADHD children grow older, girls' problems increase relative to those of boys. Cohen et al. (1993) demonstrated that the prevalence rate for ADHD amongst boys declined by nearly 20% per year between the ages of 10 and 20, while the prevalence amongst girls remained relatively constant during those ages. Costello (1990) has also noted the importance of investigating developmentally based sex differences in ADHD.

An increase in studies based on child populations in different countries, including Iceland, Hong Kong, Australia, Colombia and Brazil, has made it possible to examine the effect of cultural differences on prevalence in ADHD (Brito et al., 1995; Leung et al., 1996; Gomez et al., 1999; Magnusson et al., 1999; Pineda et al., 1999). These studies demonstrate that, generally, there are no systematic cultural effects, but differences in prevalence rates are likely to be related to differences in sample ascertainment. However, the consistent reports of an overrepresentation of boys means that the presence of sex differences in prevalence, either in clinic-referred or population samples, is not in doubt.

This chapter will attempt to determine from the scientific evidence what implications these differences in prevalence between the sexes may have. This will involve a comparison of ADHD or HKD boys with ADHD or HKD girls in order to examine whether they share the same problem and whether the same explanatory structure applies. For this reason, the published studies will be reviewed to establish whether a consensus exists. The unpublished results of our own recent study of girls will be described briefly (Taylor, personal communication, 1991; Heptinstall et al., paper presented, 1998; Taylor et al., paper presented, 1998). This study was designed as a two-stage epidemiological survey of 6–8-year-old girls attending schools in a London borough. It used the same methods as a study of boys of the same ages, living in the same area (Taylor et al., 1991). The first stage consisted of a screen of the whole population. Out of the 2285 girls registered in schools in the assigned area, full teacher ratings were obtained for 2033 girls and full parent ratings for 1687 girls. The instruments used were the Rutter A (2) and B (2) rating scales, as well as an abbreviated version of the Conners scale. Girls were characterized as 'hyperactive' or 'conduct-disordered' if they scored above the cutoff points for those scales that had been established for boys (Taylor et al., 1991). Girls were less likely to show either problems than boys; the ratio was 1 : 2.5 for hyperactive behaviour and 1 : 2.1 for CD. However, the sex ratio for emotional disorder was 1 : 1.

The second stage constituted a more detailed observational, interview and experimental study of selected groups of girls, defined by their scores on the screening questionnaires. All the hyperactive girls were included into this stage and divided into two groups: one with and one without CD. Other selected groups comprised conduct-disordered girls without hyperactivity and a random sample of control children who did not meet criteria for either hyperactivity or CD. All subjects were studied using a standardized investigator-based parent interview, a structured and standardized teacher interview, observations during a testing session, a neurological examination, reading tests, IQ tests and attention tests. The parent interview also covered details about family relationships and histories of disorder in other family members.

One of the analyses compared the deviant girls with the deviant boys. The hyperactive girls were unequivocally less active than the hyperactive boys when their movements were measured physically, directly observed or recorded through the detailed behavioural interviews. It was therefore clear that underrecognition by teachers and parents could not account for the lower prevalence in girls.

Sex differences in ADHD and HKD symptoms

Core symptoms

ADHD and HKD are characterized by overactivity, inattentiveness and impulsiveness and recognized as a disorder when these behaviours are severe, developmentally inappropriate and impair function at home and in school (Swanson et al., 1998). As Arnold (1996) has pointed out, in any consideration of sex differences in ADHD, it is important to recognize sex differences in behaviour that are 'normal' and not attributable to a differential manifestation of ADHD. A large body of literature has established that on teacher and parent rating scales girls of all ages have fewer attention problems and less hyperactivity than same-age boys – a finding that appears to be consistent across cultures (McGee et al., 1987; Bauermeister, 1992; Brito et al., 1995).

Much of the research providing evidence for the presence of core behaviour characteristics in ADHD and HKD children has concentrated on boys. Studies concentrating on girls have emphasized that, like ADHD boys, ADHD girls are more overactive, more inattentive and more impulsive than non-ADHD children (deHaas and Young, 1984; Taylor, personal communication, 1991; Gaub and Carlson, 1997; Seidman et al., 1997; Biederman et al., 1999). Several studies relying on parent and teacher reports found higher levels of hyperactive and inattentive behaviour in ADHD boys than in ADHD girls. The majority of these studies used the Conners Teacher Rating Scale to identify ADHD symptoms (Bauermeister, 1992; Brito et al., 1995). Using the Rutter B scale for teachers, McGee *et al.* (1987) also found that boys were rated as significantly more hyperactive than girls. These results were taken to indicate that teachers identify problematic behaviour more readily in boys than in girls. This possibility was supported by a study using both parent and teacher reports of behaviour (Breen and Altepeter, 1990). In a group of clinically diagnosed ADHD children, teachers regarded boys as having more severe behaviour problems than girls. In contrast, parents reported similar problems for both sexes.

Studying population-based samples of boys and girls separately in order to reduce stereotyped reports, Taylor et al. (paper presented, 1998) found a number of sex differences in psychometric measures. Although ADHD girls were less active during testing than ADHD boys, they showed more inattentive behaviour. Similar findings were reported in a metaanalysis of 18 studies directly comparing ADHD girls with ADHD boys (Gaub and Carlson, 1997). However, in clinic samples of ADHD children, Arcia and Conners (1998) and Sharp et al. (1999) found no significant differences in overactive and inattentive behaviour between boys and girls. This finding appears to support suggestions that only the most active girls with ADHD are likely to be referred.

Comorbidity

Studies of ADHD and HKD have frequently reported considerable overlap with other disorders. In an extensive review of the literature, Biederman et al. (1991a) found that ADHD children had considerable comorbidity with a variety of conditions, including CD, oppositional defiant disorder (ODD), mood disorders and anxiety disorders. Comorbidity rates between ADHD and CD were reported to be 30–50%, between ADHD and mood disorders 15–75% and between ADHD and anxiety disorders about 25%. Pliszka (1992) found high rates of anxiety disorder in ADHD children. August and Garfinkel (1993) studied ADHD in a group of primary schoolchildren and found another disruptive behaviour disorder in 25% of cases, with ODD being more common than CD.

A study carried out in the 1980s found that, in British clinics, where any diagnosis related to hyperactivity was rare, most children diagnosed as conduct-disordered met DSM-III criteria for ADHD (Taylor et al., 1986). In the Ontario Child Health study using the Achenbach Child Behavior Checklist, roughly 40% of ADHD children and adolescents aged 4–16 also had CD (Szatmari et al., 1989a). In a population study of boys identified as having behaviour problems by Rutter A and B scales, CD was found in 22% of hyperactive children (Taylor et al., 1991).

Few studies examining comorbidity in ADHD children either included girls or analysed the sexes separately. Those studies that have examined sex differential comorbidity have been inconsistent. A metaanalysis of 18 studies directly comparing ADHD girls with ADHD boys reported a greater overlap with CD in boys as compared to girls (Gaub and Carlson, 1997). However, in two separate studies of boys and girls, carried out at different times but in the same geographical area, Taylor et al. (paper presented, 1998) found CD in 58% of hyperactive boys and 61% of hyperactive girls. Gabel et al. (1996) found no difference in the pattern of comorbidity in clinic-referred children aged 6–11.

Intellectual ability and academic performance

ADHD has frequently been linked with poor educational achievement (August and Garfinkel, 1989, 1990; Frick et al., 1991). However, as has been the case with comorbidity in ADHD, relatively little attention has been paid to the overlap with learning difficulties in girls. As in the case of comorbidity, the few studies to examine sex differences in this area have been contradictory in their findings. Berry et al. (1985) claimed that referred ADHD girls showed more prominent cognitive deficits than referred ADHD boys. In particular, girls showed more severe language impairment than boys. In addition, girls had a lower mean IQ than boys. These findings correspond with those reported on a group of referred HKD children (James and Taylor, 1990). Language problems were found in 26% of boys and 66% of girls. Boys had a mean IQ of 77, while the mean IQ of girls was 67. Other studies of referred ADHD children found no sex differences in learning problems and academic performance (Gaub and Carlson, 1997; Arcia and Conners, 1998). In a small clinic-referred sample, Sharp et al. (1999) found significantly lower reading scores in ADHD girls than in ADHD boys, although the prevalence of reading disorder was low in both sexes. Gaub and Carlson (1997) found greater intellectual impairment in girls, but there were no sex differences in intellectual performance.

Very few population-based studies have found sex differences in intellectual ability and academic performance. The boys and girls studied by Taylor et al. (paper presented, 1998) showed that pure hyperactive girls had a lower mean IQ (92.0) than pure hyperactive boys (101.0). Mixed hyperactive/conduct-disordered girls also showed a lower mean IQ (89.5) than their male counterparts (95.0).

Peer relationships

A large body of literature concentrating on boys only has suggested that ADHD children have more negative relationships with their peers and fewer friends than other children (Hinshaw and Melnick, 1995; Saunders and Chambers, 1996; Hinshaw et al., 1997; Dumas, 1998; Landau et al., 1998). In a sample of over 4000 schoolchildren aged 7, 8, 11 or 12, with equal sex distribution, CD emerged as a more powerful predictor of peer isolation or rejection than hyperactivity (McArdle et al., 2000). However, despite the large numbers of girls included in the sample, the sexes were not analysed separately.

The relatively few studies including both sexes were carried out in the 1980s and reported a similar severity of peer problems in both sexes (deHaas, 1986; Horn et al., 1989), although the nature of these problems differed in boys and girls. In a referred sample, girls with ADHD were found to suffer more peer rejection, while boys with ADHD were more dominating and physically aggressive towards their peers (Berry et al., 1985). In a sample of 607 schoolchildren, boys and girls with ADHD showed similar difficulties with peer relationships, but boys were found to be more withdrawn as well as more aggressive towards their peers (Johnston et al., 1985). More recently, in a sample of schoolchildren, girls with ADHD received higher peer dislike scores than boys with ADHD (Carlson et al., 1997). Brown et al. (1991) reported that, as ADHD girls get older, they are increasingly rejected by their peers, while the peer relationships of ADHD boys did not change over time.

The parent–child relationship

Even more than in any other area of ADHD or HKD, studies of the parent–child relationship have largely concentrated on boys. Most earlier studies reported that mothers of ADHD boys were more disapproving and more directive in structured tasks compared to mothers of non-ADHD boys, while in free play they were less responsive and more controlling (Mash and Johnston, 1982; Tallmadge and Barkley, 1983).

More recent studies have tended to include parental or family functioning in their sphere of interest. Brown and Pacini (1989) compared the perceptions of parents of ADHD boys with those of parents of non-ADHD boys. The parents of ADHD boys perceived their family environment as less supportive and more stressful than did the parents in the control group. More parents in the ADHD group were divorced or separated. Barkley et al. (1992) found that the mothers of ADHD adolescents displayed more negative interactions in a neutral discussion compared with the mothers of a control group. The mothers in the ADHD group also expressed greater personal distress and less satisfaction in their marriages. This study included only eight girls, which probably explained why the sexes were not analysed separately. Johnston (1996) found more parent–child conflict and more parental disturbance in the families of 5–11-year-old ADHD children when compared with a group of families of nonproblem children. The parents of ADHD children showed a higher rate of depression and a higher rate of marital problems. Unfortunately,

Johnston gave no indication of the sexes of the children included in the study.

Unlike the previously discussed studies, Breen and Barkley (1988) included boys and girls in a study of the association between ADHD and family stress. Their findings showed no differences in parent-reported child psychopathology or parental stress.

Neuropsychological function

Cognitive deficits, in particular impairments in attention and executive function, are hypothesized to be core impairments of ADHD (Denckla, 1989; Barkley, 1997). Cognitive executive function is defined as the ability to 'maintain an appropriate problem-solving set for attainment of a future goal' (Welsh and Pennington, 1988, p. 201) and is thought to include processes responsible for allowing an individual to initiate, sustain and shift attention (Denckla, 1996).

Few studies have attempted to establish the presence of neuropsychological deficits in girls with ADHD. A study focusing on comorbidity with Tourette's syndrome included 15 girls with ADHD only, but separate analyses for the sexes by diagnosis were not reported (Schuerholz et al., 1998). A preliminary study of 43 girls aged 6–17 with ADHD and 36 comparison girls without ADHD found that ADHD girls were more impaired on estimated IQ than comparison girls, but they did not differ significantly on executive function tasks (Seidman et al., 1997). Although girls with ADHD performed less well than control girls on tests of executive function, the deficits reported in previous studies of boys with ADHD (Seidman et al., 1995a,b) were not clearly demonstrated in girls with ADHD. This study therefore raised questions about whether girls with ADHD do not have executive deficits, may be less vulnerable to such deficits, or may have a different form of executive function deficit than boys with ADHD.

Using oculomotor tasks requiring attention, working memory and response inhibition, Castellanos et al. (2000) compared 32 unmedicated girls with a DSM-IV diagnosis of ADHD with 20 control girls. Girls with ADHD performed the delayed response tasks correctly on 32% of trials, in contrast to 62% of trials for control subjects. Girls with ADHD made twice as many commission errors to no-go stimuli and three times as many intrusion errors during go–no-go tasks, compared with controls. These results would confirm that girls with ADHD exhibit similar impairments in executive function as boys with ADHD. The authors have pointed out that, in contrast with their own sample, the large majority of ADHD girls (84%) in the study by Seidman et al. (1997) had been treated with stimulant medication which may have led to an improvement in their executive function impairments.

Adolescent and adult outcome

The adolescent and adult outcome of ADHD boys is well documented. From their review of follow-up studies, Klein and Mannuzza (1991) concluded that in adolescence ADHD boys retain significant levels of restlessness and poor attention, show a greater rate of school failure and are more frequently engaged in antisocial activities than non-ADHD adolescent boys. Lilienfeld and Waldman (1990) came to similar conclusions in their review of studies following ADHD children into adulthood, but they argued that the reported persistence of antisocial behaviour may be an artefact of the overlap between ADHD and CD. Nevertheless, several studies of adult outcome of ADHD boys concluded that they were at higher risk of developing antisocial and substance-related disorders (Greene et al., 1997; Mannuzza et al., 1998) while their educational and occupational outcome was significantly lower than that of non-ADHD controls (Mannuzza et al., 1993, 1997).

In sharp contrast to ADHD boys, the adolescent and adult outcome of ADHD girls is particularly poorly researched. This is not surprising, since the majority of original studies concentrated on boys. As will be discussed in a later section, biological theories of the aetiology of ADHD lead to the expectation of a worse outcome for girls. The few studies comparing male and female adolescents reported an opposite finding. Mannuzza and Gittelman (1984) found that 42% of boys and 25% of girls with childhood ADHD received a diagnosis for the disorder at follow-up. However, the small number of ADHD girls (12) made it hard to draw firm conclusions. In addition, this study did not report on the educational achievement and the social adjustment of the ADHD children. Herrero et al. (1994) followed up 66 clinically diagnosed ADHD children over a period of 15 years and found that, although ADHD boys were at risk of developing antisocial disorders in adulthood, this did not apply to ADHD girls.

In a sample of 626 pairs of 17-year-old twins (674 girls and 578 boys), Disney et al. (1999) found no significant sex differences in the effects of ADHD and CD on substance abuse, although girls with ADHD might be at slightly higher risk of substance abuse than boys with ADHD.

Sex differences in metabolism were found by Ernst et al. (1994) in a sample of ADHD and non-ADHD adolescents. The global cerebral glucose metabolism in ADHD girls was 20% lower than in ADHD boys, while there were no differences between control boys and girls. However, the number of ADHD females in this study was very small (5).

How different are ADHD boys and girls?

The preceding review of differences in prevalence and associations of ADHD and HKD between the sexes has shown many inconsistencies and contradictions. This is not surprising, since population samples and clinic-referred samples are likely to differ in their characteristics. Furthermore, questionnaire scores in the general population and DSM clinical diagnosis in referred populations may be difficult to compare. Inconsistency is therefore to be expected and for this reason we have not attempted a metaanalysis of studies. However, it may be helpful to summarize the findings of a few recent studies which have attempted to establish similarities and differences between ADHD boys and girls on a wide variety of variables.

Gaub and Carlson (1997) carried out a metaanalysis of 18 studies directly comparing ADHD girls with ADHD boys. Studies had to include at least 10 subjects per group, aged 13 or younger and with an IQ greater than 80. Areas evaluated included primary symptomatology, intellectual and academic functioning, comorbid behaviour problems, social behaviour and family variables. No sex differences were found in impulsive behaviour, academic performance, social functioning, fine motor skills, parental education or parental depression. However, compared with ADHD boys, ADHD girls displayed greater intellectual impairment, lower levels of hyperactivity and lower rates of externalizing behaviour. The authors emphasized that some differences between the sexes were clearly mediated by the effects of referral source. ADHD girls identified from nonreferred populations displayed lower levels of inattention, internalizing behaviour problems and peer aggression than boys with ADHD. In contrast, girls and boys with ADHD identified from clinic-referred samples displayed similar levels of impairment on these variables.

Biederman et al. (1999) compared 140 clinic-referred ADHD girls with 122 non-ADHD controls. Compared with the controls, ADHD girls were characterized by prototypical core symptoms of the disorder, high levels of comorbid psychopathology, social dysfunction, cognitive impairments, educational underachievement and adversity in the family environment. These results, they argue, not only support findings documenting similarities between the sexes – they also stress the severity of the disorder in girls.

Sharp et al. (1999) compared 42 clinic-referred ADHD girls with 56 previously studied ADHD boys (Castellanos et al., 1996) on comorbid diagnoses, behaviour ratings, psychological measures, psychiatric family history and stimulant drug response. Girls with ADHD were statistically indistinguishable from the comparison ADHD boys on nearly all measures. Girls showed robust beneficial effects on both methylphenidate and dexamfetamine. The study's conclusion is therefore that ADHD girls demonstrate very similar patterns of impairment and comorbidity and identical patterns on drug response.

The nature of the sex differences in prevalence

The persistent finding that boys and girls with ADHD or HKD do not show substantial differences in their presentation raises the question of the nature of sex differences in prevalence. Several studies discussed in the previous section have suggested that sex differences in the prevalence of ADHD and HKD are due to rater bias or referral bias. However, it is not likely that the sex differences could be entirely due to rater bias. Some rater bias is likely to derive from differential adult attitudes to affected boys and girls, but if the sex differences were entirely due to rater bias, girls meeting the diagnostic criteria for ADHD would be expected to be quite different from boys meeting the diagnostic criteria, which is clearly not the case. If parents and teachers systematically underestimate the restlessness and inattentiveness of girls, one would expect to find that, when using objective test measures, girls scoring above a cutoff on their caregivers' ratings would be more overactive than boys scoring above the same cutoff. In fact, the opposite seems to be the case. Girls identified as hyperactive in a population screen were less hyperactive than boys when directly observed (Taylor et al., paper presented, 1998). This finding suggests that caregivers tend to overrate hyperactivity in girls. The true difference between the sexes is therefore likely to be greater than that estimated by screening measures and rating scales.

The factors determining the identification of children as ADHD or HKD are crucial both for the scientific understanding of identified groups and for adequate care provision, and need to be more thoroughly researched. The effects of caregivers' attitudes appear to be complex. On the one hand, parents and teachers seem to overestimate the level of ADHD characteristics of girls. On the other hand, they do not seem to regard high levels of ADHD behaviour in girls as a problem (Taylor, personal communication, 1991), which means that specialist treatment may not be sought as often as could be expected. Findings that ADHD or HKD boys are more frequently referred to clinics than ADHD or HKD girls do not mean very much without detailed information about the comparability of the sexes in terms of developmental level and severity of disorder. Future research will need to be systematic in describing the prevalence and severity of symptoms for the sexes at different levels of community identification. Caregivers might, of course, be correct in applying different standards to boys and girls. Nevertheless, even if this is the case, it would not contradict the conclusion that male predominance cannot be explained by rater effects on the recognition of inattentive, restless or hyperactive behaviour.

The second question that needs to be addressed is whether male predominance can be attributed to other conditions. Males certainly show higher levels of aggression (Eme, 1992; Gaub and Carlson, 1997) and ADHD is so much more common in children with CD that the sex difference in the prevalence of the disorder might simply be a consequence of that for antisocial behaviour. However, this assumption is refuted by the fact that the sex ratio for 'pure' ADHD (i.e. without either CD or emotional disorder) is similar to that for mixed disorders. In theory, some other disorder might be responsible for the sex difference, but it is not clear what it could be. Learning disorders are unlikely to explain the male predominance since they are more common in ADHD or HKD girls (Berry et al., 1985; James and Taylor, 1990).

A third way of explaining the sex difference involves the definition of ADHD and HKD. It has frequently been pointed out that diagnostic criteria and rating scales for CD heavily emphasize 'male' behaviours such as fighting rather than 'female' ones such as verbal cruelty and sexual precocity. As yet, there is no evidence of a specifically female pattern of ADHD or HKD which differs from the usual pattern of inattentiveness and restlessness. However, this matter could be examined more fully by establishing whether inattentiveness in psychological testing has different correlates in boys and girls.

Provisionally, therefore, we conclude that the sex differences in ADHD and HKD are not an artefact of rater or instrument effects and are not secondary to differences in other disorders. This leaves us with the question whether girls are protected against disorders in general or specific disorders involving inattentive and hyperactive behaviour in particular. The answer seems clear: not all psychological disorders are more common in girls than in boys. CD is certainly more common in boys, but we do not know whether they have the same course in both sexes.

A further question is whether girls who are protected against ADHD or HKD show general differences across the whole range of severity of hyperactive and inattentive behaviours. The simplest way to answer this question would be to exclude all cases of disorder in a population (e.g. all those scoring above a cutoff) and to determine whether a sex difference still exists. Our own studies (Taylor et al., paper presented, 1998) looked specifically at this possibility and found a sex difference amongst the controls, with boys scoring higher than girls. This makes it likely that ADHD and HKD are less common in girls because of a general protection enjoyed by the whole population of females, and not because discrete disorders involving ADHD or HKD are present less often in girls. This protection could either be a decreased variability in girls, or a resistance to ADHD or HKD. An examination of sex effects on very high levels of attentiveness and self-control would be needed to distinguish between the two types of protection.

Unfortunately, this way of considering the dimensional or categorical nature of the sex difference is not wholly reliable. It assumes that we know where a cutoff or a category should be placed. Since the distribution of ADHD and HKD appears to be continuous in the population, and the level constituting a risk is not yet defined by epidemiologically based longitudinal studies, any cutoff remains arbitrary. This reservation applies just as much to DSM-IV and ICD-10 criteria as to questionnaire scores, because they are based on committee decisions and field studies of current diagnostic practice which fail to give scientific answers to the level of definition that is required. Since the cutoff or diagnosis is arbitrary, it could be wrong. If it is wrong, it could lead to a misleading answer to an important distinction.

At a much higher level of definition – that giving the older ICD-9 category of hyperkinetic syndrome – sex differences remain much the same. However, the mixture theory analysis applied by James and Taylor (1990) provided support for the hypothesis that more than one condition was involved. A 'nondevelopmental' disorder, not characterized by a lower IQ or language delay, seemed scarcely to exist in referred hyperactive girls. On the other hand, the boy/girl ratio for 'developmental' hyperkinesis associated with a lower IQ was relatively low. Latent class analyses could now be applied to epidemiological data to test the possibility of a female protection which is of fundamental importance to understanding the nosology of the disorders. The conclusion seems to be that there is a general protective effect for females and that the possibility of a more specific protection against a subtype of disorder needs more study.

If, as we have concluded, girls' behaviour generally differs from that of boys, the question whether to apply separate standards for the sexes becomes crucial. At present, nearly all clinical practice and research apply absolute thresholds, although rater effects imply that some uncontrolled relative scaling may occur. The desirability of separate standards for the sexes would be best answered by considering outcome. If, with a lower level of ADHD or HKD, girls showed the same psychological adjustment problems as hyperactive boys, it would be necessary to apply a relative threshold for clinical diagnosis, rather than an absolute one. So far, the existing literature has only shown that hyperactive girls are less likely to remain affected in adolescence than hyperactive boys (Mannuzza and Gittelman, 1984; Herrero et al., 1994). Proponents of a relativistic approach to diagnosis would argue that an equal ADHD score for a girl and a boy at follow-up implies that the girl is more impaired because she is more deviant from the norm for her sex. Therefore, outcome needs to be assessed in terms of social adjustment rather than merely the continuation of original symptoms. As has been pointed out earlier, this type of research is as yet not available for girls.

In summary, girls are protected against the development of ADHD and HKD, and in particular against signs of neurodevelopmental delay. The full extent of the protection is obscured by adults' tendency to identify girls as ADHD or HKD on weaker behavioural grounds. Once they have reached caseness, they show behaviour which is similar to that of boys with the same disorder. Thus, there is a true sex difference that theories of aetiology must explain.

The aetiology of sex differences in prevalence

In recent years there has been considerable interest in the aetiology of sex differences in the prevalence of ADHD and HKD. During the 1990s biological explanations for the aetiology of ADHD and HKD gained momentum, which may be explained by claims that they should be regarded as neurodevelopmental disorders alongside, for example, mental retardation and autism. The main reason for this claim is that ADHD and HKD are regarded as disorders that tend to be chronic and involve a significant disturbance in the acquisition of basic skills because of neurobiological factors (Barkley, 1990; Eme, 1992).

Gualtieri and Hicks (1985) have pointed out that males are generally more frequently afflicted with neurodevelopmental disorders than females. Explanations for these sex differences are derived from two theoretical models: the constitutional variability model and the polygenetic multiple threshold model.

The constitutional variability model

The constitutional variability model is based on the assumption of a greater variability of characteristics in males. Taylor (1985) has argued that one of the most persistent features in developmental sex differences has been a greater male immaturity. Girls have been seen to be more mature than boys at all stages of development. At birth, boys are described as several weeks behind girls in maturity. The difference increases to 1 year at the time of starting school and widens to 2 years at puberty (Tanner, 1978). The sex differences in maturity have been attributed to factors on the Y chromosome, namely that males have 4–5% less chromosomal material than females. It has frequently been suggested that this relative male immaturity is at least partly responsible for a greater male susceptibility to almost any kind of physical problem because it exposes them to a greater risk of damage. Boys have more prenatal and birth complications, they are more likely to suffer from infectious disease and more frequently show neurodevelopmental abnormalities (Gualtieri and Hicks, 1985). The theory that this 'selective male affliction' can be attributed to a maternal immunoreactivity to the male fetus has been put forward by Gualtieri and Hicks (1985), but has met with some scepticism (Adinolfi et al., 1985). There is widespread agreement that, although boys are more frequently afflicted with many diseases and neurodevelopmental disorders, affected girls develop a more severe form. Taylor and Ounsted (1972) have explained this phenomenon by arguing that, because girls mature faster, they will have acquired a relatively greater degree of divergence from their norm when they cross the threshold into the pathological area and will therefore be worse affected than boys.

According to the constitutional variability model, a significant number of boys develop ADHD or HKD through the same factors that determine the range of activity and attention in the general population. In contrast, in girls ADHD or HKD may have its roots in an organic brain disorder. Support for this hypothesis was sought in a study of children with HKD (James and Taylor, 1990). HKD girls had lower IQ and significantly higher rates of language disorders and neurological disorders than HKD boys, thereby suggesting that in girls the symptoms may be caused by an atypical pathological event, such as brain damage. However, the finding that HKD girls show more developmental delays than HKD boys does not provide strong support for the theory of a general greater male susceptibility to disease. Girls may be socially and psychologically protected from the development of HKD (or ADHD), and a greater concentration of pathogenetic factors may be required to break down this protection. In addition, a study of prenatal and perinatal risk factors in clinic-referred HKD children did not provide support for a sex difference in neurological factors (Chandola et al., 1992). The results of this study suggested that these factors may be of modest aetiological importance, but no differential effects between the sexes were found.

The polygenetic multiple threshold model

The polygenetic multiple threshold model suggests that a disorder is caused by multiple genetic factors, environmental factors, or a combination of both. All genetic and environmental factors influencing an individual's risk of a disorder are considered collectively as a single variable called the *liability* (Carter, 1973).

The multiple threshold model has a number of consequences for the development of disorders in girls. First, it assumes that girls have a lower prevalence of disorders because they require a greater liability (more genetic and environmental factors) in order to develop the disorder than boys (Faraone et al., 1990). The greater liability girls need in order to develop the disorder also means that once they have reached their threshold, they will be more severely affected than boys (Tsai and Beisler, 1983). Second, because girls are less susceptible to prenatal, perinatal and postnatal difficulties than boys (Gualtieri and Hicks, 1985), they need a higher genetic loading to cross their higher threshold into disorder. Third, there should be a higher incidence of neuro-developmental disorder in the families of affected girls because the heavier dosage of genes and/or environmental factors needed to produce the disorder in girls would have as its corollary a higher frequency of the disorder amongst the relatives who would, to some extent, share the same genetic and environmental factors (DeFries, 1989).

In summary, the polygenetic multiple threshold model assumes a continuum of liability with a higher threshold for girls. Consequently, girls are predicted to be more seriously affected, to have a higher genetic loading and to have more affected relatives (Eme, 1992).

In an attempt to settle the uncertainty regarding the applicability of the multiple threshold model to hyperactive behaviour, Goodman and Stevenson (1989) used a population twin sample to test the hypothesis that twin brothers of hyperactive girls would be more frequently affected by the disorder than twin brothers of hyperactive boys. This hypothesis was not confirmed; siblings were not significantly more likely to show hyperactivity if they had an affected twin sister than if they had an affected twin brother.

The strength of the study's design appeared to cast doubt on the importance of genetic factors in causing sex differences in hyperactive behaviour. However, the age of the twins in this study (13) was rather higher than would be desirable when studying a condition such as hyperactivity, which develops at an early age and alters over time in response to external stressors. In recent years, the polygenetic multiple threshold model has been tested in a number of studies using either a familial or twin design.

Familial and genetic clustering

Family-genetic studies have consistently found that relatives of boys with ADHD were at increased risk of ADHD compared to the relatives of non-ADHD boys (Biederman et al., 1986, 1990, 1991b; Schachar and Wachsmuth,

1990). Studies testing the applicability of the polygenetic multiple threshold model on sex differences in the prevalence of ADHD and HKD have largely centred around the theory of a greater family history of ADHD in affected girls. Since it is assumed that girls with ADHD carry a higher dose of risk factors, their relatives should also have more risk factors and thus be at greater risk for ADHD than relatives of boys with ADHD. However, several studies failed to support the theory that ADHD girls have a greater family history of ADHD than relatives of ADHD boys. Mannuzza and Gittelman (1984) found a greater prevalence of ADHD in the parents of ADHD boys than in the parents of ADHD girls. James and Taylor (1990), Faraone et al. (1991) and Silverthorn et al. (1996) found no differences in the relatives of ADHD boys and girls. However, all four studies showed methodological limitations, rendering the findings inconclusive. The numbers of girls were relatively small (12, 18, 20 and 13 respectively) and DSM-III criteria were used for case identification.

It has been suggested that the genetic component in liability to ADHD is assessed more satisfactorily through the use of twin studies because these studies can differentiate the effect of nature and nurture in a way that is not possible in family studies (Rutter et al., 1999).

Rhee et al. (1999) examined 2391 twin and sibling pairs aged 3–18 in Australia. They analysed the sample on several genetic models and found quite strong evidence in their additive model of an inherited sex difference. Overall, they found probandwise concordance rates for males of 83% in monozygotic twins and 31% in dizygotic twins, compared with rates for females of 75% in monozygotic twins and 39% in dizygotic twins. Their multiple regression analysis found that sex was a significant moderator of their additive model. The heritability estimate for same-sex twins was 1.04 for boys and 0.67 for girls. On average, the cotwins of girls had a higher number of ADHD symptoms than cotwins of boys.

The findings of a lower heritability for girls and a greater severity in their cotwins does not give unequivocal support for one pattern of heritance. The results from these data suggest that there is no difference in heritability for a severe subtype. The heritability for extreme scores on ADHD symptoms is high and the differences between estimates show no sex differences. A labelling phenomenon is possible. The authors' own conclusion favours the polygenetic multiple threshold model in which girls require a higher severity of multiple liability factors to reach caseness than boys.

Other studies have reported that the finding of a lower rate of affected relatives in girls compared to boys in a severely affected clinical group is not genetically informative (James and Taylor, 1990).

Perhaps the most common finding is the similarity in heritability in boys and girls (Goodman and Stevenson, 1989; Gjone et al., 1996). However, the study by Goodman and Stevenson was limited by a small sample and has been criticized for the use of pairwise concordance rates which are said to be appropriate for diagnostic entities that are truly categorical, which does not apply to ADHD (Rhee et al., 1999). The results from the study by Gjone et al. were difficult to interpret due to a lack of sex differences in the key behaviours.

The population twin study by Eaves et al. (1997) suggested that there were strong additive genetic influences on ADHD behaviours, but there was very little evidence of sex differences in the degree of influence, or their type.

All twin studies have methodological flaws; some studies have shown marked contrast effects in which correlations in dizygotic pairs are unexpectedly low. This only applies to mothers' ratings, but not teachers' ratings (Thapar et al., 1995; Eaves et al., 1997; Simonoff et al., 1997). This finding could be due to the way in which one twin affects the other twin (as opposed to the way in which one sibling affects another sibling), or it could be an artefact of the way in which ratings are made. Modelling analysis by Simonoff et al. (1997) suggested the latter. If this is the case, it acts as a caution against basing conclusions too firmly on what may be flawed evidence.

Due to their methodological shortcomings, twin studies need to be complemented by familial studies, even if the latter are not genetically informative. Faraone et al. (2000) compared findings about biological relatives of 140 girls with ADHD and 122 girls without ADHD with a previous study of boys with and without ADHD. They found that girls with ADHD had similar rates of affected relatives as boys with ADHD. This is of course in keeping with the most common finding in twin studies concerning similar heritability.

In short, genetic studies do not contradict the notion that genetic influences on ADHD are the same for both sexes, but they do suggest that a good deal more study is needed and other forms of case identification should be used.

Implications for future research

Provisionally, the somewhat contradictory findings about the genetic influences on boys and girls need to be resolved. The most likely reason for these inconsistent findings is the differences in the identification of cases in epidemiological studies and clinic-based studies.

There has been such good progress made in identifying biological associations of ADHD, especially the DNA variants in the genetic systems coding for the dopamine D4 receptor and dopamine transporters, and in the structural and functional abnormalities of the frontal and striate parts of the brain, that it is now important to compare those in girls and boys.

There has been a striking suggestion that there are shared environmental influences in girls which are not present in boys. The studies of physical hazards of the environment, e.g. cigarette smoking, do not suggest that girls are more vulnerable than boys. It seems probable that the shared environmental variance in girls is a matter of the psychological environment. The hypothesis that girls would be a purer biological subgroup than boys has not held up. To the contrary, girls seem a very good group to study the effect of the social environment.

Another outstanding matter is the lack of satisfactory knowledge of the determinants of social adjustment in hyperactive girls. They may or may not be similar to those in boys. The different psychological meaning of puberty for boys and girls might entail a difference in course in adolescence, as might the altered reactions of teachers, parents and peers. Current knowledge suggests that mild degrees of hyperactivity either protect girls against educational failure or enhance the risk compared to boys.

The most serious gap in knowledge of girls with ADHD or HKD concerns differences in life course compared to boys. Such studies should be done on both epidemiological and referred populations. For epidemiological samples the main question to answer will be the extent to which relativistically defined ADHD would yield a group of girls who would be equally at risk as boys. If that were the case, we would revise our definition and use sex-specific norms. Another major gap concerns the differential effect of hormones on development in puberty and especially the pubertal differences between boys and girls. Third, the importance of mothers' caregiving of children means that the impact of ADHD on females should include the extent to which it impacts on their functioning as mothers.

Clinical practice for girls

Cautious clinical practice can be based on a reading of the research evidence reviewed in this chapter. The clinician following this line will not be quick to diagnose hyperactivity in a girl, but will maintain the same criteria for inattentiveness, restlessness and impulsiveness that would be applied for boys. Once diagnosed, girls will be expected to be at risk of psychological maladjustment and treatment is therefore necessary. Behavioural modification, personal counselling and stimulant medication will all have helpful short-term effects, but the use of treatments to promote psychological adjustment in the longer term will have to be based on an individual judgement about the strengths and weaknesses of a girl's development and environment. Milder degrees of hyperactive behaviour should not be given undue weight in a diagnostic formulation because the appearance of antisocial behaviour, peer relationship impairment and educational failure are likely to be more important determinants of outcome and more rewarding targets for therapy.

The effect of stimulant medication appears to be rather similar in girls and in boys. This is in keeping with the similarities in other respects between affected girls and affected boys. The main evidence for this comes from the analysis of the MTA Cooperative Group (1999) study. In this study subjects were randomly allocated to medication treatment, predominantly methylphenidate, intensive behaviour therapy, a combination of the two and community treatment, which usually included methylphenidate or other medications. This is not an ideal design for examining the responsiveness of girls to medication, because there is no placebo control. Nevertheless, the size of the study and the careful analysis give helpful information. Sex was not a moderator of the differences between the treatment groups. The superiority of stimulant treatment to behaviour therapy was present to a similar degree in boys and girls.

REFERENCES

Adinolfi, M., Polani, P.E. and Crolla, J.A. (1985). Is the sex ratio at birth affected by immune selection? *Experimental and Clinical Immunogenetics*, **2**, 54–64.

Arcia, E. and Conners, C.K. (1998). Gender differences in ADHD? *Developmental and Behavioral Pediatrics*, **19**, 77–83.

Arnold, L.E. (1996). Sex differences in ADHD: conference summary. *Journal of Abnormal Child Psychology*, **24**, 555–569.

August, G.J. and Garfinkel, B.D. (1989). Behavioral and cognitive subtypes of ADHD. *Journal of the American Academy of Child and Adolescent Psychiatry*, **28**, 739–48.

August, G.J. and Garfinkel, B.D. (1990). Comorbidity of ADHD and reading disability among clinic-referred children. *Journal of Abnormal Child Psychology*, **18**, 29–34.

August, G.J. and Garfinkel, B.D. (1993). The nosology of attention-deficit hyperactivity disorder. *Journal of the American Academy of Child and Adolescent Psychiatry*, **32**, 155–65.

Barkley, R. (1990). Attention deficit disorders: history, definition and diagnosis. In *Handbook of Developmental Psychopathology*, M. Lewis and S. Miller, eds, pp. 65–75. New York: Plenum.

Barkley, R. (1997). Behavioral inhibition, sustained attention and executive functions: constructing a unifying theory of ADHD. *Psychological Bulletin*, **121**, 65–94.

Barkley, R.A., Anastopoulos, A.D., Guevremont, D.C. and Fletcher, K.E. (1992). Adolescents with attention deficit hyperactivity disorder: mother–adolescent interactions, family beliefs and maternal psychopathology. *Journal of Abnormal Child Psychology*, **20**, 263–88.

Bauermeister, J. (1992). Factor analyses of teacher ratings of attention-deficit hyperactivity and oppositional defiant symptoms in children aged four through thirteen years. *Journal of Clinical Child Psychology*, **21**, 27–34.

Berry, C.A., Shaywitz, S.E. and Shaywitz, B.A. (1985). Girls with attention deficit disorder: a silent minority? A report on behavioral and cognitive characteristics. *Pediatrics*, **76**, 801–9.

Biederman, J., Munir, K., Knee, D. et al. (1986). A family study of patients with attention deficit disorder and normal controls. *Journal of Psychiatric Research*, **20**, 263–74.

Biederman J., Faraone, S.V., Keenan, K., Knee, D. and Tsuang, M.T. (1990). Family-genetic and psycho-social risk factors in DSM-III attention deficit disorder. *Journal of the American Academy of Child and Adolescent Psychiatry*, **29**, 526–33.

Biederman, J., Newcorn, J. and Sprich, S. (1991a). Comorbidity of attention deficit hyperactivity disorder with conduct, depressive anxiety and other disorders. *American Journal of Psychiatry*, **148**, 564–77.

Biederman, J., Faraone, S.V., Keenan, K. and Tsuang, M.T. (1991b). Evidence of familial association between attention deficit disorders and major affective disorder. *Archives of General Psychiatry*, **78**, 633–72.

Biederman, J., Faraone, S., Mick, E. et al. (1999). Clinical correlates of ADHD in females: findings from a large group of girls ascertained from pediatric and psychiatric referral sources. *Journal of the American Academy of Child and Adolescent Psychiatry*, **38**, 966–75.

Breen, M.J. (1989). Cognitive and behavioral differences in ADDH boys and girls. *Journal of Child Psychology and Psychiatry*, **30**, 711–17.

Breen, M.J. and Altepeter, T.S. (1990). Situational variability in boys and girls identified as ADHD. *Journal of Clinical Psychology*, **46**, 486–90.

Breen, M.J. and Barkley, R.A. (1988). Child psychopathology and parenting stress in girls and boys having attention deficit disorder with hyperactivity. *Journal of Pediatric Psychology*, **13**, 265–80.

Brito, G.N.O., Pinto, R.C.A. and Lins, M.F.C. (1995). A behavioral assessment scale for attention deficit disorder in Brazilian children based on DSM-IIIR criteria. *Journal of Abnormal Child Psychology*, **23**, 509–20.

Brown, R.T. and Pacini, J.N. (1989). Perceived family functioning, marital status and depression in parents of boys with attention deficit disorder. *Journal of Learning Disabilities*, **22**, 581–7.

Brown, R.T., Madan-Swain, A. and Baldwin, K. (1991). Gender differences in a clinic referred sample of attention deficit disorder children. *Child Psychiatry and Human Development*, **22**, 111–28.

Carlson, C.L., Tamm, L. and Gaub, M. (1997). Gender differences in children with ADHD, ODD and co-occurring ADHD/ODD identified in a school population. *Journal of the American Academy of Child and Adolescent Psychiatry*, **36**, 1706–14.

Carter, C.O. (1973). Multifactorial genetic disease. In *Medical Genetics*, V.A. McKusick and R. Clairborne, eds. New York: H.P. Publishing.

Castellanos, F.X., Giedd, J.N., Marsh, W.L. et al. (1996). Quantitative brain magnetic resonance imaging in attention-deficit/hyperactivity disorder. *Archives of General Psychiatry*, **53**, 607–16.

Castellanos, F.X., Fani Marvasti, F., Ducharme, J. et al. (2000). Executive function oculomotor tasks in girls with ADHD. *Journal of the American Academy of Child and Adolescent Psychiatry*, **39**, 644–50.

Chandola, C., Robling, M., Peters, T., Melville-Thomas, G. and McGuffin, P. (1992). Pre- and perinatal factors and the risk of subsequent referral for hyperactivity. *Journal of Child Psychology and Psychiatry*, **33**, 1077–90.

Cohen, P., Cohen, J., Kasen, S. et al. (1993). An epidemiological study of disorders in late childhood and adolescence – I. Age- and gender-specific prevalence. *Journal of Child Psychology and Psychiatry*, **34**, 851–67.

Costello, E.J. (1990). Child psychiatric epidemiology: implications for clinical research and practice. In *Advances in Clinical Child Psychology*, vol. 13, B.B. Lahey and A.E. Kazdin, eds, pp. 53–85. New York: Plenum.

DeFries, J. (1989). Gender ratios in children with reading disability and their affected relatives: a commentary. *Journal of Learning Disabilities*, **22**, 543–5.

deHaas, P.A. (1986). Attention styles and peer relationships of hyperactive and normal boys and girls. *Journal of Abnormal Child Psychology*, **14**, 457–67.

deHaas, P.A. and Young, R.D. (1984). Attention styles of hyperactive and normal girls. *Journal of Abnormal Child Psychology*, **12**, 531–46.

Denckla, M.B. (1989). Executive function, the overlap zone between attention deficit hyperactivity disorder and learning disabilities. *International Pediatrics*, **4**, 155–60.

Denckla, M.B. (1996). A theory and model of executive function: a neuropsychological perspective. In *Attention, Memory and Executive Function*, G.R. Lyon and N.A. Krasnegor, eds. Baltimore: Paul H. Brookes.

Disney, E.R., Elkins, I.J., McGue, M. and Iacono, W. (1999). Effects of ADHD, conduct disorder and gender on substance use and abuse in adolescence. *American Journal of Psychiatry*, **156**, 1515–21.

Dumas, M.C. (1998). The risk of social interaction problems among adolescents with ADHD. *Education and Treatment of Children*, **21**, 447–60.

Eaves, L.J., Silberg, J.L., Meyer, J.M. et al. (1997). Genetics and developmental psychopathology: 2. The main effects of genes and environment on behavioural problems in the Virginia twin study of adolescent behavioral development. *Journal of Child Psychology and Psychiatry*, **38**, 965–80.

Eme, R.F. (1992). Selective female affliction in the developmental disorders of childhood: a literature review. *Journal of Clinical Child Psychology*, **21**, 354–64.

Ernst, M., Liebenauer, L.L., King, C. et al. (1994). Reduced brain metabolism in hyperactive girls. *Journal of the American Academy of Child and Adolescent Psychiatry*, **33**, 858–68.

Faraone, S.V., Biederman, J., Keenan, K. and Ming, T.T. (1991). A family-genetic study of girls with DSM-III attention deficit disorder. *American Journal of Psychiatry*, **148**, 112–17.

Faraone, S., Kremen, W. and Tsuang, M. (1990). Genetic transmission of major affective disorders: quantitative models and linkage analyses. *Psychological Bulletin*, **108**, 109–27.

Faraone, S.V., Biederman, J., Mick, E. et al. (2000). Family study of girls with attention deficit hyperactivity disorder. *American Journal of Psychiatry*, **157**, 1077–83.

Frick, P., Kamphaus, R.W., Lacey, B.B. et al. (1991). Academic underachievement and the disruptive behavior disorders. *Journal of Consulting and Clinical Psychology*, **59**, 289–94.

Gabel, S., Schmitz, S. and Fulker, D.W. (1996). Comorbidity in hyperactive children: issues related to selection bias, gender, severity and internalizing symptoms. *Child Psychiatry and Human Development*, **27**, 15–28.

Gaub, M. and Carlson, C.L. (1997). Gender differences in ADHD: a meta-analysis and clinical review. *Journal of the American Academy of Child and Adolescent Psychiatry*, **36**, 1036–45.

Gjone, H., Stevenson, J. and Sundet, J. (1996). Genetic influence on attention problems in a general population twin sample. *Journal of the American Academy of Child and Adolescent Psychiatry*, **45**, 588–96.

Gomez, R., Harvey, J., Quick, C., Scharer, I. and Harris, G. (1999). DSM-IV AD/HD: confirmatory factor models, prevalence and gender and age differences based on parent and teacher ratings of Australian primary school children. *Journal of Child Psychology and Psychiatry*, **40**, 265–74.

Goodman, R. and Stevenson, J. (1989). A twin study of hyperactivity-II. The aetiological role of genes, family relationships and perinatal adversity. *Journal of Child Psychology and Psychiatry*, **30**, 691–709.

Goodyear, P. and Hynd, G.W. (1992). Attention-deficit disorder with (ADDH) and without (ADD/WO) hyperactivity: behavioral and neuropsychological differentiation. *Journal of Clinical Child Psychology*, **21**, 273–305.

Greene, R.W., Biederman, J., Faraone, S.V., Sienna, M. and Garcia-Jetton, J. (1997). Adolescent outcome of boys with attention-deficit/hyperactivity disorder and social disability: results from a 4-year longitudinal follow-up study. *Journal of Consulting and Clinical Psychology*, **65**, 758–67.

Gualtieri, T. and Hicks, R.E. (1985). An immunoreactive theory of selective male affliction. *Behavioral and Brain Sciences*, **8**, 427–41.

Herrero, M.E., Hechtman, L. and Weiss, G. (1994). Antisocial disorders in hyperactive subjects from childhood to adulthood: predictive factors and characterization of subgroups. *American Journal of Orthopsychiatry*, **64**, 510–21.

Hinshaw, S.P. and Melnick, S.M. (1995). Peer relationships in boys with attention-deficit hyperactivity disorder with and without comorbid aggression. *Development and Psychopathology*, **7**, 627–47.

Hinshaw, S.P., Zupan, B.A., Simmel, C., Nigg, J.T. and Melnick, S. (1997). Peer status in boys with and without attention-deficit hyperactivity disorder: predictions from overt and covert antisocial behavior, social isolation and authoritative parenting. *Child Development*, **68**, 880–96.

Horn, W.F., Wagner, A.E. and Ialongo, N. (1989). Sex differences in school-aged children with pervasive attention deficit hyperactivity disorder. *Journal of Abnormal Child Psychology*, **17**, 109–25.

James, A. and Taylor, E.A. (1990). Sex differences in the hyperkinetic syndrome of childhood. *Journal of Child Psychology and Psychiatry*, **31**, 437–46.

Jensen, P.S., Martin, D. and Cantwell, D.P. (1997). Comorbidity in ADHD: implications for research, practice and DSM-V. *Journal of the American Academy of Child and Adolescent Psychiatry*, **36**, 1065–79.

Johnston, C. (1996). Parent characteristics and parent-child interactions in families of non-problem children and ADHD children with higher and lower levels of oppositional-defiant behavior. *Journal of Abnormal Child Psychology*, **24**, 85–104.

Johnston, C., Pelham, W.E. and Murphy, H.A. (1985). Peer relationships in ADDH and normal children: a developmental analysis of peer and teacher ratings. *Journal of Abnormal Child Psychology*, **13**, 89–100.

Klein, R.G. and Mannuzza, S. (1991). Long-term outcome of hyperactive children: a review. *Journal of the American Academy of Child and Adolescent Psychiatry*, **30**, 383–87.

Lahey, B., Applegate, A., McBurnett, K. et al. (1994). DSM-IV field trials for attention-deficit hyperactivity disorder in children and adolescents. *American Journal of Psychiatry*, **151**, 1673–85.

Landau, S., Milich, R. and Diener, M.B. (1998). Peer relations of children with attention-deficit hyperactivity disorder. *Reading and Writing Quarterly: Overcoming Learning Difficulties*, **14**, 83–105.

Leung, P.W., Luk, S.L., Ho, T.P. et al. (1996). The diagnosis and prevalence of hyperactivity in Chinese schoolboys. *British Journal of Psychiatry*, **168**, 486–96.

Lilienfeld, S. and Waldman, I.D. (1990). The relationship between childhood attention-deficit hyperactivity disorder and adult antisocial behavior reexamined: the problem of heterogeneity. *Clinical Psychology Review*, **10**, 699–725.

Magnusson, P., Smari, J., Gretarsdottir, H. and Prandardottir, H. (1999). Attention-deficit/hyperactivity symptoms in Icelandic school children: assessment with the attention deficit/hyperactivity rating scale – IV. *Scandinavian Journal of Psychology*, **40**, 301–6.

Mannuzza, S. and Gittelman, R. (1984). The adolescent outcome of hyperactive girls. *Psychiatry Research*, **13**, 19–29.

Mannuzza, S., Klein, R.G., Bessler, A., Malloy, P. and Lapadula, M. (1993). Adult outcome of hyperactive boys: educational achievement, occupational rank and psychiatric status. *Archives of General Psychiatry*, **50**, 565–76.

Mannuzza, S., Klein, R.G., Bessler, A., Malloy, P. and Hynes, M.E. (1997). Educational and occupational outcome of hyperactive boys. *Journal of the American Academy of Child and Adolescent Psychiatry*, **36**, 1222–7.

Mannuzza, S., Klein, R.G., Bessler, A., Malloy P. and LaPadula, M. (1998). Adult psychiatric status of hyperactive boys grown up. *American Journal of Psychiatry*, **155**, 493–8.

Mash, E.J. and Johnston, C.A. (1982). A comparison of the mother–child interactions of younger and older hyperactive and normal children. *Child Development*, **53**, 1371–81.

McArdle, P., O'Brien, G., Macmillan, A. and Kolvin, I. (2000). The peer relations of disruptive children with reference to hyperactivity and conduct disorder. *European Child and Adolescent Psychiatry*, **9**, 91–9.

McGee, R. and Feehan, M. (1991). Are girls with problems of attention under-recognized? *Journal of Psychopathological Behavior Assessment*, **13**, 187–98.

McGee, R., Williams, S. and Silva, P.A. (1987). A comparison of girls and boys with teacher-identified problems of attention. *Journal of the American Academy of Child and Adolescent Psychiatry*, **26**, 711–17.

MTA Cooperative Group. (1999). A 14-month randomized clinical trial of treatment strategies for attention-deficit hyperactivity disorder. *Archives of General Psychiatry*, **56**, 1073–7.

Pineda, D., Ardila, A., Rosselli, M. et al. (1999). Prevalence of attention-deficit/hyperactivity disorder symptoms in 4- to 17-year-old children in the general population. *Journal of Abnormal Child Psychology*, **27**, 455–62.

Pliszka, S.R. (1992). Comorbidity of attention-deficit hyperactivity disorder and overanxious disorder. *Journal of the American Academy of Child and Adolescent Psychiatry*, **31**, 187–203.

Rhee, S.H., Waldman, I.D., Hay, D.A. and Levy, F. (1999). Sex differences in genetic and environmental influences on DSM-III-R attention-deficit/hyperactivity disorder. *Journal of Abnormal Psychology*, **108**, 24–41.

Rutter, M., Silberg, J., O'Connor, T. and Simonoff, E. (1999). Genetics and child psychiatry. II. Empirical research findings. *Journal of Child Psychology and Psychiatry*, **40**, 19–55.

Saunders, B. and Chambers, S.M. (1996). A review of the literature on attention-deficit hyperactivity disorder children: peer interactions and collaborative learning. *Psychology in the Schools*, **33**, 333–40.

Schachar, R. and Wachsmuth, R. (1990). Hyperactivity and parental psychopathology. *Journal of Child Psychology and Psychiatry*, **31**, 381–92.

Schuerholz, L.J., Singer, H.S. and Denckla, M.B. (1998). Gender study of neuropsychological and neuromotor function in children with Tourette syndrome with and without attention-deficit hyperactivity disorder. *Journal of Child Neurology*, **13**, 277–82.

Seidman, L.J., Benedict, K., Biederman, J. et al. (1995a). Performance of ADHD children on the Rey-Osterrieth complex figure: a pilot neuropsychological study. *Journal of Child Psychology and Psychiatry*, **36**, 1459–73.

Seidman, L.J., Biederman, J., Faraone, S.V. et al. (1995b). Effects of family history and comorbidity on the nerupsychology of ADHD: preliminary findings. *Journal of the American Academy of Child and Adolescent Psychiatry*, **34**, 1015–24.

Seidman, L.J., Biederman, J., Faraone, S.V. et al. (1997). A pilot study of neuropsychological function in girls with ADHD. *Journal of the American Academy of Child and Adolescent Psychiatry*, **36**, 366–73.

Sharp, W.S., Walter, J., Marsh, W.L. et al. (1999). ADHD in girls: clinical comparability of a research sample. *Journal of the American Academy of Child and Adolescent Psychiatry*, **38**, 40–7.

Silverthorn, P., Frick, P.J., Kuper, K. and Ott, J. (1996). Attention deficit hyperactivity disorder and sex: a test of two etiological models to explain the male predominance. *Journal of Clinical Child Psychology*, **25**, 52–9.

Simonoff, E., Pickles, A., Meyer, J.M. et al. (1997). The Virginia twin study of adolescent behavioral development: Influences of age, sex and impairment on rates of disorder. *Archives of General Psychiatry*, **54**, 801–8.

Still, G.F. (1902). The Coulstonian lectures on some abnormal psychical conditions in children. *Lancet*, **1**, 1008–12, 1077–82, 1163–68.

Swanson, J.M., Sergeant, J.A., Taylor, E. et al. (1998). Attention-deficit hyperactivity disorder and hyperkinetic disorder. *Lancet*, **351**, 429–33.

Szatmari, P. (1992). The epidemiology of attention-deficit hyperactivity disorder. *Child and Adolescent Psychiatric Clinics of North America*, **1**, 361–71.

Szatmari, P., Boyle, M. and Offord, D.R. (1989a). ADDH and conduct disorder: degree of diagnostic overlap and differences among correlates. *Journal of the American Academy of Child and Adolescent Psychiatry*, **28**, 865–72.

Szatmari, P., Offord, D.R. and Boyle, M.H. (1989b). The Ontario Child Health Study: prevalence of ADHD. *Journal of Child Psychology and Psychiatry*, **30**, 219–30.

Tallmadge, J. and Barkley, R.A. (1983). The interactions of hyperactive and normal boys with their fathers and mothers. *Journal of Abnormal Child Psychology*, **11**, 565–80.

Tanner, J. (1978). *Fetus into Man: Physical Growth from Conception to Maturity*. Cambridge, MA: Harvard University Press.

Taylor, D. (1985). Developmental rates is the major differentiator between the sexes. *Behavioral and Brain Sciences*, **8**, 459–60.

Taylor, D.C. and Ounsted, C. (1972). The nature of gender differences explored through ontogenetic analyses of sex ratios in disease. In *Gender Differences: Their Ontogeny and Significance*, C. Ounsted and D.C. Taylor, eds, pp. 215–40. Edinburgh: Churchill Livingstone.

Taylor, E., Everitt, B., Thorley, G. et al. (1986). Conduct disorder and hyperactivity II. A cluster analytic approach to the identification of a behavioural syndrome. *British Journal of Psychiatry*, **149**, 768–77.

Taylor, E., Sandberg, S., Thorley, G. and Giles, S. (1991). *The Epidemiology of Childhood Hyperactivity*. Maudsley Monographs, no. 33. Oxford: Oxford University Press.

Thapar, A., Hervas, A. and McGuffin, P. (1995). Childhood hyperactivity scores are highly heritable and show sibling competition effects: twin study evidence. *Behavior Genetics*, **25**, 537–44.

Thorley, G. (1984). Hyperkinetic syndrome of childhood: clinical characteristics. *British Journal of Psychiatry*, **144**, 16–24.

Tsai, L. and Beisler, J. (1983). The development of sex differences in infantile autism. *British Journal of Psychiatry*, **142**, 373–8.

Welsh, M.C. and Pennington, B.F. (1988). Assessing frontal lobe functioning in children: views from developmental psychology. *Developmental Neuropsychology*, **4**, 199–230.

5

Classification issues

Russell Schachar[1] and Joseph A. Sergeant[2]

[1]Department of Child Psychiatry, University of Toronto, Toronto, Canada; [2]Klinische Neuropsychologie, Amsterdam, the Netherlands

Introduction

Restlessness, inattention and impulsiveness are common behaviours, especially among preschool and school-age children. Adolescents and adults exhibit these traits as well but usually to a lesser extent. In the extreme, these behaviours are impairing to affected individuals and disturbing to those around them. Consequently, they are thought to define a mental disorder. The very existence of this disorder, the criteria used for diagnosis and the diagnostic label applied to it have been debated extensively. Various terms have been used to describe the syndrome of developmentally abnormal and impairing hyperactive, inattentive and impulsive behaviour. In the two most widely and currently applied diagnostic schemata in clinical child psychiatry, the *Diagnostic and Statistical Manual* of the American Psychiatric Association (DSM-IV; American Psychiatric Association, 1994), used primarily in North America, and the *International Classification of Disease* (ICD-10; World Health Organization, 1992), used primarily in Europe, the syndrome is known as attention deficit hyperactivity disorder (ADHD) and hyperkinetic disorder (HD) respectively. In this chapter, we review the evolution and scientific foundation of this category of mental illness.

Typically, the classification of psychopathology is a somewhat arcane matter of concern only to practitioners and nosologists. That is certainly not the case with hyperactivity where the diagnosis is widely discussed in the media and the lay press. It is often asserted that hyperactivity is overdiagnosed, particularly in North America. Overdiagnosis is thought to reflect both inappropriate professional practice (lax diagnostic methods, invalid diagnostic criteria and arbitrary diagnostic thresholds) interacting with consumer demand for a psychiatric diagnosis that can provide an explanation for scholastic and occupational failure in an achievement-oriented culture. The result of this overdiagnosis is supposedly the massive and inappropriate use of a psychiatric label and of stimulant medication for children, adolescents and adults who really exhibit characteristics that are within the bounds of normal or who actually have some other explanation for their disorder. According to this view, hyperactive individuals have problems that could and should be handled in a nonmedical and more appropriate way such as through psychological, social and educational interventions. In the UK and Europe, a parallel but opposite debate is evident over whether the diagnosis should be made more commonly and whether stimulant medication should be more generally available and more widely prescribed.

This chapter deals with the rationale for classification of hyperactivity as a psychiatric disorder, historical influences on the development of approaches to classifying hyperactivity, and the empirical support for the various ways of categorizing hyperactivity. We adopt the convention suggested by Taylor (1998) of using the term hyperactivity when referring to the cardinal behaviours (hyperactivity, inattention, impulsiveness) that constitute this syndrome and of using specific diagnostic terms when addressing issues relating to a particular diagnostic entity and set of criteria. Even though clinicians, scientists and authors find 'ADHD or hyperactive children' a convenient shorthand, diagnoses actually describe disorders, not individuals. People change, as do labels. In many children, disorder dissipates. In others, the manifestations of disorder vary with age and development. In this chapter, all references to hyperactive individuals should be understood as statements about disorders, not people.

Function of classification in psychiatry

Classification or diagnostic schemata, also known as taxonomies, seek to reduce the bewildering array of clinical or phenotypic manifestations of mental illness by grouping them into mutually exclusive and exhaustive categories. In doing so, this simplification hopes to facilitate communication, clinical practice and research.

A valid classification scheme has several essential characteristics. First, it must be possible to measure reliably the individual symptoms which comprise the diagnostic categories. It is unlikely that a diagnosis can be reliable, valid and clinically useful if informants and clinicians cannot agree on the definition and measurement of individual symptoms. Second, symptoms should cluster into meaningful syndromes in a consistent manner. Third, each diagnostic entity must be reliable. There is little point in a classification scheme that includes categories that cannot be applied in a consistent way by the majority of clinicians and scientists across clinical settings and countries. This is no small challenge given the global nature of communication among practitioners and scientists, differences in training and theoretical perspectives among them and variation in attitudes about behaviour and mental illness across cultures. Fourth, a diagnostic category is helpful only if it allows for valid predictions about important characteristics of affected individuals such as clinical correlates (developmental delay, cognitive deficit), causes, treatment response and outcome. Moreover, each category of mental illness should have some unique characteristics or correlates. A classification scheme that contains several categories that make identical predictions is of little use (Rutter, 1978; Quay et al., 1987). Fifth, a valid classification scheme must be mutually exclusive and exhaustive. Symptoms and individuals with a disorder should fit into few categories and there should be a category for every possible symptom or disordered individual.

A scientifically valid taxonomy may have a somewhat different intent than one that is designed primarily for clinical purposes. A scientific nosology is concerned primarily with clustering of symptoms or individuals into groups that have some common pathophysiology or aetiology. Scientific and clinical nosologies are not mutually exclusive and actually complement each other. Scientific understanding of any specific disorder depends on its accurate description and distinction from other disorders and the optimal classification scheme for clinical purposes eventually may be based on aetiology. For now, the differences in the clinical and scientific approaches depend more on the methods used to establish their validity. Clinical approaches concern themselves with the conceptual coherence of the symptoms, reliability, distinction among symptoms and prediction of clinically meaningful characteristics such as prognosis and treatment response. Scientific approaches are more often concerned with criterion or construct validity – the ability of a classification scheme to distinguish among groups of affected individuals with respect to aetiology or pathophysiology.

Historical development of diagnostic concept

Moral dyscontrol

At any point in time, a classification will embody critical hypotheses about which behaviours constitute manifestations of disorder, the clustering of these symptoms into syndromes, the distinction among categories or dimensions of psychopathology, the critical importance of particular syndromes to research and treatment and the aetiology of mental illness. Human behaviour does change but it evolves slowly, in contrast to the rapid evolution in nosology.

Much can be learned by examining the professional, scientific and social forces surrounding the development of modern notions of hyperactivity.

The historical development of the notion of hyperactivity provides a good example of the influence of social and cultural factors on medical diagnoses and nosology (see also Chapter 1 for a fuller review). In the UK, the first descriptions of the syndrome appeared in the late nineteenth century (Still, 1902; Tredgold, 1908), involving children exhibiting extremes of excitability, overactivity and aggression. These early accounts are strikingly similar to current descriptions of the syndrome. Befitting prevailing Darwinist views of society and psychopathology, the early concepts focused on a lack of sustained 'will' as the cardinal manifestation of the disorder and labelled it a syndrome of 'moral dyscontrol'. Will involved higher-order self-regulatory processes rather like theories of executive control of the late twentieth century.

At the time of the first description of the syndrome, prevailing opinions about the cause of moral dyscontrol were, however, amazingly 'modern'. The clinicians and scientists of the late nineteenth century believed that relatively minor pathogens such as minor trauma, infection or malnourishment were thought capable of causing the disorder because will, morality, sustained effort and the like were thought to be the 'highest and latest' achievements of evolution, and hence most vulnerable.

The early descriptions of moral dyscontrol were contemporaneous with dramatic alterations in social and economic life. Rapid changes in the economic order resulted in urbanization and poverty. The advent of compulsory education in the UK was, in part, a response to the resultant increase in perceived social disorder. Compulsory education led to the development of large state-run schools. Soon, it was clear that there were many children who were not easily educated or well behaved in the school setting. Also many individuals with learning and behaviour problems lived in adverse social circumstances characterized by poverty and associated disease. Nevertheless, moral dyscontrol was seen primarily as a biological disease, a perspective which reflects the prevailing philosophical and sociological inclination of the late nineteenth century to attribute extremes of behaviour, as well as poverty and its correlates such as medical illness, alcoholism and immorality, to physiological rather than psychological or social causes. From the perspective of classification, these early descriptions of the syndrome firmly established the possibility that behaviour problems such as hyperactivity could result from subtle or minimal brain damage acting on biologically and genetically predisposed individuals (Tredgold, 1908).

Following the devastating epidemic of encephalitis in 1918, attention focused on the causal role of brain injury arising from infection. The link between brain damage or dysfunction and hyperactivity persisted in various theories of hyperactivity (Kahn and Cohen, 1934; Pasamanick et al., 1956; Laufer et al., 1957; Clements, 1966), even though its name changed frequently. The link was most obvious when the disorder was known as minimal brain dysfunction (MBD; Clements, 1966), with hyperactivity, inattention and impulsiveness taken as de facto evidence of brain damage.

Since Charles Bradley (Bradley, 1937) discovered that the psychostimulant dextroamphetamine improved concentration and behaviour, the steady increase in the use of the diagnosis has also been attributed to the availability of this relatively safe and effective treatment. However, it can equally be argued that social forces rather than access to medication shaped clinical practice. After all, the sharp increase in prevalence of hyperactivity was largely a North American phenomenon with the rise in use of the diagnosis coinciding with a period of rapid changes in social and educational expectations of children and families.

Evolution of formal diagnostic criteria

Although the notion of hyperactivity has been around for over a century, formal diagnostic schemata with specified criteria and the scientific study of the taxonomic status of hyperactivity are recent phenomena. A rather bewildering array of names and aetiological concepts have been attached to the diagnosis over the years. These names reflect the prevailing notions of brain function, theories about the causes of psychopathology and opinions about the cardinal manifestations of the disorder.

When the syndrome first appeared in modern North American diagnostic classifications of mental disorders, it was known as hyperkinetic child syndrome (Laufer et al., 1957; Chess, 1960) or hyperkinetic reaction of childhood (DSM-II; American Psychiatric Association, 1968). The latter label reflected the prevailing view that psychiatric disorders represented patterns of response or reaction to psychological stress. The name of the disorder was changed to attention deficit disorder (ADD) in 1980 (DSM-III; American Psychiatric Association, 1980) to reflect the emerging opinion, particularly in North America, that cognitive deficit rather than overactivity was the cardinal manifestation of the disorder and possibly the central deficit (Douglas, 1972). Accordingly, symptoms of inattention such as difficulty concentrating and sustaining attention were added to the list of diagnostic criteria in the third revision of the DSM. As a result of this shift, 'hyperactivity' could exist even in the absence of motoric hyperactivity. Despite this change, a distinction between 'hyperactive' children with and without hyperactivity was retained (ADD and ADDH).

In 1987, the DSM-III-R changed the name of the disorder to attention deficit and hyperactivity disorder (ADHD; American Psychiatric Association, 1987) and combined all symptoms into one single dimensional category reflecting the prevailing view that inattention, restlessness and impulsiveness were related and equivalent markers of a single dimension of underlying disorder. The change in criteria embodied in DSM-III-R resulted in a loss of the distinction between 'hyperactive' children with and without hyperactivity.

Clinicians and researchers continued to feel that a distinction based on the presence of hyperactive behaviour was clinically relevant. Consequently, in 1994, the symptoms were divided once again into inattentive and hyperactive-impulsive clusters (see Table 5.1 for DSM-IV criteria; American Psychiatric Association, 1994). Current criteria allow for the diagnosis of inattentive, hyperactive-impulsive and combined subtypes of ADHD (Table 5.2).

Over the years, there was a change in the way symptoms and thresholds for diagnosis were established. The diagnostic criteria of DSM-III were developed largely through consensus among experts. DSM-III-R and DSM-IV criteria were also based largely on expert consensus. However, the results of field trials were used to establish the optimal threshold (sensitivity and specificity) for predicting a clinical diagnosis (Frick et al., 1994).

In general, the DSM-III-R criteria were less restrictive than DSM-III criteria and consequently applied to a greater proportion of the child population. The emphasis given to particular types of symptoms also changed. For example, there was a net decrease from DSM-III-R to DSM-IV in the total number of symptoms of impulsiveness. This changing emphasis seems at odds with the growing importance of impulsiveness and disinhibition to theories of hyperactivity (Barkley, 1997). Moreover, DSM-IV criteria are likely to increase the prevalence of the disorder (11.4%) in comparison with DSM-III-R (7.3%), although DSM-IV may better characterize its heterogeneity.

Diverging diagnostic practice

Rather than converging after the discovery of the effects of stimulants, clinical practice in North America and the UK diverged. In North America, the presence of the behavioural manifestations of the syndrome alone were considered sufficient for the diagnosis of MBD (Strauss et al., 1955). Coexisting disorders such as conduct disorder and learning disability were thought to be secondary manifestations of the syndrome and signs of brain damage (Clements, 1966). The diagnosis could also be made in the presence of hyperactivity that was limited to a single situation.

Clinical practice in the UK and Europe was very different. Before a diagnosis

Table 5.1. Current diagnostic criteria for attention deficit hyperactivity disorder

A. Either (1) or (2):

    (1) Six (or more) of the following symptoms of inattention have persisted for at least 6 months to a degree that is maladaptive and inconsistent with developmental level:

Inattention

    (a) often fails to give close attention to details or makes careless mistakes in schoolwork, work or other activities

    (b) often has difficulty sustaining attention in tasks or play activities

    (c) often does not seem to listen when spoken to directly

    (d) often does not follow through on instructions and fails to finish school work, chores or duties in the workplace (not due to oppositional behaviour or failure to understand instructions)

    (e) often has difficulty organizing tasks and activities

    (f) often avoids, dislikes or is reluctant to engage in tasks that require sustained mental effort (such as school work or homework)

    (g) often loses things necessary for tasks or activities (e.g. toys, school assignments, pencils, books or tools)

    (h) is often easily distracted by extraneous stimuli

    (i) is often forgetful in daily activities

A (2) Six (or more) of the following symptoms of hyperactivity-impulsivity have persisted for at least 6 months to a degree that is maladaptive and inconsistent with developmental level:

Hyperactivity

    (a) often fidgets with hands or feet or squirms in seat

    (b) often leaves seat in classroom or in other situations in which remaining seated is expected

    (c) often runs about or climbs excessively in situations in which it is inappropriate (in adolescents or adults, may be limited to subjective feelings of restlessness)

    (d) often has difficulty playing or engaging in leisure activities quietly

    (e) is often 'on the go' or often acts as if 'driven by a motor'

    (f) often talks excessively

Impulsivity

    (g) often blurts out answers before questions have been completed

    (h) often has difficulty awaiting turn

    (i) often interrupts or intrudes on others (e.g. butts into conversations or games)

B. Some hyperactive-impulsive or inattentive symptoms that caused impairment were present before age 7 years

C. Some impairment from the symptoms is present in two or more settings (e.g. at school (or work) and at home)

Table 5.1. (*cont.*)

D. There must be clear evidence of clinically significant impairment in social, academic or occupational functioning

E. The symptoms do not occur exclusively during the course of a pervasive developmental disorder, schizophrenia or other psychotic disorder and are not better accounted for by another mental disorder (e.g. mood disorder, anxiety disorder, dissociative disorder or a personality disorder)

---

of hyperkinetic disorder was made, European clinicians required evidence of documented neuropathology such as a history of head injury or seizure disorder (McKeith and Bax, 1963). They also required the presence of symptoms in various situations (i.e. pervasiveness) and the absence of significant comorbid psychopathology, especially conduct disorder. The dominant European model posited that hyperkinesis is a neuropsychological condition arising from brain abnormality (Ounsted, 1955; Rutter et al., 1970a; Gillberg and Gillberg, 1988; Sergeant and Steinhausen, 1992; Gillberg, 1998) that has two developmental waves: a preschool group of children who exhibit overactivity, impulsiveness and poor concentration and a second wave which emerges at school entry (Taylor et al., 1996).

The vast majority of hyperactive children, that is, those without clearcut neuropathology, were thought to have a nonspecific behaviour problem. Apparently, British clinicians would not make a diagnosis of hyperactivity in the presence of any degree of disruptive or antisocial behaviour because they believed that social influences such as adverse child-rearing practices rather than biological factors caused those behaviours. This belief was reflected in their preference for interventions that targeted family functioning over those involving medication.

Recent revisions of both North American (DSM-IV, American Psychiatric Association, 1994) and European (World Health Organization, 1992) criteria have resulted in a much more unified set of diagnostic criteria, although important differences remain (see below for discussion). The major change in DSM-IV was the inclusion of an explicit statement about the requirement that symptoms be pervasive, that is, be evident in more than a single setting. The major change in ICD-10 was the inclusion of a category of hyperactive conduct disorder.

Even within Europe, different diagnostic traditions are apparent. Northern European clinicians have long stressed the association of delay in motor development and psychopathology (Kalverboer, 1975; Nichols and Chen,

Table 5.2. Current diagnostic criteria for hyperkinetic disorder (HD)[a]

1. Demonstrated abnormality of attention and activity at home, for the age and developmental level of the child, as evidenced in at least three of the following attention problems:
   (a) short duration of spontaneous activities
   (b) often leaving play activities unfinished
   (c) overfrequent changes between activities
   (d) undue lack of persistence at tasks set by adults
   (e) unduly high distractibility during study, e.g. homework or reading assignment and by at least two of the following activity problems:
   (f) continuous motor activity (running, jumping, etc.)
   (g) markedly excessive fidgeting and wriggling during spontaneous activities
   (h) markedly excessive activity in situations expecting relative stillness (e.g. meal times, travel, visiting, church)
   (i) difficulty in remaining seated when required

2. Demonstrable abnormality of attention and activity at school or nursery (if applicable), for the age and developmental level of the child, as evidenced by at least two of the following attention problems:
   (a) undue lack of persistence at tasks
   (b) unduly high distractibility, i.e. often orienting toward extrinsic stimuli
   (c) overfrequent changes between activities when choice is allowed
   (d) excessively short duration of play activities and by at least two of the following activity problems:
   (e) continuous and excessive motor restlessness (running, jumping, etc.) in situations allowing free activity
   (f) markedly excessive fidgeting and wriggling in structured situations
   (g) excessive levels of off-task activity during tasks
   (h) unduly often out of seat when required to be sitting

3. Directly observed abnormality of attention or activity. This must be excessive for the child's age and developmental level. The evidence may be any of the following:
   (a) direct observation of the criteria in 1 or 2 above, i.e. the report of parent and/or teacher
   (b) observation of abnormal levels of motor activity, or off-task, behaviour, or lack of persistence in activities, in setting outside home or school (e.g. clinic or laboratory)
   (c) significant impairment of performance on psychometric tests of attention

4. Does not meet criteria for pervasive developmental disorder, mania or depressive or anxiety disorder

5. Onset before the age of 6 years

6. Duration of at least 6 months

[a]All of the criteria must be present for the ICD-10 diagnosis of hyperkinetic disorder (HD: Taylor et al., 1991; World Health Organization, 1992).

1981). The term DAMP – disorder of attention, motor control and perception – came to refer to the coincidence of deficits in attention, motor control and perception (Gillberg, 1998). Although motor clumsiness and perceptual problems are common among children with hyperkinetic disorder, they are not necessary for diagnosis as they are for the diagnosis of DAMP. Other Europeans emphasize the neuropsychological and information-processing deficits arising from various neural abnormalities to explain hyperactivity (Sergeant, 1995, 2000; Brandeis et al., 1998; Rubia et al., 1999).

A contrasting approach was found in the Mediterranean tradition where clinicians believed that hyperactivity does not actually exist. In the last decade, major changes in southern European diagnostic practice have occurred that reflect a growing empirical child psychiatry in these countries (Sergeant and Van der Meere, 1994).

What is apparent in this century-long process of diagnostic and scientific evolution is a belief that hyperactivity is a common mental illness with a biological basis. Social and cultural factors have also influenced our notions of hyperactivity. What has been slower to emerge but may now be nearer is a common set of criteria and diagnostic procedures.

Quantitative and categorical approaches to syndrome definition

There are two general traditions in the classification of hyperactivity, as there are for the classification of many other psychopathologies and medical illnesses – a categorical and a quantitative approach (Meehl, 1995). Both approaches grapple with the same problem, namely to determine whether there is some essential, nonarbitrary category or dimension of hyperactive behaviour that reflects an underlying biological or clinical reality.

In the quantitative tradition, psychopathology is conceived as a continuous dimension: normal individuals and pathological individuals are thought to differ in the extent of, rather than in the type of, behaviour on these dimensions. Moreover, important differences based on the severity of symptoms are thought to exist among both disordered and nondisordered individuals. The presence or absence of specific symptoms is less important than the extent of disturbance and categorical disorder, when diagnosed, is based on arbitrary or statistical cutoffs mapped on to these dimensions. The quantitative approach suggests that the best way to characterize the comorbidity that is common among hyperactive individuals is by describing individuals along several dimensions of psychopathology rather than by reducing the array of symptoms to a few, supposedly mutually exclusive categories.

In contrast, the categorical or qualitative approach assumes that there are important discontinuities in behavioural data. The categorical approach argues that there are important differences in behaviour, pathophysiology or aetiology between individuals who are hyperactive and those who are not. In other words, the categorical approach argues that there are important differences among hyperactive individuals even if quantitative traits do exist.

The quantitative and categorical approaches differ in their concepts of psychopathology and in their strategies for developing taxonomies. According to the categorical approach, discontinuity arises where there exists some dichotomous aetiological factor that is both necessary and sufficient for the disorder to appear (e.g. a specific gene), where a dichotomous aetiological variable exists that is necessary but not sufficient for the disease to be manifest, or where there exists a threshold effect in the relationship between exposure to the causal factor and the probability of exhibiting the syndrome.

The quantitative concept of hyperactivity is often mapped on to a particular view of aetiology, namely that hyperactivity represents a final common pathway for a multifactorial, multigenic aetiology. While a single pool of genetic and environmental factors causes hyperactivity, no single cause is necessary or sufficient and most causes are of small effect. The effect of these factors may be additive or synergistic. According to this reasoning, there is only one kind of hyperactive individual, although there may be differences in severity and clinical presentation based on the number of aetiological factors or the extent of expression of a particular genetic effect (penetrance).

Determining which of these two approaches, the quantitative or qualitative approach, is correct is a matter of considerable debate. Complexity arises from the fact that meaningful discontinuities could exist at various levels such as at the behavioural, pathological or aetiological levels, while meaningful continua could exist simultaneously at other levels.

Furthermore, in medicine, explicit definitions of disease often rely on evidence of pathology. Affected individuals manifest the supposed aetiology, say of human immunodeficiency virus (HIV); unaffected individuals do not. This is true regardless of the behavioural manifestations. For example, one can have a disease such as HIV but be asymptomatic or vary in the extent to which overt manifestations of disease are evident. Meehl (1995) points out that theoretical genetics distinguishes dominant and recessive genes, degrees of penetrance, epistatic effects and pleiotropic markers. All of these concepts presuppose that a gene can be present but its phenotypic indicators may be absent or variable. Currently, there is no established aetiology for hyperactivity to guide the separation of individuals into diseased and not diseased groups. Although a number of genetic factors are known to be associated with increased risk of hyperactivity (Chapter 9), it is also true that various biological factors, such as fetal exposure to alcohol and drugs, high lead levels and head injury, as well as various psychosocial risk factors such as early institutionalization may cause ADHD (Chapters 11 and 12). Little is known about the mechanism of these effects or their results. For example, detailed analysis of particular symptoms might reveal that various aetiological factors may generate distinct patterns of ADHD symptoms. The necessary studies have not yet been conducted.

The existence of categories or continua of psychopathology must be inferred from existing behavioural data. The existence of meaningful categories of hyperactivity does not rely on the presence of clearcut boundaries or sharp distinctions on indicator variables between affected and unaffected individuals or between hyperactive persons and those with another disorder. There are few, if any, observably sharp discontinuities in behavioural data but that does not necessarily mean that latent categories do not exist. Meehl (1995) argues that one can have a sharp latent category, defined by a specific dichotomous (present or absent) causal factor (e.g. Huntington mutation or specific micro-organism) that is indicated by quantitative variables such as age of onset or fever. According to Meehl, both the latent entity and its manifest indicators can be either qualitative or quantitative, and all degrees of overlap between quantitative indicator distributions can occur.

Quantitative approaches

The empirical taxonomic approach developed in the 1970s, following the development of behaviour rating scales or questionnaires to measure child behaviour and the advent of computers to facilitate the necessary statistical methods. Behaviour rating scales are compilations of descriptors of child behaviour such as 'restless, can't sit still', 'can't concentrate, easily distracted'. Ratings reflect the extent to which an informant such as a parent or teacher feels that these descriptors apply to a child. Typically, ratings are based on a three- or four-point scale from 'not at all' to 'very much'. These responses are given scores, for example, '0' for 'not at all' to '3' or '4' for 'very much'. These scores are the subject of analysis. Statistical techniques such as factor, cluster and latent cluster analysis are employed to assess the presence of latent variables by examining the pattern of covariation among the measurable attributes of individuals. When identified, these patterns are assumed to represent syndrome dimensions on which individuals vary. Rather than imposing a structure derived from clinical experience, this approach is presumed to allow the taxonomy of psychopathology to emerge from data on child behaviour.

Various parent and teacher rating scales have been used in the study of hyperactivity, including the Rutter Parent and Teacher Questionnaire (Rutter et al., 1970b), Conners rating scales (Conners et al., 1997) and rating scales that have been developed from DSM criteria (Burns et al., 1997). The Child Behavior Checklist (CBCL; Achenbach et al., 1989) is the most widely used and thoroughly studied.

Numerous studies of children in the general population or in clinic samples using behaviour ratings such as the CBCL confirm the existence of a dimension of hyperactive behaviour and support the essential assumption of the quantitative approach. No bimodal distribution of scores is observed. That is, there does not seem to be an obvious distinction between a group of individuals with high scores and a group with low scores. Bimodal distribution, if present, would indicate that there is both temperamental variation and the presence of a discrete 'hyperactive' group. Nevertheless, quantitative scores on checklist measures of disturbance have been translated into categorical diagnoses using thresholds. These thresholds are based on statistical considerations such as scores in excess of one or two standard deviations above the mean for a group of children of a particular age and sex. Individuals with extreme scores are more impaired than those who are not (Boyle et al., 1996).

The following examples of studies support the quantitative hypothesis. Fergusson and Horwood (1995) compared the efficacy of categorically and dimensionally scored measures of DSM-III-R diagnostic criteria in children aged 15 years in a large birth cohort. They found evidence of continuous and generally linear dose–response functions relating symptom severity and outcome risk (substance use behaviour, juvenile offending and school drop-out at age 16). They also observed that dimensionally scored variables were considerably better predictors of outcome than were measures based on a diagnostic classification (i.e. extreme scores). Levy et al. (1997) studied the extent to which ADHD is heritable using a DSM-III-R-based symptom checklist. They found ADHD to be highly heritable and estimates of heritability were similar whether ADHD was defined as part of a continuum or as a disorder with various symptom cutoffs. They concluded that ADHD is best viewed as the extreme of a behaviour that varies genetically throughout the entire population rather than as a disorder with discrete determinants.

The quantitative approach as a source of diagnostic information has been questioned on several grounds. First, latent taxonomies do not simply emerge from available evidence in the absence of the choices which one makes in conducting factor analysis or other statistical analyses. The analyst makes decisions about the sort of items that are used, the range of items included, the precise analytic method and the inferences drawn from the results. All of these factors contribute to what is 'discovered'. A recent large-scale and comprehensive evaluation of the factor structure of ratings on the CBCL collected in various countries illustrates this point persuasively. Investigators failed to confirm the factor structure assumed to exist in CBCL ratings but rather observed the existence of broad-band dimensions of internalizing and externalizing behaviours (Hartman et al., 1999).

Second, the dimensions that emerge in these factor and cluster analyses often fail to correspond to proposed or apparent clinical dimensions. For example, no syndrome or factor of ADHD or hyperactivity emerges in factor analyses of the CBCL. Instead, a factor of attention problems emerges. Also, the specific items that emerge in the CBCL attention problem factor include items that are similar to those included in DSM or in clinically derived factors (e.g. 'can't concentrate', 'can't sit still') as well as items that are not typically included in clinically derived ADHD syndrome (e.g. 'acts too young', 'confused', 'nervous'). Some items typically thought to be associated with hyperactivity such as 'talking too much' or 'talking out of turn' load on other factors such as those of aggressive behaviour.

Categorical approach

The categorical approach to diagnosis differs from the quantitative approach in various ways. Typically, the criteria that constitute the diagnosis tend to be based on clinical experience and consensus among clinicians and refined through research and experience (Frick et al., 1994) rather than on analysis of rating scales. Second, implicit in the categorical approach is the notion that judgement of the experienced clinician is better than that of the parent or the teacher in determining the presence or absence of behaviours that are developmentally abnormal, impairing and constitute symptoms of pathology. It follows that diagnostic interviewing is considered more important in the categorical tradition than in the quantitative tradition as it allows for probing of the informant's understanding of symptoms and biases. The resulting advantage of the clinical diagnostic approach is that it permits distinction among related concepts or behaviours and consequently reduces the high association among factors such as hyperactivity and conduct disorder observed in rating-scale data (Schachar et al., 1986).

One way to test the existence of a discrete entity of hyperactivity is to compare hyperactive children who have some comorbid disorder such as conduct or anxiety disorder with hyperactive children without comorbidity. The quantitative tradition argues that the correlates of hyperactivity among children with and without comorbidity should be similar and that hyperactive individuals with various manifestations such as conduct disorder exhibit either a more severe form of the disorder or some secondary manifestation of it. The categorical tradition holds that each comorbid subtype represents true hyperactivity in the behavioural sense but not necessarily in other ways such as in course, associated characteristics and treatment response. Consequently, hyperactivity among comorbid individuals may not be the same as among individuals without comorbidity. Stated another way, some hyperactivity might actually be a phenocopy of true hyperactivity.

There is evidence that ADHD children with comorbid conduct disorder differ from exclusively hyperactive children. Compared with ADHD, ADHD comorbid with conduct disorder has a different profile of cognitive test performance (Leung et al., 1996a), a worse prognosis and elevated rates of antisocial personality, nonbipolar depressive disorder and overanxious disorder among relatives (Faraone et al., 1991, 1997). Similarly, there is evidence that ADHD with comorbid reading disability may represent a phenocopy of ADHD (Pennington et al., 1993) and evidence that hyperactivity comorbid with anxiety disorder may have unique correlates and treatment response (Urman et al., 1995).

In an attempt to determine whether ADHD symptoms are continuously distributed or categorically discrete, Hudziak et al. (1998) conducted factor and latent class analysis on ADHD symptom data from a large general population of twins. Latent classes corresponding to the predominantly inattentive, predominantly hyperactive-impulsive and combined types were identified with lifetime prevalence estimates of 4.0%, 2.2% and 3.7%, respectively. Within each type, separate latent classes were evident for individuals with mild, moderate and severe symptoms. Additional research indicated that these severity classes bred true across twins. That is, identical twins of individuals who fit each class were more likely to fit the same class as their cotwin than they were to fit any of the other classes. These results support the categorical hypothesis.

Unfortunately, the categorical approach to diagnosis does not overcome all of the problems inherent in the quantitative methods. Criteria are not free from professional and cultural influences. For example, the field trials of DSM-IV suggested that a cutoff of five symptoms was optimal for prediction of a clinical diagnosis of ADHD. However, a cutoff of six symptoms was chosen for the final criteria because of the unacceptably high prevalence rate that would have resulted from a threshold of five symptoms. Moreover, the categorical approach permits development of disparate diagnostic traditions that may vary in the rules used to deal with hierarchies of disorder and comorbidity.

Reliability and validity of symptoms

The reliability and validity of the diagnoses of ADHD and HD are limited by the reliability and validity of the individual symptoms that constitute the syndrome. On one hand, there is sufficient convergence between ratings of hyperactive, inattentive and impulsive symptoms and direct measures of the same behaviours to support the general validity of hyperactivity. When observed in a playroom, for example, hyperactive children are more often off task and persist less on a particular activity than their nonhyperactive peers (Milich and Fitzgerald, 1985; Taylor et al., 1998). Hyperactive children are demonstrably more active throughout the day and in a variety of situations (Porrino et al., 1983) and less attentive in a range of laboratory situations (Sandberg et al., 1996).

On the other hand, agreement among observers about the presence of inattention, overactivity and impulsiveness tends to be rather modest. For example, agreement between individuals with similar roles, e.g. mothers and fathers, is about 0.5–0.6. Agreement between informants with different roles (e.g. parents and teachers) is much less, e.g., 0.25 (Achenbach et al., 1987).

There are many possible reasons for these modest levels of agreement. First, informants may not share a common definition of symptoms. For example, one observer might consider failure to persist in a task to be evidence of defiance, disinterest, low motivation, boredom or learning disability rather than inattention. Impulsiveness may be seen as an inability to delay responding or as evidence of conduct disturbance, that is, a lack of willingness to conform to social expectations. Second, child behaviour is a function of the demands of the setting. Parents may have less opportunity than teachers to observe children in situations that demand attention. Inattention might be particularly impairing in school and therefore salient to a teacher's judgement of psychopathology, whereas restlessness might be a more serious issue in the home. Third, the informant's mental state or expectations may influence perceptions of child behaviour. Age-appropriate levels of activity may seem particularly aversive for a depressed, socially isolated mother, for those with high expectations for academic attainment or for a teacher of a class that includes numerous children with special needs. Fourth, individuals of different cultures (Chapter 3) may differ in their sensitivity to hyperactive behaviours (Leung et al., 1996b). Leung et al. reported that parents in Hong Kong rated their children as highly hyperactive even though these children were no more hyperactive than their counterparts in the UK when behaviour was measured objectively. Fifth, informants seem to have difficulty discriminating among various dimensions of disturbance. This inability to discriminate among behaviours may result in a halo effect whereby the presence of defiance and disobedience is taken as evidence of hyperactivity (Schachar et al., 1986). Finally, parents have a tendency to exaggerate the differences among their children when making behavioural ratings (Thapar et al., 1995; Eaves et al., 1997).

Behaviour rating scales provide a valuable and simple opportunity to collect descriptions of child behaviour from various informants. Clinicians rely on these measures for teacher reports in particular. Nevertheless, rating scales present an additional source of measurement error. For example, they do not include operational criteria for individual symptoms or, in most cases, specify the setting in which the behaviour should be judged. Individual informants are left to decide what constitutes 'restlessness' or 'inability to concentrate'. No guidelines are provided about what weight to give to child behaviour at home, during completion of homework, or as reported to them by others or how to adjust ratings for the age of the child. Moreover, informants are left to determine whether these behaviours are present 'not at all', 'just a little' or 'quite a lot'. Even subtle changes in response categories ('somewhat' vs. 'just a little') may dramatically affect scores on behavioural rating scales (Woodward et al., 1989). Finally, questionnaires produce J-shaped distributions because they seek only evidence of dysfunction and provide no information on the child's strengths and psychological skills. These factors generate considerable analytic problems and may result in overestimates of prevalence (Hartman et al., 1999).

Structured diagnostic interviews have the advantage over questionnaires of providing many more probes about each behaviour and broad coverage of the range of possible syndromes. Typically, they yield reliable diagnoses (Shaffer et al., 1993). Nevertheless, decisions about the presence or absence of particular symptoms is left to the judgement of the informant rather than the interviewer. By comparison, semistructured diagnostic interviews permit probing of informant responses, consideration of the influence of informant effects on reports (bias, mental state, cultural expectations), application of operational criteria for each symptom and teasing apart of overlap among various disorders. For example, an interviewer can obtain detailed descriptions of specific instances of child behaviour in order to distinguish restlessness or inattention that is part of the syndrome of hyperactivity and similar symptoms that occur only during episodes of anxiety or depression.

Nevertheless, behaviour measures based on interviews may still pose a problem of reliability. Clinicians can differ in the specific questions that they ask, the type and number of situations about which they seek descriptions of behaviour and the criteria they apply to determine at what point a behavioural excess becomes a symptom of psychopathology. It is not surprising then that the reliability of diagnoses based on semistructured interviews may be acceptably high only for specially trained research clinicians (Prendergast et al., 1988).

The low level of convergence among various informants has implications for clinical practice. Reliance on a single source of information or failure to perceive valid differences between informants' descriptions of child behaviour can result in failure to consider important diagnostic issues that may bear on management. Moreover, failure to consider more than one informant could lead to inexact diagnoses for research. Individuals whose hyperactivity is evident at home but not at school often show oppositional behaviour and exposure to psychosocial risk, whereas individuals whose hyperactivity is primarily evident at school more commonly have language and learning difficulties. Those with pervasive hyperactivity are more likely to have language and developmental delays as well as neuropsychological dysfunction (Schachar, 1991; Taylor et al., 1991; Ho et al., 1996).

ADHD, DAMP and hyperkinetic disorder

Both ADHD in DSM-IV and HD in ICD-10 have specific diagnostic criteria that must be met for the diagnosis. DAMP, on the other hand, is less rigorously defined. ADHD and HD differ in important ways (see Tables 5.1 and 5.2 for diagnostic criteria). First, there are differences in the items included in the criteria. For example, 'talking excessively' is considered a manifestation of hyperactivity in DSM and a manifestation of impulsiveness in ICD criteria. The diagnosis of DAMP, but not ADHD or HD, requires the presence of problems in motor control and perception.

Second, ICD-10 and DSM-IV differ in their requirement for pervasiveness, i.e. evidence of disorder in more than a single setting. The requirement for pervasiveness is aimed at precluding the diagnosis for children with a history provided by a single potentially unreliable informant, with behavioural problems that arise in a single distressing environment, or with a problem that arises as an artefact of learning problems only at school. A diagnosis of HD requires that a child meet the criteria for disorder at home and at school. Symptoms must be evident on direct examination but ICD-10 does not specify the criteria for direct observation of symptoms. Directly observed behaviour depends on the specific setting, stimuli and circumstances. For example, even severely hyperactive children may behave well in a novel situation with individual attention (Tripp and Luk, 1997). However, repeated visits to the same setting, introduction of demanding tasks and increased duration of the assessment session are all likely to generate variation in behaviour that is of diagnostic significance. The field could benefit from a clinically applicable and standardized scheme for direct observation of child behaviour in the clinic environment (Kalverboer, 1993).

Despite recent attempts at harmonization, ADHD is more lenient in the requirement for pervasiveness. ADHD requires that criteria are met either at home or at school and that the person shows evidence of impairment arising from the disorder in at least two settings. The criteria for impairment are not clearly spelled out. Does impairment entail the presence of one, two or three symptoms of ADHD? Differences in the requirement for pervasiveness probably account for the majority of observed differences between ADHD and HD in prevalence and correlates. Parent- and teacher-rated hyperactivity appear to have unique correlates: school-only ADHD is characterized by learning and cognitive deficits, while home-only ADHD may be preferentially associated with psychosocial impairment (Szatmari et al., 1990; Ho et al., 1996).

Third, DSM-IV and ICD-10 permit diagnosis of different subtypes. According to DSM-IV, the diagnosis of ADHD requires the presence of six inattentive and/or six hyperactive-impulsive symptoms. As a consequence, three different subtypes of ADHD are generated: predominantly inattentive (six or more symptoms of disordered attention and fewer than six hyperactive-impulsive symptoms are present); predominantly hyperactive-impulsive (six or more hyperactive-impulsive symptoms and fewer than six symptoms of inattention are present); and combined (six or more inattentive and six or more hyperactive-impulsive symptoms present). Consequently, ADHD can be diagnosed in the virtual absence of hyperactive or impulsive behaviour. ICD-10 requires the presence of at least six inattentive, three hyperactive and one impulsive symptom for a HD diagnosis. Consequently, ICD-10 criteria ensure that some symptoms of each type are evident. This is clearly a different phenotype, cluster or category than that defined by DSM-IV.

Fourth, DSM-IV and ICD-10 classifications reflect different approaches to diagnosis in the presence of more than one coexisting disorder. DSM-IV aims to recognize all diagnoses that are present except for schizophrenia, autism and pervasive developmental delay. One only withholds the diagnosis of ADHD if some comorbid condition such as anxiety disorder better accounts for the disorder. In contrast, ICD-10, in general, discourages multiple diagnoses. In the presence of internalizing disorders such as anxiety and mood disorders, ICD-10 does not recommend the HD diagnosis. One exception to the rule occurs when both HD and conduct disorder are present: provision is made for an ICD-10 diagnostic subtype of hyperkinetic conduct disorder. This new subcategory may address the tendency of clinicians in the UK and Europe to diagnose conduct disorder over HD when both disorders are evident (Prendergast et al., 1988).

In general, DSM-IV criteria can be applied to girls (Biederman et al., 1999) and to very young children although the validity of the age-of-onset criterion has been questioned (Applegate et al., 1997; Barkley and Biederman, 1997). Neither DSM-IV nor ICD-10 has specified whether and how the criteria for diagnosis of hyperactivity should be adjusted when being applied to very young children, girls, adolescents and adults. Should a greater number of symptoms be required for a diagnosis among children younger than age 5 and fewer among adolescents and adults? In the general population, rates of hyperactivity are very high among preschoolers and much lower among adolescents and adults. Few adolescents or adults meet the full criteria for hyperactivity. Yet follow-up of affected children demonstrates that even though many individuals no longer meet full criteria for ADHD, they nevertheless experience significant impairment from their remaining symptoms (Hechtman and Weiss, 1986; Fischer at al., 1993; Mannuzza et al., 1998).

Validity of diagnostic approaches

ADHD, HD and DAMP

Differences in diagnostic practice such as those embedded in DSM-IV and ICD-10 have had a profound impact on the prevalence of the disorder and its observed clinical correlates. In the UK, for example, HD was diagnosed in only one in 1000 children. At the same time, ADHD was thought to apply to 5–10% or more of children in North America (see Buitelaar and van Engeland, 1996 for extensive review). Apparently, pervasive hyperactivity occurs in 20–50% of ADHD cases (Szatmari et al., 1989b; Swanson et al., 1998b; Tripp et al., 1999).

Considerable evidence supports the validity of both ADHD and HD. Children with ADHD diagnosed according to DSM criteria and HD diagnosed according to ICD can be distinguished from children with other disorders such as conduct disorder and differ in important ways from normally developing children on a wide range of laboratory measures of attention, social interaction and outcome (Sergeant and Van der Meere, 1994; Barkley, 1998; and covered by individual contributors to this book). Early manifestation of hyperactivity is a persistent phenomenon and an important predictor of later antisocial behaviour above and beyond the risk associated with early conduct disorder (Taylor et al., 1996).

In general, this entire volume deals with the validity of hyperactivity. No attempt will be made to summarize the predictive validity of these various definitions in each of the domains covered in the chapters of this book. The important questions from the perspective of classification is whether one set of criteria is superior to the others. Unfortunately, only a few attempts have been made to compare the predictive validity of ADHD and HD.

As a consequence of the differences in operational definitions and decision rules between ICD-10 and DSM-IV, HD constitutes a subset of ADHD (Swanson et al., 1998b; Tripp et al., 1999). HD appears to be a more severe disorder than ADHD as judged by the increased rate of important clinical correlates such as neurodevelopmental delay, poor academic and cognitive function and the presence of comorbid psychopathology (Schachar, 1991). ADHD that is not severe enough to fulfil criteria for HD is common in the general population and in many cases these children are not particularly impaired (Taylor et al., 1991). ADHD of this degree of severity may identify a group of children at high risk for the development of disturbance.

The prevalence rates are 5.3–6.9% for DAMP and 2.4–4.0% for ADHD. DAMP delineates a subset of children with ADHD. Approximately half of children with ADHD meet criteria for DAMP (Landgren et al., 1996). The prevalence of combined ADHD and DAMP is about 6% (Kadesjo and Gillberg, 1998). DAMP plus ADHD delineates a subset of children with more marked classroom dysfunction and poorer academic test scores than either ADHD or DAMP alone. By contrast, the majority of those with HD meet criteria for DAMP (Taylor et al., 1991). The validity of the concept of DAMP has been questioned because the association of neurodevelopmental abnormality and hyperactivity does not appear to be specific to hyperactivity: soft neurological signs are associated with increased risk for various behavioural abnormalities rather than for hyperactivity per se. Indeed, the strongest association appears to be between soft signs and anxiety (Shaffer, 1978).

Subtypes of ADHD and HD

Both DSM-IV and ICD-10 permit distinction of several subtypes of hyperactivity. The subtype distinction that has received the most discussion is that based on the nature of the primary symptoms. DSM-IV distinguishes hyperactive-impulsive only, inattentive only and combined hyperactive-impulsive and inattentive subtypes in ADHD. (The hyperactive-impulsive subtype is common in very young children but is less common among school-age children (2.4%).)

The inattentive and combined subtypes are about equally prevalent (5.4% and 3.6%) among school-age children (Wolraich et al., 1996). These two groups correspond to the DSM-III categories of ADD with and without hyperactivity but have no correspondence with DSM-III-R because that version of DSM did not allow for subtypes. By contrast, ICD-10 does not permit subtypes. To warrant a diagnosis of HD an individual must have symptoms of inattention, impulsiveness and hyperactivity.

Some support is found for the reliability and validity of the ADHD subtypes. ADHD subtypes emerge in latent class analysis of ADHD symptoms (Hudziak et al., 1998). Factor analysis reveals that a two-factor model such as that proposed in DSM-IV is only slightly better than a two-factor model equivalent to DSM-III (Burns et al., 1997; Gomez et al., 1999). Hyperactive and impulsive behaviour but not inattention contributes to an increased risk for criminal involvement, externalizing, delinquent and aggressive behaviours over and above the risk associated with early conduct problems alone (Babinski et al., 1999). Compared to children with ADDH or combined subtype, those with a diagnosis of inattentive subtype are more sluggish, drowsy and anxious. They have lower IQ, more abnormalities in attention and delayed language development. They are also less impulsive, aggressive, distractible, and socially disinhibited (Lahey and Carlson, 1991; Cantwell and Baker, 1992; Eiraldi et al., 1997). Taylor et al. (1991) found that the majority of attention deficits associated with inattentive subtype were artefacts of their lower IQ: differences in attention between ADD and normal children disappeared once IQ was controlled for. Genetic factors are aetiologically important in the expression of the separate dimensions of ADHD and in the covariation between them.

However, there are numerous unresolved issues with respect to the nature of these subtypes. For example, the thresholds and criteria for subtypes can be difficult to operationalize. Many individuals who clearly meet the threshold for one subtype may be just below the threshold for the other. Similarly, it is not uncommon to identify a child who meets the criteria for one subtype in school and another at home. The rules for establishing subtype status are far from clear under these circumstances. Furthermore, many children with a diagnosis of ADD or inattentive subtype may receive a diagnosis of ADHD or combined subtype on follow-up (Cantwell and Baker, 1992), suggesting that subtypes may represent developmental stages of ADHD rather than distinct entities. Finally, whereas marked differences are found among DSM-IV subtypes of ADHD in psychiatric correlates, few differences are found in cognitive or psychosocial functioning (Faraone et al., 1998b).

Another source of subtype arises from comorbidity. It appears to be the rule rather than the exception that individuals affected with hyperactivity present with a second psychiatric disorder. In many cases, more than one additional disorder is present. The most common associated disorders are oppositional (50%), conduct (20%) or anxiety disorder (20%). The cooccurrence of two or more disorders in the same individual is called comorbidity. The very fact that comorbidity is such a common phenomenon among children with a psychiatric disorder suggests that revisions in nosology may be necessary. An individual child might meet criteria for two separate disorders because the criteria for diagnosis of these disorders overlap. A classic example of diagnostic overlap is found in hyperactivity and depression. Inattention is a criterion for both disorders. The same is true for restlessness and mania (Wozniak et al., 1995). Moreover, the very high rate of comorbidity between hyperactivity and oppositional defiant disorder suggests to some that they may be part of the same syndrome.

ICD-10 identifies a subtype of HD plus conduct disorder. This category can be used by clinicians who would otherwise choose between one diagnosis or the other in the presence of both conditions. In DSM-IV there is no separate diagnosis for ADHD plus conduct disorder. This common comorbidity is handled by diagnosing two separate disorders. Typically, this common presentation is thought to be a true hybrid of hyperactivity and conduct disorder. True hybrids can arise because there is some shared underlying deficit or risk factor or because one disorder increases the risk of developing the other. This view of hyperactive conduct disorder is supported by considerable research on clinical correlates (Szatmari et al., 1989a; Schachar and Tannock, 1995). The comorbid group has both the cognitive and developmental correlates typical of hyperactivity and the social risk factors characteristic of conduct disorder. Children with comorbid hyperactive conduct disorder tend to respond to stimulants, as do hyperactive children without conduct disorder (Klein et al., 1997). Moreover, there is evidence of shared genetic risk factors in hyperactivity and conduct disorder (Nadder et al., 1998).

However, there are a surprising number of findings that dispute the hybrid notion of this comorbid condition. Instead, hyperactive conduct disorder appears to be distinct from both hyperactivity and from conduct disorder. Hyperactivity with conduct disorder has a particularly early onset, is persistent and is highly predictive of delinquency and school failure (Loeber et al., 1990; Moffitt, 1990). It does not consistently share the cognitive (Halperin et al., 1990; Moffitt, 1990; Schachar and Logan, 1990), social cognitive or familial correlates of pure hyperactivity (Faraone et al., 1997, 1998a). If hyperactive conduct disorder were simply a more severe form of disorder than hyperactivity in the absence of conduct disorder, one would have expected to see consistent evidence for greater severity of these correlates. It is possible that children with both hyperactivity and conduct disorder are referred more readily for clinical assessment because they have two less severe disorders rather than one single disorder.

It is also possible that the hyperactivity associated with conduct disorder is a phenocopy of true hyperactivity. If it were true that many children with hyperactive conduct disorder have a variant of conduct disorder rather than a variant of hyperactivity then many children may be incorrectly diagnosed as hyperactive. An incorrect diagnosis of hyperactivity may not have a large impact on clinical practice because hyperactivity of various kinds tends to respond in a similar way to the few treatments that are available currently. However, false-positive diagnoses can reduce the power of research studies to detect important aetiological factors in hyperactivity.

Anxiety disorder and Tourette syndrome are other frequent comorbidities. The nosological status of each of these combined conditions is unclear. Do these individuals have hyperactivity or does their hyperactivity have a different meaning because it has arisen in the presence of another disorder (Ozonoff et al., 1994)?

Scientific nosology and future directions

Hyperactivity presents numerous problems for scientists and clinicians. First, hyperactivity is an aetiologically diverse condition. Various factors are known to result in hyperactivity, including traumatic brain injury, genetic predisposition, exposure to toxins and extreme psychosocial adversity (Chapters 9–12). Second, the known phenotype of hyperactivity is problematic because of the uncertain reliability and validity of available measures of the constituent behaviours, developmental variation in disease expression and the possibility of phenocopies. These factors make it difficult to identify specific causes of major effect that could lead to targeted intervention. If subtypes of hyperactivity could be identified, our understanding of hyperactivity would be enhanced, our nosology made more scientifically valid and clinically relevant and the task of detecting causes with significant effects would be easier.

Advocates of newer approaches to refining the diagnosis of hyperactivity argue that it is unlikely that such a wide array of causes have exactly the same behavioural expression. Two strategies for refining the diagnosis of hyperactivity may have the potential for developing empirically validated nosologies. One approach aims to discover which symptoms in which combination of severity and pervasiveness best predict important manifestations such as clinical diagnosis, impairment, outcome, family history and treatment response. The goal of this research is to develop a nosology that would reduce the number of false-positive and false-negative cases (Tsuang et al., 1993). From a genetic perspective, for example, false positives are cases that have the ADHD phenotype but are incorrectly classified as having the genetic subform of the illness. False-negative cases are those that fail to meet criteria for hyperactivity but are affected with the genetic susceptibility. The logic is often applied to the prediction of genetic susceptibility but it can be applied to the prediction of other important characteristics such as drug response or natural history.

Milberger et al. (1996) used logistic regression to discriminate relatives of ADHD probands from relatives of normal controls in order to create a quantitative phenotype definition in relatives that combined information across psychiatric, cognitive and demographic domains. The result was not entirely satisfactory in that they observed separate models for mothers, fathers, sisters and brothers. However, they speculate that phenotype definitions based on these types of models may help elucidate features of individual cases that suggest familial transmission, and might be of benefit in weighting the contribution of individual relatives in a linkage analysis.

Faraone et al. (1993) used sensitivity and specificity analysis to identify individual ADHD symptoms and combinations of symptoms that most accurately predicted a clinical diagnosis of ADHD. They found that some symptoms were much more highly associated than others with a clinical diagnosis of ADHD. Next they used these sensitive and specific symptoms to generate a revised ADHD diagnosis for every child in their sample and each of their relatives. Individuals meeting criteria for a refined diagnosis of ADHD were many times more likely to have an affected family member than children identified with ADHD according to DSM-IV criteria, indicating that the refined phenotype was more highly heritable. Mota and Schachar (2000) used a similar approach but used impairment as the criterion for judging which individual symptoms and combinations of symptoms were most important to the diagnosis. They generated revised diagnostic algorithms in parent and teacher ratings that were much more predictive of impairment than were DSM-IV criteria. Moreover, the agreement between parents and teachers was substantially greater using the revised diagnosis than using DSM criteria. These revised criteria differed markedly from DSM in two ways. First, revised criteria were different for parent and teacher ratings. Different symptoms formed the diagnostic algorithm at home and at school. Second, the traditional subtypes of

ADHD, namely inattentive, hyperactive-impulsive and combined, were not evident (Shalev et al., 1995). Revised criteria predicted cognitive deficit better than DSM-IV criteria.

Hudziak et al. (1998) used a different approach to identifying heritable subtypes of ADHD. They used latent class analysis to identify clusters of ADHD cases. These analyses identified cases in several clusters comprised of individuals with few, moderate or severe symptoms of inattention or hyperactivity-impulsiveness. When they examined the heritability of these derived 'syndromes' among twins they discovered that they tended to breed true. That is, identical twins of individuals with few, moderate or severe symptoms were more likely to exhibit the same subtype of ADHD than one of the other subtypes.

Another potential approach would be to examine the heritability of specific symptoms of hyperactivity to develop a diagnostic algorithm to identify the most highly heritable phenotype.

A second approach aims to refine the existing phenotype through investigation of pathophysiology and aetiology. Pathophysiological indicators of hyperactivity are any anatomical, cognitive or physiological measure of brain structure or function thought to be associated with hyperactivity. A partial list of these indicators includes anatomical measurement of brain structure using neuroimaging, electrophysiological measurements, measures of cognitive function or drug response. The reasoning behind this approach is simple. It is more likely that specific aetiologies will be expressed in terms of specific brain abnormalities or dysfunction than in terms of specific behaviours. Aetiological factors that have a small effect on behaviour may have a large effect on cognition, physiology or anatomy. These intermediaries between aetiology and phenomenology are known as endophenotypes.

The example of cognitive deficit and hyperactivity will clarify the approach. On average, hyperactive individuals perform poorly on a wide range of cognitive tasks compared to their normally developing peers (Chapter 7; Swanson et al., 1998a). However, there is no cognitive or other laboratory measure on which every hyperactive individual performs poorly. This observation is very informative. On one hand, deficits in performance point toward the nature of the deficit underlying hyperactivity (Barkley, 1997). On the other hand, mean differences in performance on cognitive tasks between hyperactive and control groups obscure important variations among hyperactive individuals. This observation suggests that it may be possible that cognitive deficits of various kinds can be used to delineate aetiologically homogeneous subtypes of hyperactive individuals.

Swanson et al. (2000) used cognitive measures of inhibition taken in the laboratory to dissect the genetic aetiology of ADHD. Poor inhibition as measured in various laboratory paradigms is considered to be one of the hallmarks of hyperactivity. They demonstrated that the subgroup of ADHD subjects with poor inhibitory control were less likely to be associated with the DRD4 dopamine receptor gene even though that association has been found commonly among ADHD individuals in general. Crosbie and Schachar (2001) compared ADHD children with and without observed deficit on a laboratory measure of inhibitory control. These investigators found that ADHD individuals with poor inhibition were four times more likely to have a first-degree family member with ADHD than an otherwise similar group of ADHD individuals without poor inhibition. Taken together, these two studies suggest that deficient inhibition may be a marker for a particularly heritable subtype of ADHD but one which may not be mediated by the presence of the dopamine receptor gene abnormality. These studies also demonstrate the potential for understanding hyperactivity that can be gained from examining subgroups based on pathophysiology, cognitive deficit or other endophenotypes.

Conclusions

Hyperactivity is often portrayed as an arbitrary, unreliable and invalid diagnostic entity that adds nothing to or even obscures our understanding of children with disruptive behaviour disorders. However, available evidence supports an alternative view. The existing diagnosis, based as it has been largely on clinical observation and consensus, has proven to be quite useful for clinical practice and science. There do seem to be characteristics of hyperactive children that are not common to all individuals who behave in a disruptive, defiant and antisocial way. However, frequent changes in diagnostic criteria and thresholds indicate that the disorder and its diagnostic criteria are not well understood and that social, historical and professional factors play as significant a role in the evolution of the category as do clinical or scientific understanding.

Consequently, our current approach to diagnosis and classification may not optimally support emerging scientific developments in the study of hyperactivity as scientists search for specific causes in subgroups of affected individuals. The power to detect cause or treatment in any study of hyperactivity depends on the rigor with which the diagnostic groups are defined and selected. There are several threats to the validity of the diagnosis of hyperactivity arising from lack of reliability and validity in the measurement and definition of constituent symptoms, uncertainty in the delineation of necessary and sufficient criteria and the possibility of phenocopies arising from comorbidity and various aeti-ologies. Moreover, different diagnostic traditions have arisen and reflect par-ticular views about the balance between psychosocial and biological influences in the genesis of hyperactivity. If progress in understanding hyperactivity is to be made, new empirical approaches to establishing diagnostic criteria will be necessary. These approaches promise to yield a taxonomy based on a clearer understanding of aetiology.

The clinical and scientific approaches to classification will continue to interact. The role of future taxonomic research will be to 'bootstrap' a clinically and aetiologically valid nosology (Cronbach and Meehl, 1955). The scientific understanding of hyperactivity requires a precise and aetiologically informative method of diagnosis. Otherwise, groups of affected individuals will be so heterogeneous as to obscure potentially important connections between cause and clinical presentation. On the other hand, the development of a more informed clinical taxonomy must await a better understanding of causal fac-tors.

The debate about the categorical and quantitative views of hyperactivity has been illuminating. In the absence of clear knowledge of aetiology, the choice between discrete and continuous models of psychopathology may have to be guided by subjective and pragmatic considerations. For example, categorical approaches are effective for communications, for the development of public policy and probably for treatment planning. However, categorical approaches may obscure the presence of multiple disorders, quantitative differences among individuals (ADHD vs. HD) and the impairment found among individuals who are below potentially arbitrary diagnostic thresholds (Angold et al., 1999). Quantitative approaches may be useful in research where they are particularly powerful in data analysis. However, quantitative approaches are awkward for communications, are less effective for describing comorbidity and may obscure categorical differences among individuals.

Newer approaches such as those involving sensitivity/specificity analysis, latent cluster analysis or endophenotypes may play an increasingly important role in refining diagnostic criteria. However, these techniques are not without their limitations (Hartman et al., 1999). Until scientifically rigorous criteria are developed, progress may require an internationally agreed-upon set of diagnos-tic measures, informants and criteria for research. These criteria should require diagnosis of distinct entities rather than overlapping ones such as currently occur. For example, HD and DAMP are subsets of ADHD. Studies of ADHD will have one outcome if they include many children with HD and another one if they do not. Consequently, the results of research will be obscured if investigators do not describe their sample according to specific and agreed criteria that are mutually exclusive.

Moreover, the nature, source and reliability of the behaviour measures that subserve these diagnoses must be specified. Given current knowledge of the situational and subjective nature of hyperactivity, there seems little point in diagnostic procedures that do not include information from parents and teachers and from converging measurement procedures (questionnaires and interviews). Exactly how to combine information from multiple informants is a problem that remains to be tackled. Similarly, the diagnostic criteria and methods that are optimal for very young children, adolescents and adults are yet to be clarified (Lahey et al., 1998). Much needs to be done to improve diagnostic practice in clinical settings. Substantial variation among clinicians in diagnostic practice exists and probably leads to inconsistency in the type of individuals who receive the diagnosis (Wolraich et al., 1998; Miller, 1999).

Even though a narrowly defined syndrome of HD applies to few children, it seems to have the greatest construct validity and seems to be an important target for scientific study. However, the requirements of a scientifically informative category are not the same as those for a clinically useful one. It is not immediately clear that the narrow approach to defining hyperactivity is appropriate from a public health perspective where it may be advantageous to identify for targeted interventions all children at some degree of risk rather than the small group of children who carry the greatest risk. Nature cannot yet be carved precisely at the joints that separate all disturbed from all undisturbed individuals. Raising the threshold may be too restrictive. While it would lower the prevalence of hyperactivity, it would miss some significantly impaired children.

REFERENCES

Achenbach, T.M., McConaughy, S.H. and Howell, C.T. (1987). Child/adolescent behavioral and emotional problems: implications of cross-informant correlations for situational specificity. *Psychological Bulletin*, **101**, 213–32.

Achenbach, T.M., Conners, C.K., Quay, H.C., Verhulst, F.C. and Howell, C.T. (1989). Replication of empirically derived syndromes as a basis for taxonomy of child/adolescent psychopathology. *Journal of Abnormal Child Psychology*, **17**, 299–323.

American Psychiatric Association. (1968). *DSM-II: Diagnostic and Statistical Manual of Mental Disorders*, 2nd edn. Washington, DC: American Psychiatric Association.

American Psychiatric Association. (1980). *DSM-III: Diagnostic and Statistical Manual of Mental Disorders*, 3rd edn. Washington, DC: American Psychiatric Association.

American Psychiatric Association. (1987). *Diagnostic and Statistical Manual of Mental Disorders (DSM-III-R)*. Washington, DC: American Psychiatric Association.

American Psychiatric Association. (1994). *Diagnostic and Statistical Manual of Mental Disorders (DSM-IV)*. Washington, DC: American Psychiatric Association.

Angold, A., Costello, E.J., Farmer, E.M., Burns, B.J. and Erkanli, A. (1999). Impaired but undiagnosed. *Journal of the American Academy of Child and Adolescent Psychiatry*, **38**, 129–37.

Applegate, B., Lahey, B.B., Hart, E.L. et al. (1997). Validity of the age-of-onset criterion for ADHD: a report from the DSM-IV field trials. *Journal of the American Academy of Child and Adolescent Psychiatry*, **36**, 1211–21.

Babinski, L.M., Hartsough, C.S. and Lambert, N.M. (1999). Childhood conduct problems, hyperactivity-impulsivity, and inattention as predictors of adult criminal activity. *Journal of Child Psychology and Psychiatry*, **40**, 347–55.

Barkley, R.A. (1997). Behavioral inhibition, sustained attention, and executive functions: constructing a unifying theory of ADHD. *Psychological Bulletin*, **121**, 65–94.

Barkley, R.A. (1998). Attention-deficit hyperactivity disorder. *Scientific American*, **279**, 66–71.

Barkley, R.A. and Biederman, J. (1997). Toward a broader definition of the age-of-onset criterion for attention-deficit hyperactivity disorder. *Journal of the American Academy of Child and Adolescent Psychiatry*, **36**, 1204–10.

Biederman, J., Faraone, S.V., Mick, E. et al. (1999). Clinical correlates of ADHD in females: findings from a large group of girls ascertained from pediatric and psychiatric referral sources. *Journal of the American Academy of Child and Adolescent Psychiatry*, **38**, 966–75.

Boyle, M.H., Offord, D.R., Racine, Y. et al. (1996). Identifying thresholds for classifying childhood psychiatric disorder: issues and prospects. *Journal of the American Academy of Child and Adolescent Psychiatry*, **35**, 1440–8.

Bradley, C. (1937). The behavior of children receiving benzedrine. *American Journal of Psychiatry*, **94**, 577–85.

Brandeis, D., van Leeuwen, T.H., Rubia, K. et al. (1998). Neuroelectric mapping reveals precursor of stop failures in children with attention deficits. *Behavioural Brain Research*, **94**, 111–25.

Buitelaar, J.K. and van Engeland, H. (1996). Epidemiological approaches. In *Hyperactivity Disorders of Childhood*, S. Sandberg, ed., pp. 26–68. Cambridge: Cambridge University Press.

Burns, G.L., Walsh, J.A., Patterson, D.R. et al. (1997). Internal validity of the disruptive behavior disorder symptoms: implications from parent ratings for a dimensional approach to symptom validity. *Journal of Abnormal Child Psychology*, **25**, 307–19.

Cantwell, D.P. and Baker, L. (1992). Attention deficit disorder with and without hyperactivity: a review and comparison of matched groups. *Journal of the American Academy of Child and Adolescent Psychiatry*, **31**, 432–8.

Chess, S. (1960). Diagnosis and treatment of the hyperactive child. *New York State Journal of Medicine*, **60**, 2379–85.

Clements, S.D. (1966). *Minimal Brain Dysfunction in Children: Terminology and Identification: Phase One of a Three-Phase Project*. Washington, DC: US Department of Health, Education and Welfare.

Conners, C.K., Wells, K.C., Parker, J.D. et al. (1997). A new self-report scale for assessment of adolescent psychopathology: factor structure, reliability, validity, and diagnostic sensitivity. *Journal of Abnormal Child Psychology*, **25**, 487–97.

Cronbach, L.J. and Meehl, P.E. (1955). Construct validity in psychological tests. *Psychological Bulletin*, **52**, 281–302.

Crosbie, J.M. and Schachar, R.J. (2001). Inhibition defines a familial subgroup of attention-deficit/hyperactivity disorder. *American Journal of Psychiatry*, in press.

Douglas, V.I. (1972). Stop, look and listen: the problem of sustained attention and impulse control in hyperactive and normal children. *Canadian Journal of Behavioral Science*, **4**, 259–82.

Eaves, L.J., Silberg, J.L., Meyer, J.M. et al. (1997). Genetics and developmental psychopathology: 2. The main effects of genes and environment on behavioral problems in the Virginia Twin Study of Adolescent Behavioral Development. *Journal of Child Psychology and Psychiatry*, **38**, 965–80.

Eiraldi, R.B., Power, T.J. and Nezu, C.M. (1997). Patterns of comorbidity associated with subtypes of attention-deficit/hyperactivity disorder among 6- to 12-year-old children. *Journal of the American Academy of Child and Adolescent Psychiatry*, **36**, 503–14.

Faraone, S.V., Biederman, J., Keenan, K. and Tsuang, M.T. (1991). Separation of DSM-III attention deficit disorder and conduct disorder: evidence from a family-genetic study of American child psychiatric patients. *Psychological Medicine*, **21**, 109–21.

Faraone, S.V., Biederman, J., Sprich-Buckminster, S., Chen, W. and Tsuang, M.T. (1993). Efficiency of diagnostic criteria for attention deficit disorder: toward an empirical approach to designing and validating diagnostic algorithms. *Journal of the American Academy of Child and Adolescent Psychiatry*, **32**, 166–74.

Faraone, S.V., Biederman, J., Jetton, J.G. and Tsuang, M.T. (1997). Attention deficit disorder and conduct disorder: longitudinal evidence for a familial subtype. *Psychological Medicine*, **27**, 291–300.

Faraone, S.V., Biederman, J., Mennin, D., Russell, R. and Tsuang, M.T. (1998a). Familial subtypes of attention deficit hyperactivity disorder: a 4-year follow-up study of children from antisocial-ADHD families. *Journal of Child Psychology and Psychiatry*, **39**, 1045–53.

Faraone, S.V., Biederman, J., Weber, W. and Russell, R.L. (1998b). Psychiatric, neuropsychological, and psychosocial features of DSM-IV subtypes of attention-deficit/hyperactivity disorder: results from a clinically referred sample. *Journal of the American Academy of Child and Adolescent Psychiatry*, **37**, 185–93.

Fergusson, D.M. and Horwood, L.J. (1995). Predictive value of categorically and dimensionally scored measures of disruptive childhood behaviors. *Journal of the American Academy of Child and Adolescent Psychiatry* **34**, 477–85.

Fischer, M., Barkley, R.A., Fletcher, K.E. and Smallish, L. (1993). The adolescent outcome of hyperactive children: predictors of psychiatric, academic, social, and emotional adjustment. *Journal of the American Academy of Child and Adolescent Psychiatry*, **32**, 324–32.

Frick, P.J., Lahey, B.B., Applegate, B. et al. (1994). DSM-IV field trials for the disruptive behavior disorders: symptom utility estimates. *Journal of the American Academy of Child and Adolescent Psychiatry*, **33**, 529–39.

Gillberg, C. (1998). Hyperactivity, inattention and motor control problems: prevalence, comorbidity and background factors. *Folia Phoniatrica et Logopedica*, **50**, 107–17.

Gillberg, I.C. and Gillberg, C. (1988). Children with deficits in attention, motor control and perception (DAMP): need for specialist treatment. *Acta Paediatrica Scandinavica*, **77**, 450–1.

Gomez, R., Harvey, J., Quick, C., Scharer, I. and Harris, G. (1999). DSM-IV AD/HD: Confirmatory factor models, prevalence, and gender and age differences based on parent and teacher ratings of Australian primary school children. *Journal of Child Psychology and Psychiatry*, **40**, 265–74.

Halperin, J.M., O'Brien, J.D., Newcorn, J.H. et al. (1990). Validation of hyperactive, aggressive, and mixed hyperactive/aggressive childhood disorders: a research note. *Journal of Child Psychology and Psychiatry*, **31**, 455–9.

Hartman, C.A., Hox, J., Erol, N. et al. (1999). Syndrome dimensions of the Child Behavior Checklist and the Teacher Report Form: a critical empirical evaluation. *Journal of Child Psychology and Psychiatry*, **40**, 1095–116.

Hechtman, L. and Weiss, G. (1986). Controlled prospective fifteen year follow-up of hyperactives as adults: non-medical drug and alcohol use and anti-social behaviour. *Canadian Journal of Psychiatry*, **31**, 557–67.

Ho, T.P., Luk, E.S., Leung, P.W. et al. (1996). Situational versus pervasive hyperactivity in a community sample. *Psychological Medicine*, **26**, 309–21.

Hudziak, J.J., Heath, A.C., Madden, P.F. et al. (1998). Latent class and factor analysis of DSM-IV ADHD: a twin study of female adolescents. *Journal of the American Academy of Child and Adolescent Psychiatry*, **37**, 848–57.

Kadesjo, B. and Gillberg, C. (1998). Attention deficits and clumsiness in Swedish 7-year-old children. *Developmental Medicine and Child Neurology*, **40**, 796–804.

Kahn, E. and Cohen, L.H. (1934). Organic drivenness: a brain-stem syndrome and an experience with case reports. *New England Journal of Medicine*, **210**, 748–56.

Kalverboer, A.F. (1975). *A Neurobehavioural Study in Preschool Children*. Philadelphia: Lippincott.

Kalverboer, A.F. (1993). Neurobehavioural relationships in children: new facts, new fictions. *Early Human Development*, **34**, 169–77.

Klein, R.G., Abikoff, H., Klass, E. et al. (1997). Clinical efficacy of methylphenidate in conduct disorder with and without attention deficit hyperactivity disorder. *Archives of General Psychiatry*, **54**, 1073–80.

Lahey, B.B. and Carlson, C.L. (1991). Validity of the diagnostic category of attention deficit disorder without hyperactivity: a review of the literature. *Journal of Learning Disabilities*, **24**, 110–20.

Lahey, B.B., Pelham, W.E., Stein, M.A. et al. (1998). Validity of DSM-IV attention-deficit/hyperactivity disorder for younger children. *Journal of the American Academy of Child and Adolescent Psychiatry*, **37**, 695–702.

Landgren, M., Pettersson, R., Kjellman, B. and Gillberg, C. (1996). ADHD, DAMP and other neurodevelopmental/psychiatric disorders in 6-year-old children: epidemiology and co-morbidity. *Developmental Medicine and Child Neurology*, **38**, 891–906.

Laufer, M.W., Denhoff, E. and Solomons, G. (1957). Hyperkinetic impulse disorder in children's behavior problems. *Psychosomatic Medicine*, **19**, 38–49.

Leung, P.W., Ho, T.P., Luk, S.L. et al. (1996a). Separation and comorbidity of hyperactivity and conduct disturbance in Chinese schoolboys. *Journal of Child Psychology and Psychiatry*, **37**, 841–53.

Leung, P.W., Luk, S.L., Ho, T.P. et al. (1996b). The diagnosis and prevalence of hyperactivity in Chinese schoolboys. *British Journal of Psychiatry*, **168**, 486–96.

Levy, F., Hay, D.A., McStephen, M., Wood, C. and Waldman, I. (1997). Attention-deficit hyperactivity disorder: a category or a continuum? Genetic analysis of a large-scale twin study. *Journal of the American Academy of Child and Adolescent Psychiatry*, **36**, 737–44.

Loeber, R., Brinthaupt, V. and Green, S. (1990). Attention deficits, impulsivity, and hyperactivity with or without conduct problems: relationships to delinquency and unique contextual factors. In *Behavior Disorders of Adolescence: Research, Intervention, and Policy in Clinical and School Settings*, R.J. McMahon and R. de V. Peters, eds, pp. 39–61. New York: Plenum Press.

Mannuzza, S., Klein, R.G., Bessler, A., Malloy, P. and LaPadula, M. (1998). Adult psychiatric status of hyperactive boys grown up. *American Journal of Psychiatry*, **155**, 493–8.

McKeith, R. and Bax, M. (1963). *Minimal Cerebral Dysfunction: Papers from the International Study Group held at Oxford, September 1962*. Little Club Clinics in Developmental Medicine, no. 10. London: Heinemann.

Meehl, P.E. (1995). Bootstraps taxometrics. Solving the classification problem in psychopathology. *American Psychologist*, **50**, 266–75.

Milberger, S., Faraone, S.V., Biederman, J., Testa, M. and Tsuang, M.T. (1996). New phenotype definition of attention deficit hyperactivity disorder in relatives for genetic analyses. *American Journal of Medical Genetics*, **67**, 369–77.

Milich, R. and Fitzgerald, G. (1985). Validation of inattention/overactivity and aggression ratings with classroom observations. *Journal of Consulting and Clinical Psychology*, **53**, 139–40.

Miller, A. (1999). Appropriateness of psychostimulant prescription to children: theoretical and empirical perspectives. *Canadian Journal of Psychiatry*, **44**, 1017–24.

Moffitt, T.E. (1990). Juvenile delinquency and attention deficit disorder: boys' developmental trajectories from age 3 to age 15. *Child Development*, **61**, 893–910.

Mota, V.L. and Schachar, R.J. (2000). Reformulating attention-deficit/hyperactivity disorder according to signal detection theory. *Journal of the American Academy of Child and Adolescent Psychiatry*, **39**, 1144–51.

Nadder, T.S., Silberg, J.L., Eaves, L.J., Maes, H.H. and Meyer, J.M. (1998). Genetic effects on ADHD symptomatology in 7- to 13-year-old twins: results from a telephone survey. *Behavior Genetics*, **28**, 83–99.

Nichols, P.L. and Chen, T.-C. (1981). *Minimal Brain Dysfunction: A Prospective Study*. Hillsdale, NJ: Erlbaum.

Ounsted, C. (1955). The hyperkinetic syndrome in epileptic children. *Lancet*, **2**, 303–11.

Ozonoff, S., Strayer, D.L., McMahon, W.M. and Filloux, F. (1994). Executive function abilities in autism and Tourette syndrome: an information processing approach. *Journal of Child Psychology and Psychiatry*, **35**, 1015–32.

Pasamanick, B., Rogerrs, M.E. and Lilienfeld, A.M. (1956). Pregnancy experience and the development of behavior disorders in children. *American Journal of Psychiatry*, **112**, 613–18.

Pennington, B.F., Grossier, D. and Welsh, M.C. (1993). Contrasting cognitive deficits in attention deficit hyperactivity disorder versus reading disability. *Developmental Psychology*, **29**, 511–23.

Porrino, L.J., Rapoport, J.L., Behar, D. et al. (1983). A naturalistic assessment of the motor activity of hyperactive boys. I . Comparison with normal controls. *Archives of General Psychiatry*, **40**, 681–7.

Prendergast, M., Taylor, E., Rapoport, J.L. et al. (1988). The diagnosis of childhood hyperactivity. A US–UK cross-national study of DSM-III and ICD-9. *Journal of Child Psychology and Psychiatry*, **29**, 289–300.

Quay, H.C., Routh, D.K. and Shapiro, S.K. (1987). Psychopathology of childhood: from description to validation. *Annual Review of Psychology*, **38**, 491–532.

Rubia, K., Overmeyer, S., Taylor, E. et al. (1999). Hypofrontality in attention deficit hyperactivity disorder during higher-order motor control: a study with functional MRI. *American Journal of Psychiatry*, **156**, 891–6.

Rutter, M. (1978). Diagnostic validity in child psychiatry. *Advances in Biological Psychiatry*, **2**, 2–22.

Rutter, M., Graham, P., Yule, W. and Birch, H. (1970a). *A Neuropsychiatric Study in Childhood*. London: Spastics International Medical Publications / Heinemann Medical.

Rutter, M., Tizard, J. and Whitmore, K. (1970b). *Education, Health and Behaviour*. London: Longmans.

Sandberg, S., Day, R. and Trott, G.E. (1996). Clinical aspects. In *Hyperactivity Disorders of Childhood*, S. Sandberg, ed., pp. 69–110. Cambridge: Cambridge University Press.

Schachar, R. (1991). Childhood hyperactivity. *Journal of Child Psychology and Psychiatry*, **32**, 155–91.

Schachar, R. and Logan, G.D. (1990). Impulsivity and inhibitory control in normal development and childhood psychopathology. *Developmental Psychology*, **26**, 710–20.

Schachar, R. and Tannock, R. (1995). Test of four hypotheses for the comorbidity of attention-deficit hyperactivity disorder and conduct disorder. *Journal of the American Academy of Child and Adolescent Psychiatry*, **34**, 639–48.

Schachar, R., Sandberg, S. and Rutter, M. (1986). Agreement between teachers' ratings and observations of hyperactivity, inattentiveness, and defiance. *Journal of Abnormal Child Psychology*, **14**, 331–45.

Sergeant, J.A. (1995). Hyperkinetic disorder revisited. In *Eunethydis: European Approaches to Hyperkinetic Disorder*, J. Sergeant, ed., pp. 7–17. Zürich: Fotorator, Egg.

Sergeant, J. (2000). The cognitive-energetic model: an empirical approach to attention-deficit hyperactivity disorder. *Neuroscience and Biobehavioral Reviews*, **24**, 7–12.

Sergeant, J. and Steinhausen, H.-Ch. (1992). European perspective on hyperkinetic disorder. *European Child and Adolescent Psychiatry*, **1**, 34–41.

Sergeant, J.A. and Van der Meere, J.J. (1994). Toward an empirical child psychopathology. In *Disruptive Behavior Disorders in Childhood*, D.K. Routh, ed., pp. 59–85. New York: Plenum Press.

Shaffer, D. (1978). 'Soft' neurological signs and later psychiatric disorder – a review. *Journal of Child Psychology and Psychiatry*, **19**, 63–5.

Shaffer, D., Schwab-Stone, M., Fisher, P. et al. (1993). The Diagnostic Interview Schedule for Children – Revised Version (DISC-R): I. Preparation, field testing, interrater reliability, and acceptability. *Journal of the American Academy of Child and Adolescent Psychiatry*, **32**, 643–50.

Shalev, R., Hartman, C.A., Stavsky, M. and Sergeant, J.A. (1995). Conners rating scales of Israeli children. In *Eunethydis: European Approaches to Hyperkinetic Disorder*, J. Sergeant, ed., pp. 131–47. Zurich: Fotorator, Egg.

Still, G.F. (1902). The Coulstonian lectures on some abnormal psychical conditions in children. *Lancet*, **1**, 1008–12; 1077–82; 1163–8.

Strauss, A.A. and Lehtinen, L.E. (1947). *Psychopathology and Education of the Brain-Injured Child*, vol. I. New York: Grune and Stratton.

Strauss, A.A., Kephart, N.C., Lehtinen, L.E. and Goldenberg, S. (1955). *Psychopathology and Education of the Brain-Injured Child*, vol. II. New York: Grune and Stratton.

Swanson, J., Castellanos, F.X., Murias, M., LaHoste, G. and Kennedy, J. (1998a). Cognitive neuroscience of attention deficit hyperactivity disorder and hyperkinetic disorder. *Current Opinion in Neurobiology*, **8**, 263–71.

Swanson, J.M., Sergeant, J.A., Taylor, E. et al. (1998b). Attention-deficit hyperactivity disorder and hyperkinetic disorder. *Lancet*, **351**, 429–33.

Swanson, J., Oosterlaan, J., Murias, M. et al. (2000). Attention deficit/hyperactivity disorder children with a 7-repeat allele of the dopamine receptor D4 gene have extreme behavior but normal performance on critical neuropsychological tests of attention. *Proceedings of the National Academy of Sciences of the United States of America*, **97**, 4754–9.

Szatmari, P., Boyle, M. and Offord, D.R. (1989a). ADDH and conduct disorder: degree of diagnostic overlap and differences among correlates. *Journal of the American Academy of Child and Adolescent Psychiatry*, **28**, 865–72.

Szatmari, P., Offord, D.R. and Boyle, M.H. (1989b). Ontario Child Health Study: prevalence of attention deficit disorder with hyperactivity. *Journal of Child Psychology and Psychiatry*, **30**, 219–30.

Szatmari, P., Offord, D.R., Siegel, L.S., Finlayson, M.A. and Tuff, L. (1990). The clinical significance of neurocognitive impairments among children with psychiatric disorders: diagnosis and situational specificity. *Journal of Child Psychology and Psychiatry*, **31**, 287–99.

Taylor, E. (1998). Clinical foundations of hyperactivity research. *Behavioural Brain Research*, **94**, 11–24.

Taylor, E., Chadwick, O., Heptinstall, E. and Danckaerts, M. (1996). Hyperactivity and conduct problems as risk factors for adolescent development. *Journal of the American Academy of Child and Adolescent Psychiatry*, **35**, 1213–26.

Taylor, E., Sandberg, S., Thorley, G. and Giles, S. (1991). *The Epidemiology of Childhood Hyperactivity*. Maudsley Monographs no. 33. Oxford: Oxford University Press.

Taylor, E., Sergeant, J., Doepfner, M. et al. (1998). Clinical guidelines for hyperkinetic disorder. European Society for Child and Adolescent Psychiatry. *European Child and Adolescent Psychiatry*, **7**, 184–200.

Thapar, A., Hervas, A. and McGuffin, P. (1995). Childhood hyperactivity scores are highly heritable and show sibling competition effects: twin study evidence. *Behavior Genetics*, **25**, 537–44.

Tredgold, A.F. (1908). *Mental Deficiency (Amentia)*. New York: W. Wood.

Tripp, G. and Luk, S.L. (1997). The identification of pervasive hyperactivity: is clinic observation necessary? *Journal of Child Psychology and Psychiatry*, **38**, 219–34.

Tripp, G., Luk, S.L., Schaughency, E.A. and Singh, R. (1999). DSM-IV and ICD-10: a comparison of the correlates of ADHD and hyperkinetic disorder. *Journal of the American Academy of Child and Adolescent Psychiatry*, **38**, 156–64.

Tsuang, M.T., Faraone, S.V. and Lyons, M.J. (1993). Identification of the phenotype in psychiatric genetics. *European Archives of Psychiatry and Clinical Neuroscience*, **243**, 131–42.

Urman, R., Ickowicz, A., Fulford, P. and Tannock, R. (1995). An exaggerated cardiovascular response to methylphenidate in ADHD children with anxiety. *Journal of Child and Adolescent Psychopharmacology*, **5**, 29–37.

Wolraich, M.L., Hannah, J.N., Pinnock, T.Y., Baumgaertel, A. and Brown, J. (1996). Comparison of diagnostic criteria for attention-deficit hyperactivity disorder in a county-wide sample. *Journal of the American Academy of Child and Adolescent Psychiatry*, **35**, 319–24.

Wolraich, M.L., Hannah, J.N., Baumgaertel, A. and Feurer, I.D. (1998). Examination of DSM-IV criteria for attention deficit/hyperactivity disorder in a county-wide sample. *Journal of Developmental and Behavioral Pediatrics*, **19**, 162–8.

Woodward, C.A., Thomas, H.B., Boyle, M.H., Links, P.S. and Offord, D.R. (1989). Methodologic note for child epidemiological surveys: the effects of instructions on estimates of behavior prevalence. *Journal of Child Psychology and Psychiatry*, **30**, 919–24.

World Health Organization (1992). *ICD-10: Classification of Mental and Behavioural Disorders*. Geneva: World Health Organization.

Wozniak, J., Biederman, J., Kiely, K. et al. (1995). Mania-like symptoms suggestive of childhood-onset bipolar disorder in clinically referred children. *Journal of the American Academy of Child and Adolescent Psychiatry*, **34**, 867–76.

6

The role of attention

Jaap J. Van der Meere

Laboratory of Experimental Clinical Psychology, University of Groningen, Groningen, the Netherlands

The goal of this chapter is to present a review of research into attentional aspects of hyperactivity disorder. Before starting with the review, some issues, which are not mutually exclusive, will be discussed. The issues concern the appropriateness of the paradigms commonly used to study attention and the accuracy of the methods of identifying hyperactivity in children.

Many attempts have been made to validate the clinical concept of hyperactivity disorder in the laboratory. However, since the manifestation of the primary symptoms of hyperactivity (inattention, impulsivity and overactivity) largely depend on the types of environments in which the child is observed, the laboratory approach may be criticized because of the limited range of situations in which the child's behaviour is studied. In addition, experimental task demands may be highly sophisticated, so that extensive training is needed before the actual experiment can start. Moreover, in order to keep the child 'on the track', he or she is commonly not left to perform the task alone. When all these factors are taken into account, it could be argued that the symptoms of hyperactivity may have been 'filtered out' by the time the laboratory experiment starts. Consequently, one may question the extent to which an attention deficit in hyperactivity disorder, as indicated by teachers and parents and defined by clinical diagnostic procedures, can be accounted for by laboratory data.

Barkley (1991) examined the degree of ecological validity of laboratory experiments of hyperactivity. In his attempt to formulate a set of ecological criteria he was forced to rely primarily on parent and teacher ratings of symptoms because so few studies were available for comparing the laboratory findings with direct observations in natural settings. Since, in general, low correlations are reported between laboratory measures of attention, impulsivity and activity on the one hand and teacher and parent ratings on the other, one may conclude that laboratory experiments have little ecological validity. However this argument is not without problems.

First, it is doubtful whether parent and teacher ratings are the gold standard for ecological validity, since parents and teachers may use undifferentiated concepts in their subjective ratings. This has been demonstrated by Vaessen and Van der Meere (1990). They showed that many children rated by their teachers as hyperactive were in fact clumsy, as measured by the Test of Motor Impairment (Stott et al., 1984), or learning-disabled, as measured by a Dutch revised version of the Primary Mental Ability Test (Thurstone, 1938). Furthermore, learning-disabled and clumsy children were rated as hyperactive by their parents and/or observers during standardized laboratory observations. Hence, low correlations between laboratory measures and hyperactivity ratings by parents and teachers may reflect the heterogeneity of hyperactive samples under study instead of reflecting the degree of the ecological validity of laboratory measures per se. This brings us to the problem of the appropriateness of selection procedures. As already mentioned, key behaviours of hyperactive children vary across situations. A number of studies suggest that a child may be hyperactive at home but not at school or vice versa, or hyperactive at home and school but not in a third situation (Lambert et al., 1978; Sandberg et al., 1978; Schachar et al., 1981). If both the teacher and the parents consider the child to be hyperactive, the child may be described as showing pervasive hyperactivity. If only one of the informants considers the child hyperactive, the child is considered to show situational hyperactivity. Methodologically speaking, the degree of agreement is not obvious unless it is clear which part of the variance between teachers and parents is explained by the child's behaviour pattern and which part of the variance is accounted for by the variability and individual response bias of the teachers and parents themselves. If this requirement is met then the disagreement between sources of information is not necessarily a problem. In fact, agreement/disagreement between informants may provide important information about severity of the symptoms, and is therefore an essential factor needing to be clarified in sample selection procedures. With the exception of the study by Rapoport et al. (1986), differences between situational and pervasive hyperactivity have been reported for the age of onset of hyperactivity, neurodevelopmental immaturities, task accuracy (Sandberg et al., 1978), prognosis (Schachar et al., 1981), motor impulsivity (Cohen and Minde, 1983), activity level, attention, minor neurological deficits (Luk et al., 1991) and for stimulant drug response (Pliszka, 1989). Given these findings, the low correlations between laboratory measures and ratings of hyperactivity, as meant by Barkley, may be largely due to lack of differentiation between children with situational and pervasive hyperactivity. In order to get a better grip on the issue of situational and pervasive hyperactivity, however, we must go further than the school–home comparison which remains an oversimplification of discrimination of childhood behaviour. Following Barkley's advice (1982), it would seem more useful to refer to the occurrence of hyperactive behaviour within multiple defined settings. It is suggested here that clustering of hyperactive cases around different situational dimensions (such as highly structured vs. free play, and social interaction vs. alone) may be a way of identifying subgroups of hyperactive children.

Second, there is the problem of comorbidity and its influence on group selection. A number of studies have demonstrated that hyperactivity disorder shows considerable overlap with conduct disorder, depression and anxiety disorders (including posttraumatic stress disorder), learning disorders, Gilles de la Tourette syndrome and others. Maurer and Stuart (1980), for instance, reported that 80% of a clinical sample of children with hyperactivity disorder had at least one other psychiatric disorder. Although the extent of comorbidity is dependent on the range and reliability of the instruments used (Vaessen and Van der Meere, 1990), there is no doubt about its existence. It is reasonable to assume that the low correlations between laboratory measures and ratings of hyperactivity are at least partly due to this comorbidity. Hence the optimal design in cognitive research is the comparison of hyperactive children varying in degree of pervasiveness of the symptoms, with the type(s) of comorbidity studied clearly specified. The Research Diagnostic Criteria (RDC) as proposed by Sergeant (1988a) are a good starting point. These criteria are designed for research in which precisely defined groups are required for a meaningful interpretation of data. However, one may argue that in clinical practice it is inappropriate to select subjects on the basis of strict criteria because care should be given to all children who need it. Nevertheless, it can be argued that diagnosis for clinical as well as for research purposes will benefit from the choice of a model in which the dimensions of deviant behaviour are most clearly highlighted (Vaessen and Van der Meere, 1990).

So far, the argument has concerned the fact that correlations between laboratory measures of cognition and parent and teacher ratings of hyperactivity have generally been low because of the heterogeneity and the comorbidity of the samples used in the studies. The next question concerns the type of hyperactive behaviour that is relevant to be studied in the laboratory condition, and the appropriateness of the tasks most frequently used to study these behaviours.

As stated before, parents and teachers consider hyperactive children as inattentive, overactive and impulsive. Barkley (1990) suggests that, in ranking the importance of the primary symptoms, greater weight should be given to impulsivity and overactivity, rather than to attention, in conceptualizing the disorder. However, content overlap between items is clearly the case and it is doubtful whether entirely distinct constructs of attention, activity and impulsivity can unequivocally be operationalized in terms of observable behaviour in the laboratory (Dienske and Sanders-Woudstra, 1988). Furthermore, since parent and teacher evaluations are liable to be subjective, it may be the case that neither evaluation reflects the child's actual behaviour in the specific (school or home) situation, rather than being based on global impressions (Lambert et al., 1978), with the result that attention and activity are often indistinguishable and treated as one factor (McGee et al., 1984). Hence, it is safe to conclude that the exact relationship between activity, impulsivity and inattention is unknown for the moment. Part of this problem stems from the so-called 'lack of positive transfer' between research approaches. Overactivity has been studied using the ethological approach in a wide range of situations: at school, at home and in the laboratory (for review, see Barkley, 1990), without any reference to cognitive abilities. Cognitive abilities have been studied primarily in the laboratory, using traditional tests such as the Matching Familiar Figures (MFF) test, Porteus Mazes, Figures Embedded Test and Stroop, but again without reference to the overt behaviour of the child during experimentation. Thus, it seems that there is a gap to be bridged not only between subjective teacher and parent reports on the one hand and laboratory measures on the other, but also between research traditions themselves.

Moreover, as has been argued elsewhere (Sergeant and Van der Meere, 1989, 1990a,b) these traditional tests (MFF, Porteus Mazes, Figures Embedded Test, Stroop, etc.) can be seen as only the 'first generation' of cognitive tests. These tests measure a complex web of cognitive abilities. As a consequence, poor task performance may be caused by numerous and unknown factors which make test results difficult to interpret. The author has reason to believe that the 'information-processing approach' may be more helpful in the identification of the assumed cognitive deficits of hyperactive children. The main advantage of this approach is that cognition is unravelled in its elementary parts, thus making it possible to locate more precisely the assumed cognitive (attention) deficit in a particular clinical condition. Regarding the question of ecological validity, the author believes that the combination of attention assessments, based on the information-processing approach and online systematic behavioural observations, is required in order to make teacher and parent reports more objective compared with correlating heterogeneous measures of cognitive abilities (i.e. traditional tests) with parent and teacher hyperactivity questionnaire ratings (Kalverboer, 1990; Alberts and Van der Meere, 1992). (For a

more detailed discussion about information-processing theory and its ecological relevance the reader is referred to Sergeant and Van der Meere (1994).)

The author now wishes to proceed with a review of research into cognitive
aspects of hyperactivity disorder. The review is centred around the state/
process distinction as it is presented in recent models of information-processing
theory (Sanders, 1983; Mulder, 1986). The state/process distinction can best be
conceptualized as a continuum (Hockey et al., 1986). Processes are defined as
discrete and short-term events (elementary operations) that mediate between
stimulus and response. State fluctuations are not directly involved in information processes but modulate the elementary operations. Important state factors
are time on task, incentives, feedback and presence/absence of the experimenter. Although there are no generally agreed methods of distinguishing between
direct effects on elementary cognitive operations and indirect effects via energetic (state) mechanisms, it is assumed that basic attention abilities, such as
orienting and selective attention, are best studied if factors that influence the
subject's state are kept as constant as possible during experimentation. Hence,
tasks purporting to measure such abilities have to be short, and training as well
as the presence of the experimenter are needed (Gaillard, 1978). The results of
this type of investigation are evaluated in the first section of the review. The
concept of impulsivity in hyperactivity disorder will be discussed in the second
section. The influence of state factors on task performance is the theme of the
third section, and the fourth section reviews psychophysiological attention
research in hyperactivity disorders.

In a salutary paper by Taylor (1983), the relationship between drug response
and diagnostic validity of hyperactivity disorder was critically examined. Taylor
pointed out that methylphenidate (MPH) has not provided the favourable
outcome that one would wish to see from an effective therapy. Even in the face
of the awe-inspiring results of the USA Multicenter Study (MTA Cooperative
Group, 1999), the British perspective, as put forward by Taylor (1998), holds its
critical position. However, this drug has shown short-term effects on task
performance. If the employment of information-processing paradigms points in
a certain direction with respect to the processing deficiency of the hyperactive
child, and if drug action specifically affects this processing deficiency, then these
findings together may be considered at least as converging evidence. Therefore, in every section where an attention construct is to be discussed, the results
regarding hyperactivity disorder will be linked with MPH studies whenever
possible. (For a more indepth discussion about MPH and laboratory findings,
the reader is referred to Sergeant and Van der Meere, 1999.)

Basic attention abilities

One main characteristic of the hyperactive child is task inefficiency. Whether this task inefficiency is caused by attentional dysfunctions, such as orientation, reorientation, encoding, focused and divided attention abilities, is the central theme of this first section. For the purposes of this section, error scores and reaction times are defined as the dependent variables of the tasks.

Orientation

There is ample evidence that spatial cues are very important for organizing and guiding attention (Posner, 1988). In this type of study cues can be informative (valid), noninformative (invalid) or neutral. The typical finding is that reaction time (RT) for detection is faster on valid trials than on neutral trials, and slower on invalid trials than on neutral trials. These two effects are often referred to as the benefits and costs of allocating attention.

Studies using cuing techniques have revealed that hyperactive and control children are not different in the time taken to direct attention towards cues (Pearson and Lane, 1990). Moreover, hyperactive children show the same level of benefits in the valid cue position, and RT costs in the invalid cue position, as controls (Burke, 1990; Swanson et al., 1990). Besides varying the type of cues (valid, invalid and neutral), Burke (1990) and Swanson et al. (1990) have also varied the temporal relation between cue and target (the stimulus-onset asynchrony or SOA). Both studies reported that hyperactive children made more errors only with long SOA intervals. Hence, SOA and not cuing is the crucial factor in hyperactivity disorder. The question of SOA, i.e. presentation rate of events and hyperactivity disorder, will be further discussed in the third section of this chapter. However, Karatekin and Asarnov (1998) examining ballistic eye movements (saccadic RT) showed that attention deficit hyperactivity disorder (ADHD) children were delayed in initiating of (visual) serial search which may indicate that ADHD children are slow at moving their attention from one item to the next.

Reorientation

In the study referred to above, Pearson and Lane (1990) also compared hyperactive and nonhyperactive children for the time required to 'get back on track after switching gears' in a dichotic listening task. Subjects were instructed to detect targets in the message received by one ear and to ignore the message received by the other ear. After about 10 s, a signal instructed them either to remain on the same ear or else to reorient to the other ear. The onset of the target series varied from 0.5 to 3.5 s. Once the hyperactive children were thrown off course by the switch, they never reoriented. This was especially so at longer delay intervals. Hence, the results of this study also indicate that the rate of presentation of events is a crucial factor in studying attention deficits in hyperactivity disorder.

The effect of switching attention between modalities in hyperactive and nonhyperactive children was studied by Zahn et al. (1991). In their task, subjects were instructed to respond to a tone with the right hand and to a light with the left hand. Reaction times were sorted by preceding stimulus: ipsi-modal sequences (tone–tone; light–light) were compared to cross-modal (tone–light; light–tone) sequences. No group differences were found with respect to either type of sequence.

Information uptake

Information uptake, or encoding, can be subdivided into three types: that of codes at the physical, name and semantic level. Theoretically, each dimension forces the individual to process the stimulus at a different cognitive level, or depth, in order to perform the task accurately (Craik and Lockhard, 1972). Three types of encoding tasks have been used to study hyperactivity disorder. The first is Sternberg's (1969) stimulus degradation task. In this task, children are required to identify targets in a target-degraded and a target-nondegraded condition. Encoding time is defined as the difference in response latency between the degraded and nondegraded condition. The second is the 'depth-of-processing task' (Craik and Lockhard, 1972). Here, an incidental recall task for the stimulus words is given immediately following the encoding phase. Craik and his colleagues have argued that information which is more extensively (deeply) processed will leave a relatively stronger memory trace and is more likely to be recalled in a free recall task. It is assumed that the fewer errors, the more deeply the information has been processed. The third is Posner's letter-matching task (Posner and Mitchell, 1967). Under physical identity (PI) match-ing, subjects are instructed to indicate when two letters look exactly the same (a–a). Under name identity (NI) matching, subjects are instructed to indicate when the two letters have the same name (A–a). Encoding time is defined here as the difference in response latency between the PI and the NI conditions.

The three types of encoding tasks have failed to show differences between hyperactive and control children at the various levels of encoding (Ballinger et al., 1984; Peeke et al., 1984; Reid and Borkowski, 1984; Sergeant and Scholten, 1985a; Benezra and Douglas, 1988; Borcherding et al., 1988; Malone et al., 1988; Balthazor et al., 1991). The results can also be taken to indicate that MPH and *d*-amfetamine (the treatments of choice in hyperactivity disorder) have no effects on encoding, with only one exception (Weingartner et al., 1980). Thus, the available evidence seems to rule out encoding as the attentional deficit in hyperactivity disorder. In fact, it has been demonstrated many times that the basic abilities of encoding and retrieval of verbal and nonverbal information are intact in hyperactivity disorder (Douglas, 1983). However, there is some evidence that hyperactive children have problems in encoding stimuli presented in parallel (Wilding, 1994). Also a study by Douglas and Benezra (1990) suggested that deficits especially become apparent on word lists requiring organized and deliberate rehearsal strategies. This can be explained in terms of impaired self-regulatory processing. The matter of self-regulatory processing will be further discussed in the third section of the chapter.

Focused attention

Focused attention in the visual modality in hyperactivity disorder has been studied by Van der Meere and Sergeant (1988a). In this study the subjects were instructed to pay attention to the top-left to bottom-right (relevant) diagonal of a display but to ignore the other (irrelevant) diagonal. In half of the trials a target appeared in the relevant diagonal and a 'yes' response was required. A 'no' response was required if the target was not presented in the relevant diagonal. Foils were presented in fewer than 10% of the trials in the relevant diagonal. A focused attention deficit could be assumed if responses to foils were more pronounced in the hyperactive group than in peer controls. This was not the case: that is to say, hyperactive children responded to foils to the same extent as the control group did. Hence, this study demonstrated that hyperactive children are not abnormally distractible. In addition, an MPH study by De Sonneville et al. (1991), using the same focused attention paradigm, demonstrated that the error rate for foil signals did not improve during treatment with MPH.

Focused attention in the auditory modality has been studied using the dichotic listening task. Here, subjects are instructed to focus attention to one ear and to ignore the stimulus presented at the other ear. No differences in task performance between hyperactive and control children have been found in this type of task (Davidson and Prior, 1978; Douglas and Peters, 1979; Pelham, 1979). Only with a high event rate has the dichotic listening task differentiated hyperactive children from controls (Loiselle et al., 1980). Hence, not focused attention but, again, event rate seems to play a crucial role in the attentional performance of children with hyperactivity disorder.

In fact, there are a surprising number of failures in the attempts to show that hyperactive children are abnormally distractible (for an extensive review, see Douglas, 1983). On the contrary, many studies using external distractors (radio music, noise, etc.) have shown that hyperactive children are not hindered but may in fact benefit from this type of distraction during test performance (Browning, 1967; Zentall et al., 1978). This was confirmed by Abikoff et al. (unpublished). They reported that hyperactive children working on an arithmetic task produced significantly more correct responses under a music condition than in a speech or silence condition. The finding that hyperactive children benefit from distraction has led to the formulation of the self-stimulation hypothesis in hyperactivity disorder (Zentall and Zentall, 1983; Zentall and Meyer, 1987). This issue will be further discussed in the third section of this chapter.

Capacity

Capacity refers to the idea that the cognitive system is limited by the availability of central processing capacity. Two paradigms have been used to measure information-processing capacity in hyperactive children. The first is the double-task paradigm. Here, subjects are instructed to divide their attention between two simultaneous tasks. According to this paradigm, limitations arise when two mental tasks have to be performed at the same time. The first assumption of the paradigm is that task efficiency is positively related to the amount of available resources. The second assumption is that tasks, when performed simultaneously, will compete for processing resources. Only when groups do not differ in performance on the primary task, and when performance on the primary task does not vary as result of load manipulations on the secondary task, can performance on the secondary task be interpreted as reflecting the resources remaining after those needed for the primary task have been expended. If these requirements are met, then it is justified to interpret greater impairment of secondary task performance of the hyperactive group in terms of a smaller attentional capacity.

The dual-task paradigm has been employed in hyperactivity research by Schachar and Logan (1990a). In their study the primary task was a simple forced-choice reaction time task. The letters O and X were presented on a screen. Subjects were instructed to respond by pressing corresponding response buttons, mapped with O and X, with the fingers of the left hand. The secondary task, which involved a 55-dB tone of 100 ms duration, required the subjects to respond by pressing a third key with a finger of the right hand. The tone was generated on half of the trials. The temporal overlap between the onset of the primary and secondary task was varied. Schachar and Logan argued that the greater the temporal overlap, the less the capacity left for the secondary task and the greater the secondary task response delay. This study indicated that the extent of interference between the primary and secondary tasks, over the range of temporal overlap, was the same in hyperactive children and controls. Consequently, it was concluded that hyperactive children do not have a deficient information-processing capacity.

The dual-task paradigm has also been used in so-called ecologically relevant task conditions. In the Vaessen (1990a) study, the primary task was walking over a balance beam. The secondary task involved pressing a button attached to either the left or right thumb, in response to a high- or a low-pitched tone respectively. No difference in the secondary task performance between hyperactive and control children was observed. In another study by the same author (Vaessen, 1990b), the primary task was a traffic task. The experimental location was set up on a pavement near a road with medium to high traffic intensity (400–700 vehicles per hour). The child started at an imaginary curb and had to cross over a distance of 9 m to the other curb, representing the opposite side of the imaginary road. The latter curb was at a safe distance of 4 m from the real road. The child had an adequate view of the traffic on the real road. Hence, real traffic was used as stimulus material, and the child had to cross the imaginary street in the same way and with the same time interval as when crossing the real street. The secondary task was a digit recall task. The digits had to be memorized during the period in which the child had to observe the traffic and detect a suitable gap. The digits were to be repeated by the child on reaching the other side of the imaginary road. It was emphasized that the child should cross as soon as the last car he or she had been waiting for had passed. It appeared that, particularly in a difficult recall condition, hyperactive children consistently accepted shorter gaps in the traffic to cross the street. The results could be interpreted as indicating that the primary task interacted with the secondary task, and therefore, the requirements of the dual-task paradigm were not fully met in this study. Consequently, no direct conclusions in terms of capacity limitations may be drawn from this particular experiment.

Another capacity measure employed in hyperactivity research is the Sternberg (1969) memory recognition task. Here subjects are instructed to divide attention between simultaneously presented input. Increasing the cognitive load (consonant letters) will lead to slower processing. This is reflected in a linear increase in reaction time. This increase, in turn, is an index of the information-processing capacity (Sanders, 1983). Following this paradigm, a limitation in capacity could be assumed in hyperactivity disorder if, because of cognitive overload, the increase in reaction time and errors were more pronounced in the hyperactive group than in peer controls. With one exception (Leung and Connolly, 1994) a number of studies have indicated that this is not the case with children either currently suffering from hyperactivity or with those with a past diagnosis of hyperactivity disorder (Sergeant and Scholten, 1983, 1985a; Coons et al., 1987; Van der Meere and Sergeant, 1987; Van der Meere et al., 1989).

One reason why studies have failed to show that ADHD children have difficulty processing high loads may be due to a floor effect, i.e. the task complexity has generally been low with memory or visual search loads of up to four items. In this respect, a study by Bergman et al. (1999) is of importance. Here ADHD children (free from medication) were compared with a normal control group on a high-load Sternberg memory search task with memory loads of one, two and four items and visual search loads of four, nine and 16. However, in spite of the high cognitive load, this study also failed to demonstrate that complexity is a crucial factor in ADHD. The findings are consistent with results from the above-mentioned studies using the Sternberg paradigm.

Evidence in favour of the idea that children with ADHD are not hindered by limited attentional capacity is also provided by Hazell et al. (1999). The researchers used automatic and effortful cognitive tasks of parallel and sequential processing described by Treisman and Gelade (1980). They showed that ADHD children do have attentional capacity in reserve, enabling them to improve on their performance under feedback and reward conditions. Only children with learning difficulties appeared to have a reduced attentional capacity. The same conclusion was drawn by Van der Meere and colleagues using the Sternberg paradigm: LD children have a divided attention deficit, whereas ADHD children have poor response organization processes (Van der Meere et al., 1989).

Consequently, three different paradigm findings demonstrate that hyperactive children have no capacity problem. Two MPH studies have likewise indicated that capacity measures, as defined in terms of both the dual-task paradigms and the Sternberg paradigm, are not affected by the stimulant drug (Carlson et al., 1991; De Sonneville et al., 1991). In contrast to this negative finding, the afore-mentioned study of Bergman et al. (1999) indicated that a wide range of MPH doses helped children to improve accuracy with no cost to RT, whereas on high loads, higher MPH doses improved error rates while slowing RT. Hence, MPH enabled ADHD children to adapt differently to high and low loads.

In summary, the majority of studies have failed to demonstrate that children suffering from hyperactivity disorder have an inability in orienting, reorienting, encoding, focused attention or divided attention. The argument that it is the paradigm itself that may account for the negative findings does not hold, given that cuing techniques (Akhtar and Enns, 1989), distraction tasks (Enns and Girgus, 1985), and capacity measures (Kail, 1990) are sensitive to age. The work in this area has also brought to light information-processing deficits in various clinical groups other than those suffering from hyperactivity. (For a review see Sergeant and Van der Meere (1990a,b).)

Motor-related processes

There is some evidence that task inefficiency of hyperactive children is caused by dysfunctional processes located at the output (motor) side of information processing. Sergeant and Van der Meere (1988) reported that during a visual search task, hyperactive children corrected their errors as frequently as the control children did but failed to adjust their response speed after a mistake. In a subsequent visual search study by Van der Meere et al. (1989), hyperactive children were instructed to react either in the direction of the target location (i.e. a compatible response) or in the opposite direction from the target location (i.e. an incompatible response). The finding of delayed incompatible responses of hyperactive children was interpreted in terms of a motor decision problem. Also, the finding that presentation rate of stimuli play a crucial role in the attentional performance of children with hyperactivity disorder points in the direction of a motor-related dysfunction given that motor timing/preparation is more difficult with either a fast or a slow event rate of stimuli. Event rate has been shown to play a crucial role during orientation, reorientation and dichotic listening tasks (discussed above) and in paired associate learning tasks (Dalby et al., 1977; Conte et al., 1986), and visual search tasks (Chee et al., 1989; Van der Meere et al., 1992, 1995a). Also, the study by Zahn et al. (1991) revealed that hyperactive children have difficulties with motor timing/preparation. In this study reaction times were examined while varying the length and regularity of the preparatory intervals. The results showed that, in the regular series, reaction times were delayed more at long intervals for the hyperactive group. In the irregular series, an additional effect was reported. The findings indicate a greater lack of preparation of the hyperactive group on trials on which a shorter interval is followed by a long interval. Problems of motor timing/preparation of hyperactive children have also been reported by Cappella et al. (1977).

Since experimental findings using RT paradigms point in the direction of an information-processing deficiency in hyperactivity disorder being located at the output side of the information processing, it is important to note first, that a positive influence by MPH on response processes has been demonstrated by

Frowein (1981) in adults and by De Sonneville et al. (1991) in children, and second, that in order to get some grip on the nature of the cognitive deficits associated with ADHD and related disorders, it is extremely important that instruments are used which are able to differentiate between cognitive input and output processes. This argument may be illustrated by discussing a paper of Leung and Connolly (1996). The researchers intended to investigate distractibility in ADHD and conduct-disordered children. For this purpose, they used a modified version of the Stroop test. Leung and Connolly admitted that the process underlying the Stroop effect is still the subject of debate (i.e. the Stroop interference effect may be located at the stimulus input side or motor output side (response competition)). Therefore, two types of distractors were used: distractors that evoke response competition and distractors that were believed not to evoke response competition because there were no corresponding keys for them. It appeared that ADHD children reacted slower and were more variable to stimuli during both types of distraction. Consequently, the design of the study did not allow the researchers to disentangle input- from output-related processes. Having said this, the 'motor hypothesis' highlights the admonishment by Douglas (1983) that researchers should not neglect the long history of clinical and research interest in motor control deficiencies in hyperactive children. Motor control and impulsivity is the theme of the next section.

Motor control and impulsivity

Impulsivity is a loosely defined concept in the literature concerning hyperactivity disorder. The concept includes, among others, social responsibility, risk taking and task-inappropriate responding (Taylor, 1989). The present review focuses on the concept of task-inappropriate responding.

Many procedures for operationalizing impulsivity in terms of task-inappropriate responding have been developed in the laboratory. A current operationalization of impulsivity consists of fast but inaccurate responding on tests such as the MFF Test, the Children's Embedded Figure test, The Wisconsin Card Sorting Test, the Porteus Mazes, the Stroop and errors of commission on the Continuous Performance Test (CPT). As stated earlier, these tests are not appropriate measures in describing the mechanisms underlying task inefficiency (defined here as fast but inaccurate responding). That is to say, poor performance on these tests may reflect any combination of poor quality of information processing such as hasty scanning of the stimulus material, rapid decision making or lack of planning and/or difficulties in response inhibition per se. In addition, the test findings are rather inconsistent (for review, see

Barkley et al., 1992). Many information-processing studies show that hyperactive children are slow-inaccurate performers rather than fast-inaccurate performers (Van der Meere and Sergeant, 1987, 1988a,b,c; Van der Meere et al., 1989, 1991, 1992). Moreover, hyperactive children tend to slow down even when they are asked to perform as quickly as possible (Stevens et al., 1970; Pelham, 1979; Kalverboer and Brouwer, 1983; Milich and Kramer, 1985; Sergeant and Scholten, 1985b). Hence, impulsivity defined as fast-inaccurate responding has little validity in hyperactivity disorder.

The ability to withhold responses to distractors

With some exceptions (McIntyre et al., 1978; Rosenthal and Allen, 1980; Zentall and Shaw, 1980; Ceci and Tisman, 1984), the plethora of studies using external distractors (radio music, noise, colour discrepancy, peripheral pictures, foils, etc.) have failed to show that hyperactive children are unable to withhold responses to distractors (for review, see Douglas, 1983; Van der Meere and Sergeant, 1988a). On the contrary, task performance of hyperactive children may even improve in the presence of a distractor (see the section on focused attention, above). Consequently, the concept of impulsivity, defined in terms of distractibility, has little validity in hyperactivity disorder. In addition, the findings suggest that hyperactive children are able to generate an internal stop signal and subsequently withhold responding, if required.

Ability to inhibit a response after a stop signal

In children suffering from hyperactivity disorder this ability has been measured using the stop task of Logan et al. (1984). This involves engaging the subjects in a forced-choice letter discrimination task with the need to respond to an occasional stop signal. The signal instructs the subjects to inhibit their response. The main independent variable of the stop task is the interval between the stop signal and response signal. If the stop signal occurs early enough, all subjects are able to inhibit. Plotting the probability of inhibition against the stop signal delay generates an 'inhibition function'. Schachar and Logan (1990b) were the first in a row to publish demonstrating that the slope of the inhibition function is much flatter in hyperactive children than in the controls. This finding was confirmed by seven other studies using the stop signal paradigm. Oosterlaan et al. (1998) carried out a metaanalysis concerning these studies and argued that it is unlikely that poor response inhibition in externalizing disorders (ADHD and conduct disorder) is associated with intellectual functioning. MPH has been shown to improve response inhibition in the stop task (Tannock et al., 1989).

The stop signal paradigm has produced interesting findings. However, it is questionable whether the stop task findings reflect an inability to withhold responding in hyperactive children. The stop signal paradigm assumes a race between the response signal process and the stop signal process. Stopping or responding depends upon which process will win the race. The proportion of responses which escape inhibition increases with the stop signal delay. Consequently, the stop signal findings in studies of hyperactive children may be explained in terms of a slow motor inhibition instead of a failure to inhibit responding per se. There are three reasons to assume that this possibility is more likely. First, there is increasing evidence that children with hyperactivity disorder are slow motor processors (see the first section). Second, there is increasing evidence that hyperactive children are able to withhold responses to distractors (see above). And third, experimental findings indicate that hyperactive children, like their peer controls, are able to inhibit automatized responses if they are instructed to do so (Van der Meere and Sergeant, 1988a). Further evidence that it is more appropriate to interpret the stop signal findings in terms of slow motor processing than inhibition comes from a subsequent study of Van der Meere et al. (1996). In this study, the author and his colleagues investigated whether children are able to stop and change a response set if required. This executive control function was examined using a variant of Sternberg's memory search paradigm which includes a response bias. The task consisted of two response probability conditions – a baseline condition and a response bias condition. In the baseline condition the target probability was 50%. In the response bias condition the target probability was 30%. Subjects were required to press a 'yes' response button if a target appeared on a screen. Otherwise a 'no' response was required. Specifically, the response bias condition required executive control involving both the ability to adjust a response set towards the most frequent response type, while at the same time being able to stop and change the response set if the infrequent response type was required. If hyperactive children lack executive control then fast inaccurate responding would be expected in the response bias condition. This was not the case. The findings indicate that, although slower, children with hyperactivity were comparable with their controls in their ability to stop and change their response set in the response bias condition. Hence, this study gave no indication of hasty scanning or difficulty in the 'stop and change' response set in the hyperactive group. This finding is comparable with the findings of the reorienting and dual task experiments, as discussed earlier, which have indicated no problems in switching from one course of action to another.

In summary, the repeated finding that ADHD children show a low probability of inhibition while executing the stop signal paradigm may be due either to slowness of processing the stop signal or slowness of reacting to the stop signal which, in turn, are both reflections of the motor output hypothesis in ADHD (see section on motor-related processes, above). This suggestion was adopted by Rubia et al. (1998) and Oosterlaan and Sergeant (1998), when interpreting their stop signal findings.

Ability to withhold responding in order to receive reinforcement

The Differential Reinforcement of Low-rate responding (DRL) procedure was devised to measure this construct (Gordon, 1979). In this test the subjects are instructed to respond after a set time interval in order to receive reinforcement. Gordon (1979) and McClure and Gordon (1984) showed that hyperactive children are unable to withhold responding, as evidenced by the large number of anticipatory responses. However, Daugherty and Quay (1991) and Loge et al. (1990) reported no differences in DRL performance between hyperactive and normal children. Apart from such inconsistencies in findings, one may question how far the anticipatory responding of hyperactive children totally reflects an inability to delay gratification. If it does, then hyperactive children may be expected to make more anticipatory responses during reinforcement than during response cost conditions. Solanto (1990) showed, however, that the number of anticipatory responses during DRL in hyperactive and in control children is equally affected by reinforcement and response costs. Furthermore, it has been suggested that hyperactive children delay averse responses rather than are impulsive or reward-maximizers (Sonuga-Barke et al., 1992). The findings of Roth et al. (1991) are also of importance with respect to this issue. In order to measure the efficacy of inhibitory motor processes they used the Delayed Motor Reaction Time Task (Leubuscher and Roth, 1983). Like the DRL, this task requires the suppression of an immediate response to an imperative signal. After presentation of a visual signal (white bar) on the video screen, a delayed (800 ms) motor response is required. Correctness of the delay is fed back by auditory signals. The more accurate the delay of the motor response, the smaller the time window becomes (range 600–150 ms). The results indicated that children with signs of allergy (about half of the sample showing symptoms of hyperactivity disorder) performed with less temporal stability than the controls. However, it is to be noted that since less temporal stability of performance was observed in the absence of reinforcement, the results are at odds with the delayed gratification hypothesis but are compatible with the motor deficiency hypothesis as put forward by the author and his colleagues. Last but not least, a stop signal study by Oosterlaan and Sergeant (1998) also showed that ADHD children were equally impaired in their capability to inhibit motor responses in both a reward and response costs condition, suggesting that ADHD seems to involve a fundamental motor organization deficit, and that reward is not a crucial factor in this respect.

The sensation-seeking component of impulsivity seems to offer a more promising explanation. Daugherty and Quay (1991) administered a response perseveration task and the DRL task to groups of children with hyperactivity and related disorders. The performance of the subjects differed on the perseveration task but not on the DRL. The perseveration task consisted of a series of doors presented sequentially in a preprogrammed order of winning and losing doors. The probability of a winning door appearing decreased by 10% with each succeeding set of 10 doors. The dependent measure was the total number of doors opened before giving up. The results supported the hypothesis that subjects suffering from conduct disorder or conduct disorder with hyperactivity would perseverate while responding to a game in which the probability of winning decreases as the game is played. For a review of the inability to withhold responding in so-called risk-taking conditions in hyperactivity disorder, see Douglas (1983).

In summary, the studies reviewed seem to indicate that it is rather questionable whether hyperactive children, strictly speaking, suffer from an inability to withhold responses. Given the findings that hyperactive children are delayed in their response-related processes, it may be concluded that the motor hypothesis is not covered by the impulsivity concept of fast-inaccurate responding. The author and his colleague Sergeant (Sergeant and Van der Meere, 1989, 1990a,b) have argued that a state regulation problem may account for loss of motor control. The findings of Daugherty and Quay (1991) may also be interpreted in terms of a state regulation dysfunction. The concept of state regulation dysfunction in children suffering from hyperactivity disorder is the theme of the following section.

The concept of state

A nonoptimal arousal state has a long tradition as a physiological mechanism underlying hyperactivity (for review, see Douglas, 1983). According to this theory, in order to normalize their arousal level, hyperactive children require stimulants, benefit from extraneous distraction and are sensation seekers (Zentall and Zentall, 1983). However, it requires to be pointed out here that the 'unitary state' concept in cognitive psychology has in the past been criticized for the following two main reasons. First, the unidimensionality and nonspecificity of arousal cannot explain the lack of correlation between different measures of energy mobilization. Second, the unitary state concept of arousal gives no clarification of the different patterns of autonomic activity observed in subjects during different tasks (Lacey, 1967). This dissatisfaction has led to the postulation of a variety of cognitive multistate models. Although there remain a fundamental set of questions concerning the basis of energetical constructs in psychophysiology, anatomy and biochemistry of the brain and the nervous system (Hockey et al., 1986), there are strong arguments for distinguishing arousal and activation as different physiological states. Tucker and Williamson (1984) have suggested that arousal and activation are concerned respectively with the alerting effect of sensory activity and the control of motor readiness. Arousal is located in the frontolimbic forebrain and activation in the basal ganglia (Pribram and McGuinness, 1975). Important neurotransmitters in the arousal system are noradrenaline (norepinephrine) and serotonin. The primary neurotransmitters in the activation system are dopamine and acetylcholine (Tucker and Williamson, 1984). In addition, arousal and activation are affected by different drugs, e.g. barbiturates affect arousal whereas amfetamine affects activation (Frowein, 1981).

Pribram and McGuinness (1975), Mulder (1986) and Sanders (1983) have postulated a third energetic system – the effort system. This system, in turn, is under the control of an evaluation system (Sanders, 1983). The latter mechanism scans the subject's arousal and activation state. A suboptimal state as identified by the evaluation mechanism may be compensated for by effort. The hippocampus is believed to be involved in such compensatory control (Pribram and McGuinness, 1975; Gray, 1982). The effort mechanism is influenced by motivational factors such as knowledge of results, absence/presence of the experimenter and payoff. Figure 6.1 presents the Sanders model.

The model has received support from the results of neural network simulation studies (Molenaar and Van der Molen, 1986), developmental studies (Van der Molen, 1990) and psychophysiological studies (Mulder, 1986; see section on psychophysiological measures, below). Therefore, the multistate approach may be of great value in future studies since it may help to specify the assumed cognitive deficits in hyperactivity disorder (Sergeant and Van der Meere, 1989, 1990a,b).

Using the model of Sanders (Figure 6.1), task inefficiency in children with hyperactivity disorder may be considered to be caused by limitations located at the elementary level of information processing, or at the state level, or in a combination of both levels. In the first section of this chapter, a variety of tasks

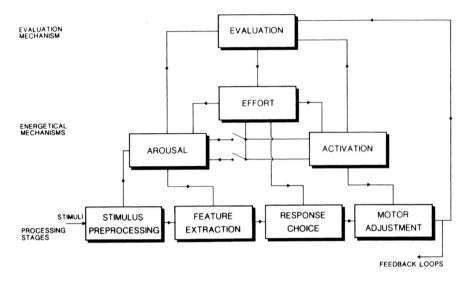

EVALUATION
MECHANISM

ENERGETICAL
MECHANISMS

STIMULI

PROCESSING
STAGES

FEEDBACK LOOPS

Figure 6.1   The Sanders model.

considered to measure the efficiency of information processing at the first level of the model were discussed. These tasks are characterized by short duration, lack of use of incentives and by children working in the presence of an experimenter. Hence, it may be assumed that in these experiments the influence of state factors has been kept as constant as possible. The evidence available so far suggests that hyperactive children have a deficit on the motor side of the information-processing chain. The motor-processing deficit manifests itself as slow-inaccurate responding, instead of fast-inaccurate responding. These are unexpected findings in so-called impulsive children (see section on motor control and impulsivity, above). Consequently, another explanation is needed to account for the hypothesized motor-processing dysfunction in hyperactive children. The author believes that the postulation of deficit in the regulation of activation/effort is a good working hypothesis. As can be seen from Figure 6.1, the Sanders model connects motor processes with the effort/ activation state of the subject. Hence, in terms of the model, it is possible that the motor dysfunction in hyperactive children actually involves an activation/ effort dysfunction. This would mean that hyperactive children respond slowly and inaccurately because of a 'state' condition which is inadequate. Four types of state manipulations will be discussed: time on task, presentation rate of stimuli, payoff and absence/presence of the experimenter.

State regulation and sustained attention

A deficit in sustained attention is considered to be the prime characteristic of hyperactivity disorder (Douglas, 1983). The consistent finding of poor performance on a CPT, characterized by the detection of fewer targets and more omissions, is generally considered as proof of the assumed sustained attention deficit. However, as the author has pointed out elsewhere (Van der Meere and Sergeant, 1988b), the main argument against this interpretation is that an 'overall' CPT performance difference between hyperactive and control children is not sufficient for validation, since a sustained attention deficit implies a deficit originating during the course of the task. Consequently, a sustained attention deficit is only demonstrated when hyperactive children show a greater decline in performance over a period of time than the controls do.

According to the literature on vigilance (for review, see Van der Meere and Sergeant, 1988b) there are two different types of sustained attention deficits, depending on whether time on task exerts its influence on arousal or activation. The factor considered responsible for the performance decline depends in turn on the task parameters of the vigil. If the subject is required to discriminate a target from a nontarget represented in working memory at a high event rate, then arousal is affected. If few working memory processes are involved and the event rate is low, the performance decrement is thought to result from changes in the activation level.

CPTs with a fast event rate of stimuli

So far, the majority of CPT studies in hyperactivity disorder have employed a high event rate. Hence, in terms of the vigilance paradigm these studies have tested the arousal hypothesis. With four exceptions (Sykes et al., 1973; Dykman et al., 1979; Seidel and Joschko, 1990; Hooks et al., 1994), the plethora of studies show that in a wide variety of prolonged tasks, initial differences in task accuracy between hyperactive children and controls are present right from the beginning; however, more important is the finding that hyperactive children do not differ from the controls in terms of decline in task performance in the course of the task (Michael et al., 1981; Nuechterlein, 1983; O'Dougherty et al., 1984, 1988; Prior et al., 1985; Schachar et al., 1988; Sergeant, 1988b; Van der Meere and Sergeant, 1988b; Kupietz, 1990; Leung and Connolly, 1994; McLaren, unpublished; Solanto et al., unpublished). The findings of Rapoport et al. (1980) are also important with respect to this issue. They reported a comparable time decrement effect and improvement in performance by *d*-amfetamine in hyperactive, control children and college students over time.

Hence, according to the model of Sanders, hyperactive children do not suffer from a sustained attention deficit in terms of an inadequate arousal state.

So far, sustained attention abilities have been discussed in terms of the extent of decline in task efficiency over time under conditions with a fast presentation rate of stimuli. However, the finding that, in conditions with a fast presentation rate of stimuli, hyperactive children and controls do not differ in either the rate of acquisition of a divided attention skill in a testing period of 6 h (Van der Meere and Sergeant, 1988c) nor in the rate of changing that skill measured in focused attention conditions (Van der Meere and Sergeant, 1988a) is at odds with the assumed sustained attention deficit in hyperactivity disorder. Furthermore, school-like paper-and-pencil tasks which are self-paced have failed to differentiate between hyperactive and normal children in terms of performance decline in the course of the task (Van der Meere et al., 1991; Gunning, 1992).

CPTs with a slow presentation rate of stimuli

The author and his colleagues have tested the underactivation hypothesis in hyperactivity disorder using a slow event rate vigilance task. In our first experiment, the task was performed during experimenter-present and experimenter-absent conditions. Two hypotheses were proposed. First, if hyperactive children have a sustained attention deficit, they will exhibit a greater decrement in performance over time than the control group. Second, if motivational factors are responsible for the deficit, the decrement in task performance will be minimal during the experimenter-present condition and maximal during the experimenter-absent condition. Both hypotheses were confirmed in this experiment. That is to say, the sustained attention deficit was prominent in hyperactive children, especially while working in the absence of the experimenter. This finding supports the underactivation/effort hypothesis in hyperactivity disorder and underlines the need for external control in such children (Barkley, 1991). The same study demonstrated that the deficit disappears when hyperactive children are placed on MPH medication (Van der Meere et al., 1995c). Using the same CPT, a positive effect of MPH on sustained attention was found with epileptic children with ADHD (Gross-Tsur et al., 1997). Studies by Draeger et al. (1986) and Power (1992) have likewise reported that the task efficiency (and activity) level of hyperactive children is sensitive for experimenter presence/absence. However, the drawback of the former study was that it did not examine the effects of experimenter presence and absence over a noninterrupted period of time. The latter study did not include a control group, and hence, it cannot be known whether the reported findings are specific for hyperactivity disorder. Gomez and Sanson (1994) compared attentional performance of hyperactive children with and without conduct disorder on a cancellation task under three conditions: when performing the task alone, with mother present and with the experimenter present. Results indicated that attentional scores of hyperactive children with conduct disorder were normalized when the experimenter was present; this was not so marked for hyperactive children without conduct disorder. Unfortunately, no reference was made concerning time on task, but this study also underlines the importance of external control in hyperactivity.

In the second experiment of the author and his colleagues, hyperactive children with and without conduct disorder were compared on the slow event rate vigilance task performed under reward and nonreward conditions. Both groups of children were receiving medication: MPH was the predominant medication in the pure hyperactive group, whereas tricyclics, lithium and carbamazepine were more frequently used in the mixed group. The results indicated that, in spite of the active treatment, the children suffering from the mixed disorder showed a deficit of sustained attention in the nonreward condition. In the reward condition the deficit disappeared for a short period of time. This finding suggests that children with a mixed hyperactivity-conduct disorder suffer from an activation/effort disturbance. No difference in task performance was found between children with a pure hyperactivity disorder and the controls. It can therefore be argued that MPH improved the CPT performance of the hyperactive children to the level found in normal children (Van der Meere et al., 1995b).

In summary, whether the CPT is a valuable research tool for use with children with ADHD (Corkum and Siegel, 1993) depends on a few factors: the evidence available so far indicates that hyperactive children do not suffer from a sustained attention deficit in prolonged task conditions when stimuli are presented at a high rate of sequence, or when the children are allowed to adapt their own speed of performing. According to the model of Sanders, these negative findings do not support the presence of an arousal deficiency in hyperactivity disorder. However, a sustained attention deficit does emerge in hyperactive children in CPT conditions when a slow presentation rate is used. In children with hyperactivity without conduct disorder, this is especially the case in conditions of experimenter absence. In children with a mixed hyperactivity and conduct disorder, this is especially the case in the absence of reward. According to the model of Sanders, these positive findings are in favour of a nonoptimal activation state as a physiological basis of hyperactivity disorder and support the idea that the motor hypothesis in hyperactive children, as discussed in the first section, is in fact reflecting a nonoptimal activation state.

With respect to the discriminant validity of the above-mentioned findings, it must be emphasized that children with an early treated congenital hypo-thyroidism show poor sustained attention abilities irrespectively of specific CPT characteristics, which seems to be the case in ADHD children (Kooistra et al., 1996). A CPT study in which RT performance of children with a nonverbal learning disability were compared with ADHD children without a learning deficit showed that the sustained attention problems in ADHD children prog-ressed over time, whereas the RT performance of the learning-disabled group was poor right from the start of the CPT, indicating that the mental steps needed to fulfil the test requirements are badly organized independently of energetical factors (Landau et al., 1999).

So far, the focus of this section has been on changes of task accuracy over time. The theme of the next section is changes of activity level over time.

Activity level during CPT performance

Unfortunately, observational studies of hyperactive children's behaviour dur-ing CPT are scarce. Sykes et al. (1971) reported an increased restlessness between first and second test sessions in hyperactive children when compared to controls. Their results seem to suggest that hyperactive children are more restless when required to perform the same task twice. It is, however, not possible to know whether the increased activity in the second session was due to difficulties in sustained attention or due to differences in recovery of activity level between the sessions. Draeger et al. (1986) reported that, in the absence of the experimenter, task accuracy was lower and activity level higher in the hyperactive group. Unfortunately, the activity level was not measured in a noninterrupted condition, but, as in the study by Sykes et al. between success-ive conditions. Hence, studies have failed to show that hyperactive children become more restless in the course of a noninterrupted period. Alberts and Van der Meere (1992) presented behavioural observation data of hyperactive and control children during a 36-min CPT task. Five categories of body activity were measured: automanipulations, arm, leg and trunk movements and posi-tion shifts. Visual behaviour was measured in terms of frequency and duration of looking away from the screen. The data indicated that bodily activity tended to be more pronounced in hyperactive children than in controls. More import-ant, however, was the finding that both groups showed the same increase in body movements and the same decrease in task efficiency in the course of the experiment. However, in the course of the experiment, hyperactive children did start to look away more frequently from the monitor than the controls did. An analysis of the temporal relations between (the onset and offset of) periods of looking away and the occurrence of omission errors indicated that looking away did not negatively interfere with the task performance. The authors speculated that looking away from the screen may have reflected self-stimulation in order to compensate for the assumed nonoptimal activation state of hyperactive children. This speculation was tested by Börger and van der Meere (2000b). In this study, ADHD and normal children carried out two CPTs: one with a regular Interstimulus Interval (ISI), and the other with an irregular ISI. Children were instructed to push a response button when a target stimulus was presented on the monitor. The children's visual behaviour was recorded and scored offline. A microanalysis of the visual behaviour indicated that the ADHD children timed their looking-away behaviour in the regular CPT: i.e. they looked away from the monitor and back in the interval between two succeeding stimuli. As a result, they did not miss stimuli. Timing of looking away was less possible in the CPT with the irregular ISI. In this condition, looking away interfered with the ADHD children's task accuracy. In sum, looking-away behaviour had a negative effect on the accuracy of test performance of the ADHD children when stimuli were unpredictable. Looking-away behaviour was not associated with the slower reaction times of the ADHD children. Hence, the often-reported slowness of ADHD children is not to be explained by their visual behaviour.

State regulation and impulsiveness in ADHD

Today the hallmark of ADHD seems to be a deficiency in the ability to inhibit behaviour (Barkley, 1997). A series of studies will be discussed showing that ADHD children are, in principle, able to inhibit their ongoing activities, and that the term 'poor impulse control' is best put under the umbrella of a state regulation deficit.

The first study (Van der Meere and Stemerdink, 1999) focused on the developmental trajectory of state regulation and impulse control in normal children in the age range of 7–12 years. For this purpose we developed a go–no-go test which is derived from Sanders' (1983) theory of state regulation (Figure 6.1). In this task, children were instructed to press a response button when the letter P appeared on the screen. No response was required when the letter R appeared on the monitor. Responses towards the letter R were considered an index of response inhibition. The trials were presented in three conditions with a stimulus density of 1 s (fast condition), 4 s (medium condition) and 8 s (slow condition).

According to Sanders' theory, the signal density of the go–no-go signals may alter the behavioural state of the subject, i.e. compared to the medium condition, the fast condition may induce 'overactivation', resulting in fast-inaccurate responding, whereas the slow condition may induce 'underactivation', resulting in slow-inaccurate responding. Therefore, to counteract a decrement in task efficiency, subjects have to correct their state in the fast and slow conditions. It was hypothesized that if younger children do not effectively change their state then task inefficiency will be most pronounced in the fast and slow conditions, wherein state regulation is assumed to be essential; whereas the effect of signal density on task performance will be less pronounced in older children who effectively correct their state. The hypothesis was confirmed: the effect of signal density on response inhibition was most pronounced in the youngest age group of 7–8 years. Hence, state regulation, operationalized in terms of the go–no-go measure, develops during the elementary school years, which is an important finding in view of the growing consensus that knowledge of normal developmental processes is essential to understand the nature of childhood behaviour disorders.

The second study (Van der Meere and Stemerdink, 1999) compared ADHD children without a tic disorder (TD), ADHD children with a comorbid condition and a normal control group, using our go–no-go measure. Findings indicated that ADHD children with and without TD made more errors of commission (i.e. responses to the no-go stimuli) than the normal group. This result is not new and is congruent with the results of others (Trommer et al., 1988; Shue and Douglas, 1989; Milich et al., 1994). More interesting was the finding that the task-inefficient behaviour of ADHD children, in particular those without a comorbid TD, was related to the signal rate. That is, children made many errors of commission in the fast and slow conditions, but not in the medium condition. Hence, children's lack of response inhibition reflected their inability to modulate their state according to task and situational demands. The effect of signal density on the number of errors of commission was less pronounced in the ADHD group with TD. Consequently, the inability to inhibit a response in ADHD children with TD could not be explained in terms of poor state control.

A comparison of the developmental data with the outcome of the ADHD go–no-go study of Van der Meere and Stemerdink (1999) indicated that the ability to regulate the behaviour state is delayed (2 years at least) in ADHD children.

The third study (Stemerdink et al., 1995) compared children with early and continuously treated phenylketonuria (PKU) with a normal control group. Relative to the controls, the PKU group made more errors of commission. In addition, a positive correlation was found between the task inefficiency and phenylalanine levels in the first 4 years in the PKU group. These results underscored the frontal lobe hypothesis in early-treated PKU patients, as formulated elsewhere (Stemerdink et al., 1994, 1999, 2000). For the purpose of the present chapter, the finding that the task inefficiency of the PKU children was not related to the signal density was more relevant, indicating that PKU is fairly restricted to dysfunctions in executive functioning other than the intensive part, which is the case in ADHD children.

The aim of the fourth study (Van de Meer et al., submitted), was to evaluate the association between state regulation measure and IQ. It must be underlined that IQs of the ADHD groups who participated in the studies were – although in the normal range – lower than those of the controls. Consequently, if the construct of poor state regulation in ADHD is to have any utility, then it must offer valid information regarding an individual's behaviour, beyond that which can be predicted by IQ. For this purpose, a group of mildly mentally retarded (MMR) children with and without externalizing disorders (conduct disorder and ADHD, with a mean IQ of 66) was compared with a normal peer control group using the go–no-go test.

The findings clearly demonstrate that the effect of presentation rate of signals on task performance was the same in the MMR group without externalizing disorders and in the control group, indicating that MMR is not related to a deficit in state regulation and poor response inhibition. This negative finding, in turn, indicates that the postulated state regulation deficit in ADHD is a deficit over and above the level of intelligence. Even more important was the finding that the MMR plus externalizing disorders showed poor response inhibition which was independent of the presentation rate of the go–no-go stimuli. Hence, the impulsiveness in MMR children with externalizing disorders does not mirror impulsiveness in the ADHD child with an IQ level in the normal range.

A fifth study (Van der Meere et al., 1999) evaluated the effects of MPH and clonidine in children with ADHD in terms of the go–no-go task, which may provide insight into the mechanisms of drug action. Kinsbourne (1990) distinguishes two competing hypotheses as to how medication works: normalizing and stimulus level shifts. The normalizing hypothesis proposes that deficient performance benefits from medication, while adequate performance remains unchanged. It was expected that children with ADHD would perform well during the medium condition and worse during the fast and slow conditions. Hence, according to the normalizing hypothesis, medication should have its beneficial effects specifically on performance during the fast and slow conditions without affecting the performance on the medium condition. The stimulus level shift hypothesis proposes that medication raises the baseline activation level. Consequently, according to this hypothesis, it may be expected that medication enables the children to do well during the slow condition, whereas task performance declines on the medium condition and in particular on the fast condition, which is the most activating condition.

The most important finding of the study was that the task performance of ADHD children receiving placebo, clonidine or MPH did not differ significantly. Only in the slow condition was there a (slight) beneficial effect of MPH compared to clonidine (not to placebo) for response speed (not for response accuracy). This was the case irrespective of age, IQ, type of comorbidity and the clinical response of the child (here defined in terms of opinions of parent and teacher). Consequently, the study suggests that the state regulation problem in ADHD may be resistant to MPH and clonidine. This underlines Taylor's critical position in relation to MPH and ADHD (Taylor, 1998).

In summary, there is growing evidence that the quality of impulse control of ADHD children with a normal intelligence is related to the presentation rate of go–no-go signals on display: with a fast presentation rate, children are easily overactivated; with a slow presentation rate, children are easily underactivated. Both over- and underactivation result in poor response inhibition. This finding has been interpreted in terms of poor state regulation in ADHD.

The hypothesis that a suboptimal activation level can be held responsible for poor response inhibition in externalizing disorders has recently been replicated by others (Scheres et al., 2001), in another laboratory (Amsterdam not Groningen), using another inhibition paradigm (the stop signal paradigm). In their research, the stop paradigm (discussed above in the section on ability to inhibit a response after a stop signal) was administered in three event rate conditions similar to the earlier discussed go–no-go paradigm, with signals presented every 1 s, every 4 s and every 8 s. Given the consistency in findings between the two laboratories, it is unlikely that Van der Meere evoked a Hawthorn effect when he reported that presentation rate of stimuli is an important factor in ADHD, not response inhibition per se. That state regulation not response inhibition per se is the key problem in ADHD has also been suggested by behaviour genetic research. On the basis of a twin study, Kuntsi and Stevenson (2001) showed that a state regulation problem mediates the genetic effects on hyperactive behaviour, not findings produced by the stop paradigm. In a subsequent study by Stevenson and colleagues (Kuntsi et al., 2001), the researchers concluded that the stop failure of ADHD children with the stop task reflects a general slowing down of responses. This conclusion fits well with Van der Meere et al. (1996) and Oosterlaan and Sergeant (1998) who used a response bias and a response reengagement test, respectively, and the routine finding that ADHD children are deficient in their motor presetting (see sections on motor-related processes and motor control and impulsivity, above).

To summarize the evidence dealt with so far, it is to be noted that task performance of hyperactive children is sensitive for event rate manipulations during tasks involving orienting, reorienting dichotic listening, paired associate learning and visual search, as pointed out in the first section of this chapter. Also the CPT findings, discussed above, indicate that event rate is a crucial factor in the performance of hyperactive children. These findings, together with behavioural observations, lead to the suggestion that hyperactive children have a nonoptimal activation/effort state: their task performance decreases when the stimulus rate or event rate decreases or when the experimenter is absent, and conversely, their task performance increases when the presentation rate of stimuli increases or when the experimenter is sitting beside the child. Using a metaphor, the engine is intact (i.e. the basic information-processing capacity is intact) but there is a problem with the petrol supply (i.e. the utilization of the cognitive capacity depends on state factors such as incentives, event rate and presence/absence of the experimenter). Consequently, this review strongly supports the sensation-seeking concept as a relevant factor in hyperactivity disorder, as formulated by Zentall and Zentall (1983), and the suggestion made by Douglas and Peters (1979) that hyperactive children have an inability to modulate their physiological state according to task and situation demands. However, the concept of a 'nonoptimal state' in hyperactivity disorder, as put forward by the author and his coworkers, differs in an important way from its previous definitions in that it is more precisely based on the theoretical model by Sanders. That is, slow and inaccurate responses of hyperactive children are caused by a nonoptimal activation/effort state which manifests itself in slow motor preparation and execution processes. Whether MPH has a positive effect on state regulation is still to be seen.

ADHD and mental retardation

With respect to the comorbidity issue, it may be said that the majority of cognitive research has concentrated on ADHD with or without conduct disorder/learning disabilities. With respect to ADHD with conduct disorder plus mental retardation, a different picture emerges: a dearth of research. There are four reasons why such children with a mental handicap deserve more attention. First, the prevalence of ADHD with conduct disorder in children with mental retardation is considerably higher (ranging from 9 to 18%) compared to ADHD with conduct disorder children with IQs in the normal range

(3–5%: Epstein et al., 1986; American Psychiatric Association, 1994). Second, it is likely that cognitive problems in cases with a dual diagnosis are more pronounced compared to cases with a single diagnosis (in this case, ADHD children with a normal intelligence). Third, children diagnosed as ADHD but without mild or moderate mental retardation are likely to be behind in their intellectual development: for instance, they score an average of 7–15 points below their own siblings on standardized intelligence tests (Barkley, 1991). Thus, a low IQ is very much part of the ADHD disorder, and may give a clue about the 'core' deficit, given that such children are more likely than children with other psychiatric disorders to show intellectual retardation or subtler forms of mental delay. Fourth, children with an externalizing disorder plus low IQ deserve scientific attention in order to improve the efficacy of treatment. Consequently, the nature of ADHD in normally intelligent subjects and its relationship to that in mentally retarded individuals should be a major question in our field of interest.

Within this perspective, a study by Pearson et al. (1996) is of importance. Here, the relationship between ADHD and mental retardation was explored. For this purpose, Pearson and colleagues compared mentally retarded children with and without ADHD on a CPT, patterned after Rosvold et al. (1956: the X-only version). They reported that children with the dual diagnosis committed four times as many errors of commission compared to children with mental retardation only. The authors concluded that the children with the dual diagnosis had poor impulse control. However, this conclusion may be premature because CPT commission errors do not comprise a unitary measure indicative of a single deficit (e.g. impulsivity). Other psychological processes such as attention are operative as well. With this in mind, one of our research projects focused on ADHD with conduct disorder plus mental retardation in an attempt to distinguish more clearly between the constructs of inattention and impulsivity or response inhibition. The findings of three studies indicated that such children have no problems with different attention abilities, such as dividing attention between simultaneously presented visual and auditive stimuli, engagement/reengagement of attention, and sustained attention (van de Meer et al., submitted). However, children demonstrated high levels of impulsive behaviour. This impulsive behaviour could not be explained in terms of poor state regulation, which happened to be the case in ADHD children with an IQ level within the normal age range. Consequently, the results altogether suggest that the cognitive problems seen in pure ADHD children compared to children with the dual diagnosis MMR plus externalizing disorders are qualitatively different (van de Meer et al., submitted).

So far, the review has largely concentrated on interpreting the research on inattention in terms of reaction time measures (the second generation of cognitive tests). How far the nonoptimal motor activation state and effort allocation hyperactivity disorder is supported by psychophysiological measures (the third generation of cognitive tests) is the topic of the next section.

Psychophysiological measures

Heart rate deceleration: measure of motor activation

In the period between the warning and the imperative signal, a triphasic heart rate response has been observed. This response consists of an initial deceleration followed first by an acceleration and then by a second deceleration which reaches a minimum at the time of presentation of the reaction time signal. It is suggested that this final cardiac deceleration is related to both stimulus anticipation and motor preparation. The anticipatory deceleration has been extensively studied to investigate preparatory processes in information processing tasks (for reviews see Pribram and McGuinness, 1975; McGuinness and Pribram, 1980; Van der Molen et al., 1987).

In terms of the cardiac response, there is evidence that ADHD is associated with a poor motor activation state. That is to say, a smaller anticipatory deceleration in combination with a normalization of the cardiac response after the administration of MPH has been reported in hyperactivity and related disorders (Sroufe et al., 1973; Porges et al., 1975; Zahn et al., 1978; Porges and Smith, 1980; Dykman et al., 1983; Porges, 1984; O'Dougherty et al., 1988).

Heart rate deceleration and impulsiveness

Psychophysiological research also suggests that inhibition failures of ADHD children are associated with a nonoptimal effort/activation. Using the stop paradigm, Jennings et al. (1997) indexed heart rate changes in ADHD and normal boys. Changes in cardiac interbeat interval during task performance were used to assess an inhibitory process assumed to occur during both anticipation of reaction time stimuli and inhibition of responses. They studied in particular the heart rate deceleration during the anticipation of the go signal and also in response to the stop signal. According to earlier research, they claimed that anticipatory cardiac deceleration before the go–no-go signal is an index of inhibition of motor action at the central nervous system level. It appeared that ADHD children induced a similar degree of cardiac deceleration on all trials, suggesting that this degree of inhibition is intact in ADHD.

According to the researchers, the heart rate results were most consistent with an alternative hypothesis: when appropriately motivated ADHD children may compensate for deficits by allocating more attention to a task.

Evaluating the same cardiac motor inhibition index as Jennings et al. did, Börger and Van der Meere (2000a) found no difference in heart rate deceleration between ADHD and control children when go–no-go stimuli were presented rapidly. However, group differences were found when the presentation rate was slow: groups differed with respect to their heart rate deceleration preceding go and no-go stimuli, but groups did not differ in heart rate deceleration in the period after a no-go stimulus was presented! This suggests that ADHD is associated with delayed motor activation (not motor inhibition) which becomes manifest in conditions with a slow presentation rate of stimuli. This finding may be seen to validate the earlier discussed RT data concerning ADHD impulsiveness.

Heart rate variability and state regulation

As stated earlier, the author considers the CPT paradigm, and its performance decrement, an excellent paradigm to evaluate state regulation in children with ADHD. This test merely requires the child to display a simple motor response on a button when a target letter is presented on the monitor. The task duration is generally 25–30 min without any breaks. It is obvious that children will demonstrate a performance decline as the task duration progresses. This decline in performance over time may be explained as follows.

The factor, time on task, induces a state of underactivation in the child, which in turn results in a decrement in task efficiency as the task continues. To counteract this decrement in performance, children may change their actual (underactivated) state in the direction of the required state by allocating extra effort across the CPT. Hence, we may hypothesize task efficiency to be 'optimal' at the beginning of the CPT, but minimal at the end of the test, in those who do not allocate extra effort in the course of the CPT. The performance data, as discussed earlier (see section on state regulation and sustained attention, above), suggest that ADHD children are not able to allocate extra effort in order to adjust their underactive state in the course of the CPT. This hypothesis was recently tested in our laboratory using the 0.10 Hz component of the heart rate variability. The component is considered to be a psychophysiological index of effort (Jorna, 1992; Mulder et al., 1992): the more effort the subject allocates, the smaller the variability of the 0.10 Hz component. The component was related with on- and off-task behaviour of ADHD and normal children while performing a CPT with a slow presentation rate without supervision. Again, a rapid decline in task performance was demonstrated by the ADHD group compared to the normal group, validating our former findings. More important, however, was the finding that the 0.10 Hz component was related to performance decline, indicating that controls were allocating extra effort over time in order to fulfil the task requirements (Börger et al., 1999).

Evoked potentials

It has been claimed that various (endogenous) components of the evoked reaction on potentials (ERP) reflect more precisely the timing and duration of cognitive processing than does RT (Mulder, 1986). Four components which are important in hyperactivity disorder will be discussed here: the N2, P3b, contingent negative variation (CNV) and the Nd. The N2 is a negative peak starting around 200 ms after stimulus onset. Two negative components can be distinguished in this range: the mismatch negativity (MMN) and the N2b (Näätänen and Gaillard, 1983). The MMN is modality-specific and reflects an automatic mismatch process between input and template. The N2b is not modality specific and occurs only when the stimulus is attended to. It has been suggested that this component reflects an early process related to sensory encoding (Van Dellen et al., 1984).

The P3b latency indexes the stimulus evaluation time and is relatively independent of response selection and production (Brookhuis et al., 1981; Mulder et al., 1984). The CNV is a slow negative shift, developing over the foreperiod of a stimulus presentation and consisting of two negative components: the early CNV or O (for orientation)-wave, and the terminal CNV or E (for expectancy)-wave (Gaillard, 1977, 1978). The terminal CNV seems to reflect the level of motor preparation and is similar to the readiness (Bereitschaft) potential preceding voluntary movements (Deecke et al., 1976). The Nd is obtained by subtracting ERPs to unattended stimuli from ERPs to attended stimuli. The Nd also contains two separate components, an early phase (Nde) with a sensory-specific maximum and a later phase (Ndl) with a more anterior (frontal) distribution (Näätänen and Michie, 1979). This Ndl may reflect the further ongoing stimulus evaluation.

In an extension of Sanders' model, Mulder (1986) considers amplitude variations as measures of arousal, effort and activation. Peak latencies are measures of the duration of basic (input, central and output) processing. For a critical discussion of Mulder's model, presented in Figure 6.2, the reader is refered to Kok (1990).

The RT research has directed us to an output activation/effort-related

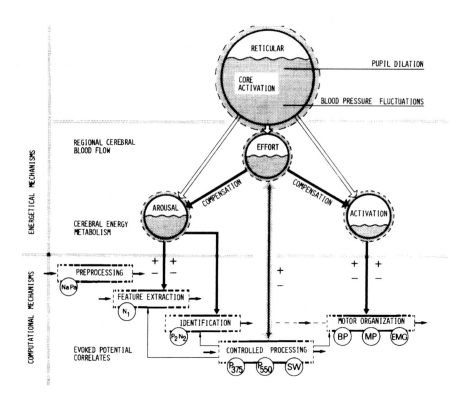

Figure 6.2   Mulder's model. BP, Bereitschaftspotential (readiness potential); MP, motor potential; EMG, electromyogram; SW, slow wave.

problem in the hyperactive child. This section deals with different measures thought to reflect arousal, activation and effort in an attempt to assess whether conclusions based on RT measures hold for electrophysiological measures in terms of Mulder's model.

The (input) arousal hypothesis

Grunewald-Zuberbier et al. (1975, 1978) reported a great α-attenuation (i.e. measure of phasic arousal) after warning signals in hyperactive children. In addition, smaller N2 amplitudes have also been reported (Satterfield and Braley, 1977; Satterfield and Schell, 1984; Camman, 1985; Satterfield et al., 1988). Moreover, Satterfield et al. (1988) reported an abnormal processing negativity (Nd) in hyperactivity disorder. Larger negative slow waves over frontal sites in children with attentional problems were reported by Friedman et al. (1986). Given these findings, an (arousal) selective attention deficit may not be excluded from further consideration. Also, a neuroelectric mapping study by Brandeis et al. (1998) suggests that an input deficit in ADHD cannot be excluded. Using the stop paradigm, this state-of-the-art study indicated that both stop failures and stop successes of the ADHD child are at least partly related to increased variability in an early automatically induced form of orienting to stimuli. This argues in favour of input deficiency but is against a response inhibition problem of ADHD children.

The (output) activation hypothesis

A series of ERP studies point in the direction of an output-related dysfunction in hyperactivity disorder. With some exceptions (Loiselle et al., 1980; Holcomb et al., 1985; Brumaghim et al., 1987), the majority of studies indicate that hyperactive and control children differ with respect to post-P3b (motor-related) processes. In addition, these studies show that MPH affects post-P3b processes (Hink et al., 1978; Klorman et al., 1979; Coons et al., 1981, 1987; Callaway, 1983, 1984; Peloquin and Klorman, 1986; Brumaghim et al., 1987; Fitzpatrick et al., 1988).

With respect to CNV findings, it appeared that hyperactive children have a smaller CNV after a warning signal (Grunewald-Zuberbier et al., 1978). The finding that the amplitude of the CNV (motor preparation) has been increased by stimulant administration (Kopell et al., 1974; Coons et al., 1981) confirms the output-related hypothesis.

The effort hypothesis

The consistent finding that hyperactive children have a smaller P3b amplitude (Loiselle et al., 1980; Holcomb et al., 1985, 1986) is consistent with the effort hypothesis. The fact that MPH increases the P3b amplitude (Coons et al., 1981; Michael et al., 1981; Strauss et al., 1984) confirms this hypothesis.

Neurochemical level

Neurochemical studies lend further support to the motor output deficiency hypothesis in hyperactivity (see Chapter 10 for a more detailed account). The basal ganglia, particularly the corpus striatum, is involved in the organization of motor behaviour (activation) (Sanders, 1983; Mulder, 1986). Most brain dopamine is found within the nigrostriatal system and both dopamine and noradrenaline are associated with frontostriatal circuits (Tucker and Williamson, 1984). There is evidence that hyperactivity is associated with a dysfunction of the frontostriatal system. Neurochemical studies have led to explanations of hyperactivity that are based on dysfunction of monoaminergic systems, especially dopamine (Shaywitz et al., 1977), and perhaps to a lesser extent noradrenaline (Zametkin and Rapaport, 1987; Sagvolden and Archer, 1989).

Schneider and Roeltgen (1991) observed poor attention and hyperactivity in animals who received chronic low doses (CLD) of 1-methyl–4-phenyl–1,2,3,6-tetrahydropyridine (MPTP). MPTP is a neurotoxin that selectively damages dopaminergic innervation of the dorsal striatum and disrupts the functioning of the frontostriatal axis. A reduced glucose metabolism of the striatum has been reported in children with hyperactivity disorder (Lou et al., 1989, 1990). (See Zametkin et al. (1990) for further discussion on this issue.)

However, altered metabolism of serotonin, which is an important neuro-transmitter in the arousal system (Tucker and Williamson, 1984), has also been suggested as a potential aetiology of hyperactivity (Zametkin and Rapaport, 1987). Thus, an altered metabolism of a single neurotransmitter does not seem to be an adequate explanation of hyperactivity.

In summary, the interpretation of heart rate and evoked potential studies in terms of Mulder's model leads to the conclusion of an activation effort dysfunction in hyperactivity. However, the arousal hypothesis is not to be dismissed. Also, neurochemical studies point in the direction of an output-related dysfunction (i.e. a dysfunction of monoaminergic systems) but, again, the arousal hypothesis (i.e. an altered metabolism of serotonin) is not to be dismissed.

State regulation and the effects on the environment

In summary, there is growing evidence that hyperactive children are delayed in cognitive processes just preceding the overt motor action, i.e. response decision and response organization processes. It is probably of interest to the present argument that the later the cognitive stage is in the suggested sequence of cognitive stages, the more its active processes refer to 'presetting the stage' prior to the presentation of the stimulus (Sanders, 1983). Hence, the output-related processing disturbance may also hinder the hyperactive child in the execution of so-called input-related processes such as orientation and reorienta-tion. In this chapter, an attempt has so far been made to explain the motor output hypothesis in terms of a state regulation (activation and effort) problem. It is obvious that an instability in behavioural states affects the caretaker's ability to interact properly with an ADHD child. This is the central theme of the following sections.

State regulation and development

Infant studies have shown that state regulation is essential immediately after birth, providing the newborn with the opportunity for information processing and social interaction (Colombo and Horowitz, 1987). Gaze behaviour is considered to be one of the earliest indicators of state control in newborns: they avert the gaze to reduce input when confronted with stimuli that are too intensive (Stifter and Moyer, 1991; see also Chapter 8 for a review of developmental aspects). At first, the infant's ability to regulate state depends largely on the quality of the caretaker's behaviour, stimulating the baby when underaroused, and reducing stimulation when the baby is overaroused (Field, 1987; Stifter and Moyer, 1991; Gable and Isabella, 1992). During development, the majority of infants begin to exert control over their state, and the regulation process becomes internalized (Field, 1977). Some infants, however, do not develop state control and may cycle through various states quite rapidly. Thoman and Whitney (1990) argued that a lack of state control in the infant has predictive validity for (ab)normal central nervous system development, and that poor state regulation during infancy constitutes a serious risk for current and later development (DiPietro and Porges, 1991). Within this perspective, ADHD (DSM-IV) may be considered to be a state deficit in the elementary school years. It is obvious that a lack of state control places high demands on the quality of the social environment because, now internal state control is lacking, the environment has to control the behaviour state of the ADHD child. This is the subject of the next section.

State regulation and social interactions

Many studies of interaction between ADHD children and their mothers have reported directive behaviour of the mothers towards ADHD children. The mothers were found to be more directive and controlling, more disapproving, more encouraging and they made more suggestions about impulse control. In sum, the social behaviour of ADHD children in interaction with their mother may be interpreted as different forms of structure-seeking behaviour: they talk more to themselves, they make more requests for feedback from their mothers, and they are less compliant. The mothers, in turn, seem to provide more structure in interaction with ADHD children, relative to control dyads (for a review, see Barkley, 1991). Campbell et al. (1977) were the first to introduce the concepts of structure-seeking and structure-providing behaviour in respect to the ADHD child and the caretaker (see Chapter 11 for a fuller discussion).

It has been suggested that, due to previous experiences, a mother of an ADHD child may have developed a certain emotional attitude towards her child, which may have influenced the development of a certain interaction pattern. Keeping this in mind, it is surprising that to date few studies have observed the social behaviour of ADHD children in interaction with a strange adult who has no former experience with ADHD behaviour. Recently, Stroes et al. (submitted) tested whether ADHD children display structure-seeking behaviour in interaction with a stranger (student) and whether they trigger structure-providing behaviour in the student who was not informed that his or her behaviour was part of the study as well.

Behaviour elements of both child and student were observed in two conditions: an interview and free play. Especially in the free-play situation, the ADHD children and students interacted differently with one another, compared to the control dyads. The ADHD children talked more, their verbal reactions to the student's speech were faster, and they looked at the student longer and more frequently. In addition, when there was no verbal communication, they monitored the student more frequently, and when the student spoke, the ADHD children and students looked at each other more than was the case with the control dyads. Taken together, these behaviours give the impression that the ADHD children directed more attention to the student than did the control children. Second, the ADHD children talked more to themselves than did the control children. This talking to themselves consisted of making comments on their free-play activity (building a tower), and of thinking aloud. As mentioned earlier, the students also behaved differently when interacting with the ADHD children than with the normal children. With respect to noncompliance, it was remarkable that the students were forced to repeat their requests only in interactions with the ADHD children. In addition, the students praised the ADHD children more frequently than the control children on their building activities. These findings suggest that, during their first encounter with a stranger, ADHD children trigger structure-providing behaviour.

In sum, the present findings parallel a series of mother–ADHD child dyad studies: ADHD children direct more attention to the student than the controls do, they talk more to themselves than the controls do, and their behaviour leads the student to repeat requests. Overall, these behaviours may be interpreted in terms of the concept of structure-seeking behaviour in ADHD children suffering from a state regulation deficit.

State regulation and the experimental test condition

An important issue to discuss concerns the potential implications for how CPTs should be administered in the field of developmental neuropsychopathology, and in particular to children suspected as having ADHD. During the last decade, many computer software programs have been developed for research purposes, such as the Gordon diagnostic system, the test of variable attention and the stop paradigm. The tests have in common that they measure ability factors. State fluctuations of the subject during testing are considered here to be a confounding factor that precludes a firm conclusion about a subject's true cognitive potential. However, evidence accumulates that the CPT perform-ance of ADHD children is mainly determined by state factors such as presenta-tion rate of stimuli, time on task, reward and external control, and not by ability factors per se. Since state factors, not ability factors, are argued to be at the core of the difficulty exhibited by ADHD children, it is recommended that the effects of state factors on cognitive functioning are investigated instead of treating state fluctuation as a confounding factor in cognitive research. A complete picture of the ADHD child's abilities requires consideration of a broader range of states.

To be very specific, the time now seems to be ripe for implementing functional magnetic resonance imaging (MRI) measures in our ADHD field wisely. It would be a pity if all future MRI studies were gathering data while ADHD children are in an optimal state and executing cognitive tests tapping task difficulty. What is needed are MRI data comparing the moment when an ADHD child is in an optimal state with the moment when he or she is not. This can be achieved by altering the presentation rate of stimuli, which has been the heart of this chapter.

Conclusions

The term 'state regulation' is still loosely defined and deserves more investiga-tion using a chain of approaches: the behavioural observation approach, the reaction time approach, the electrophysiological approach, the neurochemical approach and the metabolic approach (functional MRI). The term may also be nonspecific. By this is meant that cognitive dysfunctions found in clinical groups other than those involving hyperactivity may also be explained in terms of a dysfunction in the energetical regulation of motor control (Sergeant and Van der Meere, 1990a). Further research, especially that based on longitudinal data, is needed to help clarify these issues. The present theoretical review of the role of attention in ADHD can hopefully be used to make specific predictions about the patterns of deficits encountered.

The final important question to answer is how to relate the laboratory findings as reviewed here with the clinical concept of hyperactivity disorder. The diagnostic label is derived from behavioural descriptions by parents, teachers and clinicians that are highly subjective and imprecise. Laboratory findings show that children with a so-called attention deficit are able to orient, reorient, divide and focus their attention. In addition, such children do not differ from controls with respect to the rate of the acquisition of attentional skills. These are unexpected findings in children with a so-called attention deficit. However, laboratory findings indicate that the task efficiency of hyperactive children is highly sensitive to state manipulations, such as presentation rate and external control. So, the first conclusion to be drawn is that the diagnostic term is incorrect and should be changed to the label of state regulation deficit. Whether this state regulation deficit is due to a suboptimal arousal, activation or effort level is an important issue, but the issue is unimportant with respect to this conclusion.

The second conclusion to be drawn is that we may present parents and teachers with the wrong questions. The question is not whether a hyperactive child is easily distracted or not, or whether the child is able to sustain his or her attention for a long period. The question is whether the symptoms of hyperactivity disorder emerge in conditions which are believed to tap the state of the child. The author's experience with parents of hyperactive children is that they describe that the symptoms are manifested in boring conditions. Thus, their claim is that if the child is really motivated, the symptoms will disappear to a large extent. Such a decription perfectly fits the majority of laboratory findings. In summary, the trait of the hyperactive child is state regulation deficit!

REFERENCES

Akhtar, N. and Enns, J.T. (1989). Relations between covert orienting and filtering in the development of visual attention. *Journal of Experimental Child Psychology*, **48**, 315–34.

Alberts, E. and Van der Meere, J.J. (1992). Observations of hyperactive behaviour during vigilance. *Journal of Child Psychology and Psychiatry*, **33**, 1355–64.

American Psychatric Association. (1994). *Diagnostic and Statistical Manual of Mental Disorders*, 4th edn. Washington, DC: American Psychiatric Association.

Ballinger, C.T., Varley, C.K. and Nolen, P.A. (1984). Effects of methylphenidate on reading in children with attention deficit disorder. *American Journal of Psychiatry*, **141**, 1590–3.

Balthazor, M., Wagner, R.K. and Pelham, W.E. (1991). The specificity of the effects of stimulant medication on classroom learning-related measures of cognitive processing for attention deficit disorder children. *Journal of Abnormal Child Psychology*, **19**, 35–52.

Barkley, R.A. (1982). Guidelines for defining hyperactivity in children. In *Advances in Clinical Child Psychology*, vol. 5, ed. B.B. Lahey and A.E. Kazdin eds, pp. 95–137. New York: Plenum.

Barkley, R.A. (1990). *Attention Deficit Hyperactivity Disorder: A Handbook for Diagnosis and Treatment*. New York: Guilford Press.

Barkley, R.A. (1991). The ecological validity of laboratory and analogue assessment methods of ADHD symptoms. *Journal of Abnormal Child Psychology*, **19**, 149–78.

Barkley, R.A. (1997). Behavioral inhibition, sustained attention, and executive functions: constructing a unifying theory of ADHD. *Psychological Bulletin*, **121**, 65–94.

Barkley, R.A., Grodzinsky, G. and Du Paul, G.J. (1992). Frontal lobe functions in attention deficit disorder with and without hyperactivity: a review and research report. *Journal of Abnormal Psychology*, **20**, 163–88.

Benezra, E. and Douglas, V.I. (1988). Short-term serial recall in ADDH, normal, and reading disabled boys. *Journal of Abnormal Child Psychology*, **16**, 511–26.

Bergman, T., Douglas, V.I. and Barr. R.G. (1999). Effects of methylphenidate on complex cognitive processing in attention deficit hyperactivity disorder. *Journal of Abnormal Psychology*, **108**, 90–105.

Borcherding, B., Thompson, K., Kruesi, M. et al. (1988). Automatic and effortful processing in attention deficit hyperactivity disorder. *Journal of Abnormal Child Psychology*, **16**, 333–46.

Börger, N.A. and Van der Meere, J.J. (2000a). Motor control and state regulation in children with ADHD: a cardiac response study. *Biological Psychology*, **51**, 247–67.

Börger, N.A. and Van der Meere, J.J. (2000b). Visual behaviour of ADHD children during an attention test: an almost forgotten variable. *Journal of Child Psychology and Psychiatry*, **41**, 525–32.

Börger, N.A., Van der Meere, J.J., Ronner, A. et al. (1999). Heart rate variability and sustained attention in ADHD children. *Journal of Abnormal Child Psychology*, **27**, 25–33.

Börger, N.A., Wiersema, R.J. and Van der Meere, J.J. (2000). 0.10 Hz heart rate variability component and sustained attention. *Journal of Psychophysiology*, **14**, 260–1.

Brandeis, D., Van Leeuwen, T.H., Rubia, K. et al. (1998). Neuroelectric mapping reveals precursor of stop failures in children with attention deficits. *Behavioural Brain Research*, **94**, 111–25.

Brookhuis, K.A., Mulder, G., Mulder, L.J.M. et al. (1981). Late positive components and stimulus evaluation time. *Biological Psychology*, **13**, 107–23.

Browning, R.M. (1967). Effects of irrelevant peripheral visual stimuli in minimally brain damaged children. *Journal of Consulting Psychology*, **31**, 371–6.

Brumaghim, J.T., Klorman, R., Strauss, J., Lewine, J.D. and Goldstein, M.G. (1987). Does methylphenidate affect information processing? Findings from two studies on performance and P3b latency. *Psychophysiology*, **24**, 361–73.

Burke, R.S. (1990). A cognitive-developmental approach to studying attention deficits. In *The Development of Attention: Research and Theory*, J.T. Enns, ed., pp. 365–81. Amsterdam: Elsevier Science.

Callaway, E. (1983). The pharmacology of human information processing. *Psychophysiology*, **20**, 359–70.

Callaway, E. (1984). Human information-processing: some effects of methylphenidate, age, and scopolamine. *Biological Psychiatry*, **19**, 649–62.

Camman, L. (1985). Evoked potentials in children with impaired and normal powers of concentration. In *Psychophysiological Approaches to Human Information Processing*, F. Klix, R. Näätänen and K. Zimmer, eds., pp. 269–78. Amsterdam: Elsevier Science.

Campbell, S.B., Endman, M.W. and Bernfeld, G. (1977). A three-year follow-up of hyperactive preschoolers into elementary school. *Journal of Child Psychology and Psychiatry*, **18**, 239–50.

Cappella, B., Gentile, J.R. and Juliano, D.B. (1977). Time estimation by hyperactive and normal children. *Perceptual and Motor Skills*, **44**, 787.

Carlson, C.L., Pelham, W.E., Swanson, J.M. and Wagner, J.L. (1991). A divided attention analysis of the effects of methylphenidate on the arithmetic performance of children with attention deficit hyperactivity disorder. *Journal of Child Psychology and Psychiatry*, **32**, 463–71.

Ceci, S.J. and Tisman, J. (1984). Hyperactivity and incidental memory: evidence for attentional diffusion. *Child Development*, **55**, 2192–203.

Chee, P., Logan, G., Schachar, R., Lindsay, P. and Wachsmuth, R. (1989). Effects of event rate and display time on sustained attention in hyperactive, normal, and control children. *Journal of Abnormal Child Psychology*, **17**, 371–91.

Cohen, N.J. and Minde, K. (1983). The hyperactive syndrome in kindergarten children: comparison of children with pervasive and situational symptoms. *Journal of Child Psychology and Psychiatry*, **24**, 443–55.

Colombo, J. and Horowitz, F.D. (1987). Behavioral state as a lead variable in neonatal research. *Merill-Palmer Quarterly*, **33**, 423–37.

Conte, R., Kinsbourne, M., Swanson, J., Zirk, H. and Samuels, M. (1986). Presentation rate effects on paired associate learning by attention deficit disordered children. *Child Development*, **57**, 681–7.

Coons, H.W., Peloquin, L.J., Klorman, R., et al. (1981). Effects of methylphenidate on young adults: vigilance and event-related potentials. *Electroencephalography and Clinical Neurophysiology*, **51**, 373–87.

Coons, H.W., Klorman, R. and Borgstedt, A.D. (1987). Effects of methylphenidate on adolescents with a childhood history of attention deficit disorder: 2. *Journal of the American Academy of Child Psychiatry*, **26**, 368–74.

Corkum, P.V. and Siegel, L.S. (1993). Is the continuous performance task a valuable research tool for use with children with attention deficit hyperactivity disorder? *Journal of Child Psychology and Psychiatry*, **34**, 1217–39.

Craik, F.I.M. and Lockhard, R.S. (1972). Levels of processing: a framework for memory research. *Journal of Verbal Learning and Verbal Behavior*, **11**, 671–84.

Dalby, D.T., Kinsbourne, M., Swanson, J.M. and Sobel, M.P. (1977). Hyperactive children's use of learning time: correlation by stimulant treatment. *Child Development*, **48**, 1448–53.

Daugherty, T.K. and Quay, H.C. (1991). Response pervasiveness and delayed responding in childhood behavior disorders. *Journal of Child Psychology and Psychiatry*, **32**, 453–61.

Davidson, E.M. and Prior, M.R. (1978). Laterality and selective attention in hyperactive children. *Journal of Abnormal Child Psychology*, **6**, 475–81.

Deecke, L., Grzinger, B. and Kornhuber, H.H. (1976). Voluntary finger movement in man: cerebral potentials and theory. *Biological Cybernetics*, **23**, 99–119.

De Sonneville, L.M.J., Njiokiktjien, C. and Hilhorst, R.C. (1991). Methylphenidate-induced changes in ADDH information processors. *Journal of Child Psychology and Psychiatry*, **32**, 285–95.

Dienske, H. and Sanders-Woudstra, J.A.R. (1988). A critical and conceptual consideration of attention deficit and hyperactivity from an ethological point of view. In *Attention Deficit Disorder: Criteria, Cognition, Intervention*, L.M. Bloomingdale and J.A. Sergeant, eds, pp. 43–64. Oxford: Pergamon Press.

DiPietro, J.A. and Porges, S.W. (1991). Relations between neonatal states and 8-month developmental outcome in preterm infants. *Infant Behavior and Development*, **14**, 441–50.

Douglas, V.I. (1983). Attentional and cognitive problems. In *Developmental Neuropsychiatry*, M. Rutter, ed., pp. 280–328. New York: Guilford Press.

Douglas, V.I. and Benezra, E. (1990). Supraspan verbal memory in attention deficit disorder with hyperactivity, normal and reading disabled boys. *Journal of Abnormal Child Psychology*, **18**, 617–38.

Douglas, V.I. and Peters, K.G. (1979). Toward a clearer definition of the attentional deficit of hyperactive children. In *Attention and the Development of Cognitive Skills*, G.A. Hale and M. Lewis, eds, pp. 173–247. New York: Plenum Press.

Draeger, S., Prior, M.R. and Sanson, A.V. (1986). Visual and auditory attention performance in hyperactive children: competence or compliance. *Journal of Abnormal Child Psychology*, **14**, 411–24.

Dykman, R.A., Ackerman, M.A. and Oglesby, D.M. (1979). Selective and sustained attention in learning disabled and normal boys. *Journal of Nervous and Mental Disease*, **167**, 288–97.

Dykman, R.A., Ackerman, P.T., Holcomb, P.J. and Boudreau, A.Y. (1983). Physiological manifestations of learning disabilities. *Journal of Learning Disabilities*, **16**, 46–53.

Enns, J.T. and Girgus, J.S. (1985). Developmental changes in selective and integrative visual attention. *Journal of Experimental Child Psychology*, **40**, 319–37.

Epstein, M.H., Cullinan, D. and Gadow, K. (1986). Teacher ratings of hyperactivity in learning-disabled, emotionally disturbed, and mentally retarded children. *Journal of Special Education*, **22**, 219–29.

Field, T.M. (1977). Effects of early separation, interactive deficits, and experimental manipulations of infant–mother face-to-face interaction. *Child Development*, **48**, 763–71.

Field, T.M. (1987). Interaction and attachment in normal and atypical infants. *Journal of Consulting and Clinical Psychology*, **55**, 853–9.

Fitzpatrick, P., Klorman, R., Brumaghim, J.T. and Keefover, R.W. (1988). Effects of methylphenidate on stimulus evaluation and response processes: evidence from performance and event-related potentials. *Psychophysiology*, **25**, 292–304.

Friedman, D., Cornblatt, B., Vaughan, H. and Erlenmeyer-Kimling, L. (1986). Event-related potentials in children at risk for schizophrenia during two versions of the continuous performance test. *Psychiatric Research*, **18**, 161–77.

Frowein, H.W. (1981). *Selective Drug Effects on Information Processing*. Thesis. Enschede: Sneldruk Boulevard.

Gable, S. and Isabella, R.A. (1992). Maternal contributions to infant regulation of arousal. *Infant Behavior and Development*, **15**, 95–107.

Gaillard, A.W.K. (1977). The late CNV wave: preparation versus expectancy. *Psychophysiology*, **14**, 563–8.

Gaillard, A.W.K. (1978). The evaluation of drug effects in laboratory tasks. In *Psychopharmacology and Reaction Time*, I. Hindmarch, B. Aufdembrinke and H. Ott, eds., pp. 15–24. Chichester: John Wiley.

Gomez, R. and Sanson, A.V. (1994). Effects of experimenter and mother presence on the attentional performance and activity of hyperactive boys. *Journal of Abnormal Child Psychology*, **22**, 517–29.

Gordon, M. (1979). The assessment of impulsivity and mediating behaviors in hyperactive and nonhyperactive children. *Journal of Abnormal Child Psychology*, **7**, 317–26.

Gray, J.A. (1982). *The Neurophysiology of Anxiety: An Enquiry into the Functions of the Septo-Hippocampal System*. New York: Oxford University Press.

Gross-Tsur, V., Manor, O., Van der Meere, J.J., Joseph, A. and Shalev, R. (1997). Epilepsy and ADHD: is methylphenidate safe and effective? *Journal of Pediatrics*, **130**, 40–4.

Grunewald Zuberbier, E., Grunewald, G. and Rasche, A. (1975). Hyperactive behavior and EEG arousal reactions in children. *Electroencephalography and Clinical Neurophysiology*, **38**, 149–59.

Grunewald-Zuberbier, E., Grunewald, G., Rasche, A. and Netz, J. (1978). Contingent negative variation and alpha attenuation responses in children with different abilities to concentrate. *Electroencephalography and Clinical Neurophysiology*, **44**, 37–47.

Gunning, B. (1992). *A Controlled Trial of Clonidine in Hyperkinetic Children*. Thesis. Rotterdam: Erasmus University.

Hazell, P.L., Carr, V.J., Lewin, T.J. et al. (1999). Effortful and automatic information processing in boys with ADHD and specific learning disorders. *Journal of Child Psychology and Psychiatry*, **40**, 275–86.

Hink, R.F., Fenton, W.H., Tinklenberg, J.R., Pfefferbaum, A. and Kopell, B.S. (1978). Vigilance and human attention under conditions of methylphenidate and secobarbital intoxication. *Psychophysiology*, **15**, 116–25.

Hockey, G.R.J., Coles, M.G.H. and Gaillard, A.W.K. (1986). Energetical issues in research on human information processing. In *Energetics and Human Information Processing*, G.R.J. Hockey, A.W.K. Gaillard and M.G.H. Coles, eds, pp. 3–22. Dordrecht: Martinus Nijhoff.

Holcomb, J.P., Ackerman, P.T. and Dykman, R.A. (1985). Cognitive event related brain potentials in children with attention and reading deficits. *Psychophysiology*, **6**, 656–67.

Holcomb, P.J., Ackerman, P.T. and Dykman, R.A. (1986). Auditory event related potentials in attention and reading disabled boys. *International Journal of Psychophysiology*, **3**, 263–73.

Hooks, K., Milich, R. and Pugzles Lorch, L. (1994). Sustained and selective attention in boys with attention deficit hyperactivity disorder. *Journal of Clinical Child Psychology*, **23**, 69–77.

Jennings, J.R., Van der Molen, M.W., Pelham, W., Brock Depski, K. and Hoza, B. (1997). Inhibition in boys with attention deficit hyperactivity disorder as indexed by heart rate change. *Developmental Psychology*, **33**, 308–18.

Jorna, P.G.A.M. (1992). Spectral analysis of heart rate and psychological state: a review of its validity as a workload index. *Biological Psychology*, **34**, 237–57.

Kail, R. (1990). More evidence for a common, central constraint on speed of processing. In *The Development of Attention Research and Theory*, J.T.Enns, ed., pp. 159–73. Elsevier Science Publishers B.V. (North-Holland).

Kalverboer, A.F. (1990). Introduction: developmental biopsychology and the study of behavioral deviance in childhood. In *Developmental Biopsychology. Experimental and Observational Studies in Children at Risk*, A.F. Kalverboer, ed., pp.1–17. Ann Arbor: University of Michigan Press.

Kalverboer, A.F. and Brouwer, W.H. (1983). Visuomotor behaviour in preschool children in relation to sex and neurological status. *Journal of Child Psychology and Psychiatry*, **24**, 65–88.

Karatekin, C. and Asarnov, R.F. (1998). Components of visual serach in childhood-onset schizophenia and attention deficit hyperactivity disorder. *Journal of Abnormal Child Psychology*, **26**, 367–80.

Kinsbourne, M. (1990). Testing models for attention deficit hyperactivity disorder in the behavioral laboratory. In *Attention Deficit Hyperactivity Disorder*, K. Conners and M. Kinsbourne, eds, pp. 51–69. Munich: Medizin Verlag.

Klorman, R., Brumaghim, J.T., Salzman, L.F. et al. (1979). Effects of methylphenidate on attention deficit hyperactivity disorder with and without aggressive/noncompliant features. *Journal of Abnormal Child Psychology*, **16**, 413–22.

Kooistra, L., Van der Meere, J.J., Vulsma, T. and Kalverboer, A.F. (1996). Sustained attention problems in children with early-treated congenital hypothyroidism. *Acta Pediatrica*, **85**, 425–9.

Kok, A. (1990). Internal and external control: a two factor model of amplitude change of event-related potentials. *Acta Psychologica*, **74**, 203–35.

Kopell, B.S., Wittner, W.K., Lunde, D.T., Wolcott, L.J. and Tinklenberg, J.R. (1974). The effects of methamphetamine and secobarbital on the contingent negative variation amplitude. *Psychopharmacologia*, **34**, 55–62.

Kuntsi, J. and Stevenson, J. (2001). Psychological mechanisms in hyperactivity: II The role of genetic factors. *Journal of Child Psychology and Psychiatry*, **42**, 211–19.

Kuntsi, J., Oosterlaan, J. and Stevenson, J. (2001). Psychological mechanisms in hyperactivity: I Response inhibition deficit, working memory impairment, delay aversion or something else? *Journal of Child Psychology and Psychiatry*, **42**, 199–210.

Kupietz, S.S. (1990). Sustained attention in normal and in reading disabled youngsters with and without ADDH. *Journal of Abnormal Child Psychology*, **18**, 357–72.

Lacey, J.I. (1967). Somatic response patterning and stress: some revisions of activation theory. In *Psychological Stress*, M.H. Appley and R. Turnbull, eds, pp. 14–42. New York: Appleton Century Crofts.

Lambert, N.M., Sandoval, J. and Sassone, D. (1978). Prevalence of hyperactivity in elementary school children as function of social system definers. *American Journal of Orthopsychiatry*, **48**, 446–63.

Landau, Y.E., Gross-Tsur, V., Auerbach, J., Van der Meere, J.J. and Shalev, R.S. (1999). Attention deficit hyperactivity disorder and nonverbal learning disabilities: congruence and incongruence of cognitive and behavioral aspects of attention. *Journal of Child Neurology*, **14**, 299–303.

Leubuscher, H.J. and Roth, N. (1983). A computer-controlled conditioning procedure in man. In *Psychophysiology*, R. Sinz and M. Rosenzweig, eds, pp. 151–7. Jena: Fischer Verlag.

Leung, P.W.L. and Connolly, K.J. (1994). Attentional difficulties in hyperactive and conduct-disordered children: a processing deficit. *Journal of Child Psychology and Psychiatry*, **35**, 1229–45.

Leung, P.W.L. and Connolly, K.J. (1996). Distractibility in hyperactive and conduct disordered children. *Journal of Child Psychology and Psychiatry*, **37**, 305–12.

Logan, G.D., Cowan, W.B. and Davis, K.A. (1984). On the ability to inhibit simple and choice reaction time responses: a model and a method. *Journal of Experimental Psychology: Human Perception and Performance*, **10**, 276–91.

Loge, D.V., Staton, R.D. and Beatty, W.W. (1990). Performance of children with ADHD on tests sensitive to frontal lobe dysfunction. *Journal of the American Academy of Child and Adolescent Psychiatry*, **29**, 540–5.

Loiselle, D.L., Stamm, J.S., Maitinsky, S. and Whipple, S. (1980). Evoked potential and behavioural signs of attentive dysfunctions in hyperactive boys. *Psychophysiology*, **17**, 193–201.

Lou, H.C., Henriksen, L., Bruhn, P., Brner, H. and Nielsen, J.B. (1989). Striatal dysfunction in attention deficit and hyperkinetic disorder. *Archives of Neurology*, **46**, 48–52.

Lou, H.C., Henriksen, L. and Bruhn, P. (1990). Focal cerebral dysfunction in developmental disabilities. *Lancet*, **338**, 8–11.

Luk, S.L., Leung, P.W.L. and Yuen, J. (1991). Clinic observations in the assessment of pervasiveness of childhood hyperactivity. *Journal of Child Psychology and Psychiatry*, **32**, 833–50.

Malone, M.A., Kershner, J.R. and Siegel, L. (1988). The effects of methylphenidate on levels of processing and laterality in children with attention deficit disorder. *Journal of Abnormal Child Psychology*, **16**, 379–96.

Maurer, R.G. and Stuart, M.A. (1980). Attention deficit without hyperactivity in a child psychiatric clinic. *Journal of Clinical Psychiatry*, **41**, 232–3.

McClure, F.D. and Gordon, M. (1984). Performance of disturbed hyperactive and non-hyperactive children on an objective measure of hyperactivity. *Journal of Abnormal Child Psychology*, **12**, 561–72.

McGee, R., Williams, S. and Silva, P.A. (1984). Background characteristics of aggressive, hyperactive and aggressive-hyperactive boys. *Journal of the American Academy of Child Psychiatry*, **23**, 280–4.

McGuinness, D. and Pribram, K.H. (1980). The neuropsychology of attention; emotional and motivational controls. In *The Brain and Psychology*, M.C. Wittrock, ed., pp. 95–139. New York: Academic Press.

McIntyre, C.W., Blackwell, S.L. and Denton, C.L. (1978). Effects of noise distractability on the spans of apprehension of hyperactive boys. *Journal of Abnormal Psychology*, **6**, 483–92.

Michael, B.M., Klorman, R., Salzman, L.F., Borgstedt, A.D. and Dainer, K.B. (1981). Normalizing effects of methylphenidate on hyperactive children's performance and evoked potentials. *Psychophysiology*, **18**, 665–71.

Milich, R. and Kramer, J. (1985). Reflections on Impulsivity: an empirical investigation of impulsivity as a construct. In *Advances in Learning and Behavioral Disabilities*, vol. 3, K.D. Gadow and I. Bialer, eds, pp. 57–94. Greenwich, CT: JAI Press.

Milich, R., Hartung, C.M., Martin, C.A. and Haigler, E.D. (1994). Behavioral disinhibition and underlying processes in adolescents with disruptive behavior disorders. In *Disruptive Behavior Disorders in Childhood*, D.K. Routh, ed., pp. 109–38. New York: Plenum.

Molenaar, P.C.M. and Van der Molen, M. (1986). Steps to a formal analysis of the cognitive-energetic model of stress and human performance. *Acta Psychologica*, **62**, 237–61.

MTA Cooperative Group. (1999). A 14-month randomized trial of treatment strategies for attention-deficit/hyperactivity disorder. *Archives of General Psychiatry*, **56**, 1073–86.

Mulder, G. (1986). The concept and measurement of mental effort. In *Energetics and Human Information Processing*, G.R.J. Hockey, A.W.K. Gaillard and M.G.H. Coles, eds, pp. 175–98. Dordrecht: Martinus Nijhoff.

Mulder, G., Gloerich, A.B.M., Brookhuis, K.A., Van Dellen, H.J. and Mulder, L.J.M. (1984). Stage analysis of the reaction process using brain-evoked potentials and reaction time. *Psychological Research*, **46**, 15–32.

Mulder, L.J.M., Veldman, J.P.B., Van der Veen, F.M. et al. (1992). On the effects of mental task performance on heart rate, blood pressure and its variability measures. In *Blood Pressure and Heart Rate Variability*, M. di Rienzo, G. Mancia, G. Parati, A. Pedotti and A. Zanchetti, eds, pp. 153–66. Amsterdam: IOS Press.

Näätänen, R. and Gaillard, A.W.K. (1983). The orientation reflex and the N2 deflection of the event-related potential (ERP). In *Tutorials in Event-related Potential Research: Endogenous Components*, A.W.K. Gaillard and W. Ritter, eds, pp. 119–41. Amsterdam: Elsevier North Holland.

Näätänen, R. and Michie, P.T. (1979). Early selective attention effects on the evoked potential: a critical review and reinterpretation. *Biological Psychology*, **8**, 81–136.

Nuechterlein, K.H. (1983). Signal detection in vigilance tasks and behavioural attributes among offspring of schizophrenic mothers and among hyperactive children. *Journal of Abnormal Psychology*, **92**, 4–28.

O'Dougherty, M., Neuchterlein, K. and Drew, B. (1984). Hyperactive and hypoxic children: signal detection, sustained attention and behaviour. *Journal of Abnormal Psychology*, **93**, 178–91.

O'Dougherty, M., Berntson, G.G., Boysen, S.T., Wright, F.S. and Teske, D. (1988). Psychophysiological predictors of attentional dysfunction in children with congenital heart defects. *Psychophysiology*, **25**, 305–15.

Oosterlaan, J. and Sergeant, J.A. (1998). Response inhibition and response re-engagement in attention-deficit/hyperactivity disorder, disruptive, anxious and normal children. *Behavioural Brain Research*, **94**, 33–43.

Oosterlaan, J., Logan, G.D. and Sergeant, J.A. (1998). Response inhibition in AD/HD, CD, comorbid AD/HD + CD, anxious, and control children: a meta-analysis of studies with the stop task. *Journal of Child Psychology and Psychiatry*, **39**, 411–25.

Pearson, D.A. and Lane, D.M. (1990). Reorientation in hyperactive and non-hyperactive children: evidence for developmentally immature attention? In *The Development of Attention: Research and Theory*, J.T. Enns, ed., pp. 345–63. Amsterdam: Elsevier Science.

Pearson, D.A., Yaffee, L.S., Loveland, K.A. and Lewis, K.R. (1996). Comparison of sustained and selective attention in children who have mental retardation with and without attention deficit. *American Journal on Mental Retardation*, **6**, 592–607.

Peeke, S., Halliday, R., Callaway, E., Prael, R. and Reus, V. (1984). Effects of two doses of methylphenidate on verbal information processing in hyperactive children. *Journal of Clinical Psychopharmacology*, **4**, 82–8.

Pelham, W.E. (1979). Selective attention deficits in poor readers. Dichotic listening, speeded classification, and auditory and visual and incidental learning tasks. *Child Development*, **50**, 1050–61.

Peloquin, L.J. and Klorman, R. (1986). Effects of methylphenidate on normal children's mood, event-related potentials, and performance in memory scanning and vigilance. *Journal of Abnormal Psychology*, **95**, 88–98.

Pliszka, S.R. (1989). Effect of anxiety on cognition, behaviour, and stimulant response in ADHD. *Journal of the American Academy of Child and Adolescent Psychiatry*, **28**, 882–7.

Porges, S.W. (1984). Physiological correlates of attention: a core process underlying learning disorders. *Pediatric Clinics of North America*, **31**, 371–85.

Porges, S.W. and Smith, K.M. (1980). Defining hyperactivity: psychophysiological and behavioral strategies. In *Hyperactive Children: The Social Ecology of Identification and Treatment*, C.K. Whalen and B. Henker, eds, pp. 75–84. New York: Academic Press.

Porges, S.W., Walter, G.F., Korb, R.J. and Sprague, R.L. (1975). The influence of methylphenidate on heart rate and behavioural measures of attention in hyperactive children. *Child Development*, **46**, 727–33.

Posner, M.I. (1988). Structures and functions of selective attention. In *Clinical Neuropsychology and Brainfunction: Research, Assessment*, T. Boll and D.K. Bryant, eds, pp. 173–202. Washington, DC: American Psychiatric Association.

Posner, M.I. and Mitchell, R.F. (1967). Chronometric analysis of classification. *Psychological Review*, **74**, 392–409.

Power, T.J. (1992). Contextual factors in vigilance testing of children with ADHD. *Journal of Abnormal Child Psychology*, **20**, 579–95.

Pribram, K.H. and McGuinness, D. (1975). Arousal, activation and effort in the control of attention. *Psychological Review*, **2**, 116–49.

Prior, M., Sanson, A., Freethy, C. and Geffen, G. (1985). Auditory attentional abilities in hyperactive children. *Journal of Child Psychology and Psychiatry*, **26**, 289–304.

Radosh, A. and Gittelman, R. (1981). The effect of appealing distractors on the performance of hyperactive children. *Journal of Abnormal Child Psychology*, **9**, 179–89.

Rapoport, J.L., Buchsbaum, M.S., Weingartner, H. et al. (1980). Dextroamphetamine – its cognitive and behavioral effects in normal and hyperactive boys and normal men. *Archives of General Psychiatry*, **37**, 933–43.

Rapoport, J.L., Donnely, M., Zametkin, A. and Carrougher, J. (1986). Situational hyperactivity in a US clinical setting. *Journal of Child Psychology and Psychiatry*, **27**, 639–46.

Reid, M.K. and Borkowski, J.G. (1984). Effects of methylphenidate (Ritalin) on information processing in hyperactive children. *Journal of Abnormal Child Psychology*, **12**, 169–86.

Rosenthal, H.R. and Allen, T.W. (1980). Intratask distractibility in hyperkinetic and nonhyperkinetic children. *Journal of Abnormal Child Psychology*, **8**, 175–87.

Rosvold, H.E., Mirsky, A.F., Sarason, I. and Beck, L. (1956). A continuous performance test of brain damage. *Journal of Consulting Psychology*, **20**, 343–50.

Roth, N., Beyreiss, J., Schlenzka, K. and Beyer, H. (1991). Coincidence of attention deficit disorder and atopic disorders in children: empirical findings and hypothetical background. *Journal of Abnormal Child Psychology*, **19**, 1–13.

Rubia, K., Oosterlaan, J., Sergeant, J.A., Brandeis, D. and Van Leeuwen, T. (1998). Inhibitory dysfunction in hyperactive boys. *Behavioural Brain Research*, **94**, 25–32.

Sagvolden, T. and Archer, S (1989). *Attention Deficit Disorder. Clinical and Basic Research*. Hillsdale, NY: Lawrence Erlbaum.

Sandberg, S.T., Rutter, M. and Taylor, E. (1978). Hyperkinetic disorder in clinic attenders. *Developmental Medicine and Child Neurology*, **20**, 279–99.

Sanders, A.F. (1983). Toward a model of stress and human performance. *Acta Psychologica*, **53**, 61–97.

Satterfield, J.H. and Braley, B.W. (1977). Evoked potentials and brain maturation in hyperactive and normal children. *Electroencephalography and Clinical Neurophysiology*, **43**, 43–51.

Satterfield, J.H. and Schell, A.M. (1984). Childhood brain function differences in delinquent and non-delinquent hyperactive boys. *Electroencephalography and Clinical Neurophysiology*, **57**, 199–207.

Satterfield, J.H., Schell, A.M., Nicholas, T. and Backs, R.W. (1988). Topographic study of auditory event-related potentials in normal boys and boys with attention deficit disorder with hyperactivity. *Psychophysiology*, **25**, 591–606.

Schachar, R. and Logan, G. (1990a). Are hyperactive children deficient in attentional capacity? *Journal of Abnormal Child Psychology*, **18**, 493–513.

Schachar, R. and Logan, G.D. (1990b). Impulsivity and inhibitory control in normal development and childhood psychopathology. *Developmental Psychology*, **26**, 710–20.

Schachar, R., Rutter, M. and Smith, A. (1981). Characteristics of situationally and pervasively hyperactive children: implications in syndrome definition. *Journal of Child Psychology and Psychiatry*, **22**, 375–92.

Schachar, R., Logan, G.D., Wachsmuth, R. and Chajczyk, D. (1988). Attaining and maintaining preparation: a comparison of attention in hyperactive, normal, and disturbed control children. *Journal of Abnormal Child Psychology*, **16**, 361–70.

Scheres, A., Oosterlaan, J. and Sergeant, J.A. (2001). Response execution and inhibition in children with AD/HD and other disruptive disorders: the role of behavioral activation. *Journal of Child Psychology and Psychiatry*, **42**, 347–57.

Schneider, J.S. and Roeltgen, D.P. (1991). Chronic low dose MPTP-induced cognitive impairments in primates: a possible model for the cognitive disturbances of attention deficit disorders. *Journal of Child Neurology*, **6**, 82–9.

Seidel, W.T. and Joschko, M. (1990). Evidence of difficulties in sustained attention in children with ADDH. *Journal of Abnormal Child Psychology*, **18**, 217–9.

Sergeant, J.A. (1988a). RDC for hyperactivity/attention disorder. In *Attention Deficit Disorder: Criteria, Cognition, Intervention*, L.M. Bloomingdale and J.A. Sergeant, eds, pp. 1–8. Oxford: Pergamon Press.

Sergeant, J.A. (1988b). From DSM attentional deficit disorder to functional defects. In *Attentional Deficit Disorder: Criteria, Cognition, Intervention*, L.M. Bloomingdale and J.A. Sergeant, eds, pp. 183–98. Oxford: Pergamon Press.

Sergeant, J.A. and Scholten, C.A. (1983). A stages of information approach to hyperactivity. *Journal of Child Psychology and Psychiatry*, **24**, 49–60.

Sergeant, J.A. and Scholten, C.A. (1985a). On data limitations in hyperactivity. *Journal of Child Psychology and Psychiatry*, **26**, 111–24.

Sergeant, J.A. and Scholten, C.A. (1985b). On resource strategy limitations in hyperactivity: cognitive impulsivity reconsidered. *Journal of Child Psychology and Psychiatry*, **26**, 97–109.

Sergeant, J.A. and Van der Meere, J.J. (1988). What happens after a hyperactive commits an error? *Psychiatric Research*, **24**, 157–64.

Sergeant, J.A. and Van der Meere, J.J. (1989). The diagnostic significance for ADD(H) classification, a future DSM. In *Attention Deficit Disorder and Hyperkinetic Syndrome*, T. Sagvolden, H.M. Borggrevink and T. Archer, eds, pp. 149–63. New York: Lawrence Erlbaum.

Sergeant, J.A. and Van der Meere, J.J. (1990a). Convergence of approaches in lokalizing the hyperactivity deficit. In *Advances in Clinical Child Psychology*, B.B. Lahey and A.E. Kazdin, eds, pp. 207–46. New York: Plenum Press.

Sergeant, J.A. and Van der Meere, J.J. (1990b). Additive factor method applied to psychopathology with special reference to childhood hyperactivity. *Acta Psychologica*, **74**, 277–96.

Sergeant, J.A. and Van der Meere, J.J. (1994). Towards an emperical child psychopathology. In *Disruptive Behaviour Disorders in Childhood*, D.K. Routh, ed., pp. 59–78. New York: Plenum Press.

Sergeant, J.A. and Van der Meere, J.J. (1999). Ritalin: an energetical factor? In *Ritalin. Theory and Practice*, L.L. Greenhill and B.B. Osman, eds, pp. 321–40. New York: Mary Ann Liebert.

Shaywitz, B.A., Cohen, D.J. and Bowers, M.B. (1977). CFS monoamine metabolites in children with minimal brain dysfunction – evidence for alteration of brain dopamine. *Journal of Pediatrics*, **90**, 67–71.

Shue, K. and Douglas, V.I. (1989). Attention deficit hyperactivity disorder, normal development, and frontal lobe syndrome. *Canadian Psychology*, **30**, 498–512.

Solanto, M.V. (1990). The effects of reinforcement and response cost on a delayed response task in children with attention deficit hyperactivity disorder: a research note. *Journal of Child Psychology and Psychiatry*, **31**, 803–8.

Sonuga-Barke, E.J.S., Taylor, E., Sembi, S. and Smith, J. (1992). The effect of delay of choice. *Journal of Child Psychology and Psychiatry*, **33**, 387–98.

Sroufe, L.A. Sonies, B.C., West, W.D. and Wright, F.S. (1973). Anticipatory heart rate deceleration and reaction time in children with and without referral for learning disability. *Child Development*, **44**, 267–73.

Stemerdink, B.A, Van der Molen, M.W., Kalverboer, A.F. et al. (1994). Information processing deficits in children with early and continuously treated phenylketonuria. *Acta Pediatrica*, **407**, 106–8.

Stemerdink, B.A., Van der Meere, J.J., Van der Molen, M.W. et al. (1995). Information processing in patients with early and continuously treated phenylketonuria. *European Journal of Pediatrics*, **154**, 739–46.

Stemerdink, B.A., Van der Molen, M.W., Kalverboer, A.F. et al. (1999). Prefrontal dysfunction in early and continuously treated phenylketonuria. *Developmental Neuropsychology*, **15**, 29–57.

Stemerdink, B.A., Kalverboer, A.F., Van der Meere, J.J. et al. (2000). Behaviour and school achievement in patients with early and continuously treated phenylketonuria. *Journal of Inherited Metabolic Disease*, **23**, 548–62.

Sternberg, S. (1969). Discovery of the processing stages: extensions of the Donder's method. In

Attention and Performance, vol. 2, W.G. Kosters, ed., pp. 276–315. Amsterdam: Noord Holland.

Stevens, D.A., Stover, C.F. and Backus, J.T. (1970). The hyperkinetic child: effects of incentives on the speed of rapid tapping. *Journal of Consulting and Clinical Psychology*, **34**, 56–9.

Stifter, C.A. and Moyer, D. (1991). The regulation of positive affect: gaze aversion activity during mother–infant interaction. *Infant Behavior and Development*, **14**, 111–23.

Stott, D.H., Moyes, F.A. and Henderson, S.E. (1984). *Test of Motor Impairment*. Guelph, Ontario, Canada: Brook Educational.

Strauss, J., Lewis, J.L., Klorman, R. et al. (1984). Effects of methylphenidate on young adults' performance and event related potentials in a vigilance and a paired-associates learning test. *Psychophysiology*, **21**, 609–61.

Stroes, A., Alberts, E. and Van der Meere, J.J. (submitted). ADHD children in social interaction with a stranger: an observational study.

Swanson, J.M., Shea, C., McBurnett, K. et al. (1990). Attention and hyperactivity. In *The Development of Attention: Research and Theory*, J.T. Enns, ed., pp. 383–403. Amsterdam: Elsevier Science.

Sykes, D.H., Douglas, V.I., Weiss, G. and Minde, K.K. (1971). Attention in hyperactive children and the effect of methylphenidate (Ritalin). *Journal of Child Psychology and Psychiatry*, **12**, 129–39.

Sykes, D.H., Douglas, V.I. and Morgenstern, G.L. (1973). Sustained attention in hyperactive children and the effect of methylphenidate (Ritalin). *Journal of Child Psychology and Psychiatry*, **14**, 129–39.

Tannock, R., Schachar, R.J., Carr, R.P., Chajczyk, D. and Logan, G.D. (1989). Effects of methylphenidate on inhibitory control in hyperactive children. *Journal of Abnormal Child Psychology*, **17**, 473–91.

Taylor, E. (1983). Drug response and diagnostic validation. In *Developmental Neuropsychiatry*, M. Rutter, ed., pp. 348–68. New York: Guilford Press.

Taylor, E. (1989). Some research issues in attention deficit. In *Attention Deficit Disorder. Current Concepts and Emerging Trends in Attentional and Behavioral Disorders of Childhood*, L.M. Bloomingdale and J. Swanson, eds, pp. 313–33. Oxford: Pergamon Press.

Taylor, E. (1998). Clinical foundations of hyperactivity research. *Behaviour and Brain Research*, **94**, 11–24.

Thoman, E.B. and Whitney, M.P. (1990). Behavioral states in infants: individual differences and individual analyses. In *Individual Differences in Infancy: Reliability, Stability, Prediction*, J. Colombo and J. Fagen, eds, pp. 113–35. Hillsdale, NJ: Lawrence Erlbaum.

Thurstone, L.L. (1938). Primary mental abilities. *Psychometric Monographs*, **1**, ix–121.

Treisman A. and Gelade, G.C. (1980). A feature integration theory of attention. *Cognitive Psychology*, **12**, 97–136.

Trommer, B.L., Hoeppner, J.B., Lorber, R. and Armstrong, K.J. (1988). The go–no go paradigm in attention deficit disorder. *Annals of Neurology*, **24**, 610–14.

Tucker, D.M. and Williamson, P.A. (1984). Asymmetric neural control systems in human self-regulation. *Psychological Review*, **91**, 185–215.

Vaessen, W. (1990a). *Ecological Validity of Hyperactivity Studies. Two Field Experiments with*

Carefully Selected Hyperactive and Clumsy Children. Thesis. The Netherlands: University of Groningen.

Vaessen, W. (1990b). Performance of hyperactive children in a traffic task: a validation study. In *Developmental Biopsychology: Experimental and Observational Studies in Children at Risk*, A.F. Kalverboer, ed., pp. 95–114. Ann Arbor: University of Michigan Press.

Vaessen, W. and Van der Meere, J.J. (1990). Issues in the selection of hyperactive/ADD(H) children for experimental clinical studies. In *Developmental Biopsychology: Experimental and Observational Studies in Groups 'At Risk'*, A.F. Kalverboer, ed., pp. 21–37. Ann Arbor: University of Michigan Press.

Van Dellen, H.J., Brookhuis, K.A., Mulder, G., Okita, T. and Mulder, L.J.M. (1984). Evoked potential correlates of practice in a visual search task. In *Clinical and Experimental Neuro-psychophysiology*, D. Papakostopoulos, S. Butler and L.Martin, eds, pp. 132–56. London: Croom Helm.

Van de Meer, D.J., Van der Meere, J.J., Kunert, H.J. and Kalverboer, A.F. (submitted). A series of cognitive experiments in children with MMR plus or minus ADHD and conduct disorder.

Van der Meere, J.J. and Sergeant, J.A. (1987). A divided attention experiment with pervasively hyperactive children. *Journal of Abnormal Child Psychology*, **15**, 379–91.

Van der Meere, J.J. and Sergeant, J.A. (1988a). A focused attention experiment in pervasively hyperactive children. *Journal of Abnormal Child Psychology*, **16**, 627–39.

Van der Meere, J.J. and Sergeant, J.A. (1988b). Controlled processing and vigilance in hyperactivity: time will tell. *Journal of Abnormal Child Psychology*, **16**, 641–55.

Van der Meere, J.J. and Sergeant, J.A. (1988c). Acquisition of attention skill in pervasively hyperactive children. *Journal of Child Psychology and Psychiatry*, **29**, 301–10.

Van der Meere, J.J. and Stemerdink, B.A. (1999). The normal development of state regulation in school-aged children: an indirect comparison with ADHD. *Developmental Neuropsychology*, **16**, 213–25.

Van der Meere, J.J., Van Baal, M. and Sergeant, J.A. (1989). The additive factor method: a differential diagnostic tool in hyperactive and learning disability. *Journal of Abnormal Child Psychology*, **17**, 409–22.

Van der Meere, J.J., Wekking, E. and Sergeant, J. (1991). Sustained attention and pervasive hyperactivity. *Journal of Child Psychology and Psychiatry*, **32**, 275–84.

Van der Meere, J.J., Vreeling, H.J. and Sergeant, J.A. (1992). A motor presetting experiment in hyperactive, learning disabled and control children. *Journal of Child Psychology and Psychiatry*, **33**, 1347–54.

Van der Meere, J.J., Gunning W.B. and Stermerdink, B.A. (1995a). The effect of presentation rate on task perfromance in ADHD with and without tics. *Journal of Perceptual and Motor Skills*, **81**, 259–62.

Van der Meere, J.J., Hughes, K.A., Borger, N. and Sallee, F.R. (1995b). The effect of reward on sustained attention in ADHD children with and without CD. In *Eunethydia: European Aproaches to Hyperkinetic Disorder*, J.A. Sergeant, ed., pp. 239–52. Zurich: Trumphimportuer.

Van der Meere, J.J., Shalev, R.S., Börger, N. and Gross-Tsur, V. (1995c). Sustained attention, activation and MPH in ADHD. *Journal of Child Psychology and Psychiatry*, **36**, 697–703.

Van der Meere, J.J., Hughes, K., Börger, N.A. and Sallee, R. (1995d). The effect of reward on sustained attention in children with ADHD with and without CD. In *European Approaches to Hyperkinetic Disorder*, J.A. Sergeant, ed., pp. 241–53. Zurich: Trumphimporteur.

Van der Meere, J.J., Shalev, R., Gross-Tsur, V. and Börger, N.A. (1995e). Sustained attention, motivation, and MPH in ADHD. *Journal of Child Psychology and Psychiatry*, **36**, 697–703.

Van der Meere, J.J., Gunning, B. and Stemerdink, N. (1996). Changing a response set in normal development and in ADHD children with and without tics. *Journal of Abnormal Child Psychology*, **24**, 767–86.

Van der Meere, J.J., Gunning, B. and Stemerdink, B.A. (1999). The effect of methylphenidate and clonidine on state regulation in ADHD children. *Journal of Abnormal Child Psychology*, **40**, 291–8.

Van der Molen, M.W. (1990). Energetics of cognitive development. In *Developmental Psychology Behind the Dikes*, W. Koops and H. Soppe, eds, pp. 123–40. Delft: Eburon.

Van der Molen, M.W., Somsen, R.J.N., Jennings, J.R., Nieuwboer, R.T. and Orlebeke, J.F. (1987). A psychophysiological investigation of cognitive-energetical relations in human information processing: a heart rate / additive factors approach. *Acta Psychologica*, **66**, 251–89.

Weingartner, H., Rapoport, J.L., Buchsbaum, M.S. et al. (1980). Cognitive processes in normal and hyperactive children and their response to amphetamine treatment. *Journal of Abnormal Psychology*, **89**, 25–37.

Wilding, J. (1994). Attentional problems in the classroom and parallel processing ability. *British Journal of Developmental Psychology*, **12**, 539–53.

Zahn, T.P., Little, B. and Wender, (1978). Pupillary and heart rate reactivity in children with minimal brain dysfunction. *Journal of Abnormal Child Psychology*, **6**, 135–47.

Zahn, T.P., Kruesi, M.J.P. and Rapoport, J.L. (1991). Reaction time indices of attention deficit in boys with disruptive behavior disorders. *Journal of Abnormal Child Psychology*, **19**, 233–52.

Zametkin, A.J. and Rapaport, J.L. (1987). The neuropharmacology of attention deficit disorder with hyperactivity: where have we come in 50 years? *Journal of the American Academy of Child and Adolescent Psychiatry*, **26**, 676–86.

Zametkin, A.J., Nordahl, T.E. and Gross, M. (1990). Cerebral glucose metabolism in adults with hyperactivity of childhood onset. *New England Journal of Medicine*, **323**, 1361–6.

Zentall, S.S. and Meyer, M.J. (1987). Self-regulation of stimulation for ADD-H children during reading and vigilance task performance. *Journal of Abnormal Child Psychology*, **15**, 519–36.

Zentall, F.S. and Shaw, J.H. (1980). Effects of classroom noise on performance and activity of second-grade hyperactives and control children. *Journal of Educational Psychology*, **71**, 830–40.

Zentall, S.S. and Zentall, T.R. (1983). Optimal stimulation: a model of disordered activity and performance in normal and deviant children. *Psychological Bulletin*, **94**, 446–71.

Zentall, S.S., Zentall, T.R. and Barack, R.B. (1978). Distraction as a function of within-task stimulation for hyperactive and normal children. *Journal of Learning Disabilities*, **11**, 13–21.

7

Cognitive aspects and learning

Erika Hagemann[1], David A. Hay[1] and Florence Levy[2]

[1]School of Psychology, Curtin University of Technology, Perth, Western Australia; [2]Avoca Clinic, Princess of Wales Hospital and University of New South Wales, Sydney, NSW, Australia

Introduction

The psychopathology of attention deficit hyperactivity disorder (ADHD) consists of the behavioural symptoms of inattention, overactivity and impulsiveness, is well recognized in children and adolescents, and is reported as one of the most frequently seen problems in child psychiatry (Toone and Van der Linden, 1997; Taylor, 1998). However, there is significant heterogeneity among individuals presenting with behavioural problems of inattention, overactivity and impulsiveness. Different diagnostic traditions have evolved different conceptualizations of the essential features associated with such behaviour by both clinicians and researchers (Ostrander et al., 1998). Heterogeneity between individuals and diagnostic classification systems contributes to much of the conflicting evidence over the cognitive functioning or dysfunctioning in ADHD.

The main diagnostic classifications for such psychopathology are:

- Attention deficit hyperactivity disorder (ADHD) in the *Diagnostic and Statistical Manual of Mental Disorders* (DSM-IV) by the American Psychiatric Association (APA: American Psychiatric Association, 1994)
- Hyperkinetic disorder (HKD) in the *International Classification of Mental and Behavioural Disorders* (ICD-10) by the World Health Organization (WHO: World Health Organization, 1993).

Until recently, the classification of childhood psychopathology of hyperactivity by the APA and WHO differed in three key respects – the symptoms they emphasized, the importance they placed on symptom pervasiveness and their treatment of comorbid disorders (Tripp et al., 1999). However, the fourth edition of the DSM (APA, 1994) brought the APA and WHO systems for classifying childhood hyperactivity closer (Tripp et al., 1999). Tripp et al. (1999) compared the overlap in identification, core features and the neurodevelopmental, academic and cognitive correlates of children identified according to

ICD-10 HKD and DSM-IV ADHD. Although there was significant overlap in the cases identified by the two diagnostic systems, with the majority of children diagnosed with HKD meeting criteria for ADHD, the DSM-IV criteria did identify a broader group of children than the ICD-10 definition. The ICD-10 description of HKD was identifying a more seriously impaired and younger subset of the population of children who met criteria for ADHD. This is consistent with HKD requiring separate informants on behaviour in at least two settings, whereas the DSM-IV criteria of impairment in at least two situations can be based on a single informant. But for any discussion of cognition in ADHD, probably a more significant issue concerns differences in patterns of symptomatology.

DSM-IV divided the symptomatology into two independent dimensions of symptoms, namely inattention and hyperactivity-impulsivity (Lahey et al., 1998; Ostrander et al., 1998; Tannock, 1998a; Gomez et al., 1999). Many studies have confirmed the validity of this bidimensional division of ADHD symptomatology (Ostrander et al., 1998; Gomez et al., 1999). Burns et al. (1997) and Wolraich et al. (1996) utilized parent and teacher ratings and confirmed the independence of the two dimensions by means of confirmatory factor analysis, as did a discriminant validity study by Lahey et al. (1998). Based on these separate dimensions, DSM-IV recognizes three subtypes of ADHD: one with mainly inattentive symptoms (the 'predominantly inattentive type', ADHD;PI), one with hyperactive-impulsive symptoms (the 'predominantly hyperactive-impulsive type', ADHD;HI), and one with symptoms from both dimensions (the 'combined type', ADHD;CT; Lahey et al., 1998). In contrast, HKD requires the presence of symptoms from all three categories. Subsequent to the DSM-IV field trials, several studies have sought to clarify the nosological validity of the DSM-IV subtypes of ADHD. The subtypes differ in associated neuropsychological, cognitive and behavioural features (Gaub and Carlson, 1997; Houghton et al., 1999), comorbidity (Eiraldi et al., 1997; Faraone et al., 1998b; Lalonde et al., 1998) and severity of impairment (Wood, 1999).

Tripp et al. (1999) suggested that children with HKD were closer to the ADHD;CT but not ADHD;PI or ADHD;HI. Conversely, results from studies including ADHD;PI or ADHD;HI will not necessarily apply to children with HKD. To date, few studies have investigated the topics of this chapter – cognition and learning in relation to the DSM-IV subtypes – and inconsistencies remain in identifying differences between subtypes. Many recent studies have obtained data with diagnostic systems prior to DSM-IV and the term 'ADHD' can often be assumed to refer to DSM-III-R diagnoses where the criterion was eight of 14 inattentive, hyperactive and impulsive symptoms.

Cognitive functioning

General intelligence

Intelligence tests provide a very broad index of higher cortical functioning and have predictive validity for school achievement and diagnostic utility for clinical populations such as learning disorders (Kaufman, 1999). Although there has been concern about the utility of IQ tests in ADHD (Barkley, 1995), the psychometric properties of intelligence tests remain robust for the clinical group of ADHD (Tannock, 1998b). McGee et al. (1989) proposed a general cognitive deficit correlated with ADHD. Tannock (1998b) reported that ADHD is typically associated with lower full-scale IQ and deficits on some specific subtests, but the mean levels of intellectual functioning fall well within the normal range. These findings generally apply even after controlling for the presence of comorbid disorders, considered later in this chapter.

In relation to the bidimensional division of ADHD symptomatology and the resulting subtypes recognized in DSM-IV, Barkley (1997) proposed that any evidence of a general cognitive deficit is more likely to be reflective of the ADHD;PI subtype. This is consistent with Gaub and Carlson (1997), Semrud-Clikeman et al. (1992), and Hinshaw (1992), whose results suggested that the intellectual profile may be a correlate of inattention rather than hyperactivity-impulsiveness. However, such suggestions are not conclusive, with some studies finding no differences between the subtypes (e.g. Morgan et al., 1996) on IQ measures, and others (e.g. Eiraldi et al., 1997) not finding significant differences once the effects of socioeconomic status (SES) were taken into account. Such results are not easy to interpret, given the long history of genetic analyses of the association between SES and intelligence test performance (Hay, 1985).

Neuropsychological function

The term 'neuropsychological' is used informally to refer to tests commonly used in neuropsychology, such as Stroop, Trail-making and Verbal Fluency, which provide indices of a wide variety of cognitive functions that afford presumed insights into brain function and brain behaviour relationships (Tannock, 1998b; Nigg et al., 1999). Such tests are sensitive to subtle deficits that interfere with learning and achievement (Tannock, 1998b). Such a circumspect definition of neuropsychological assessment is appropriate with ADHD, given that almost every test, including conventional intelligence tests, has been given the label 'neuropsychological'. With the long history of labelling ADHD as 'minimal brain damage' or 'minimal brain dysfunction', the use of the term 'neuropsychological' warrants caution, especially as so much of the work has been atheoretical rather than testing a particular model of brain functioning. Previous research on neuropsychological functioning in children with ADHD suggests that there are deficits specific to ADHD (Seidman et al., 1997; Nigg et al., 1998) with more recent convergence on the broad domain of executive functions as the relevant functional arena (Nigg et al., in press).

Executive functioning

No overall agreement exists as to the best definition of executive function. Formal definition and measurement (particularly in children) remains elusive (Tannock, 1998b) and the problem is compounded by the paucity of adequate age norms for most neuropsychological measures. Executive functions are not always adequately specified nor studied under the rubric of a single measure or function (Pennington and Ozonoff, 1996; Nigg et al., in press). They may be conceptualized as regulation of response to context and maintenance of behaviour towards a goal (Nigg et al., 1999), rather than being concerned with processing, perception or storage, or 'what we know'. Executive functioning focuses on information utilization or 'how we use what we know', that is, planning, organizing and self-monitoring in order to act upon knowledge or produce from a store of knowledge (Reader et al., 1994). Executive function facilitates future-oriented behaviour by allowing for planning, flexible strategy employment, impulse control and organized search (Welsh et al., 1991).

The construct of executive functions overlaps closely, but is not identical to theories of prefrontal cortical function, given clinical and empirical evidence identifying the role of this brain region in executive functioning (Weyandt and Willis, 1994; Barkley, 1997; Tannock, 1998a). It has been argued that defective executive functioning plays a key role in the cognitive and behavioural deficits and symptomatology associated with ADHD (Douglas and Benezra, 1990; Shelton and Barkley, 1994; Ehlers et al., 1997; Tannock, 1998a).

Executive functions generally include planning, impulse control, cognitive flexibility and self-monitoring. Pennington and Ozonoff (1996) reviewed the neuropsychological measures used in 18 studies of ADHD, classifying executive function (EF) and nonexecutive function (non-EF) measures, and identified significant differences between ADHD subjects and controls on EF measures in 15 of the 18 studies. The largest effect sizes and consistency of differences from controls were found for the Wisconsin Card Sorting Test (WCST) Perseverations, Trail-making Test B, Matching Familiar Figures, Errors and Time, Stroop Time, Tower of Hanoi (TOH), and Motor Inhibition Tasks. Across the

18 studies reviewed, ADHD subjects fairly consistently exhibited poorer performance on measures of EF and vigilance/perceptual speed, whereas they exhibited normal performance on a variety of verbal and nonverbal measures. The authors interpreted their findings as suggesting a core deficit, possibly in response inhibition, consistent with Barkley (1997).

Executive functioning and DSM-IV subtypes

It is important to consider domains of EF in relation to DSM-IV subtypes of ADHD, although very few studies of EF in ADHD have looked at the DSM-IV diagnostic definitions. There are two different approaches, one based around Barkley's (1997) model which emphasizes a developmental continuum from the hyperactive-impulsive to the combined type, and one based on a much more straightforward comparison between the DSM-IV subtypes.

Barkley (1997) proposed a unifying theory of ADHD, which involves a central deficit in response inhibition. This deficit is secondarily linked to five neuropsychological functions, namely prolongation/working memory, internalization of speech, self-regulation of affect, reconstitution and motor control/fluency, thought to be broadly representative of the more general concept of EF. He suggested the inattentive (ADHD;PI) subtype may represent a separate disorder, with more problems with selective attention, sluggishness and memory retrieval, as well as problems with mathematics, language and reading (Taylor et al., 1991). However, some of the comorbidity studies discussed later do not show more problems in ADHD;PI than in ADHD;CT.

To date, only a limited number of studies have investigated the implications of Barkley's hypothesis for ADHD subtypes. Klorman et al. (1999) evaluated EF in children classified as ADHD;CT or ADHD;PI, using the WCST and TOH. At first sight their chief findings supported Barkley's hypothesis, namely, EF deficits characterized only ADHD children with hyperactivity-impulsivity. ADHD;CT subjects performed poorly on the TOH (solving fewer problems and violating more rules) compared with both ADHD;PI and non-ADHD children.

The results are not really so clear. The authors report that the TOH reflects planning as well as working memory and spatial skills, and so much more is being tapped than just EF. This fits with their finding of no differences between ADHD subtypes or non-ADHD children on WCST perseverative errors, possibly reflecting limited sensitivity of the WCST. On the other hand ADHD;CT children, independent of age, made more nonperseverative errors than ADHD;PI children and marginally more than non-ADHD subjects. Interestingly, there were comparable EF deficits in ADHD subjects with and without reading disorder (RD), despite lower IQ in the latter case with the difference between ADHD with or without RD being the same in ADHD;PI and ADHD;CT. Comorbidity with oppositional defiant disorder (ODD) was common but did not influence the findings for ADHD.

Vaughn et al. (unpublished work) report a somewhat contrasting set of results. They compared children with ADHD;CT and ADHD;PI on a number of working memory tasks, including the WCST, Clinical Evaluation of Language Fundamentals – Revised (CELF-R; Semel et al., 1987) Oral Directions and Recall of Sentences subtests, and the Wechsler Intelligence Scale for Children – Third Edition (WISC-III; Wechsler, 1991). From Barkley's (1997) predictions it was expected that ADHD groups would not differ from normal controls on simple rote memory tasks, but would show significant impairments on more complex memory tasks (WISC-III arithmetic, CELF-R oral directions and recall of sentences and WCST trials to set and failure to maintain set). It was expected that the ADHD;CT group would be more impaired than the ADHD;PI group due to greater deficits with inhibitory control. They covaried for verbal ability in the analyses of memory to control for group differences in verbal IQ but chose to use the verbal comprehension composite from the WISC rather than the full verbal IQ since the latter includes arithmetic. Along with digit span and coding, these three tests comprise the Freedom from Distractibility factor and so this is confounded with attention. The ADHD;PI subtype performed significantly below normal controls on the WCST cognitive index. However, stepwise discriminant analyses showed the cognitive index and verbal comprehension were poor predictors of group membership. The authors interpreted their findings as indicating limitations in Barkley's unifying theory of ADHD and queried the rationale for excluding children with ADHD;PI from a unifying theory of ADHD.

The question of how best to covary for intelligence is not easy. Wood (1999) compared ADHD;PI and ADHD-CT and controls on the Intradimensional and Extradimensional (ID/ED) attentional set shifting tasks from the Cambridge Neuropsychological Test Automated Battery (CANTAB; Robbins et al., 1994), as well as the WISC-III. The ID/ED task is similar in cognitive demands to the WCST. The ADHD;CT did worse on the symbol search and the coding subtests of the WISC-III than children with ADHD;PI and controls. There were no significant group differences on the ID/ED attentional set shifting task when full-scale IQ was used as a covariate.

Some other studies provide preliminary evidence on differential patterns of executive function according to ADHD subtype. Reader et al. (1994) proposed that executive dysfunction might be more common in children who meet criteria for ADHD with hyperactivity than those who meet criteria for ADHD without hyperactivity. This coincides with Houghton et al. (1999), who found significant impairments in EF in children with ADHD compared with non-ADHD children were mediated by DSM-IV ADHD subtype. Children with ADHD;CT and not those with ADHD;PI were more impaired on a number of measures of the WCST and the Stroop Color–Word test. However, the effect sizes were small and on many measures the ADHD;PI scores were actually closer to those of the ADHD;CT than of the controls. Nigg et al. (in press) also suggested that executive functioning problems were specific to DSM-IV ADHD subtype. The ADHD;PI showed some executive deficits, but these were not the same as those for the combined type. The ADHD;CT had a deficit in behavioural inhibition, whereas the ADHD;PI had a deficit in tasks that required mental but not behavioural control, in particular set-shifting and, to a lesser degree, planning.

The above studies used somewhat different measures of EF and working memory, and could also have been influenced by ascertainment bias. For example, the ADHD;PI group in the Vaughn et al. (unpublished work) study had a mean IQ of 93.4 (standard deviation (SD) 9.1) compared with 105.45 (SD 11.6) in the Klorman et al. (1999) study. The varying findings also reflect the variety of measures incorporated in the EF concept, many of which no longer show group differences when IQ is covaried. It is unlikely that consistent group differences will be shown until measures used to define concepts like working memory and inhibition are standardized and distinguished from their role in IQ. It is clear that at present some studies are covarying out the very attentional components that are their focus of study.

Nigg et al. (in press) suggested that neuropsychological research using the DSM-IV subtypes of ADHD faces several challenges, such as explaining the theorized executive or other cognitive deficit in ADHD;PI, demonstrating that executive deficits are independent of reading ability and IQ, and showing specific/differential executive deficits. Their finding of different executive deficits for the ADHD;PI and CT subtypes argue against a 'general deficit' model of ADHD executive dysfunction, in favour of a 'specific deficit' model. In a general deficit model, the ADHD;CT would have problems in all types of control processes while the ADHD;PI would have deficits in only some of these processes. This model was not supported because the combined type had a deficit only in behavioural inhibition.

However, it is imperative that comorbidity and other general and specific cognitive abilities are taken into account, since these differ so much between subtypes. Failure to consider comorbidity is a frequent problem in the ADHD neuropsychological literature. As suggested by Nigg et al. (in press), it is necessary to clarify whether deficits observed in ADHD are actually due to comorbid problems, such as learning disorder (Nigg et al., 1999). We have already mentioned Klorman et al.'s (1999) finding of lower IQ scores on ADHD;PI and ADHD;CT in the presence of comorbid reading disability.

Comorbidity and ADHD

Comorbidity, the cooccurrence of two or more separate disorders, is common in psychopathology. It is emerging as a major issue for both clinical practice and research that must be taken into account for understanding the aetiology, course and treatment of disorders (Nigg and Goldsmith, 1998; Angold et al., 1999). The recent text by Pliszka et al. (1999) has focused attention on the role of comorbidity in ADHD.

Comorbidity can occur for many reasons beyond the scope of this review, including methodological artefacts, such as referral bias, sampling bias, rater expectancy or halo effects (Faraone et al., 1998a; Angold et al., 1999; Caron and Rutter, 1991). Alternatively there could be overlapping diagnostic criteria, artificial subdivisions of syndromes, one disorder representing an early manifestation of another, or one disorder being part of another (Caron and Rutter, 1991). Several rather different underlying processes need to be considered in the case of true comorbidity, such as the following:

(1) Disorders share the same risk factor or factors
(2) One disorder creates an increased risk for another
(3) The comorbid pattern constitutes a meaningful syndrome, that is, comorbid cases are due to a separate third disorder

Neale and Kendler (1995) developed several formal genetic models for comorbidity based on these different underlying processes, on which critical hypotheses relevant to both research and clinical practice can be investigated. Although these are only now starting to be applied to ADHD, the value of the genetic approach is such that we have included a section on the genetics of comorbidity.

As many as two-thirds of elementary-school-age children with ADHD who are referred for clinical evaluation have at least one other diagnosable psychiatric disorder (Cantwell, 1996). The major comorbid conditions of ADHD include learning disorders, communication disorders, conduct and oppositional defiant disorder, anxiety disorders, mood disorders and Tourette syndrome or chronic tics (Goldman et al., 1998; Zametkin and Ernst, 1999). The actual comorbid conditions and their prevalence rates vary across different types of samples, depending on whether the sample is clinical or population-based, and whether a clinical sample is paediatric or psychiatric. For example, while rates of learning disorders are higher in paediatric samples, conduct and oppositional defiant disorder are reported more often in psychiatric samples (Cantwell, 1996).

Learning disorders and ADHD

DSM-IV (APA, 1994) emphasizes that many individuals with ADHD also have learning disorders. Numerous studies have reported that children with ADHD symptomatology are at increased risk for poor cognitive functioning and school failure as measured by grade repetitions, academic underachievement, placement in special classes and need for remedial tutoring (Hinshaw, 1992; Semrud-Clikeman et al., 1992; Faraone et al., 1996; Velting and Whitehurst, 1997; Tannock, 1998b). In addition, learning disorders have been associated with a broad range of internalizing and externalizing disorders (Prior et al., 1999).

Comorbidity rates of ADHD and learning disorders vary from 10 to 92% (Jensen et al., 1997). This large range reflects the diagnostic confusion that not only surrounds the classification of ADHD discussed earlier, but also which plagues learning disorders. This confusion is associated with variable selection criteria, sampling procedures, measurement instruments, operationalization of ADHD and learning disorders, and hence variable comorbidity rates among studies (Faraone et al., 1996).

There is ongoing debate over how best to define specific learning difficulties (Spear-Swerling and Sternberg, 1998). Although DSM-IV introduced the term 'learning disorder', few scientific publications have used this terminology, preferring and substituting terms such as 'learning disabilities', 'learning difficulties' or 'learning deficits' instead (Beitchman and Young, 1997). In addition, the IQ/achievement discrepancy criterion that is adopted in DSM-IV and most often used to identify individuals with learning disorders/disabilities, has been contested (Prior et al., 1999). This is because it may overidentify underachievement in individuals with above-average intelligence, underidentify individuals with below-average intelligence, and provides little insight into the individual's learning difficulties (Spear-Swerling and Sternberg, 1998; Wood, 1999). Here and neutrally the term 'learning disorder' will represent a group of cognitive disorders reflecting circumscribed handicaps in one or more basic cognitive processes manifested as disorders of literacy and numeracy.

The most common, and consequently best researched, type of learning disorder is RD (Beitchman and Young, 1997). Reading is the primary problem in around 80% of children with a diagnosed learning disorder (Plomin et al.,

1997). Given its importance and prominence, the remainder of this section focuses on the comorbidity of ADHD with RD and the associated language problems.

Comorbidity between reading disability/disorder (RD) and ADHD is found in both clinical and epidemiological samples (Felton and Wood, 1989; Douglas and Benezra, 1990; Pennington et al., 1993; Lombardino et al., 1997). The question of overlapping EF problems has been addressed through studies of verbal memory. Felton and Wood (1989) reported deficits in verbal learning and memory as a function of ADHD rather than RD. Douglas and Benezra (1990) reported that both children with ADHD and children with RD experience deficits in verbal memory, but children with ADHD exhibit most pronounced deficits on memory tasks requiring organized, deliberate rehearsal strategies, whereas children with RD show more generalized verbal/memory deficits. Similarly, Frost et al. (1989) suggested that the deficits in children with ADHD become most apparent when more complex information must be held in mind, especially over a lengthy delay period. These studies suggest the possibility that higher-order cognitive processes involved in organization are the predominant cognitive correlate of ADHD.

Some evidence exists that early ADHD increases the risk of reading problems (Shelton and Barkley, 1994) and/or intensifies the severity of reading and other learning problems (Mayes and Calhoun, 2000). There is no doubt that a substantial proportion of children with ADHD meet criteria for a diagnosis of RD (Semrod-Clikeman et al., 1992; Faraone et al., 1993; Purvis and Tannock, 1997). Beitchman and Young (1997) reported that one of the most common comorbid conditions in childhood is that of RD and ADHD.

But it is important to take the issue further to that of causation (Hinshaw, 1992; Stevenson, 2001). Does ADHD lead to the development (and hence comorbidity) of RD, or alternatively, may RD lead to the development (and hence comorbidity) of ADHD? Where does the EF deficit theory of ADHD straddle these two behavioural problems? For example, Pennington et al. (1993) compared subjects with ADHD only, RD only, a comorbid (ADHD and RD) group and control group on measures of EF and of a separate cognitive domain, namely phonological processing. They found a double dissociation. The ADHD-only group showed significant impairment in EF but no impairment in phonological processing, the RD-only group showed an impairment in phonological processing but no impairment in EF, and the comorbid (ADHD and RD) group resembled the RD-only group, with intact EF skills.

Pennington et al. (1993) concluded from their study that the comorbid condition of ADHD and RD might arise as a phenocopy of RD, that is, ADHD

Table 7.1. Comorbidity of attention deficit hyperactivity disorder (ADHD) and other disorders in same-sex twin pairs in the Australian Twin ADHD Project

ADHD category	Reading therapy	Speech therapy	Conduct disorder	Separation anxiety
No diagnosis	338	386	41	642
($n = 2644$)	12.8%	14.6%	1.6%	24.3%
Inattention	103	61	17	94
($n = 239$)	43.1%	25.5%	7.1%	39.3%
Hyperactivity-impulsivity	12	14	5	36
($n = 82$)	14.6%	17.1%	5.2%	43.9%
Combined type	64	39	36	68
($n = 134$)	47.8%	29.1%	26.9%	50.7%

may be a secondary consequence of RD. More recent cross-sectional and longitudinal studies have failed to support the notion that the comorbidity of ADHD and RD arises via a phenocopy mechanism. Stevenson (2001) concluded that there is little evidence that reading and spelling disability contributes at the phenotypic level to the onset of ADHD, or convincing evidence that ADHD leads to RD. Rather, he suggested that ADHD symptomatology may exacerbate reading and spelling difficulties. The possibility of common genetic influences underlying the comorbidity of RD and ADHD is discussed in the section on the genetics of comorbidity, below.

Less is known about the association of ADHD subtypes with RD. Table 7.1 illustrates some of the subtype differences from our Australian Twin ADHD Project (ATAP), which is described more fully in Hay et al. (2001). The measures of speech and reading here are very crude, namely whether the children have received formal intervention for such problems, and there are many social and other issues that may cloud whether or not children have access to such intervention. But the differences between the subtypes are striking, with the ADHD;PI and the ADHD;CT having much higher rates of speech and reading problems than the ADHD;HI. The groups were all of similar ages and this counters the Barkley view of ADHD;HI as a developmental precursor to the ADHD;CT and the associated possibility that the ADHD;HI may be too young to have warranted reading intervention. This group is qualitatively different from the other ADHD subtypes, with no higher rates of intervention than the control children with no ADHD problems. DSM-IV requires impairment as well as just the number of symptoms. The rates of the three subtypes in the Australian girls in this sample were very similar to the 'severely impaired' categories in the Hudziak et al. (1998) study of American adolescent female twins. To be in these categories, the girls had to have significant problems in at least two of home, school and social situations.

Table 7.1 shows that there are significant comorbidities with other psychiatric conditions – a point that has also been made by Willcutt et al. (1999). Their finding of higher rates of depressive symptomatology in the ADHD;CT and PI groups may well impact on cognitive functioning and to date no one has tried to isolate these effects of other comorbid conditions on cognition from the direct association of the subtypes with cognition and learning. The problem may be even more complex. Wood et al. (1999) showed that there were no clear effects of comorbidity on several laboratory-based measures of attention, the Covert Orienting of Visuospatial Attention Task (COVAT) and the Continuous Performance Task (CPT), but not all tasks showed subtype differences. So, one has the potential for a three-way interaction of ADHD subtypes × comorbidities × measures of EF and other neuropsychological tasks.

Table 7.1 has identified subtype differences in speech and language at the crude level of 'who gets therapy?' but what other data are there on the association with language development?

Language disorders and ADHD

Expressive language disorder, mixed receptive-expressive language disorder and phonological disorder are recognized in the DSM-IV category of communication disorders. These disorders are often comorbid with behavioural disorders, irrespective of whether one samples from a psychiatric population or, conversely, from a speech- and language-impaired population (Shelton and Barkley, 1994; Beitchman and Brownlie, 1996; Cohen et al., 1998b). Epidemiological studies indicate that approximately half of the children who present to speech and language clinics have a psychiatric disorder and a similar proportion of children who attend psychiatric outpatient clinics have speech and/or language impairments (Vallance et al., 1998). A high rate (40% in a study by Cohen et al., 1998a) of children who present for psychiatric services have undiagnosed language impairments, with estimates of cooccurrence rates for ADHD and language learning disabilities (LLD) ranging from 10% to 80% (Javorsky, 1996). LLD is recognized as a significant deficit in expressive and/or receptive language abilities. Javorsky (1996) discussed the possibility that LLD share a significant relationship with ADHD, given increasing evidence that many students who are initially diagnosed with communication disorders are later also diagnosed with ADHD. Similarly, there is evidence from several studies that a greater percentage of children with ADHD are somewhat delayed in the onset of talking (6–35%) than children without ADHD (2–5.5%; Westby and Cutler, 1994). Taylor (1998) reported that children with HKD revealed more frequent language delays in early development than other groups.

Beitchman et al. (1996b) suggested that the association between speech and language impairments and psychiatric disorders is complex, and the effects may be mediated through the operation of many different factors. For example, do individuals with speech and language impairments develop psychiatric disorders only in the presence of additional risk factors such as low SES? Alternatively, speech and language impairments may act secondarily through phenomena such as school failure, specific learning disabilities or peer and social rejection, and in turn lead to behavioural disturbance and psychiatric disorder. It may be that cognitive impairments, based on the speech and language impairment, may limit the individual's ability to use language to modulate emotions, express feelings and ideas, delay action, and control his or her own and other people's behaviour. Alternatively, neurodevelopmental immaturity may act as an antecedent variable responsible for the cooccurrence of psychiatric disorders and speech and language impairment.

Despite recognition of the significant relationship between speech and language impairments and psychiatric disorder, the mechanisms that mediate this association are poorly understood. ADHD has long been associated with communication disorders (Beitchman and Brownlie, 1996; Purvis and Tannock, 1997; Cohen et al., 1998b; Oram et al., 1999), especially expressive language and mixed receptive-expressive language disorders (APA, 1994). Relative to unaffected peers, children with ADHD symptomatology have been found in clinical studies to have particular difficulties in formulating sentences (Oram et al., 1999) and producing oral narratives (Zentall, 1988; Tannock et al., 1993; Purvis and Tannock, 1997). These problems occur most notably in situations which require organization, deliberate planning and monitoring (Zentall, 1988; Douglas and Benezra, 1990; Tannock et al., 1993; Carte et al., 1996; Purvis and Tannock, 1997). These expressive language difficulties specifically represent a problem with pragmatics, as opposed to difficulties in syntax and semantics (Purvis and Tannock, 1997; Oram et al., 1999). Numerous investigators have hypothesized that the reported language difficulties may result from underlying deficits in EF, mediated by the frontal lobes (Tannock et al., 1993; Carte et al., 1996).

However, other hypotheses have been presented. Riccio et al. (1994) suggested that central auditory processing may be an underlying factor in the cooccurrence of language difficulties and behaviours associated with ADHD. It is evident that more research is required to investigate communication behaviour in individuals with ADHD disorders (Oram et al., 1999). Many questions remain unanswered. For example, although there is evidence showing an association of speech and language impairment with ADHD, Beitchman and Brownlie (1996) identified that it is not yet known if this association is specific to a younger population or if it also applies to adolescents and adults. There is a need to attain a better understanding of individuals who present with both ADHD and communication disorders, to determine whether there are unique diagnostic and intervention issues raised by the cooccurrence of these two disorders, and why this comorbidity occurs (Oram et al., 1999).

Research in relation to the specific communication disorders and the nature of the language deficits most commonly exhibited by children with ADHD is in its infancy. Javorsky (1996) provided support for the differentiation of children with ADHD and concomitant LLD from children with pure ADHD on measures of syntax. This finding suggests that the comorbid language deficits exhibited by children with ADHD may be more likely to represent an expressive language disorder than a mixed receptive-expressive language disorder.

One other view is that learning disorders, such as reading or language disorders, commonly converge on a diagnosis of ADHD as the individual matures. That is, they are merely developmental markers of ADHD. There is a view that some comorbid conditions may represent developmental sequences of unitary underlying developmental psychopathological processes, at least in some individuals (Angold et al., 1999). Levy et al. (1996b) showed that speech and language difficulties (symptomatology of communication disorders) predicted the persistence of ADHD. Early speech and language impairments have been found to be associated with high rates of psychiatric disorder, such as ADHD, in later development (Beitchman and Brownlie, 1996). They reported that middle childhood and young adolescent outcome of early language impairment show an increased risk of psychiatric and behavioural problems. This risk may be increased when receptive language (as opposed to expressive language) is more severely compromised (Baker and Cantwell, 1987), although this issue warrants further study (Beitchman et al., 1996a). The risk is still evident even when children's speech and language impairment apparently resolves. Rates of disorder have not been found to be significantly higher for children who remain speech- and language-impaired compared with children whose speech and language status has improved at follow-up (Beitchman and Brownlie, 1996). It is a key question as to why early speech and language problems are associated with later psychiatric disorder even when these verbal problems have improved.

Learning disorders, such as RD, are also associated with communication disorders (Beitchman and Brownlie, 1996). For some time it has been observed that young children with speech and language impairments go on to demonstrate learning and reading disabilities in the early school grades. A large body of research now provides strong empirical support for these observations (Catts, 1993; Schachter, 1996). Considerable research has shown that language impairments underlie most reading problems (Cohen, 1996). It is of interest to determine to what extent speech and language impairment in early childhood constitutes a risk for the later development of RD and, potentially, ADHD. Beitchman and Brownlie (1996) reported that 90% of language-impaired children showed some form of RD at follow-up 3–4 years later at the age of 12. In Baker and Cantwell's (1987) study, 71% of children who developed a learning disorder had a language disorder initially. Specifically, children with receptive language impairment were most likely to develop a learning disorder. Several investigators have noted that the more pervasive the speech and language impairment, the worse the academic outcome in terms of reading ability tends to be (Beitchman and Brownlie, 1996). Longitudinal studies that report the presence of language delay or impairment preceding academic difficulty have led to the suggestion of a causal mechanism in the development of RDs from communication disorders (Schachter, 1996). A recent view (Hohnen and Stevenson, 1999) is that specific RD is a developmental language disorder and children who suffer from reading problems have an underlying language deficit that manifests itself differently with age. During the preschool years, these children have problems with spoken language, such as syntactical and morphological problems. They have phonological processing difficulties during the school years, when their problems in acquiring literacy skills are also manifest.

Thus we have three lines of evidence linking ADHD with RD, LLD with ADHD and LLD with RD. Is there a common basis to all three?

Genetics of comorbidity

Genetic studies have been proposed as a powerful way of examining comorbidity (Taylor, 1998). Traditionally, human behavioural genetic research has combined data from twin, adoption and family studies to elucidate the importance of genetics, and establish the magnitude of genetic contribution to variability in a trait or disorder in a population (Neale and Cardon, 1992; Nigg and Goldsmith, 1998). Modern statistical methods have taken behavioural genetic research far beyond the estimation of heritability to the elucidation of multiple genetic components of variation as well as various environmental components and interactions between components (Neale and Cardon, 1992).

Table 7.2. Comorbidity and concordance of attention deficit hyperactivity disorder (ADHD) and reading disorder in twin pairs in the Australian Twin ADHD Project

	Reading pairs	ADHD	Reading and ADHD
Concordant pairs			
Monozygotic twins	63	51	31
Dizygotic twins	41	24	12
Discordant pairs			
Monozygotic twins	34	53	9
Dizygotic twins	103	119	57

Contemporary behavioural genetic methodology can now be used to address key questions that often arise in psychopathology, such as comorbidity. For example, multivariate genetic methodology allows one to examine whether the genetic overlap between disorders such as ADHD and reading problems may be responsible for their cooccurrence. That is, the question is not whether one causes the other but rather whether they share a common genetic aetiology.

Conversely, it has been proposed that comorbidity may be a vital clue for genetic research, in that genes may operate on much more distinct phenotypes than our current broad diagnostic classifications (Neale and Kendler, 1995). Table 7.2 illustrates the methodology, using data from the ATAP (Levy et al., 1996a). The conventional approach has been to consider the extent of genetic overlap between conditions. A different way of interpreting the same information is to ask if there are twin pairs who have a genetic liability to reading problems, another group with liability to ADHD and a third group with a propensity to both? What we see in Table 7.2 is a group of monozygotic twins (31/40) pairs who are concordant for both reading and ADHD, compared with only 12/69 diozygotic pairs. The methods developed by Neale and Kendler (1995) allow us to consider if this is a third group and not simply the product of the separate liabilities to reading and ADHD.

Comorbidity offers an opportunity for understanding better the development of psychopathology and is a potential tool for improving nosology (Angold et al., 1999), especially when incorporated in genetic analysis. Most studies to date (summarized in Levy and Hay, 2001) suggest that the significant contribution of comorbid conditions often occurs because of common genetic influences to comorbidity with ADHD. One exception is comorbid depression which shows little genetic overlap (Nigg and Goldsmith, 1998).

Despite the wide variability in definitions and samples, recent studies suggest that comorbid RD and ADHD are due at least in part to heritable influences (Beitchman and Young, 1997). The first attempt to identify shared genetic influences for reading and spelling difficulties and ADHD came from Gilger et al. (1992), though the power of the study was insufficient to support their idea of shared genetic effects. More recently, their colleagues (discussed in Nigg and Goldsmith, 1998) fitted a bivariate biometric twin model to data from the Colorado reading project, relying on dimensional (as opposed to categorical) measures of hyperactivity and RD. They reported that approximately 70% of the covariation in RD and hyperactivity scores were attributable to genetic influences. The association between RD and ADHD has been replicated in studies from the ATAP. Hay and Levy (1996) proposed a very strong genetic overlap between DSM-III-R ADHD and reading problems, caused less by one causing the other than by both resulting from a common genetic influence. The prime evidence was that for monozygotic twins: one twin's ADHD score correlated as highly with the cotwin's reading (0.44) as with his or her own reading score (0.47). For dizygotic twins the corresponding correlations were 0.40 and 0.19, so the association of ADHD and reading was only half as strong, consistent with additive genetic expectations.

Rice (1997) postulated that some individuals included in genetic studies of RD (dyslexia) could be unidentified cases of specific language impairment and went further to suggest that the two conditions, RD and language impairment, may in fact share a common, inherited aetiological component. Further to this, it is feasible that reading, language and ADHD all share some common inherited aetiological component. Indeed, our own unpublished multivariate genetic analyses have shown that there is a set of genes influencing speech, reading and ADHD, contributing to approximately 40% of variance in ADHD. One problem with developing such models came in 1994 with the DSM-IV recognition of three ADHD subtypes and the differential comorbidity of these, already discussed in Table 7.1. Thus, any genetic modelling becomes much more complex and the sample size much larger if differences in susceptibility are to be reliably identified.

This model (Figure 7.1) confirms and extends the existing evidence on the relationship of reading to dimensional measures of inattention and hyperactivity-impulsivity. It was not possible to get an adequately fitting model that incorporated speech as well. The methods for understanding such diagrams in behaviour genetics are described in Hay et al. (2001). There are additive genetic effects that are common to all measures, but the association is strongest between inattention and reading. In fact, there are no genes determining inattention that are not also associated with reading, whereas hyperac-

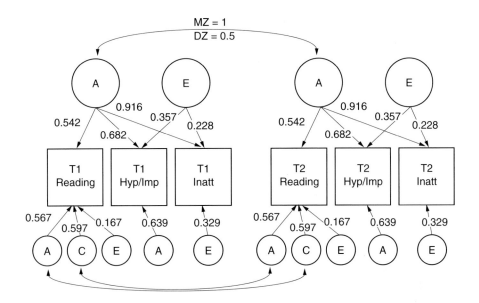

Figure 7.1   The best-fitting genetic model for the relationship between inattention (Inatt), hyperactivity-impulsivity (Hyp/Imp) and a history of formal reading intervention (Reading) in the Australian Twin Attention Deficit Hyperactivity Disorder (ADHD) Project. In the middle row in the squares are the observed variables for each twin. Above are latent additive genetic (A) and specific environmental (E) traits common to all three measures and estimated from the data. Below are the estimates of A and E specific to each variable. In addition for the model to fit, it was necessary to include a common family environmental effect (C) for reading. MZ, monozygotic; DZ, dizygotic; T1, twin 1; T2, twin 2. $\chi^2(23) = 32.103$; $P < 0.098$; root mean squared error approximation = 0.012.

tivity-impulsivity has some specific genetic determinants. This is what would be anticipated from the previous discussion of the greater association of inattention symptoms with RD. Reading problems have their specific genetic influences that are probably associated with IQ, though it has not been explicitly modelled here, as well as some common family environmental effects. These could reflect family attitudes to reading or even some twin-specific features of the environment, such as shared language delay and the so-called 'secret language of twins'.

The familial transmission of ADHD will turn out to be complex, given that many family studies have shown that relatives of children with ADHD have higher risk for many psychiatric disorders, including anxiety disorders, depression, conduct disorder and substance abuse (Thapar et al., 1999). There has not been space here to review the neurodevelopmental model that posits a specific association of ADHD and anxiety in one group of children who often respond poorly to stimulant medication (Vance and Luk, 1998). A comprehensive model that links these with the array of language, learning and cognitive impairments in ADHD will demand very large and probably collaborative studies.

Conclusions

Even though this is the second edition of this text, the situation regarding cognition and learning is more complex than at the time of the first edition. With the introduction of DSM-IV and its subtypes of ADHD, plus the refinement in ICD-10 of HKD, studies applying these new definitions of ADHD to cognition are only just now being published. Complicating the situation further has been the increasing rate of diagnosis of attentional problems, especially in the UK (Taylor, 1998). The children have not changed, but referral and diagnostic practices have. Apart from the concern that children who previously may have been in the control groups for studies would now be in the diagnosed groups, the main concern is that we are really dealing with a very different view of cognitive and learning problems.

No longer is the question that of which problems occur in children with attentional disorders. Much more it is which problems occur in particular attentional disorders? The question of the heterogeneity of attentional problems has become a key issue. It was one main reason why DSM-IV moved from a unitary to a three-way classification, but research is still catching up with classification. In terms of what should be happening, there are at least four issues that must be addressed:

(1)   Clearer delineation of cognitive and learning problems in DSM-IV subtypes, recognizing there is heterogeneity. Barkley (1997) provided one model for dealing with differences between subtypes, but this may have been premature, given the admittedly limited evidence to date. His assertion of two disorders, the hyperactive leading into the combined type, and a separate inattention disorder, does not fit with the more recent cognitive and learning data discussed here.

It may be premature to be testing a theoretical model of cognition in ADHD. An alternative approach is offered by Conners (1997), who advocated cluster analysis of large groups tested on objective measures such as neuroimaging or neuropsychological tests rather than 'a vague and poorly operationalised set of symptoms'. He used multiple measures from the Rey–Osterrieth Complex Figure to define four groups of ADHD children, who in turn were found also to differ on symptom patterns. There are two obvious difficulties with this approach. It may be too atheoretical and the clusters may be too remote from existing knowledge – though the process of identifying clusters on symptom number provides some concurrent validation. Second, the strength of the clustering is only as good as the measures that are used to identify these. It is clear many of the measures routinely used in ADHD research, such as the WCST, show complex and often equivocal patterns of differentiation between subtypes.

(2)   Intelligence. While there is growing evidence of intelligence test performance differences between subtypes, the trends are not consistent and may reflect sampling differences. But this remains a key issue both in itself and in the related area of covariance. There is a fundamental problem in covarying for a variable that reliably distinguishes between groups and then interpreting differences that do remain after this procedure. Covariance approaches may be fine within one group, but their application to intergroup differences needs careful consideration. A related issue is that of covarying for what? As discussed by Barkley (1995), there is a real problem in identifying just which components of such standard intelligence measures as the WISC-III are affected by attentional problems. Certainly, if one were to covary on the total WISC score, one is also covarying for some effects specific to attention, making clear discrimination impossible.

An additional problem, so clearly identified in the Klorman et al. (1999) study, is that comorbidity may be associated with lower intelligence test scores. It is not clear if this is just an ascertainment bias, in that lower-ability children may be more likely to be seen in clinics, but it does emphasize that much more is needed in ADHD research than just collecting IQ data for the purposes of covariance.

(3)   Comorbidity. How much of the effects of attentional disorders are specific and how much are due to comorbid problems? In this chapter we have emphasized some of the genetic studies that explicitly seek – and do find – a common basis to attentional and learning problems. But there is still limited agreement on whether there are specific cognitive profiles associated with specific subtypes. Some of the differences that have been found may just achieve statistical significance but it is not clear whether these are large enough to have clinical significance and to guide best practice in the future. Making it more difficult is the question of the direct relationship of comorbid conditions to cognition and learning problems. A good analogy would be the ongoing debate as to whether there is any relationship between ADHD and substance abuse or whether it is all mediated by the frequently comorbid conduct disorder. In the area of

cognition, it is only RD that has so far received much emphasis, rather than the many other comorbidities with ADHD. There is no doubt this will be the key issue for ADHD in the next decade.

(4)   The final point is the growing focus on identifying the effects of stimulant medication on cognition (Berman et al., 1999). There are obvious limitations in combining a research design with what are often routine clinical interventions. The children being seen at centres that conduct ADHD research protocols may not be typical of those being seen and prescribed medication by paediatricians, but this is a vital area of research. If we are claiming specific cognitive profiles are associated with ADHD and probably also with the dopamine pathways (Levy, 1989), then any model needs to take into account clinical perturbations of this system.

The situation is likely to be more complex, as we increasingly recognize potential limitations of a direct medication-behavioural response pathway. Problems may happen at the level of comorbid conditions, as already mentioned in the case of anxiety (Vance and Luk, 1998). Now there is some evidence (in need of corroboration) that polymorphisms in the dopamine transporter gene may be associated with response to methylphenidate (Winsberg and Comings, 1999); genetic factors complicate the picture even further.

A parting point concerns the practical implications for the very unclear picture we have outlined here. There are lots of ideas and some supportive evidence about models for what may be occurring at the level of cognition in the increasingly complex entity that is ADHD. But we do have to consider what is needed among families and professionals, as the heterogeneity within the label 'ADHD' is better appreciated. This review has certainly demonstrated that best practice in management of a child with ADHD should include assessment of cognition as well as of many of the potentially comorbid conditions. But we are far from having any theoretical model of the role of cognition that may guide intervention.

REFERENCES

American Psychiatric Association. (1994). *Diagnostic and Statistical Manual of Mental Disorders*, 4th edn. Washington, DC: American Psychiatric Association.

Angold, A., Costello, E.J. and Erkanli, A. (1999). Comorbidity. *Journal of Child Psychology and Psychiatry*, **40**, 57–87.

Baker, L. and Cantwell, D.P. (1987). A prospective psychiatric follow-up of children with speech/language disorders. *Journal of the American Academy of Child and Adolescent Psychiatry*, **26**, 546–53.

Barkley, R.A. (1995). A closer look at the DSM-IV criteria for ADHD: some unresolved issues. *ADHD Report*, **3**, 1–5.

Barkley, R.A. (1997). Behavioural inhibition, sustained attention, and executive functions: constructing a unifying theory of ADHD. *Psychological Bulletin*, **121**, 65–94.

Beitchman, J.H. and Brownlie, E.B. (1996). Childhood speech and language disorders. In *Do They Grow out of it? Long-term Outcomes of Childhood Disorders*, L. Hechtman, ed., pp. 225–53. Washington, DC: American Psychiatric Press.

Beitchman, J.H. and Young, A.R. (1997). Learning disorders with a special emphasis on reading disorders: a review of the past 10 years. *Journal of the American Academy of Child and Adolescent Psychiatry*, **36**, 1020–32.

Beitchman, J.H., Brownlie, E.B., Inglis, A. et al. (1996a). Seven-year follow-up of speech/language impaired and control children: psychiatric outcome. *Journal of Child Psychology and Psychiatry*, **37**, 961–70.

Beitchman, J.H., Brownlie, E.B. and Wilson, B. (1996b). Linguistic impairment and psychiatric disorder: pathways to outcome. In *Language, Learning, and Behavior Disorders: Developmental, Biological, and Clinical Perspectives*, J.H. Beitchman, N.J. Cohen, M.M. Konstantareas and R. Tannock, pp. 493–514. New York: Cambridge University Press.

Berman, T., Douglas, V.I. and Barr, R.G. (1999). Effects of methylphenidate on complex cognitive processing in attention-deficit hyperactivity disorder. *Journal of Abnormal Psychology*, **108**, 90–105.

Burns, G.L., Walsh, J.A., Patterson, D.R. et al. (1997). Internal validity of the disruptive behavior disorder symptoms: implications from parent ratings for a dimensional approach to symptom validity. *Journal of Abnormal Child Psychology*, **25**, 307–19.

Cantwell, D.P. (1996). Attention deficit disorder: a review of the past 10 years. *Journal of the American Academy of Child and Adolescent Psychiatry*, **35**, 978–87.

Caron, C. and Rutter, M. (1991). Comorbidity in child psychopathology: concepts, issues and research strategies. *Journal of Child Psychology and Psychiatry*, **32**, 1063–80.

Carte, E.T., Nigg, J.T. and Hinshaw, S.P. (1996). Neuropsychological functioning, motor speed, and language processing in boys with and without ADHD. *Journal of Abnormal Child Psychology*, **24**, 481–98.

Catts, H.W. (1993). The relationship between speech-language impairments and reading disabilities. *Journal of Speech and Hearing Research*, **36**, 948–58.

Cohen, N.J. (1996). Unsuspected language impairments in psychiatrically disturbed children: developmental issues and associated conditions. In *Language, Learning, and Behavior Disorders: Developmental, Biological, and Clinical Perspectives*, J.H. Beitchman, N.J. Cohen, M.M. Konstantareas and R. Tannock, eds, pp. 105–27. New York: Cambridge University Press.

Cohen, N.J., Barwick, M.A., Horodezky, N.B., Vallance, D.D. and Im, N. (1998a). Language, achievement, and cognitive processing in psychiatrically disturbed children with previously identified and unsuspected language impairments. *Journal of Child Psychology and Psychiatry*, **39**, 865–77.

Cohen, N.J., Menna, R., Vallance, D.D. et al. (1998b). Language, social cognitive processing, and behavioral characteristics of psychiatrically disturbed children with previously identified and unsuspected language impairments. *Journal of Child Psychology and Psychiatry*, **39**, 853–64.

Conners, C.K. (1997). Is ADHD a disease? *Journal of Attention Disorders*, **2**, 3–17.

Douglas, V.I. and Benezra, E. (1990). Supraspan verbal memory in attention deficit disorder with hyperactivity normal and reading-disabled boys. *Journal of Abnormal Child Psychology*, **18**, 617–38.

Ehlers, S., Nyden, A., Gillberg, C. et al. (1997). Asperger syndrome, autism and attention disorders: a comparative study of the cognitive profiles of 120 children. *Journal of Child Psychology and Psychiatry*, **38**, 207–17.

Eiraldi, R.B., Power, T.J. and Nezu, C.M. (1997). Patterns of comorbidity associated with subtypes of attention-deficit/hyperactivity disorder among 6- to 12-year-old children. *Journal of the American Academy of Child and Adolescent Psychiatry*, **36**, 503–14.

Faraone, S.V., Biederman, J., Krifcher Lehman, B. et al. (1993). Intellectual performance and school failure in children with attention deficit hyperactivity disorder and in their siblings. *Journal of Abnormal Psychology*, **102**, 616–23.

Faraone, S.V., Biederman, J. and Kiely, K. (1996). Cognitive functioning, learning disability, and school failure in attention deficit hyperactivity disorder: a family study perspective. In *Language, Learning, and Behaviour Disorders: Developmental, Biological, and Clinical Perspectives*, J.H. Beitchman, N.J. Cohen, M.M. Konstantareas and R. Tannock, eds, pp. 247–71. New York: Cambridge University Press.

Faraone, S.V., Biederman, J., Mennin, D., Russell, R. and Tsuang, M.T. (1998a). Familial subtypes of attention deficit hyperactivity disorder: a 4-year follow-up study of children from antisocial-ADHD families. *Journal of Child Psychology and Psychiatry*, **39**, 1045–53.

Faraone, S.V., Biederman, J., Weber, W. and Russell, R.L. (1998b). Psychiatric, neuropsychological, and psychosocial features of DSM-IV subtypes of attention-deficit/hyperactivity disorder: results from a clinically referred sample. *Journal of the American Academy of Child and Adolescent Psychiatry*, **37**, 185–93.

Felton, R.H. and Wood, F.B. (1989). Cognitive deficits in reading disability and attention deficit disorder. *Journal of Learning Disabilities*, **22**, 3–14.

Frost, L.A., Moffitt, T.E. and McGee, R. (1989). Neuropsychological correlates of psychopathology in an unselected cohort of young adolescents. *Journal of Abnormal Psychology*, **98**, 307–13.

Gaub, M. and Carlson, C.L. (1997). Behavioural characteristics of DSM-IV ADHD subtypes in a school-based population. *Journal of Abnormal Child Psychology*, **25**, 103–11.

Gilger, J.W., Pennington, B.F. and DeFries, J.C. (1992). A twin study of the etiology of comorbidity: attention-deficit hyperactivity disorder and dyslexia. *Journal of the American Academy of Child and Adolescent Psychiatry*, **31**, 343–8.

Goldman, L.S., Genel, M., Bezman, R.J. and Slanetz, P.J. (1998). Diagnosis and treatment of attention-deficit/hyperactivity disorder in children and adolescents. *Journal of the American Medical Association*, **279**, 1100–7.

Gomez, R., Harvey, J., Quick, C., Scharer, I. and Harris, G. (1999). DSM-IV AD/HD: confirmatory factor models, prevalence, and gender and age differences based on parent and teacher ratings of Australian primary school children. *Journal of Child Psychology and Psychiatry*, **40**, 265–74.

Hay, D.A. (1985). *Essentials of Behaviour Genetics*. Oxford: Blackwell Scientific.

Hay, D.A. and Levy, F. (1996). The differential diagnosis of ADHD. *Australian Educational and Developmental Psychologist*, **13**, 69–78.

Hay, D.A., McStephen, M. and Levy, F. (2001). Introduction to the genetic analysis of attentional disorders. In *Attention, Genes and ADHD*, eds. F. Levy and D. Hay, pp. 7–34. London: Brunner-Routledge.

Hinshaw, S.P. (1992). Externalizing behavior problems and academic underachievement in childhood and adolescence: causal relationships and underlying mechanisms. *Psychological Bulletin*, **111**, 127–55.

Hohnen, B. and Stevenson, J. (1999). The structure of genetic influences on general cognitive, language, phonological, and reading abilities. *Developmental Psychology*, **35**, 590–603.

Houghton, S., Douglas, G., West, J. et al. (1999). Differential patterns of executive function in children with attention-deficit hyperactivity disorder according to gender and subtype. *Journal of Child Neurology*, **14**, 801–5.

Hudziak, J.J., Heath, A.C., Madden, P.F. et al. (1998). Latent class and factor analysis of DSM-IV ADHD: a twin study of female adolescents. *Journal of the American Academy of Child and Adolescent Psychiatry*, **37**, 848–57.

Javorsky, J. (1996). An examination of youth with attention-deficit/hyperactivity disorder and language learning disabilities: a clinical study. *Journal of Learning Disabilities*, **29**, 247–58.

Jensen, P.S., Martin, D. and Cantwell, D.P. (1997). Comorbidity in ADHD: implications for research, practice, and DSM-V. *Journal of the American Academy of Child and Adolescent Psychiatry*, **36**, 1065–80.

Kaufman, A.S. (1999). Genetics of childhood disorders: II. Genetics and intelligence. *Journal of the American Academy of Child and Adolescent Psychiatry*, **38**, 626–8.

Klorman, R., Hazel-Fernandez, L.A., Shaywitz, S.E. et al. (1999). Executive functioning deficits in attention-deficit/hyperactivity disorder are independent of oppositional defiant or reading disorder. *Journal of the American Academy of Child and Adolescent Psychiatry*, **38**, 1148–55.

Lahey, B.B. and Willcutt, E.G. (1998). *Current Diagnostic Schema/Core Dimensions* (abstract). *NIH Consensus Development Conference on Diagnosis and Treatment of Attention Deficit Hyperactivity Disorder*, 25–31. Available at http://odp.od.nih.gov/consensus/cons/110/110_abstract.pdf (22 February 1999).

Lahey, B.B., Pelham, W.E., Stein, M.A. et al. (1998). Validity of DSM-IV attention-deficit/hyperactivity disorder for younger children. *Journal of the American Academy of Child and Adolescent Psychiatry*, **37**, 695–703.

Lalonde, J., Turgay, A. and Hudson, J.I. (1998). Attention-deficit hyperactivity disorder subtypes and comorbid disruptive behaviour disorders in a child and adolescent mental health clinic. *Canadian Journal of Psychiatry*, **43**, 623–8.

Levy, F. (1989). CNS stimulant controversies. *Australian and New Zealand Journal of Psychiatry*, **23**, 497–502.

Levy, F. and Hay, D. (2001). *Attention, Genes and ADHD.* London: Brunner-Routledge.

Levy, F., Hay, D., McLaughlin, M., Wood, C. and Waldman, I. (1996a). Twin-sibling differences in parental reports of ADHD, speech, reading and behaviour problems. *Journal of Child Psychology and Psychiatry*, **37**, 569–78.

Levy, F., Hay, D.A. and Rooney, R. (1996b). Predictors of persistence of symptoms: preliminary report. *ADHD Report*, **4**, 12.

Lombardino, L.J., Riccio, C.A., Hynd, G.W. and Pinheiro, S.B. (1997). Linguistic deficits in children with reading disabilities. *American Journal of Speech-Language Pathology*, **6**, 71–8.

Mayes, S.D. and Calhoun, S.L. (2000). Prevalence and degree of attention and learning problems in ADHD and LD. *ADHD Report*, **8**, 14–16.

McGee, R., Williams, S., Moffitt, T. and Anderson, J. (1989). A comparison of 13-year-old boys with attention deficit and/or reading disorder on neuropsychological measures. *Journal of Abnormal Child Psychology*, **17**, 37–53.

Morgan, A.E., Hynd, G.W., Riccio, C.A. and Hall, J. (1996). Validity of DSM-IV ADHD predominantly inattentive and combined types: relationship to previous DSM diagnoses/subtype differences. *Journal of the American Academy of Child and Adolescent Psychiatry*, **35**, 325–33.

Neale, M.C. and Cardon, L.R. (1992). *Methodology for Genetic Studies of Twins and Families.* Dordrecht: Kluwer Academic.

Neale, M.C. and Kendler, K.S. (1995). Models of comorbidity for multifactorial disorders. *American Journal of Human Genetics*, **57**, 935–53.

Nigg, J.T. and Goldsmith, H.H. (1998). Developmental psychopathology, personality, and temperament: reflections on recent behavioral genetics research. *Human Biology*, **70**, 387–412.

Nigg, J.T., Carte, E.T., Hinshaw, S.P. and Treuting, J.J. (1998). Neuropsychological correlates of childhood attention-deficit/hyperactivity disorder: explainable by comorbid disruptive behavior or reading problems? *Journal of Abnormal Psychology*, **107**, 468–80.

Nigg, J.T., Quamma, J.P., Greenberg, M.T. and Kusche, C.A. (1999). A two-year longitudinal study of neuropsychological and cognitive performance in relation to behavioral problems and competencies in elementary school children. *Journal of Abnormal Child Psychology*, **27**, 51–63.

Nigg, J.T., Blaskey, L., Huang-Pollock, C. and Rappley, M.D. (in press). Neuropsychological executive functions and ADHD DSM-IV subtypes. *Journal of the American Academy of Child and Adolescent Psychiatry.*

Oram, J., Fine, J., Okamoto, C. and Tannock, R. (1999). Assessing the language of children with attention deficit hyperactivity disorder. *American Journal of Speech-Language Pathology*, **8**, 72–80.

Ostrander, R., Weinfurt, K.P., Yarnold, P.R. and August, G.J. (1998). Diagnosing attention deficit disorders with the behavioral assessment system for children and the child behavior checklist: test and construct validity analyses using optimal discriminant classification trees. *Journal of Consulting and Clinical Psychology*, **66**, 660–72.

Pennington, B.F. and Ozonoff, S. (1996). Executive functions and developmental psychopathology. *Journal of Child Psychology and Psychiatry*, **37**, 51–87.

Pennington, B.F., Groisser, D. and Welsh, M.C. (1993). Contrasting cognitive deficits in attention deficit hyperactivity disorder versus reading disability. *Developmental Psychology*, **29**, 511–23.

Pliszka, S.R., Carlson, C.L. and Swanson, J.M. (1999). *ADHD with Comorbid Disorders: Clinical Assessment and Management*. New York: Guilford Press.

Plomin, R., DeFries, J.C., McClearn, G.E. and Rutter, M. (1997). *Behavioral Genetics*, 3rd edn. New York: W.H. Freeman.

Prior, M., Smart, D., Sanson, A. and Oberklaid, F. (1999). Relationships between learning difficulties and psychological problems in preadolescent children from a longitudinal sample. *Journal of the American Academy of Child and Adolescent Psychiatry*, **38**, 429–36.

Purvis, K.L. and Tannock, R. (1997). Language abilities in children with attention deficit hyperactivity disorder, reading disabilities, and normal controls. *Journal of Abnormal Child Psychology*, **25**, 133–44.

Reader, M.J., Harris, E.L., Schuerholz, L.J. and Denckla, M.B. (1994). Attention deficit hyperactivity disorder and executive dysfunction. *Developmental Neuropsychology*, **10**, 493–512.

Riccio, C.A., Hynd, G.W., Cohen, M.J., Hall, J. and Molt, L. (1994). Comorbidity of central auditory processing disorder and attention-deficit hyperactivity disorder. *Journal of the American Academy of Child and Adolescent Psychiatry*, **33**, 849–57.

Rice, M.L. (1997). Specific language impairments: in search of diagnostic markers and genetic contributions. *Mental Retardation and Developmental Disabilities Research Reviews*, **3**, 350–7.

Robbins, T.W., James, M., Owen, A.M. et al. (1994). Cognitive deficits in progressive supranuclear palsy, Parkinson's disease, and multiple system atrophy in tests sensitive to frontal lobe dysfunction. *Journal of Neurology, Neurosurgery and Psychiatry*, **57**, 79–88.

Schachter, D.C. (1996). Academic performance in children with speech and language impairment: a review of follow-up research. In *Language, Learning, and Behaviour Disorders: Developmental, Biological, and Clinical Perspectives*, J.H. Beitchman, N.J. Cohen, M.M. Konstantareas and R. Tannock, eds, pp. 515–29. New York: Cambridge University Press.

Seidman, L.J., Faraone, S.V., Biederman, J., Weber, W. and Ouellette, C. (1997). Toward defining a neuropsychology of attention deficit-hyperactivity disorder: performance of children and adolescents from a large clinically referred sample. *Journal of Consulting and Clinical Psychology*, **65**, 150–61.

Semel, E., Wiig, E. and Secord, W. (1987). *Clinical Evaluation of Language Fundamentals – Revised*. Toronto: Harcourt Brace Jovanovich.

Semrud-Clikeman, M., Biederman, J., Sprich-Buckminster, S. et al. (1992). Comorbidity between ADHD and learning disability: a review and report in a clinically referred sample. *Journal of the American Academy of Child and Adolescent Psychiatry*, **31**, 439–48.

Shelton, T.L. and Barkley, R.A. (1994). Critical issues in the assessment of attention deficit disorders in children. *Topics in Language Disorders*, **14**, 26–41.

Spear-Swerling, L. and Sternberg, R.J. (1998). Curing our 'epidemic' of learning disabilities. *Phi Delta Kappan*, **79**, 397–401.

Stevenson, J. (2001). Comorbidity of reading/spelling disability and ADHD. In *Attention, Genes and ADHD*, F. Levy and D. Hay, eds, pp. 99–114. London: Brunner-Routledge.

Tannock, R. (1998a). Attention deficit hyperactivity disorder: advances in cognitive, neurobiological, and genetic research. *Journal of Child Psychology and Psychiatry*, **39**, 65–99.

Tannock, R. (1998b). *Cognitive and behavioral correlates* (abstract). *NIH Consensus Development*

Conference on Diagnosis and Treatment of Attention Deficit Hyperactivity Disorder, 43–51. Available at http://odp.ad.nih.gov/consensus/cons/110/110_abstract.pdf (22 February 1999).

Tannock, R., Purvis, K.L. and Schachar, R.J. (1993). Narrative abilities in children with attention deficit hyperactivity disorder and normal peers. *Journal of Abnormal Child Psychology*, **21**, 103–17.

Taylor, E. (1998). Clinical foundations of hyperactivity research. *Behavioural Brain Research*, **94**, 11–24.

Taylor, E., Sandberg, S., Thorley, G. and Giles, S. (1991). *The Epidemiology of Childhood Hyperactivity Disorder*. Institute of Psychiatry Maudsley monograph. London: Oxford University Press.

Thapar, A., Holmes, J., Poulton, K. and Harrington, R. (1999). Genetic basis of attention deficit and hyperactivity. *British Journal of Psychiatry*, **174**, 105–11.

Toone, B.K. and Van der Linden, J.H. (1997). Attention deficit hyperactivity disorder or hyperkinetic disorder in adults. *British Journal of Psychiatry*, **170**, 489–91.

Tripp, G., Luk, S.L., Schaughency, E.A. and Singh, R. (1999). DSM-IV and ICD-10: a comparison of the correlates of ADHD and hyperkinetic disorder. *Journal of the American Academy of Child and Adolescent Psychiatry*, **38**, 156–64.

Vallance, D.D., Cummings, R.L. and Humphries, T. (1998). Mediators of the risk for problem behavior in children with language learning disabilities. *Journal of Learning Disabilities*, **31**, 160–71.

Vance, A.L.A. and Luk, E.S.L. (1998). Attention deficit hyperactivity disorder and anxiety: is there an association with neurodevelopmental deficits? *Australian and New Zealand Journal of Psychiatry*, **32**, 650–7.

Velting, O.N. and Whitehurst, G.J. (1997). Inattention-hyperactivity and reading achievement in children from low-income families: a longitudinal model. *Journal of Abnormal Child Psychology*, **25**, 321–31.

Wechsler, D. (1991). *Wechsler Intelligence Scale for Children*, 3rd edn. San Antonio: Psychological Corporation.

Welsh, M.C., Pennington, B.F. and Groisser, D.B. (1991). A normative-developmental study of executive function: a window on prefrontal function in children. *Developmental Neuropsychology*, **7**, 131–49.

Westby, C.E. and Cutler, S.K. (1994). Language and ADHD: understanding the bases and treatment of self-regulatory deficits. *Topics in Language Disorders*, **14**, 58–76.

Weyandt, L.L. and Willis, W.G. (1994). Executive functions in school-aged children: potential efficacy of tasks in discriminating clinical groups. *Developmental Neuropsychology*, **10**, 27–38.

Willcutt, E.G., Pennington, B.F., Chhabildas, N.A., Friedman, M.C. and Alexander, J. (1999). Psychiatric comorbidity associated with DSM-IV ADHD in a nonreferred sample of twins. *Journal of the American Academy of Child and Adolescent Psychiatry*, **38**, 1355–62.

Winsberg, B.G. and Comings, D.E. (1999). Association of the dopamine transporter gene (DAT1) with poor methylphenidate response. *Journal of the American Academy of Child and Adolescent Psychiatry*, **38**, 1474–7.

Wolraich, M.L., Hannah, J.N., Pinnock, T.Y., Baumgaertel, A. and Brown, J. (1996). Comparison of diagnostic criteria for attention-deficit hyperactivity disorder in a county-wide sample. *Journal of the American Academy of Child and Adolescent Psychiatry*, **35**, 319–24.

Wood, C. (1999). *DSM-IV ADHD – Predominantly Inattentive and Combined Types: A Comparative Study*. Unpublished PhD. Melbourne: La Trobe University.

Wood, C., Maruff, P., Levy, F., Farrow, M. and Hay, D. (1999). Covert orienting of visual spatial attention in attention deficit hyperactivity disorder: does comorbidity make a difference? *Archives of Clinical Neuropsychology*, **14**, 179–89.

World Health Organization. (1993). *The ICD-10 Classification of Mental and Behavioural Disorders: Diagnostic Criteria for Research*. Geneva: World Health Organization.

Zametkin, A.J. and Ernst, M. (1999). Problems in the management of attention-deficit-hyperactivity disorder. *New England Journal of Medicine*, **340**, 40–6.

Zentall, S.S. (1988). Production deficiencies in elicited language but not in the spontaneous verbalizations of hyperactive children. *Journal of Abnormal Child Psychology*, **16**, 657–73.

8

Developmental perspectives

Sheryl Olson

Department of Psychology, University of Michigan, Ann Arbor, MI, USA

There is a growing consensus that knowledge of normal developmental processes is essential for understanding the nature of childhood behaviour disorders (Sroufe and Rutter, 1984; Cicchetti and Cohen, 1995; Sameroff, 2000). In
this chapter, developmental perspectives are brought to bear on questions
concerning the ontogenesis and course of childhood hyperactivity. Despite the
fact that hyperactivity is one of the most densely researched childhood behaviour disorders, its developmental precursors are poorly understood. We are
only beginning to disentangle the complex tapestries of biological, emotional,
cognitive-developmental, familial and social-ecological factors that mark individual pathways to this disorder and to its multiform outcomes in later life.

The term 'developmental perspectives' refers to a rich set of concepts
derived from the study of normal and abnormal development. The most
basic context for understanding childhood disorders is the age or cognitive-
developmental level of the child. Normal processes of development involve
complex quantitative and qualitative transformations in children's physical,
cognitive, emotional and behavioural functioning, with increasing differentiation and hierarchical integration as age progresses (Sroufe and Rutter, 1984).
Thus, atypical or 'deviant' development can only be defined in relation to what
is known to be normal for a given age group. For example, negativism, temper
tantrums and attention seeking, relatively commonplace in toddlers, would
have very different meaning in school-age children or adolescents. Once a
behaviour disorder is defined, the age of the child affects how it is perceived and
interpreted by adults, the manner in which symptomatic behaviours are
expressed, and the probable course of the disorder (Campbell, 2000). Moreover,
the developing cognitive emotional and behavioural characteristics of the child
determine what types of clinical interventions may be optimally effective (Coie
et al., 2000).

Beyond concern with normative, age-related trends, developmental perspectives also encompass questions of individual development that are vitally

important to the psychopathologist. The concept of developmental issues or tasks is useful for examining continuities in individual adaptation over the course of time (Sroufe and Rutter, 1984). At each different age period, there are adaptational challenges that are central to the development of competent social and emotional functioning. Successful adaptation provides the child with increased behavioural flexibility, providing a foundation for the growth of normal competence (Block and Block, 1980; Waters and Sroufe, 1983). Conversely, adaptational failures at any level may predispose the child to develop behaviour disorders at later stages of development, although this progression is far from inevitable and is unlikely to occur in a simple, linear manner (Sroufe et al., 2000). Also, the manner in which adaptational failures mark pathways to specific childhood behaviour disorders is not well understood.

Finally, the process of individual development is characterized by complex transactions between child and environment. Current models stress that behavioural deviance is the product of a continuous, dynamic interplay between qualities that individual children bring to their social interactions and characteristics of the immediate caregiving environment and its broader social-ecological context (Sameroff and Chandler, 1975; Sameroff, 1995). Concepts of risk (factors which increase the chance of developing behaviour disorders), vulnerability (factors which intensify the effects of risk) and protection (factors which ameliorate risk) are important for understanding the individual paths that children take in developing behaviour disorders (Rutter, 1987; Sameroff, 2000).

In the current chapter, these concepts are applied to our knowledge of the early developmental precursors and course of childhood hyperactivity. First, however, defining features of the hyperactive syndrome will be briefly outlined in the following section.

Overview of clinical and associated features

Historically, diagnostic concepts of hyperactivity have undergone many major transitions (Barkley, 1996; Chapter 5). The publication of the third edition of *Diagnostic and Statistical Manual of Mental Disorders* (DSM-III: American Psychiatric Association, 1980) marked the increasing consensus that deficits in attention or concentration were central features of hyperactivity, together with age-inappropriate levels of impulsivity and overactivity. In the latest revision of the DSM (DSM-IV; American Psychiatric Association, 1994), there are two broad groups of primary symptoms: inattention (e.g. fails to attend to details; has difficulty sustaining attention in task or play; is easily distracted) and hyperactivity-impulsivity (e.g. fidgety; often out of seat; highly active and talkative; often interrupts; has difficulty waiting turn). To receive a diagnosis of attention deficit and hyperactivity disorder (ADHD), children must show at least six symptoms from either the inattention or hyperactivity-impulsivity groups. In addition, symptoms of ADHD must appear before the age of 7 and persist for a minimum of 6 months. Moreover, these symptoms must be present in at least two different settings, and there must be clear evidence of significant impairment in social or academic functioning. Hyperactivity has been consistently found to be overrepresented in boys, by ratios of approximately 3 : 1 in clinical samples (Szatmari et al., 1989).

Primary characteristics

The primary or core features of ADHD have been well established clinically, and in numerous research studies comparing hyperactive children with normal peers (see reviews by Hinshaw, 1994; Barkley, 1996). One primary characteristic is that of overactivity. Hyperactive children are often described by parents and teachers as fidgety, 'always on the go', restless and accident-prone (Whalen, 1989). Qualitative features are paramount, in that the overactivity of ADHD children appears disorganized, haphazard and contextually inappropriate in contrast to the goal-directed behaviour of highly active but normal peers. However, these behavioural difficulties are more evident in some settings than others. Generally, children with ADHD are more likely to manifest problems with overactivity in highly structured task situations than in more relaxed or informal settings (Porrino et al., 1983), making the school classroom environment an ideal context for observing symptomatic behaviour.

Attentional problems comprise a second primary characteristic of ADHD. Parents of children with ADHD complain that they never listen, and have difficulty playing alone and sticking to single activities. Teachers complain that children with ADHD are frequently 'off task' in classroom situations, and that they have difficulty following directions and completing assignments. Due to the multidimensional nature of the attention construct and to subtleties involved in the measurement of attentional processes, however, efforts to pinpoint specific attentional deficits in hyperactivity are ongoing (Chapter 6). It is unclear whether these difficulties primarily reflect distractibility (Leung and Connolly, 1996), difficulty sustaining attention over long time periods (Douglas, 1983; Losier et al., 1996) or other problems of attentional regulation (see review by Taylor, 1999). Moreover, in both natural settings and on sustained attention tasks in the laboratory, it is very difficult to separate attentional deficits from problems of motivation, cooperation or fluctuations in mood (Sonuga-Barke et al., 1996).

Finally, deficiencies in inhibitory control comprise the third core characteristic of ADHD. Problems of impulse control manifest themselves in diverse situations; the hyperactive child may intrude upon the games of peers, have difficulty waiting for a turn to play, behave in 'silly' ways that are situationally inappropriate, interrupt others, call out answers before the question is finished, or even run into traffic to retrieve a wayward toy. Currently, deficiencies in impulse control are conceptualized as central deficits in ADHD, with problems of attentional and activity regulation viewed as secondary manifestations (Barkley, 1997a,b; Quay, 1997; Schachar et al., 2000). However, as with the concept of inattention, impulsivity is a complex, multidimensional construct that has proven difficult to operationalize: different laboratory measures of impulsivity typically show modest levels of convergence with one another and with reports of hyperactive symptoms by teachers and parents (Milich and Kramer, 1984; Olson, 1989; Olson et al., 1999). An additional complication is that impulsivity problems are common to many different types of childhood behaviour problems (Biederman et al., 1991), most notably disturbances of conduct.

Associated characteristics

Conduct problems

Conduct disorders have been found to cooccur frequently with ADHD (Hinshaw, 1987; Szatmari et al., 1989; August et al., 1996). For example, Hinshaw (1987) reviewed studies that had classified children into subtypes, and concluded that 30–90% of children who were classified as having ADHD also received diagnoses of conduct disorder. The high degree of correspondence between these two disorders, coupled with lack of evidence indicating that ADHD and conduct disorders show distinctive aetiological patterns or longterm prognoses, has led some to question whether ADHD is a distinct syndrome (Prior and Sanson, 1986). One approach to this problem has been to subdivide youngsters with ADHD according to the presence and severity of concomitant conduct problems (Lahey et al., 1988; Hinshaw and Melnick, 1995). Generally, children with combined symptom patterns have more broadranging and severe adaptational problems than children with 'pure' ADHD (Barkley, 1997a,b), whereas the latter subdiagnosis has been more strongly associated with cognitive and neurodevelopmental difficulties (Pennington and Ozonoff, 1996).

Academic problems

Academic failure and underachievement are common problems of children with ADHD, as evidenced by poor grades and low achievement test scores, low teacher evaluations, placement in special classes and failure to be promoted to the next grade (Hinshaw, 1992). Specific learning disabilities have been found to be overrepresented among hyperactive children (Schachar, 1991; Faraone et al., 1996); however, estimates of the proportion of hyperactive children who are also learning-disabled vary widely between studies, reflecting heterogeneity in sample composition and diagnostic criteria (Shaywitz and Shaywitz, 1988; Semrud-Clikeman et al., 1992; Chapter 7). Although the presence of learning and academic problems in hyperactive children has been well-established, it is unclear whether these problems are attributable to deficits in motivation, attention, impulse control, problem solving, or some combination of these factors (McGee and Share, 1988; Pennington et al., 1993).

Problems in social relationships

Children with ADHD tend to show pervasive problems in social adjustment (Whalen et al., 1990; Hinshaw, 1994). Relative to other children, they have few friends and experience high rates of peer rejection (Whalen et al., 1990; Erhardt and Hinshaw, 1994). Several studies have suggested that the behaviour of hyperactive children catalyses negative interactions with others. For example, sibling dyads that contain a hyperactive child show more negative interaction than others (Mash and Johnston, 1990); similar patterns have been found for peer interactions with and without the presence of a hyperactive child (Madan-Swain and Zentall, 1990). Similarly, teachers and parents tend to be more directive and controlling with hyperactive children than with normal children (Whalen et al., 1990). However, adults' responses to hyperactive children become less controlling and more positive as ADHD symptoms improve with either age (Barkley et al., 1985) or stimulant medication (Hinshaw and McHale, 1991), indicating that the negative response styles of adults are 'elicited' in part by difficult or annoying child behaviour.

Several potential explanations for the social maladjustment of hyperactive children have been proposed, including specific deficits in social knowledge, attributional style and social reasoning (Whalen et al., 1990). Current studies suggest that problems in social goal setting and in emotional regulation (e.g. poor frustration tolerance), as well as cooccurring aggressive behaviour, may play important roles in the poor peer adjustment of children with ADHD (Hinshaw and Melnick, 1995).

Hyperactivity: a disorder of self-regulation

In summary, hyperactive children show considerable heterogeneity in their symptom pictures, and their adaptational difficulties tend to span many different life contexts. The pervasiveness of these problems, coupled with their task and situational variability, has led many to question whether hyperactive children possess a generalized deficit in the integration of cognitive, affective and motor functions in response to varying situational demands. An emerging consensus is that the diverse problems of adaptation shown by hyperactive children share a common thread; they all reflect deficits in self-regulation (Douglas, 1983; Barkley, 1997a,b; Quay, 1997). Self-regulation is a complex, superordinate construct that encompasses many different component processes. One approach focuses upon affect regulation, particularly regulation of fear and anger (Rothbart, 1989; Thompson, 1994). Infants show clear individual differences in emotional arousability and intensity which remain moderately stable through early development (Kagan et al., 1984; Fox and Calkins, 1993). Moreover, emotional arousability and intensity have been associated with aggressive and disruptive behaviour in children (Brody et al., 1988; Teglasi and McMahon, 1990; Fabes and Eisenberg, 1992), suggesting that modulation of strong emotional arousal is an important component of social competence (Eisenberg et al., 1994). Another major approach to understanding self-regulation emphasizes aspects of cognitively mediated behavioural inhibition, assessed using specific laboratory tasks. For example, self-control has been variously operationalized as the ability to inhibit immediate responding to achieve a goal or comply with a request (Schachar et al., 1993; Kochanska et al., 1996), ability to wait for a desired object or goal (Mischel et al., 1989; Barkley, 1994) and ability to behave in a 'socially approved' manner in the absence of external controls (Kopp, 1989; Kochanska and Murray, 2000). As Kopp (1987) has noted, common to all definitions is the requirement that children flexibly adapt to life situations that have different standards of conduct associated with them: 'Thus it is permissible to shout in a playground but not in a classroom, to run across a meadow but not a street, and to respect another's possessions whether the person is present or absent (p. 34)'. Similarly, Barkley (1997a,b) has argued that children with ADHD have a generalized deficit in rule-governed behaviour, defined as the ability of language or other symbol systems to serve as discriminative stimuli for contextually appropriate responding. Hence, their behaviour is under the control of immediately occurring contingencies, not rules, which could explain the poor problem solving, impulsivity, noncompliance and socially inappropriate behaviour so commonly observed in these children. In the following sections, the construct of self-regulation will be used as a context for examining earliest developmental precursors of hyperactivity.

Early developmental precursors

It is widely believed that hyperactivity has its onset in early childhood, even though the majority of cases are not diagnosed until the school-age years. Indeed, a requirement of diagnosis is that symptoms appear before the age of 7 (American Psychiatric Association, 1980, 1987, 1994). Ironically, however, the early development of hyperactivity has been grossly underresearched. Relatively little is known about developmental pathways in infancy and early childhood which lead to full expression of the syndrome in later life. One way to approach this question is by examining the early development of self-regulatory competence. As discussed above, there are cogent arguments for viewing hyperactivity as a disorder of self-regulation. Thus, knowledge of factors which influence the normal and abnormal development of self-regulatory skills can provide a foundation for exploring early developmental pathways to hyperactivity.

Normative development of self-regulation

Achieving flexible levels of self-control is a major developmental task for the preschool-age child (Flavell, 1977, 1985; Block and Block, 1980; Kopp, 1982; Sroufe, 1983). Self-regulation provides an important foundation for the growth of normal social and academic competence. Young children who have difficulty managing their impulses, appraising the demands of different life situations and organizing environmental stimuli efficiently are at risk for a host of behavioural and learning problems in the school-age period, chief among them the attention deficit disorders (Campbell and Ewing, 1990; Campbell, 1995). Despite the clear importance of the construct, however, we know relatively little about the development of self-regulation in young children at risk for ADHD.

In a review article integrating diverse theoretical and empirical perspectives, Kopp (1982) placed the antecedents of self-regulation in a developmental framework. The most salient feature of her model is that the development of self-regulation is closely linked to the growth of higher-order cognitive processes. Self-regulatory competence emerges gradually in a series of discontinuous developmental phases which parallel the maturation of different cognitive skills. The role of the caregiving environment is also critical, in that it mediates the extent to which the child successfully negotiates developmental challenges inherent in each different phase. Because issues relative to each phase have different implications for understanding how normal development can go awry, these challenges will be briefly reiterated here.

(1)   Neurophysiological maturation (0–3 months). In the earliest months of life,

'control' takes the form of modulation of arousal states. Individual infants differ in the capacity to modulate arousal: for example, some infants are easily distressed, and have difficulty self-soothing or being soothed by caregivers. Caregivers can facilitate effective arousal modulation by responding sensitively to the child's communications (e.g. adjusting their behaviour to the state of the child), and by providing a routine which marks transitions between different states of arousal.

(2)   Sensorimotor modulation (3–12 months). During this phase, infants are capable of adjusting their voluntary motor behaviour in response to environmental stimuli, e.g. reaching for an interesting toy, or responding to the vocalizations and smiles of caregivers. According to Kopp, these modulations help infants efficiently organize their interactions with the social and physical world, which sets the stage for more complex levels of control with advancing age. The ability to modulate sensorimotor behaviour is thought to reflect individual differences in biological predispositions (such as activity levels) as well as patterns of caregiver stimulation and the availability of play objects.

(3)   Control (12–18 months). Towards the end of the first year, there is an important transitional phase in the development of self-regulation. Because of their rapidly maturing cognitive and motoric abilities, infants become aware of social demands and are able to adjust their behaviour accordingly. For example, although control is limited to the immediate stimulus environment, infants of this age are capable of complying with simple caregiver requests ('give Mummy a kiss') and prohibitions ('no, baby!'). The child's increased capacity for locomotion and intense need to explore the environment leads to a natural escalation in caregiver demands. During this critical transition phase, individual differences in control may be facilitated by caregiver sensitivity to the child's preferred style of engaging the social and physical environment; for example, if the child is highly active, to what extent can the caregiver 'channel' this activity into constructive rather than conflicted interactions? Caregivers of toddlers also differ in their efficacy as teachers. For example, adults can facilitate the development of attention and comprehension skills by providing verbal instructions for compliance (Schaffer, 1984), and by using multiple cues and age-appropriate language to reinforce a point (Kopp, 1987).

(4)   Self-control (24+ months). With the development of representational (symbolic) thought and recall memory, the child is increasingly able to delay immediate gratification of desires and to engage in self-initiated monitoring of behaviour as a consequence of remembered information. Moreover, self-consciousness begins to solidify during this phase, as a result of the child's increasing capacity to differentiate self from others. Thus, both struggles with

caregivers over autonomy issues and pride in self-help behaviours become normative. The child's behavioural flexibility in adapting to new situations is still quite limited, however, as is capacity for delay.

As cognitive skills mature into the preschool years, children become increasingly capable of self-monitoring their behaviour in response to diverse situational demands. More complex cognitive processes play an important role in self-regulatory behaviour at this age, such as internalized, self-guiding speech (Luria, 1961; Vygotsky, 1962) and self-generated strategies aimed at reducing frustration (Mischel et al., 1989). It is this expanded and flexible repertoire of coping responses that marks the achievement of true self-regulatory competence.

Although Kopp's framework focuses upon normative developmental transitions, it provides a good basis for raising the question of how individual differences in self-regulatory competence arise. Perhaps the most obvious theme is that the development of self-regulation is firmly entrenched in the caregiving system. At each different phase of early development, caregiver behaviours may facilitate or retard the child's progress in achieving internal controls, either through direct social interaction or the manner in which the caregiver structures the physical environment. To the extent that it has a disorganizing effect upon the caregiving system, environmental stress may play an important role in the early development of self-regulation. A second, less obvious theme concerns individual differences in infants' biological predispositions. Individual infants vary considerably in the ability to modulate arousal, the earliest hallmark of self-regulation (see, for example, Thompson, 1994). At later ages, biologically based differences in behavioural tempo and emotional expression may have an important impact upon the development of self-regulatory competence, especially if the child's interactional style leads to conflicts with caregivers and peers (Teglasi and McMahon, 1990; Eisenberg et al., 1994; Rothbart and Bates, 1998). Thus, constructs of temperament are critical to an understanding of the early development of self-regulation. In the following sections, these constructs are used to examine the development of individual differences in self-regulation among infants and toddlers.

Early caregiving relationships

Through processes of social interaction with their infants and the ways in which they structure the physical environment, caregivers are thought to play a critical role in the development of self-regulation (Sander, 1975; Kopp, 1982, 1987; Sroufe, 1991; Calkins, 1994; Kochanska, 1997). However, due to a paucity of research, we are only beginning to understand the complex relationships between early caregiving systems and the development of individual differences in children's self-regulatory competence. Several different approaches to this question are discussed below.

Caregiver–infant synchrony

The quality of early caregiver–infant relationships has been construed as a 'primary learning environment' for the development of self-regulatory competence (Field, 1994). Through early development, there is a general progression from reliance on caregivers for regulation of arousal to self-regulation (Sroufe, 1996; Derryberry and Rothbart, 1997; Calkins et al., 1998). Thus, in early infancy, regulation of negative states of arousal (such as emotional distress or physical discomfort) is achieved through responsive caregiving. Mother–infant relationships have been found to differ in the extent of 'synchrony' or 'attunement', concepts that refer to smooth-flowing, reciprocal, behaviourally co-ordinated mother–infant exchanges, usually observed in the context of face-to-face interaction (Stern, 1983; Tronick, 1989; Field, 1992). The optimal maternal role involves correctly 'reading' the infant's signals and providing appropriate levels of responsive communication; sensitive, responsive caregiving, in turn, helps the baby modulate states of negative arousal, permitting positive social exchanges (Sroufe, 1996). Dysregulation, marked by the absence of synchronous interaction, can result from a variety of factors including insensitive caregiving (e.g. overstimulation of the infant), unresponsive caregiving, physical disruptions in caregiving (such as separations) and also from endogenous infant variables such as developmental immaturity or irritable temperament (Calkins, 1994; Field, 1994).

Failure to develop effective self-regulatory skills during infancy is hypothesized to be linked to poor attention and emotional regulation strategies (Rothbart and Bates, 1998) and to problems in later behavioural adjustment (Thompson and Calkins, 1996). Thus, infants who experience frequent dysregulated interactions with caregivers may be a risk for delays or impairments in the development of self-regulatory competence (Emde, 1992). Longitudinal studies have provided preliminary empirical support for this notion. For example, Zeanah and associates (1997) found that infants who experienced chronically poorly regulated interactions with primary caregivers had higher rates of emotional and behavioural adjustment problems in early childhood. Similarly, Feldman et al. (1999) measured individual differences in maternal responsiveness to microshifts in infant affect at 3 and 9 months, and found that synchronous interactions predicted self-regulatory competence at age 2, even when the effects of infant temperament and infant cognitive maturity were controlled. Finally, Wakschlag and Hans (1999) examined maternal responsive-ness to infant behaviour in a high-risk sample of families. Early maternal unresponsiveness was found to be a good predictor of disruptive behaviour disorders in adolescence, but not attention problems.

Caregiver–infant attachment relationships

As discussed above, the most important developmental task of infancy is the establishment of a positive, smoothly functioning relationship with primary caregivers. According to Bowlby (1982), early attachment relationships provide a critical context for the development of physical and emotional security. Attachment refers to a specific, enduring and reciprocal bond between infant and caregiver. Bowlby conceived of attachment relationships as homeostatic systems which function to ensure the safety and security of the infant through regulation of physical proximity to the caregiver. Thus, if the infant is fright-ened or distressed, the caregiver provides protection and soothing. On the psychological level of the attached child, the availability and responsiveness of the caregiver lead to feelings of emotional security and attraction to the relationship (Bowlby, 1982). Although the formation of attachment bonds is considered to be a species universal, individual attachment relationships show qualitative variations that are of clinical relevance.

In their classic studies on the Strange Situation, a laboratory paradigm designed to measure the infant's trust in the physical and emotional availability of the caregiver, Ainsworth and her colleagues (Ainsworth et al., 1971; Ain-sworth et al., 1978) distinguished three qualitatively different patterns of attachment. Following brief separations from the caregiver, 'secure' 1-year-old infants were able quickly to reestablish and maintain positive contact with the caregiver. A substantial minority (approximately one-third in this study) were deemed 'insecure' or 'anxiously attached' in that they either ignored the caregiver on her return (insecure-avoidant) or mixed proximity seeking with angry, ambivalent behaviour (insecure-resistant). Consistent with the hypoth-esis that these patterns reflect qualities of antecedent mother–infant interac-tion, caregiver sensitivity and responsiveness during the first year have been empirically linked to secure attachment at 1 year of life (see review and metaanalysis by DeWolff and van IJzendoorn, 1997). However, emerging conceptualizations of attachment stress that caregiver sensitivity is one compo-nent of a dynamic relationship system that reflects infant, caregiver and broader environmental influences (Seifer and Schiller, 1999).

How, specifically, can knowledge of early attachment relationships inform our understanding of the development of self-regulation? One hypothesis is that quality of caregiver–infant interaction is linked to the development of cognitive/affective schemata which mediate the emergence of basic attentional, motivational and problem-solving skills (Cassidy, 1994). As Bretherton (1985) stated:

Confidence in the mother's physical and psychological availability appears to lay the groundwork for autonomous exploration and problem solving coupled with the expectation that help will be forthcoming when needed. Thus attention span and persistence, which have often been regarded as traitlike, perhaps constitutionally based, qualities, may at least be in part a product of particular relationship systems (p. 21).

Assuming (as Kopp has argued) that compliance is an emergent characteristic of self-regulation, security of attachment has been empirically related to toddlers' willingness to comply with the mother and engage in constructive problem solving (Matas et al., 1978; Londerville and Main, 1981). For example, Matas et al. demonstrated that children who were rated securely attached at 18 months tended to function more competently than others in a 24-month dyadic problem-solving task. In a laboratory setting, mother and toddler were given four puzzles of increasing difficulty; the most difficult tasks were only solvable with maternal assistance. Securely attached toddlers were found to be more compliant, enthusiastic, persistent and attentive to maternal suggestions than insecurely attached children. Similarly, Frankel and Bates (1990) found that toddlers who had been rated securely attached at 13 months spent more time 'on task' and showed less aggression and verbal negativism than insecurely attached toddlers. However, the groups did not differ in compliance with the mother, or in expressions of frustration and whiny affect. Frustration on the part of the child was closely linked to maternal directiveness; the most frustrated toddlers had mothers who issued frequent commands. Further analyses revealed that this type of dyadic interaction was linked to a generalized pattern of conflicted mother–child interaction: children who were frustrated in problem solving tended to be demanding and troublesome at home, and had mothers who exerted high degrees of restrictive, punitive control. As infants, these children were observed to be more socially demanding than others and their mothers tended to show low levels of positive involvement with them during the first year of life.

In other studies, quality of mother–infant interaction behaviour and attachment have been viewed as antecedents of later externalizing-type behaviour problems. In a large prospective study of socially disadvantaged families (the Minnesota High Risk Study), Erickson et al. (1985) found that children who had anxious-avoidant attachments to their mothers at 12 and 18 months were rated by preschool teachers as more impulsive and hostile than others. The latter ratings comprised a broad dimension of negative behaviour; a narrower hyperactivity scale did not differentiate the groups. The overall pattern of findings appeared to fit a 'multipathway' model of transmission, in that the prediction of behaviour problems from early attachment status was mediated by later aspects of parenting. For example, secure infants who eventually developed behaviour problems evidenced suboptimal patterns of mother–child interaction in the early preschool years. Cognitive characteristics of children were also important in accounting for group differences: children who showed behaviour problems in preschool had lower scores than others on measures of cognitive competence at 24 months and language ability at 42 months, irrespective of attachment status. Similarly, follow-up assessments in the early school-age period (Renken et al., 1989) and in preadolescence (Urban et al., 1991) have shown that at-risk children who have insecure early attachments tended to have poorer peer relationships and greater problems with depression and aggression than those with secure early attachments. In all cases, these predictive relationships were stronger for boys than for girls. Evidence for a multipathway model has also been reported by Shaw and his colleagues, who examined caregiver–infant attachment relationships as possible precursors of early-appearing externalizing problems among socioeconomically disadvantaged children (Shaw et al., 1998).

However, other longitudinal studies have been inconsistent in supporting a link between insecure attachment and later problems of impulsivity and aggression. Lewis et al. (1984) found that quality of attachment at 12 months predicted mother reports of internalizing problems at 6 years of age, but only for boys. There was a marginal relationship between early attachment status and later externalizing problems in boys, and no relationship between early attachment status and any kind of psychopathology in girls. Further, predictions between attachment security and later adjustment were moderated by many different factors; insecurely attached boys who were unplanned, second-born children and had experienced elevated rates of family stress were most highly at risk for later negative outcomes.

Fagot and Kavanagh (1990) assessed security of attachment in 18-month-old children and related it to parents' reports of problem behaviours at 24, 27, 30 and 42 months. Children were also observed at 18 and 30 months in the home and in toddler play groups. No relationships were found between insecure attachment status and later indices of problem behaviour, although girls who had been classified insecure-avoidant at 18 months were viewed by teachers and observers as more difficult to manage and more incompetent with peers than others.

Similarly, Bates et al. (1985) found that attachment security in 13-month infants was unrelated to maternal and secondary caregivers' reports of behaviour problems at age 3, and to maternal reports of behaviour problems at age 5 and 6 (Bates and Bayles, 1988). Boys' externalizing problems were related to mothers' early reports of temperamental difficultness and resistance to control, whereas girls' externalizing problems were related to the same temperament variables and to a general lack of early positive involvement with their mothers, as observed in the home.

Thus, attempts to link early attachment status to global measures of externalizing problems have been inconsistent, failing to support a simple linear association between insecure attachment and child behaviour problems, especially in low-risk samples. The most consistent links between insecure parent–infant attachment and later disruptive child behaviour have been found in studies of multirisk families (DeMulder and Radke-Yarrow, 1991; Lyons-Ruth, 1996). This pattern converges with a large body of prior research showing that single indices of risk have been proven much less reliable predictors of later child deviance than multiple and cumulative indices (Sameroff, 2000).

Two later reports from the Bloomington and Minnesota groups indicate that choice of predictor and outcome measures is important in examining links between early experience and children's later impulse control deficits. Reporting from the Bloomington Longitudinal Study, Olson et al. (1990) found that specific self-control deficits in 6-year-old children were associated with prior attachment history and with other antecedent mother–infant interaction variables. In this prospective study of 80 mother–child dyads, quality of mother–infant interaction was assessed in the home at age 6, 13 and 24 months, and security of attachment was assessed using a subsample at age 13 months. Measures of infant temperament and cognitive competence were also collected during the first 2 years, and related to later outcome status. At 6 years of age, children participated in a series of laboratory procedures designed to measure different aspects of self-regulatory competence. These included tests of cognitive impulsivity, motor inhibition and delay of gratification, as well as indexes of off-task behaviour and resistance to temptation assessed during a 30-min structured observation paradigm. Boys who were rated insecurely attached in infancy tended to show inferior cognitive impulse control and delay ability at age of 6 years. Patterns of early maternal control also predicted later self-control in boys: those who engaged in restrictive, punitive interactions with their mothers at age 2 tended to perform more poorly on a measure of cognitive inhibition than others. For both sexes, ability to stay task-focused during the observation was predicted by antecedent patterns of enriched mother–child verbal communication during the second year. Finally, measures of child cognitive competence at 24 months predicted a broad range of self-control competencies at follow-up, including delay ability, inhibitory control and task orientation.

Jacobvitz and Sroufe (1987), reporting from the Minnesota High Risk Study, observed mother–child interaction at 6 months in feeding and play situations. Their main hypothesis was that early maternal intrusiveness might interfere with infants' abilities to modulate their arousal states, thus creating a risk condition for the later difficulties in regulation of arousal to meet situational demands. When children were 42 months old, levels of distractibility, inattention and impulsivity were assessed using a laboratory barrier box paradigm, and mother–child interaction was again observed during a teaching task. At 6 years, teachers rated children for symptoms of attention deficit disorder, and two extreme groups (hyperactive and control) were designed. In addition, a variety of early health status and temperament variables were assessed between 0 and 30 months and related to age 42 month and 6-year outcomes. As hypothesized, hyperactive and control children differed according to qualities of early caregiving. As infants, children in the hyperactive group had mothers who scored highly on a rating measure of maternal intrusiveness/interference, which indexed the extent to which mothers disrupt infants' ongoing activities rather than adapting their responses to the infant's state, mood and interests. Distractibility at 42 months was also moderately correlated with early intrusiveness, and with later hyperactivity ratings. Surprisingly, however, measures of early health status and temperament did not differentiate the groups. Very similar findings were reported by Carlson et al. (1995) in relation to the prediction of hyperactivity in middle childhood.

In summary, although relevant empirical studies have been sparse and inconsistent, aspects of early caregiving have been prospectively linked to children's later self-regulatory capabilities. Even so, associations between early caregiving and later impulse control problems have been quite modest, and their clinical relevance is uncertain. In addition, the reasons for these associations remain unclear. Sroufe's hypothesis (Sroufe, 1991) that intrusive caregiving interferes with early modulation of arousal deserves further attention, as it is consistent with theories of self-regulation (Kopp, 1982) and hyperactivity (Douglas, 1983). It is puzzling that aspects of temperament did not relate to hyperactivity in this study, as many of the temperament measures included by the Minnesota groups bore direct relevance to the construct of arousal modulation. Only linear relationships between early temperament and later hyperactivity were examined, indicating the importance of searching for interactional or transactional effects in further work.

In addition, it is necessary to specify how maternal intrusiveness might affect the risk of later hyperactivity. Sroufe (1991) has argued that insensitive maternal care is a primary causal agent in developmental pathways to hyperactivity, disrupting the child's ability to learn effective techniques for modulating arousal and sustaining attention. As the child grows, he or she may perceive little control over emotionally arousing situations, which in turn may account for later difficulties in attention modulation. However, this theory focuses upon only one aspect of the hyperactive syndrome, inattention. It is unclear how problems of impulsivity and overactivity might result from early intrusive maternal care, particularly in the absence of temperamental vulnerabilities that the child brings to his or her caregiving interactions.

Qualities of early caregiving could also be associated with childrens' self-regulatory abilities because they stimulate the development of cognitive and linguistic competence. For example, in the Olson et al. (1990) study, the patterns of verbally stimulating and nonrestrictive caregiving that predicted children's later self-control were closely related to superior child cognitive competence at earlier age levels (Olson et al., 1984, 1986). Moreover, cognitive and linguistic deficits have been found to covary with problems of hyperactivity and aggression in young children (Campbell et al., 1982; Richman et al., 1982; Bates et al., 1985; Erickson et al., 1985; Moffitt, 1990; Pianta and Caldwell, 1990), suggesting that the extent to which early verbal competence mediates children's attentional and impulse control capabilities is an important topic for further research. Cognitive immaturity is usually conceptualized as a secondary correlate of hyperactivity, but it may play a primary role in its early development.

Finally, an intriguing new direction in attachment research has been the identification of the 'disorganized' pattern of attachment (Main and Solomon, 1990). The disorganized subtype is one of several 'atypical' patterns of attachment that do not fit previously defined categories (Barnett and Vondra, 1999). Infants with disorganized attachment relationships lack a consistent strategy for organizing security seeking following the stress of maternal separation. This pattern is most prevalent in high-risk samples (Vondra et al., 1999). Several studies now indicate that infants with disorganized attachment patterns are at elevated risk for later disruptive behaviour problems (see review by Lyons-Ruth, 1996). Likewise, 'controlling-disorganized' attachment patterns have been linked to aggressive behaviour in clinic-referred preschoolers (Greenberg et al., 1991). In high-risk samples, disorganized attachment patterns have been linked to lack of maternal responsiveness (Lyons-Ruth et al., 1993) and to signs of early neuropsychological impairment in the infant (Vondra and Barnett, 1999). Thus, further research attention should be given to possible links between patterns of disorganized attachment and the development of ADHD.

To conclude, much further work is needed before we understand the role of early caregiving in the development of hyperactivity. Refinements in attachment research, such as the development of new methods for assessing attachment constructs (Waters et al., 1999) and of new categories of insecure attachment (Barnett and Vondra, 1999), may facilitate these efforts. Clearly, however, there is a need to go beyond attachment constructs by incorporating socioecological influences, broader patterns of family relationships (e.g. fathers, peers, siblings) and biological contributions to parent–child relationships.

Parent–toddler control interactions

Achieving a sense of independent mastery is a major developmental task issue for toddlers. In this period of rapid cognitive, social and motor growth, it is normal for toddlers to test parental limits and resist control (MacFarlane et al., 1954; Richman et al., 1982). As Kopp (1982) has argued, toddlerhood marks a critical transition period in the development of self-regulation, due to these very developmental changes. The manner in which parents and toddlers resolve these normative issues may forecast continuing problems in self-regulation.

A substantial body of research indicates that highly directive, negatively toned parent–toddler interactions are associated with noncompliance and other early manifestations of self-control problems. For example, the work of Lytton and his colleagues has shown that highly directive, controlling interactional styles are associated with noncompliance and escalating cycles of conflict between parents and toddlers (Lytton, 1979). These findings coincide with those of other recent investigators who have reported links between highly directive maternal behaviour in task situations and toddler noncompliance and task disengagement (Feldman and Sarnat, 1986; Crockenberg and Litman, 1990; Frankel and Bates, 1990; Silverman and Ragusa, 1992; Arnold et al., 1993; O'Leary et al., 1999). Moreover, although most previous studies have been conducted with normal samples, Campbell and her colleagues (1986b) have shown that this dyadic pattern also characterizes clinically relevant populations of young children. Campbell et al. studied a group of 3-year-old children who were identified by their parents as excessively overactive, noncompliant and inattentive. Mother–child dyads were observed during free play at initial assessment and again 1 year later. Relative to controls, dyadic interactions between referred children and their mothers were characterized by less positive affect, more conflict and greater directiveness. At 1-year follow-up, mothers were less directive in play than at intake, but those with complaints about their children continued to provide more direction than mothers of controls. Finally, mothers showed high levels of individual stability in style of interaction: those who were initially most directive tended to remain so 1 year later.

These combined findings have a clear analogue in studies of older hyperactive children and their parents. Generally, social interactions between hyperactive children and their mothers have been characterized by greater conflict than is seen in normal mother–child dyads (Mash and Johnston, 1990). Relative to controls, hyperactive children have shown higher degrees of noncompliant, negativistic and off-task behaviour during interactions with their mothers, particularly in highly structured task situations. Mothers of hyperactive children, in turn, have been found to be more directive, intrusive and less positively reinforcing in these situations than mothers of normal children. However, interactions between mothers and younger hyperactive children tend to be more directive and controlling than those between dyads containing older children (Barkley et al., 1985). Further, hyperactive boys who receive stimulant medication are less negativistic and more compliant with their mothers in task situations, and mothers respond in kind by becoming less directive and critical (Hinshaw and McHale, 1991). Thus, directive, conflicted interactions between mothers and their hyperactive children are in part a response to high levels of difficult child behaviour: when these levels decrease developmentally or as a result of medication, interactions become less restrictive and more positively toned. On the other hand, restrictive, controlling maternal behaviour towards infants and toddlers has been identified as a stable individual difference dimension in previous research (Clarke-Stewart, 1973; Olson et al., 1984; Pettit and Bates, 1984; Campbell et al., 1996; O'Leary et al., 1999), suggesting that it would be premature to dismiss the parent's contribution as an 'epiphenomenon' of difficult child behaviour. Indeed, Silverman and Ragusa (1992) reported that maternal negative control vis-à-vis toddlers in a structured task situation predicted disruptive behaviour problems at age 4 even when earlier levels of negative child behaviours were statistically controlled. Similar findings were reported by O'Leary et al. (1999) in their longitudinal study of hard-to-manage toddlers. Clearly, a transactional model is needed.

A study by Lee and Bates (1985) illustrates the importance of examining complex transactional relationships between maternal and child behaviour in the genesis of self-regulatory problems. These authors found that 2-year-old children perceived as difficult by their mothers were more likely to have conflicted mother–child interactions than others. In the home setting, difficult children were more negative and resistant to maternal control attempts than others. Mothers of difficult children, in turn, tended to use intrusive control strategies. The more difficult the child, the more likely there would be conflict after maternal control responses, resulting in extended episodes of negative interaction. Most significantly, these troubled relationship patterns had antecedents in earlier maternal ratings of temperamental difficultness: infants who were viewed as extremely irritable and difficult to manage at 6 and 13 months were at risk for conflicted mother–child interactions at age 2. It is noteworthy that most of the toddlers in the difficult group were boys, even though the number of difficult boys and girls was relatively even at earlier age points. Similarly, Campbell et al. (1991) found that a combination of negative, noncompliant and overactive child behaviour strongly predicted negative maternal control toward preschool-age boys.

In summary, there is a substantial body of literature linking maternal directiveness and problems of noncompliance in toddlers. Some theorists might view the difficulties as early precursors of later behaviour disorders. For example, according to Patterson (1982), noncompliance is a form of coercive child behaviour that is maintained by inept parental control techniques. Early conflicts around noncompliance may place children at risk for escalating cycles of coercive interactions with parents and siblings, perhaps eventuating in later patterns of peer rejection, academic failure and delinquency (Patterson et al., 1989). However, in many cases it is both normal and healthy for toddlers to show noncompliance vis-à-vis their parents. As Kuczynski et al. (1987) have emphasized, noncompliance can serve many positive developmental functions, e.g. by providing a context for the development of socially appropriate expressions of autonomy and independence. Qualitative features of noncompliance may provide a key to understanding its clinical relevance. In a longitudinal study of parent–toddler interaction, Kuczynski and Kochanska (1990) examined multiple dimensions of child noncompliance which ranged from unskilful (angry, reactive, defiant behaviour) to skilful (active negotiation with parent) in quality. Only unskilful forms of resistance were predictive of children's behaviour problems at age 5, suggesting that these distinctions are important to consider in future research. Similarly, Crockenberg and Litman (1990) found that defiance, compliance and self-assertion were separate dimensions of behaviour in 1-year-old children, in that they loaded on different factors and showed distinctive relationships with mother–child interaction in a teaching task. Child defiance was a strong and consistent correlate of maternal negative control, but this association did not hold true for other dimensions of child noncompliance.

As with the research on mother–infant attachment and children's behaviour disorders, it is unclear how conflicted mother–toddler relationships relate to emerging self-regulatory difficulties in young children, and whether these problems generalize to other socializing agents and/or situational contexts. For example, recent studies have shown that the caregiving behaviours of mothers and fathers may be differentially related to the development of behaviour problems in young children (Belsky et al., 1998), and that high levels of family stress have strong effects on the stabilization of early-appearing problem behaviours (Campbell et al., 1996). Moreover, again paralleling the attachment studies, these dyadic patterns of maternal overcontrol/child negativity appear to be risk markers for generalized patterns of behavioural maladjustment in young children. Their specific relevance to hyperactivity remains to be demonstrated.

Finally, many of the studies discussed above have indicated that 'difficult' child behaviour tends to elicit upper-limit control responses from socializing agents. As suggested by the Lee and Bates (1985) study, it is quite plausible that the child's behaviour reflects early-appearing temperamental traits. Therefore, the role of early temperament as an antecedent of children's self-regulatory competence is considered in the following section.

Temperament and self-regulation

The construct of temperament encompasses individual differences in responsiveness to the environment which appear early in life, show evidence of heritability and remain relatively stable within developmental periods (Bates, 1987; Rothbart and Bates, 1998). Temperamental differences are thought to play an important role in the early development of self-regulation (Thompson, 1994; Rothbart and Bates, 1998). Moreover, the aetiology of hyperactivity is believed to be at least partly rooted in diverse organic factors (Barkley, 1997a) which may find expression in temperamental traits. Surprisingly, however, there is a paucity of evidence linking early temperament to individual differences in self-regulatory competence, or to the later development of impulse control disorders. Two aspects of temperament have received the most attention in this regard: the global concept of difficultness and the narrower concept of activity level. In addition, recent research has focused on a third set of constructs involving individual differences in cognitive regulation of behaviour.

Difficultness

The concept of temperamental difficultness was introduced by Thomas et al. (1968) to explain early-appearing patterns of hyperirritability and biological irregularity. The most central feature of difficultness is a generalized pattern of negative emotional arousal in the young infant (Bates, 1980, 1987). Thus, 'difficult' infants fuss and cry excessively, and are resistant to caregivers' attempts to soothe them. They may also be slow to adapt to changes in daily routine, and irregular in sleep and feeding habits. Clearly, these infants show difficulties in the modulation of arousal, which is considered a critical early antecedent of self-regulation.

There are two sources of evidence linking temperamental difficultness in infancy to later problems of self-regulation. First, retrospective reports have indicated that some hyperactive children manifest early difficulties with emotional arousal and regulation (Ross and Ross, 1982). For example, Lambert (1982) examined evidence of infant temperamental difficultness among school-age hyperactive children and controls, using retrospective interviews with parents. Dimensions of difficult infant temperament, such as negative mood, unadaptability, low persistence and high activity level, differentiated hyperactive children from controls at the 0.01 level of significance. Similarly, Campbell et al. (1982) studied a group of 2–3-year-old children identified by parents as overactive, inattentive, aggressive and noncompliant. In a structured interview, mothers of 'problem' children reported more difficulties during the early infant period than other mothers. As infants, the clinical group was described as highly active, hyperirritable, unsoothable and resistant to changes in feeding routines. The reports are intriguing, but methodological problems preclude any firm conclusions. Obviously, retrospective reports are highly vulnerable to selective distortion and bias, i.e. mothers of problem children may tend to recall selectively or exaggerate negative infant characteristics. Moreover, not all hyperactive children have been described as 'difficult' in infancy. Finally, difficultness is a nonspecific risk condition that may predispose children to a wide variety of later behavioural and emotional problems, not just hyperactivity (Bates, 1987; Bates et al., 1991).

Second, several prospective longitudinal studies have revealed associations between measures of infant difficultness and later child externalizing behaviour. For example, consistent evidence for a link between infant difficultness and later behaviour problems has come from the Bloomington Longitudinal Study of Bates and his colleagues (1982). In a large prospective study of normal infants and their families, temperamental difficultness was assessed using a maternal report questionnaire at age 6 months (Bates et al., 1979), with age-adjusted forms at 13 and 24 months of age. Observational measures of difficult temperament were also collected by visiting homes to assess levels of infant and toddler irritability, as were measures of parent–child interaction at each different assessment point. Two different aspects of early difficultness were salient as predictors: global scores, which indexed frequent and intense expressions of negative affect, and a narrow 'temperament-like' dimension involving toddler activity management problems and resistance to maternal control. Early irritability and resistance to control, as reported by mothers, were the best predictors of maternal ratings of aggression and hyperactivity in the preschool years (Bates et al., 1985; Bates and Bayles, 1988). More recently, these predictive patterns were found to generalize to mother-reported behaviour problems at age 8 (Bates et al., 1991). Observational indices of irritability were relatively weak predictors of these outcomes, as were measures of parent–infant and parent–toddler interaction. Mothers' perceptions of early activity management problems predicted later externalizing but not internalizing problems. However, global ratings of negative emotionality predicted internalizing problems as well, necessitating further differentiation of this broad construct.

More recently, other investigators have reported associations between early assessments of difficult child behaviour and externalizing problems in later childhood and/or adolescence (Biederman et al., 1990; Hagekull, 1994; Keenan and Shaw, 1994; Caspi et al., 1995; Shaw et al., 1998). These reports suggest that early indices of negative emotionality and difficult behaviour may forecast later behaviour problems, particularly in the context of the mother–child relationship. The predictive associations are quite modest, however, and their clinical relevance is unclear. Moreover, other longitudinal reports have failed to substantiate a link between early temperament and children's later impulse control problems. Olson et al. (1990), drawing upon the Bloomington database, correlated mothers' ratings of difficult temperament at 24 months with a diverse set of laboratory and observational measures of impulsivity assessed at age 6 years. No relationship was found between early temperamental difficultness and later measures of self-control, nor did temperament interact with qualities of the caregiving environment to predict impulsive responding. Similarly, in their prospective study of high-risk families, Jacobvitz and Sroufe (1987) assessed individual differences in temperamental difficultness during the newborn period using nurses' ratings, and at 3, 6 and 30 months using maternal ratings. No relationships were found between the various temperament measures and teacher assessments of hyperactivity at age 6. Very similar findings were reported in relation to temperamental predictors of hyperactive behaviour in older school-age children (Carlson et al., 1995).

Thus, relevant research is both sparse and inconsistent on the role of temperamental difficultness in the development of ADHD. Although hyperactive children have often been described as 'difficult infants' in retrospective reports, prospective longitudinal studies have provided little support for a linear association between early difficultness and later problems of impulse control. However, difficultness may be an early marker of more general patterns of behavioural maladjustment, especially oppositional behaviour in the context of the mother–child relationship.

Due to limitations in the measurement and conceptualization of temperament, the relationship between early difficultness and self-regulatory problems remains an open and highly researchable question. Several points are worth noting. First, temperament is not an 'immutable' characteristic of individuals: temperamental traits show only modest to moderate stability within developmental periods, indicating the importance of examining sources of discontinuity as well as continuity (Rothbart and Bates, 1998). The extent to which temperamental traits remain stable and predict important developmental outcomes depends upon how they transact with qualities of the caregiving environment (Sameroff, 2000). The prevailing model of temperament–environment interaction is a 'goodness of fit' model (Lerner et al., 1989), stressing that lack of mutual accommodation between child and caregiver, not isolated characteristics of individuals, predicts negative developmental outcomes. The amount of stress vs. support resources in the broader social environment also plays an important role in this process. It is easy to imagine how an extremely irritable infant might overwhelm the caregiving resources of a chronically stressed parent who possesses few social or economic resources, yet be quite manageable for a parent with adequate support.

In addition, it is necessary to question how interactions between difficult children and their parents might foster problems of distractibility, aggression and impulsivity. Although few researchers have addressed this question, the Lee and Bates (1985) study (discussed above) showed that difficult infants, especially boys, were at risk for highly conflicted mother–toddler interactions that may presage the development of conduct problems. Indeed, recent research has indicated that developmental pathways to externalizing problems may differ for boys and girls, perhaps reflecting variations in family socialization practices (McFayden-Ketchum et al., 1996; Keenan and Shaw, 1997; Belsky et al., 1998). This is an important question for further longitudinal research.

Lambert and Hartsough (1984) have argued that an additive model of risk

best explains the apparent relationship between early temperamental difficultness and later hyperactivity. They studied 97 5–11-year-old children who were
identified as pervasively hyperactive and compared their developmental progress to that of 93 matched controls. Based on retrospective interviews with
parents and concurrent assessments of family functioning, the hyperactive
children were found to have higher incidences of pre- and perinatal risk factors,
greater evidence of early health and temperamental problems, and less optimal
parental relationships (e.g. more punitive, less educationally stimulating) than
the controls. All three sets of risk factors made independent contributions to
diagnoses of hyperactivity, but an aggregated set of predictors explained more
variance in diagnostic status than either predictor set alone. Thus, temperamental difficultness was one of many risk factors which accumulate to predict
later hyperactivity, necessitating a multifactorial and longitudinal approach to
this problem. However, the additive model still leaves us questioning how
constitutional vulnerabilities transact with other risk conditions to potentiate
hyperactivity.

Finally, there is a need to identify specific indices of temperament that place
children at risk for hyperactivity. Difficultness is probably too broad a construct
to use as a risk marker for specific behaviour disorders. For example, as Bates
(1987) has noted, there are many reasons why infants may fuss and cry
excessively: some may be seeking stimulation, whereas others may be seeking
reductions in stimulation due to autonomic overactivity. The former pattern is
most convergent with concepts of conduct and impulsivity problems.

Activity level
Activity level is commonly regarded as a dimension of temperament (Buss and
Plomin, 1984), even though there has been inconsistent evidence for its stability
in the first year of life (Bates, 1987). Evidence linking early activity levels to
clinical manifestations of hyperactivity is lacking, but several studies have
shown that highly active toddlers and preschoolers have elevated rates of
conflicted/coercive interactions with parents and peers. Analysing data from
the Fels Longitudinal Study, Battle and Lacey (1972) identified a group of
3–6-year-old 'hyperactive' children using observation-based ratings of impulsive and highly active behaviour. Active boys and girls were less compliant
towards adults and more domineering and physically aggressive towards peers
than others. Billman and McDevitt (1980) found that highly active preschoolers, as rated by parents and teachers, were involved in more coercive
interactions with peers than others. Similarly, Halverson and Waldrop (1973)
found that highly active toddlers, identified using actometer ratings, tended to

play more vigorously and become involved in more negative peer interactions than others. Finally, Buss et al. (1980) found that highly active 3-year-olds, identified by actometer ratings, were less compliant, more resistant to adult control, more domineering with peers and more impulsive than others. In a follow-up study, Buss (1981) found that activity level assessed at age 3 predicted quality of parental control at age 5: highly active children tended to have more conflicted interactions with parents than others, as evidenced by greater use of physical control and expressions of hostility and impatience on the part of parents.

Additionally, two research teams have reported prospective links between activity level in infancy and later child conduct problems. In a small subsample, Rothbart et al. (1994) found that infant activity level during laboratory testing predicted school-age ratings of aggression and negativity. Similarly, Hagekull (1994) found that children who were rated as highly active during the toddler period tended to receive relatively high ratings of externalizing problem behaviour several years later.

However, the association of early activity level with later hyperactivity is questionable: stability coefficients are only in the moderate range, and it is unclear whether highly active-aggressive children are manifesting early onset of hyperactivity or more generalized patterns of negativistic behaviour (Bates, 1987). As with the construct of difficultness, longitudinal research is needed to identify specific markers of the hyperactivity syndrome (perhaps using more qualitative indices of overactivity), then examine how they change over time as a consequence of being filtered through different social systems.

Attention and effortful control

Recently, higher cognitive processes involved in the executive control of behaviour have been conceptualized as having strong temperamental (Rothbart and Bates, 1998) and/or neurophysiological (Taylor, 1999) underpinnings. Because executive control systems play an increasingly central role in theories of ADHD (Barkley, 1997a,b; Quay, 1997; Taylor, 1999), relevant research on the early development of these systems will be briefly discussed.

Individual differences in reactive attentional processes can be assessed in early infancy (Ruff and Rothbart, 1996). For example, young infants differ in how long they fixate on novel objects, and individual differences in fixation times are relatively stable through the first year of life (Rothbart, 1988). During the latter half of the first year, a self-regulative form of attention, effortful control, begins to develop (Posner and Rothbart, 1994). The development of effortful control is thought to underlie children's increasing capacities for behavioural control and planning. A third attention system develops in later infancy and is related to alerting responses (Posner and Petersen, 1990). This attentional system, activated under conditions requiring sustained vigilance, has been linked to ADHD (Posner and Raichle, 1994).

The sustained attention and effortful control systems are interrelated, and both develop rapidly over the preschool years (Reed et al., 1984; Kochanska et al., 1997). Recent longitudinal studies have focused on the construct of effortful control, defined as the ability to inhibit a dominant response in order to perform a subdominant response (Rothbart, 1989). During the toddler and preschool periods, individual differences in inhibitory capacity have been linked to the child's ability to internalize standards of conduct (Kochanska et al., 1997). In normal samples, individual differences in inhibitory capacity are moderately stable across early development (Olson, 1989; Kochanska et al., 1996), and across the school-age years (Olson et al., 1999). Finally, individual differences in early inhibitory capacity have been prospectively linked to externalizing problems in adolescence (Mischel et al., 1989; Olson et al., 1999).

Longitudinal research on the development of inhibitory processes may eventually lead to a fuller understanding of the early development of children with ADHD. For example, Barkley (1997a) has hypothesized that generalized dysfunctions in mechanisms of inhibition underlie most of the cognitive and behavioural manifestations of ADHD. Likewise, Quay (1997) has proposed that a more specific problem in inhibitory control, diminished responsivity to conditioned stimuli on which punishment is contingent, is the primary deficit in ADHD. In support of these hypotheses, children with ADHD tend to perform poorly on laboratory paradigms such as go–no-go tasks (Shue and Douglas, 1992), stop tasks (Schachar and Logan, 1990) and Stroop tasks (Gorenstein et al., 1989; Grodzinsky and Diamond, 1992) and patterns of poor inhibitory control have differentiated children with ADHD from those with related diagnoses (Quay, 1997). A dissenting opinion has been offered by Sonuga-Barke and his associates (Sonuga-Barke, 1995), who have argued that children with ADHD often manifest motivational problems that appear to be deficits in inhibitory control. Continued study of these important issues promises to enrich our understanding of the early behavioural development of children who later receive diagnoses of ADHD. In addition, this research area provides a natural link to research on neurobiological mechanisms involved in inhibitory processes. As yet, these linkages are poorly understood (Taylor, 1999).

Developmental course

Preschool predictors of hyperactivity

As children progress through the preschool years, the number of referrals for hyperactivity rises sharply; Barkley (1996) has estimated that 50% of hyperactive children manifest significant behaviour problems by the time they are 3. Although studies of hyperactive symptoms in preschoolers have been relatively rare, there is an emerging consensus that the primary features of hyperactivity can be identified at these early ages (Campbell, 1995; Barkley, 1997a). However, diagnosis and prognosis are complicated by a host of developmental and definitional factors.

In one of the earliest studies, Schliefer et al. (1975) examined 28 children who were referred for symptoms of 'hyperactivity'; according to their parents, these children were unresponsive to discipline, inattentive, overactive and unable to play by themselves. The clinical group was compared with 26 matched controls on measures of impulsive responding assessed in the laboratory, and measures of social and task-relevant behaviour assessed in home and preschool settings. In the preschool setting, only 11/28 children manifested problems of hyperactivity, and thus the clinical group was subdivided into 'true' and 'situational' subgroups. Relative to controls, hyperactive children were more impulsive on a test of reflection-impulsivity, and manifested more overactive, inattentive behaviour in the preschool, but only during structured task situations. Elevated rates of physical and verbal aggression were also found in the hyperactive group. Parents of children with 'true' hyperactivity reported more parenting stress than parents of children with 'situational' hyperactivity and controls, and were observed to use more physical punishment than others. At 2-year follow-up, children in the hyperactive group continued to evidence conflicts with parents (Campbell et al., 1977b). Finally, in a 3-year follow-up, Campbell et al. (1977a) examined the self-esteem and classroom behaviours of these children using teacher reports and direct observation. Children who were designated hyperactive (both subtypes) in preschool continued to show problems in elementary school: they were more disruptive and, to a slight degree, had lower self-esteem than controls. Children who had been designated 'true' hyperactives in preschool manifested more out-of-seat and off-task behaviour than the 'situationals'. Thus, although the groups were very small, these findings indicated that hyperactive symptoms could be identified early in life, and persisted across the transition to elementary school.

Similar conclusions have been reached by Campbell and her colleagues on the basis of their programmatic efforts to identify preschoolers at elevated risk for hyperactivity. In their initial study, Campbell et al. (1982) identified a group of 46 2–3-year-old children whose parents complained of high motor activity, distractibility, tantrums, defiance and difficulty playing alone. These children were compared with controls on a broad range of measures, including parent rating questionnaires and laboratory measures of impulsivity and inattention. Not surprisingly, parents' complaints centred upon problems in social relationships: referred children were described as highly attention seeking, resistant to discipline and aggressive with peers and siblings. On the Behar Problem Behaviour Questionnaire, referred children were rated highly on both the hyperactivity and aggression scales. Maternal reports of hyperactive symptoms were validated by the results of laboratory tests: during structured observations, the clinical group switched activities more often and spent less time on single activities; during structured tasks, they were more often out of seat and off-task, and showed poorer ability to delay gratification than controls. Finally, these problems generalized to other situational contexts: Campbell and Cluss (1982) observed a subsample of subjects who attended preschool and found that they were more aggressive with peers during free play and less compliant in response to teacher directives than controls.

In short, parental complaints about these children were analogous to symptoms of hyperactivity in older, clinically defined groups. As Campbell has repeatedly emphasized, however, identification of 'hyperactivity' in the preschool period is complicated by significant developmental and definitional issues (Campbell, 1995). The chief difficulty concerns the normative nature of early 'problem' behaviours. Many of the problems that parents in her study complained of, such as restlessness, defiance and tantrums, are common during this developmental period. Thus, it was unclear how many of these problems reflected true precursors of the disorder, rather than more transient manifestations of age-specific issues. Additionally, referred children showed considerable heterogeneity in their symptom pictures, and so it was uncertain whether these problems were precursors of hyperactivity per se, or more generalized patterns of conduct disturbance.

A series of follow-up reports by the Campbell group have illuminated some of these questions. Although there were general improvements in symptom levels over time, at 1-year follow-up parent-referred children continued to exhibit more active, inattentive and impulsive behaviour than controls (Campbell et al., 1984). At age 6, problems of aggression and hyperactivity were found to be strongly related to earlier assessments of negative behaviour, and symptom severity was predicted by a constellation of factors, particularly low socioeconomic status (SES) and highly conflicted, directive mother–child interaction (Campbell et al., 1986b). In addition, children who were identified as hard-to-manage at age 4 continued to differ from normal peers on laboratory measures of impulsivity and activity (Campbell et al., 1994). Since half of the referred group continued to show chronic problems, Campbell and associates (Campbell et al., 1996; Marakovitz and Campbell, 1998) have searched for antecedent variables that discriminated those who improved from those who persisted in their maladjustment. Children with persistent problems were rated by mothers as more inattentive, disobedient and maladjusted in their peer relations (e.g. disliked, aggressive) than others. Across the age range, children with persistent problems were rated higher on measures of antisocial behaviour than those who improved, whereas children who improved tended to show steady decrements in levels of externalizing symptoms over time. At age 9, children in the persistent problems group were more likely than others to receive DSM-III diagnoses of attention deficit disorder, oppositional disorder and/or conduct disorder (Campbell and Ewing, 1990) and, relative to controls, showed higher levels of activity and lower levels of efficient task orientation (Marakovitz and Campbell, 1998). Moreover, teachers evaluated them as having significant problems with core symptoms of hyperactivity, and with peer adjustment. Once again, continuing problems of aggression and hyperactivity, as reported by mothers, had multiple antecedents, including reports of difficult temperament in infancy, high levels of preschool externalizing problems, conflicted mother–child interaction at age 3 and 4, and elevated levels of family stress (Campbell et al., 1996). Finally, early levels of family stress and laboratory measures of inattention and overactivity were predictive of later teacher ratings of externalizing problems.

These combined findings suggest several tentative conclusions. First, symptoms of hyperactivity can be identified early in life, and they persist at moderate levels across the transition to middle childhood. Although the Montreal and Pittsburgh studies were limited by very small sample sizes, their findings are consistent with other reports showing moderately high persistence of externalizing symptoms from preschool to the school-age years (Richman et al., 1982; Fischer et al., 1984; Achenbach et al., 1987; Rose et al., 1989). For example, in their epidemiological survey of 3-year-old children living in a London borough, Richman et al. (1982) identified a subgroup who showed serious behaviour problems. When children were 8 years of age, 62% of the initial problem group remained disturbed, compared with 22% of a matched control group. Among those who persisted in their maladjustment, temper tantrums, negativism, antisocial behaviour, restlessness, overactivity and poor social relationships were salient concerns. Boys were far more likely than girls to show problem persistence, especially in the area of antisocial behaviour. Consistent with Campbell et al.'s (1986b) findings, boys with persistent problems were more difficult to manage, restless and overactive as preschoolers. As preschoolers, they also had more symptoms in general, and lower levels of language competence than others.

Moderate levels of stability in symptomatic behaviour exist despite developmental changes in primary problem areas such as overactivity, inattention and disruptiveness. Numerous studies have shown that hyperactive and normal children show clear decrements in activity level between the age of 3 and 9 (Routh et al., 1974; Abikoff et al., 1977; Milich, 1984). Sustained attention and motor inhibition also increase over the same time period (Levy, 1980; Milich, 1984; Schachar and Logan, 1990; Olson et al., 1999). Apparently, children who begin with the highest number and most severe initial symptoms fail to 'catch up' with their peers (Richman et al., 1982; Mash and Johnston, 1990; Campbell, 1995), evidencing patterns of cognitive and social functioning characteristic of much younger children.

However, a substantial number of 'difficult' children do not manifest behaviour problems in later childhood. The presence of chronic family adversity, such as maternal distress, mother–child conflict and marital discord, is a powerful predictor of problem persistence in preschoolers (Richman et al., 1982; McGee et al., 1984; Egeland et al., 1990; Campbell, 1990; Shaw et al., 1994; Campbell, 1995; Campbell et al., 1996). These reports are consistent with current systems models which stress that persistent maladjustment is most likely to occur in the context of continuously and pervasively negative child–environment interactions (Sameroff, 2000).

Problem persistence can also be viewed from the perspective of adaptational failures. The transition to preschool requires that young children adapt to structured routines, conform to the authority of adults other than parents, and share resources and adult attention with many other peers. Hence, establishing flexible levels of self-control and positive peer relationships are central developmental tasks for the preschool-age child (Sroufe, 1979; Sroufe and Rutter, 1984). For example, preschoolers at risk for continued maladjustment show pervasive deficits in self-regulatory competence and, perhaps as a consequence, experience disharmonious relationships with peers (Richman et al., 1982; Allesandri, 1992; Campbell et al., 1994). Similarly, studies of nonreferred preschool children have shown that impulsive and disruptive behaviour tends to cooccur with peer rejection (Milich et al., 1982; Olson and Brodfeld, 1991; Olson, 1992) and predicts social maladjustment in the school-age years (Olson, 1989; Olson and Hoza, 1993; Campbell, 1995). These early patterns may represent one developmental pathway to the pervasive patterns of social maladjustment that often characterize school-age hyperactive children.

Finally, the issue of symptom heterogeneity within the broad externalizing spectrum remains unresolved. Preschoolers at risk for persistent maladjustment show a mix of negativistic and aggressive features in addition to the 'classic' characteristics of hyperactivity (Richman et al., 1982; Campbell, 1995; Keenan and Wakschlag, 2000). These symptom patterns forecast later diagnoses of attention deficit disorder, conduct disorder, oppositional disorder and combinations of these problems (Campbell and Ewing, 1990). Small sample sizes have precluded efforts to examine the long-term developmental sequelae of preschool subtypes, but a growing consensus is that a combination of hyperactive and aggressive features places children at greatest risk for serious and persistent maladjustment (Campbell, 1995). This is an important issue for further systematic study.

Long-term outcome and predictors

Although hyperactivity was once thought to reflect a maturational disorder that children 'outgrew' in adolescence, accumulating evidence from follow-up studies of school-age children with ADHD has put this notion to rest. It is abundantly clear that hyperactive children are at elevated risk for a host of adaptational difficulties in later life, ranging from problems in self-esteem and social relationships to serious criminality (Weiss and Hechtman, 1993).

Longitudinal studies have shown that the 'core' symptoms of hyperactivity clearly persist into adolescence and early adulthood (Barkley et al., 1990b; Fischer et al., 1990; Weiss and Hechtman, 1993; Biederman et al., 1996; Chapter 14) but diminish in severity over time (Thorley, 1984; Hill and Schoener, 1996). Behavioural manifestations of core symptoms also differ between childhood and adolescence; for example, the unfocused overactivity so commonly reported in hyperactive children tends to be expressed as sedentary restlessness in later life (Gittelman and Mannuzza, 1985; Weiss and Hechtman, 1993). However, the most salient concerns of hyperactive adolescents and young adults do not centre upon core symptoms, but upon global patterns of educational, occupational and interpersonal maladjustment.

For example, the greatest long-term mental health risk for hyperactive children appears to be in the area of antisocial spectrum disorders. Hence, the relationship between initial hyperactivity and later antisocial outcomes has been the focus of several follow-up reports. Gittelman and her colleagues (Gittelman et al., 1985; Mannuzza et al., 1991) followed 101 16-year-old male adolescents who had received a childhood diagnosis of hyperactivity. Follow-up assessments were conducted by the interviewers who were blind to subjects' early diagnostic status. Although there was a gradual attrition in the severity of symptoms over time, 31% of the probands were given a DSM-III diagnosis of ADD, in comparison with 3% of the controls. Both conduct disorder and substance use disorders were overrepresented in the clinical group, and tended to aggregate with continued symptoms of hyperactivity. The most interesting aspect of this report concerned a developmental progression in patterns of comorbidity: boys whose symptoms of hyperactivity had not remitted were four times more likely to develop conduct disorder in adolescence than others. Moreover, two-thirds of those who eventually developed conduct disorders progressed to drug and/or alcohol abuse.

Satterfield et al. (1982, 1994) also reported high rates of antisocial behaviour in adolescents with a childhood history of hyperactivity. Following a group of 110 young adults (mean age 17) who had received a childhood diagnosis of hyperactivity and 88 normal controls, Satterfield and colleagues found striking differences between probands and controls in rates of adjudicated antisocial behaviour. Only serious offences, defined as 'robbery', 'burglary', 'grand theft auto', and 'assault with a deadly weapon', were examined. Since the control group had higher SES levels than the probands, comparisons were made with SES groups. The percentage of hyperactive individuals arrested at least once for a serious offence ranged from 38% to 58% across SES groups, in comparison with 2–11% for the controls. Moreover, probands had multiple arrest rates of 25–45% across SES groups, in comparison with 0–6% for controls. Finally, 25% of the probands had been admitted in institutions for delinquent behaviour, compared with only one subject in the control group.

Reporting from a large longitudinal study of New Zealand boys, Moffitt (1990) also found important differences between hyperactive children with and without histories of antisocial behaviour. At the age of 13, four groups were identified on the basis of self-reported delinquent behaviour and a professional diagnosis of hyperactivity: hyperactive + delinquent, hyperactive only, delinquent only and nondisordered. Correlates of delinquency, such as antisocial behaviour problems, verbal IQ deficits, reading problems and family adversity, were traced across childhood. The mixed hyperactivity-delinquent group showed the highest rates of aggressivity, family adversity and neurophysiological deficits, along with the greatest potential for sustained antisocial behaviour. Children with symptoms of hyperactivity alone showed only mild antisocial behaviour at follow-up, and had normal IQs, reading scores and family backgrounds. In comparing patterns of adaptation across time, Moffitt found that the mixed-symptom group had a distinctive developmental trajectory. Antisocial behaviour and symptoms of hyperactivity were present in the preschool years, escalated at school entry and remained stable into adolescence. Patterns of antisocial behaviour consistently covaried with verbal IQ deficits, reading failure at school and a cumulative index of family adversity. In contrast, the delinquent-only group had no verbal IQ deficits, and did not evidence antisocial behaviour or family adversity before the age of 11. These interesting findings should be viewed with caution, given that the mixed hyperactive-delinquent group was very small. However, they are consistent with other reports suggesting that boys with symptom comorbidity are at very high risk for persistent and serious antisocial behaviour (Hinshaw, 1987; Farrington et al., 1990; Magnusson and Bergman, 1990), and they suggest new information concerning the long-term developmental trajectories of at-risk children.

In summary, although risk of later psychiatric disorder loads into the antisocial spectrum, rates of actual antisocial behaviour in hyperactive individuals vary considerably between studies, reflecting heterogeneity in both initial sample selection and diagnostic criteria at follow-up (see review by Lynam, 1996).

Given the substantial variability in later life outcomes among hyperactive children, what factors differentiate those who improve from those who continue to evidence maladjustment? Because childhood hyperactivity is associated with pervasive problems of interpersonal and educational adjustment, it is unclear whether adolescent and adult outcomes are attributable to antecedent symptoms of hyperactivity, associated features such as family dysfunction, conduct disorder or learning disabilities, or some combination of these factors (Cantwell, 1986). Indeed, predictive studies of long-term outcome status (Loney et al., 1981; Hechtman et al., 1984; Taylor et al., 1996; Babinski et al., 1999) have consistently identified very global antecedent correlates of poor outcomes such as low IQ, low SES, childhood aggression and family instability. For example, Taylor et al. (1996) followed a sample of school-age boys who had been identified as pervasively hyperactive on the basis of parent and teacher ratings. Lack of parental warmth and high parental hostility predicted the long-term course of these problems, particularly which boys identified as 'hyperactive' would manifest symptoms of conduct disorder in adolescence.

Based on analyses of their long-term follow-up data, Weiss and Hechtman (1993) concluded that particular adult outcomes are not well predicted by specific antecedent variables, but by additive combinations of personal and social-familial characteristics. Moreover, different combinations of predictors appear to be salient for different outcome measures. For example, academic status was best predicted by a combination of childhood IQ, SES, initial measures of hyperactive symptoms and child-rearing practices, whereas emotional adjustment was predicted by mental health status of family members in combination with low frustration tolerance and emotional instability in childhood. Similarly, in her extensive analyses of long-term predictors of outcome status in hyperactive children, Lambert (1988) concluded that there are general characteristics of hyperactive children (such as severity of initial symptoms and concomitant aggression) that predispose children to maladjustment in later life, but also specific pathways to educational, mental health, conduct and substance use outcomes. Lambert and her colleagues have adopted an expanded developmental approach to the prediction of later life outcomes by considering infancy and preschool predictors as well as those characterizing the school-age period. Different pathways to outcome within the same disorder were marked by differentially weighted combinations of individual, environmental and developmental factors. For example, factors operating during infancy and preschool, such as the presence of difficult temperament and poor health status, were more important predictors of adolescent mental health status than those operating during the school-age years. Conversely, home environment and family interaction during the elementary school years were superior predictors of later academic achievement.

Finally, the search for predictors of long-term adaptation in hyperactive individuals has focused on negative outcomes. Given that as many as 25–50% of hyperactive children are judged to be functioning normally in later life, it would be worthwhile to search for factors that ameliorate risk and lead to positive psychosocial outcomes (Whalen, 1989). In the context of assessing treatment effects, Weiss and Hechtman (1993) asked their adult subjects to identify what was most helpful to them in their childhood years. Caring, positive relationships with significant others emerged as consistent themes. Most often these relationships were with parents, but teachers, tutors, counsellors and friends were also mentioned. Social support and caring family relationships have been repeatedly identified as general protective factors in children at risk for a broad range of adverse psychiatric outcomes (Rutter, 1987; Werner and Smith, 1992). Recently, Hinshaw et al. (1997) found that firm parental discipline combined with high levels of parental warmth and support were associated with positive social adjustment in boys with ADHD. Further research is needed to specify how interpersonal support affects long-term outcomes in hyperactive children.

In conclusion, risk factors associated with negative outcome in hyperactive individuals appear to be additive within developmental periods and cumulative across time (Lambert, 1988). However, more complex analyses of risk should also be conducted, such as examining whether certain factors (e.g. the presence of antisocial behaviour and family adversity) combine multiplicatively rather than additively in the prediction of later outcome status (Rutter, 1987). The picture that is emerging is that there are multiple developmental pathways to hyperactivity, and to later life outcomes once a diagnosis has been made. Explaining inter- and intraindividual variability in the life paths of hyperactive children is a critical direction for further research.

REFERENCES

Abikoff, H., Gittleman-Klein, R. and Klein, D. (1977). Validation of a classroom observation code for hyperactive children. *Journal of Consulting and Clinical Psychology*, **45**, 772–83.

Achenbach, T.M., Edelbrock, C. and Howell, C. (1987). Empirically-based assessment of the behavior problems of 2–3 year old children. *Journal of Abnormal Child Psychology*, **15**, 629–50.

Ainsworth, M.D.S., Bell, S.M. and Stayton, D.J. (1971). Individual differences in strange situation behavior of one year olds. In *The Origins of Human Social Relations*, H.R. Schaffer, ed., pp. 17–57. London; Academic Press.

Ainsworth, M.D.S., Blehar, M.C., Waters, E. and Wall, S. (1978). *Patterns of Attachment: A Psychological Study of the Strange Situation*. Hillsdale, NJ: Erlbaum.

Allesandri, S.M. (1992). Attention, play, and social behavior in ADHD preschoolers. *Journal of Abnormal Child Psychology*, **20**, 289–302.

American Psychiatric Association. (1980). *DSM-III: Diagnostic and Statistical Manual of Mental Disorders*, 3rd edn. Washington, DC: American Psychiatric Association.

American Psychiatric Association. (1987). *DSM-III-R: Diagnostic and Statistical Manual of Mental Disorders*, 3rd edn revised. Washington, DC: American Psychiatric Association.

American Psychiatric Association. (1994). *DSM-IV: Diagnostic and Statistical Manual of Mental Disorders*, 4th edn. Washington, DC: American Psychiatric Association.

Arnold, D.S., O'Leary, S.G., Wolff, L.S. and Acker, M.M. (1993). The Parenting Scale: a measure of dysfunctional parenting in discipline situations. *Psychological Assessment*, **5**, 137–44.

August, G., Realmuto, G.M., MacDonald, A.W., Nugent, S.M. and Crosby, R. (1996). Prevalence of ADHD and comorbid disorders among elementary school children screened for disruptive behavior. *Journal of Abnormal Child Psychology*, **24**, 571–96.

Babinski, L.M., Hartsough, C.S. and Lambert, N.M. (1999). Childhood conduct problems, hyperactivity-impulsivity, and inattention as predictors of adult criminal activity. *Journal of Child Psychiatry and Psychology*, **40**, 347–55.

Barkley, R.A. (1994). Impaired delayed responding: a unified theory of attention deficit disorder. In *Disruptive Behavior Disorders: Essays in Honor of Herbert Quay*, D.K. Routh, ed., pp. 11–57. New York: Plenum.

Barkley, R.A. (1996). Attention-deficit hyperactivity disorder. In *Child Psychopathology*, E. Mash and R.A. Barkley, eds, pp. 63–112. New York: Guilford Press.

Barkley, R.A. (1997a). Behavioral inhibition, sustained atttention, and executive functions: constructing a unifying theory of ADHD. *Psychological Bulletin*, **121**, 65–94.

Barkley, R.A. (1997b). *ADHD and the Nature of Self-control*. New York: Guilford Press.

Barkley, R.A., Karlsson, J. and Pollard, S. (1985). Effects of age on the mother–child interactions of ADD-H and normal boys. *Journal of Abnormal Child Psychology*, **13**, 631–8.

Barkley, R.A., DuPaul, G.J. and McMurray, M.B. (1990a). Comprehensive evaluation of attention deficit disorder with and without hyperactivity as defined by research criteria. *Journal of Consulting and Clinical Psychology*, **58**, 775–89.

Barkley, R.A., Fischer, M., Edelbrock, C.S. and Smallish, L. (1990b). The adolescent outcome of hyperactive children diagnosed by research criteria: An 8-year follow-up study. *Journal of the American Academy of Child and Adolescent Psychiatry*, **29**, 546–57.

Barnett, D. and Vondra, J. (1999). Atypical patterns of early attachment: theory, research, and current directions. *Monographs of the Society for Research in Child Development*, **64**, 1–24.

Bates, J.E. (1980). The concept of difficult termperament. *Merrill-Palmer Quarterly*, **26**, 299–319.

Bates, J.E. (1987). Temperament in infancy. In *Handbook of Infant Development*, 2nd edn, J.D. Osofsky, ed., pp. 1101–49. New York: Wiley.

Bates, J.E. and Bayles, K. (1988). The role of attachment in the devleopment of behaviour problems. In *Clinical Applications of Attachment*, J. Belsky and T. Nezworski, eds, pp. 253–99. Hillsdale, NJ: Lawrence Erlbaum.

Bates, J.E., Freeland, C.A.B. and Lounsbury, M.L. (1979). Measurement of infant difficultness. *Child Development*, **50**, 794–803.

Bates, J.E., Olson, S.L., Pettit, G. and Bayles, K. (1982). Dimensions of individuality in the mother–infant relationship at 6 months of age. *Child Development*, **53**, 445–61.

Bates, J.E., Bayles, K., Bennett, D., Ridge, B. and Brown, M. (1991). Origins of externalizing behaviour problems at eight years of age. In *Development and Treatment of Childhood Aggression*, D. Pepler and K. Rubin, eds, pp. 93–120. Hillside, NJ: Erlbaum.

Bates, J.E., Maslin, C.A. and Frankel, K. (1985). Attachment security, other-child interaction, and temperament as predictors of behaviour problem ratings at age three years. *Monographs of the Society for Research in Child Development*, **50**, 167–93.

Bates, J.E., Bayles, K., Bennett, D., Ridge, B. and Brown, M.B. (1991). Origins of externalizing behavior problems at eight years of age. In *Development and Treatment of Childhood Aggression*, D. Pepler and K. Rubin, eds, pp. 93–120. Hillsdale, NJ: Erlbaum.

Battle, E.S. and Lacey, B. (1972). A context for hyperactivity in children over time. *Child Development*, **43**, 757–73.

Belsky, J., Hsieh, K.-H. and Crnic, K. (1998). Mothering, fathering, and infant negativity as antecedents of boys' externalizing problems and inhibition at age 3 years: differential suscepti-bility to rearing experience? *Development and Psychopathology*, **10**, 301–19.

Biederman, J., Rosenbaum, J.F., Hirshfeld, D.R. et al. (1990). Psychiatric correlates of behavioral inhibition in young children of parents with and without psychiatric disorders. *Archives of General Psychiatry*, **47**, 21–6.

Biederman, J., Newcomb, J. and Sprich, S.E. (1991). Comorbidity of ADHD. *American Journal of Psychiatry*, **148**, 564–77.

Biederman, J., Faraone, S., Milberger, S. et al. (1996). Predictors of persistence and remissions of ADHD into adolescence: results from a four-year prospective follow-up. *Journal of the American Academy of Child and Adolescent Psychiatry*, **35**, 343–51.

Billman, J. and McDevitt, S.C. (1980). Convergence of parent and observer ratings of temperament with observations of peer interaction in nursery school. *Child Development*, **51**, 395–400.

Block, J.H. and Block, J. (1980). The role of ego control and ego resiliency in the organization of development. *Minnesota Symposia on Child Psychology*, vol. 13, W.A. Collins, ed., pp. 39–101. Hillsdale, NJ: Erlbaum.

Bowlby, J. (1982). *Attachment and Loss:* vol. 1: *Attachment*, 2nd edn. New York: Basic.

Bretherton, I. (1985). Attachment theory: Retrospect and prospect. *Monographs of the Society for Research in Child Development*, **50**, 3–35.

Brody, G.H., Stoneman, Z. and Burke, M. (1988). Child temperament and parental perceptions of individual child adjustment: an intrafamilial analysis. *American Journal of Orthopsychiatry*, **58**, 532–42.

Buss, D.M. (1981). Predicting parent–child interactions from children's activity level. *Developmental Psychology*, **17**, 59–65.

Buss, A.H. and Plomin, R. (1984). *Temperament: Early Developing Personality Traits*. Hillsdale, NJ: Erlbaum.

Buss, D.M., Block, J.H. and Block, J. (1980). Preschool activity level: personality correlates and developmental implications. *Child Development*, **51**, 401–8.

Calkins, S.D. (1994). Origins and outcomes of individual differences in emotion regulation. *Monographs of the Society for Research in Child Development*, **59**, pp. 53–72.

Calkins, S.D., Smith, C.L., Gill, K.L. and Johnson, M.C. (1998). Maternal interactive style across contexts: relations to emotional, behavioral, and physiological regulation during toddlerhood. *Social Development*, **7**, 350–69.

Campbell, S.B. (1990). *Behavior Problems in Preschool Children: Clinical and Developmental Issues*. New York: Guilford Press.

Campbell, S.B. (1995). Behavior problems in preschool children: a review of recent research. *Journal of Child Psychology and Psychiatry*, **36**, 113–49.

Campbell, S.B. (2000). Attention deficit hyperactivity disorder: a developmental view. In *Handbook of Developmental Psychopathology*, 2nd edn, A.J. Sameroff, M. Lewis and S.M. Miller, eds, pp. 383–402. New York: Wiley.

Campbell, S.B., Breaux, A.M., Ewing, L.A. and Szumowski, E.K. (1984). A one-year follow-up study of parent-referred 'hyperactive' preschoolers. *Journal of the American Academy of Child Psychiatry*, **23**, 243–9.

Campbell, S.B. and Cluss, P. (1982). Peer relations in young children with behaviour problems. In *Peer Relationships and Social Skills in Childhood*, K.H. Rubin and H.S. Ross, eds, pp. 323–53. New York: Springer-Verlag.

Campbell, S.B. and Ewing, L.J. (1990). Follow-up of hard-to-manage preschoolers: adjustment at age 9 and predictors of continuing symptoms. *Journal of Child Psychology and Psychiatry*, **31**, 871–89.

Campbell, S.B., Endman, M. and Bernfeld, G. (1977a). A three year follow-up of hyperactive preschoolers into elementary school. *Journal of Child Psychology and Psychiatry*, **18**, 239–50.

Campbell, S.B, Schleifer, M., Weiss, G. and Perlman, T. (1977b). A two-year follow-up of hyperactive preschoolers. *American Journal of Orthopsychiatry*, **47**, 149–62.

Campbell, S.B., Szumowski, E.K., Ewing, L.J., Gluck, D. and Breaux, A.M. (1982). A multidimensional assessment of parent-identified behavior problem toddlers. *Journal of Abnormal Child Psychology*, **10**, 569–629.

Campbell, S.B., Breaux, A.M., Ewing, L.A. and Szumowski, E.K. (1986a). Correlates and predictors of hyperactivity and aggression: a longitudinal study of parent-referred problem preschoolers. *Journal of Abnormal Child Psychology*, **14**, 217–34.

Campbell, S.B. Ewing, L.J., Breaux, A.M. and Szumowski, E.K. (1986b). Parent-referred problem three-year-olds: follow-up at school entry. *Journal of Child Psychology and Psychiatry*, **27**, 473–88.

Campbell, S.B., Pierce, E., March, C. and Ewing, L.J. (1991). Noncompliant behavior, overactivity, and family stress as predictors of negative maternal control in preschool children. *Development and Psychopathology*, **3**, 175–90.

Campbell, S.B., Pierce, E., March, C., Ewing, L.J. and Szumowski, E.K. (1994). Hard-to-manage preschool boys: symptomatic behavior across contexts and time. *Child Development*, **65**, 836–51.

Campbell, S.B., Pierce, E., Moore, G., Marakovitz, S. and Newby, K. (1996). Boys' externalizing problems at elementary school age: pathways from early behavior problems. Maternal control, and family stress. *Development and Psychopathology*, **8**, 701–19.

Cantwell, D.P. (1986). Attention deficit disorder in adolescents. *Clinical Psychology Review*, **6**, 237–47.

Carlson, E.A., Jacobvitz, D. and Sroufe, L.A. (1995). A developmental investigation of inattentiveness and hyperactivity. *Child Development*, **66**, 37–54.

Caspi, A., Henry, B., McGee, R.O., Moffitt, T.E. and Silva, P.A. (1995). Temperamental origins of child and adolescent behavior problems: from age three to age fifteen. *Child Development*, **66**, 55–68.

Cassidy, J. (1994). Emotion regulation: influences on attachment relationships. *Monographs of the Society for Research in Child Development*, **59**, 228–49.

Cicchetti, D. and Cohen, D. (1995). Perspectives in developmental psychopathology. In *Developmental Psychopathology*, vol. 1: *Theory and Methods*, D. Cicchetti and D. Cohen, eds, pp. 3–20. New York: Wiley.

Clarke-Stewart, K.A. (1973). Interactions between mothers and their young children: characteristics and consequences. *Monographs of the Society for Research in Child Development*, **38**, no. 153.

Coie, J.D., Miller-Jackson, S. and Bagwell, C. (2000). Prevention science. In *Handbook of Developmental Psychopathology*, 2nd edn, A.J. Sameroff, M. Lewis and S.M. Miller, eds, pp. 93–108. New York: Wiley.

Crockenberg, S.B. and Litman, C. (1990). Autonomy as competence in 2-year-olds: maternal correlates of child defiance, compliance, and self-assertion. *Developmental Psychology*, **26**, 961–71.

DeMulder, E.K. and Radke-Yarrow, M. (1991). Attachment with affectively ill and well mothers: concurrent behavioral correlates. *Development and Psychopathology*, **3**, 227–42.

Derryberry, D. and Rothbart, M.K. (1997). Reactive and effortful processes in the organization of temperament. *Development and Psychopathology*, **9**, 633–52.

DeWolff, M.S. and van IJzendoorn, M. (1997). Sensitivity and attachment: a meta-analysis on parental antecedents of infant attachment. *Child Development*, **68**, 571–91.

Douglas, V.I. (1983). Attention and cognitive problems. In *Developmental Neuropsychiatry*, M. Rutter, ed., pp. 280–329. New York: Guilford Press.

Egeland, B., Kalkoske, M., Gottesman, N. and Erickson, M.F. (1990). Preschool behaviour problems: stability and factors accounting for change. *Journal of Child Psychology and Psychiatry*, **31**, 891–909.

Eisenberg, N., Fabes, R.A., Nyman, M., Bernzweig, J. and Pinnuelas, A. (1994). The relations of emotionality and regulation to children's anger-related reactions. *Child Development*, **65**, 109–28.

Emde, R.N. (1992). Amae, intimacy, and the early moral self. *Infant Mental Health Journal*, **13**, 34–42.

Erhardt, D. and Hinshaw, S.P. (1994). Initial sociometric impressions of attention-deficit hyperactivity disorder and comparison boys: predictions from social behaviors and from nonverbal variables. *Journal of Consulting and Clinical Psychology*, **62**, 833–42.

Erickson, M.F., Sroufe, L.A. and Egeland, B. (1985). The relationship between quality of attachment and behavior problems in preschool in a high-risk sample. *Monographs of the Society for Research in Child Development*, **50**, 147–65.

Fabes, R.A. and Eisenberg, N. (1992). Young children's coping with interpersonal anger. *Child Development*, **63**, 116–28.

Fagot, B. and Kavanagh, K. (1990). The prediction of antisocial behavior from avoidant attachment classifications. *Child Development*, **61**, 864–73.

Faraone, S.V., Biederman, J. and Kiely, K. (1996). Cognitive functioning, learning disability, and school failure in attention deficit hyperactivity disorder: a family study perspective. In *Language, Learning, and Behavior Disorders*, J.H. Beitchman, N.J. Cohen, M.M. Konstantareas and R. Tannock, eds, pp. 247–71. New York: Cambridge University Press.

Farrington, D.P., Loeber, R. and Van Kammen, W.B. (1990). Long-term criminal outcomes of hyperactivity-impulsivity-attention deficit and conduct problems in childhood. In *Straight and Devious Pathways from Childhood to Adulthood*, L.N. Robins and M. Rutter, eds, pp. 62–81. Cambridge: Cambridge University Press.

Feldman, S. S. and Sarnat, L. (1986). Israeli town and kibbutz toddlers' compliance and adults, control attempts. *Merrill-Palmer Quarterly*, **32**, 365–82.

Feldman, R., Greenbaum, C.W. and Yirmiya, N. (1999). Mother–infant affect syncrony as an antecedent of the emergence of self-control. *Developmental Psychology*, **35**, 223–31.

Field, T. (1992). Infants of depressed mothers. *Development and Psychopathology*, **4**, 49–66.

Field, T. (1994). The effects of mother's physical and emotional availability on emotion regulation. *Monographs of the Society for Research in Child Development*, **59**, 208–27.

Fischer, M., Rolf, J., Hasazi, J.E. and Cummings, L. (1984). Follow-up of a preschool epidemiological sample: cross-age continuities and predictions of later adjustment with internalizing and externalizing dimensions of behavior. *Child Development*, **55**, 137–50.

Fischer, M., Barkley, R.A., Edelbrock, C.S. and Smallish, L. (1990). The adolescent outcome of hyperactive children diagnosed by research criteria. II: Academic, attentional, and neuropsychological status. *Journal of Clinical and Consulting Psychology*, **58**, 580–8.

Flavell, J.H. (1977). *Cognitive Development*. Engelwood Cliffs, NJ: Prentice-Hall.

Flavell, J.H. (1985). *Cognitive Development*, 2nd edn. Engelwood Cliffs, NJ: Prentice-Hall.

Fox, N. and Calkins, S. (1993). Pathways to aggression and social withdrawal: interactions among temperament, attachment, and regulation. In *Social Withdrawal, Inhibition, and Shyness in Childhood*, K.H. Rubin and J.B. Asendorpf, eds, pp. 81–100. Hillsdale, NJ: Lawrence Erlbaum.

Frankel, K. and Bates, J.E. (1990). Mother–toddler problem solving: antecedents in attachment, home behavior, and temperament. *Child Development*, **61**, 820–31.

Gittelman, R. and Mannuzza, S. (1985). Diagnosing ADD-H in adolescents. *Psychopharmocology Bulletin*, **21**, 237–42.

Gittelman, R., Manuzza, S., Shenker, R. and Bonagura, N. (1985). Hyperactive boys almost grown up: psychiatric status. *Archives of General Psychiatry*, **42**, 937–47.

Gorenstein, E.E., Mammato, C.A. and Sandy, J.M. (1989). Performance of inattentive-overactive children on selected measures of prefrontal-type function. *Journal of Clinical Psychology*, **45**, 619–34.

Greenberg, M.T., Speltz, M.L., DeKlyen, M. and Endriga, M.C. (1991). Attachment security in preschoolers with and without externalizing problems. *Development and Psychopathology*, **3**, 413–30.

Grodzinsky, G.M. and Diamond, R. (1992). Frontal lobe functioning in boys with attention-deficit hyperactivity disorder. *Developmental Neuropsychology*, **8**, 427–45.

Hagekull, B. (1994). Infant temperament and early childhood functioning: possible relations to the five-factor model. In *The Developing Structure of Temperament and Personality*, C.J. Halvorsen and R.P. Martin, eds, pp. 227–40. Hillsdale, NJ: Erlbaum.

Halverson, C.F. and Waldrop, M. (1973). The relations of mechanically recorded activity level to varieties of preschool play behavior. *Child Development*, **44**, 678–81.

Hechtman, L., Weiss, G., Perlman, T. and Amsel, R. (1984). Hyperactives as young adults: initial predictors of adult outcome. *Journal of the American Academy of Child Psychiatry*, **23**, 250–61.

Hill, J.C. and Schoener, E.P. (1996). Age-dependent decline of attention deficit hyperactivity disorder. *American Journal of Psychiatry*, **153**, 1143–6.

Hinshaw, S.P. (1987). On the distinction between attentional deficits/hyperactivity and conduct problems/aggression in child psychopathology. *Psychological Bulletin*, **101**, 443–63.

Hinshaw, S.P. (1992). Externalizing behavior problems and academic underachievement in childhood/adolescence: causal relationships and underlying mechanisms. *Psychological Bulletin*, **111**, 127–55.

Hinshaw, S.P. (1994). *Attention Deficits and Hyperactivity in Children*. Thousand Oaks, CA: Sage.

Hinshaw, S.P. and McHale, J.P. (1991). Stimulant medication and the social interactions of hyperactive children. In *Personality, Social Skills, and Psychopathology: An Individual Differences Approach*, D.G. Gilbert and J.J. Connolly, eds, pp. 229–53. New York: Plenum Press.

Hinshaw, S.P. and Melnick, S.M. (1995). Peer relationships in boys with attention-deficit hyperactivity disorder with and without co-morbid aggression. *Development and Psychopathology*, **7**, 627–47.

Hinshaw, S.P., Zupan, B.A., Simmel, C., Nigg, J. and Melnick, S. (1997). Peer status in boys with and without attention-deficit hyperacitivty disorder: predictions from overt and covert anti-social behavior, social isolation, and authoritative parenting beliefs. *Child Development*, **68**, 880–96.

Jacobvitz, D. and Sroufe, L.A. (1987). The early caregiver–child relationships and attention deficit disorder with hyperactivity in kindergarten: a prospective study. *Child Development*, **58**, 1496–504.

Kagan, J., Reznick, J.S., Clarke, C., Snidman, N. and Garcia-coll, C. (1984). Behavioral inhibition to the unfamiliar. *Child Development*, **55**, 2212–25.

Keenan, K. and Shaw, D.S. (1994). The development of aggression in toddlers: a study of low-income families. *Journal of Abnormal Child Psychology*, **22**, 53–77.

Keenan, K. and Shaw, D.S. (1997). Developmental and social influences on young girls' early problem behaviors. *Psychological Bulletin*, **121**, 95–113.

Keenan, K. and Wakschlag, L. (2000). More than the terrible twos: The nature and severity of behavior problems in clinic-referred preschool children. *Journal of Abnormal Child Psychology*, **28**, 33–46.

Kochanska, G. (1997). Multiple pathways to conscience for children with different temperaments. *Developmental Psychology*, **33**, 228–40.

Kochanska, G. and Murray, K. (2000). Mother–child mutually responsive orientation and conscience development: from toddler to early school age. *Child Development*, **71**, 417–31.

Kochanska, G., Murray, K., Jacques, T.Y., Koenig, A. and Vandegeest, K.A. (1996). Inhibitory control in young children and its role in emerging internalization. *Child Development*, **67**, 490–507.

Kochanska, G., Murray, K. and Coy, K.C. (1997). Inhibitory control as a contributor to conscience in childhood: from toddler to early school-age. *Child Development*, **68**, 263–77.

Kopp, C.B. (1982). Antecedents of self-regulation: a developmental perspective. *Developmental Psychology*, **18**, 199–214.

Kopp, C.B. (1987). The growth of self-regulation: caregivers and children. In *Contemporary Topics in Developmental Psychology*, N. Eisenberg, ed., pp. 34–56. New York: Wiley.

Kopp, C.B. (1989). Regulation of distress and negative emotions: a developmental view. *Developmental Psychology*, **25**, 343–54.

Kuczynski, L. and Kochanska, G. (1990). Development of children's noncompliance strategies from toddlerhood to age 5. *Developmental Psychology*, **26**, 398–408.

Kuczynski, L., Kochanska, G., Radke-Yarow, M. and Girnius-Brown, O. (1987). A developmental interpretation of young children's noncompliance. *Developmental Psychology*, **23**, 799–806.

Lahey, B.B., Piacentini, J.C., McBurnett, K. et al. (1988). Psychopathology in the parents of children with conduct disorder and hyperactivity. *Journal of the American Academy of Child and Adolescent Psychiatry*, **27**, 163–170.

Lambert, N.M. (1982). Temperament profiles of hyperactive children. *American Journal of Orthopsychiatry*, **52**, 458–67.

Lambert, N.M. (1988). Adolescent outcomes for hyperactive children: perspectives on general and specific patterns of childhood risk for adolescent educational, social, and mental health problems. *American Psychologist*, **43**, 786–99.

Lambert, N.M. and Hartsough, C.S. (1984). Contribution of predispositional factors to the diagnosis of hyperactivity. *American Journal of Orthopsychiatry*, **54**, 97–109.

Lee, C.L. and Bates, J.E. (1985). Mother–child interaction at age two years and perceived difficult temperament. *Child Development*, **56**, 1314–25.

Lerner, J.V., Nitz, K., Talwar, R. and Lerner, R.M. (1989). On the functional significance of temperament and mental individuality: a developmental contextual view of the concept of goodness of fit. In *Temperament in Childhood*, G.A. Kohnstamm, J.E. Bates and M. Rothbart, eds, pp. 509–22. New York: Wiley.

Leung, P.W.L. and Connolly, K.J. (1996). Distractibility in hyperactive and conduct-disordered children. *Journal of Child Psychology and Psychiatry*, **37**, 305–32.

Levy, F. (1980). The development of sustained attention (vigilance) and inhibition in children. Some normative data. *Journal of Child Psychology and Psychiatry*, **21**, 77–84.

Lewis, M., Feiring, C., McGuffog, C. and Joskir, J. (1984). Predicting psychopathology in six-year-olds from early social interactions. *Child Development*, **55**, 123–36.

Londerville, S. and Main, M. (1981). Security of attachment, compliance, and maternal training methods in the second year of life. *Developmental Psychology*, **17**, 289–99.

Loney, J., Kramer, J. and Milich, R. (1981) The hyperkinetic child grows up: predictors of symptoms, delinquency, and achievement at follow-up. In *Psychosocial Aspects of Drug Treatment for Hyperactivity*, K.D. Gadow and J. Loney, eds, pp. 381–415. Boulder, CO: Westview Press.

Losier, B.J., McGrath, P.J. and Klein, R.M. (1996). Error patterns on the continuous performance test in non-medicated and medicated samples of children with and without ADHD. *Journal of Consulting and Clinical Psychology*, **37**, 971–87.

Luria, A.R. (1961). *The Role of Speech in the Regulation of Normal and Abnormal Behaviour*. New York: Liveright.

Lynam, D.K. (1996). Early identification of chronic offenders: who is a fledgling psychopath? *Psychological Bulletin*, **120**, 209–34.

Lyons-Ruth, K. (1996). Attachment relationships among children with aggressive behavior problems: the role of disorganized early attachment patterns. *Journal of Consulting and Clinical Psychology*, **64**, 64–73.

Lyons-Ruth, K., Alpern, L. and Repacholi, B. (1993). Disorganized infant attachment classification and maternal psychosocial problems as predictors of hostile-aggressive behavior in the preschool classroom. *Child Development*, **64**, 572–85.

Lytton, H. (1979). Disciplinary encounters between young boys and their mothers and fathers: is there a contingency system? *Developmental Psychology*, **15**, 256–68.

MacFarlane, J.W., Allen, L. and Honzik, M.P. (1954). *A Developmental Study of the Behavior Problems of Normal Children Between Twenty-one Months and Fourteen Years.* Berkeley: University of California Press.

Madan-Swain, A. and Zentall, S.S. (1990). Behavioral comparisons of liked and disliked hyperactive children in play contexts and the behavioral accomodations by their classmates. *Journal of Consulting and Clinical Psychology,* **58**, 197–209.

Magnusson, D. and Bergman, A. (1990). A pattern approach to the study of pathways from childhood to adulthood. In *Straight and Devious Pathways from Childhood to Adulthood,* L. Robins and M. Rutter, eds, pp. 101–15. Cambridge, UK: Cambridge University Press.

Main, M. and Solomon, J. (1990). Procedures for identifying infants as disorganized/disoriented during the Ainsworth Strange Situation. In *Attachment in the Preschool Years: Theory, Research, and Intervention,* M. Greenberg, D. Cicchetti and E.M. Cummings, eds, pp. 339–425. Chicago: University of Chicago Press.

Mannuzza, S., Klein, R.G. and Addalli, K.A. (1991). Young adult mental status of hyperactive boys and their brothers: a prospective follow-up study. *Journal of the American Academy of child and Adolescent Psychiatry,* **30**, 743–51.

Marakovitz, S.E. and Campbell, S.B. (1998). Inattention, impulsivity, and hyperactivity from preschool to school-age: performance of hard-to-manage boys on laboratory measures. *Journal of Child Psychology and Psychiatry,* **39**, 841–51.

Mash, E.J. and Johnston, C. (1990). Determinants of parenting stress: illustrations from families of hyperactive children and families of physically abused children. *Journal of Clinical Child Psychology,* **19**, 331–8.

Matas, L., Arend, R.A. and Sroufe, L.A. (1978). Continuity of adaptation in the second year: the relationship between quality of attachment and later competence. *Child Development,* **49**, 547–56.

McFayden-Ketchum, S.A., Bates, J.E., Dodge, K.A. and Pettit, G.S. (1996). Patterns of change in early childhood aggressive-disruptive behavior: gender differences in predictions from early coercive and affectionate mother–child interactions. *Child Development,* **61**, 2417–33.

McGee, R. and Share, D.L. (1988). Attention deficit disorder-hyperactivity and academic failure: what comes first and what should be treated? *Journal of the American Academy of Child and Adolescent Psychiatry,* **27**, 318–25.

McGee, R., Silvan, P.A. and Williams, S. (1984). Perinatal, neurological, environmental and developmental characteristics of seven-year-old children with stable behaviour problems. *Journal of Child Psychology and Psychiatry,* **25**, 573–86.

Milich, R. (1984). Cross-sectional and longitudinal observations of activity level and sustained attention in a normal sample. *Journal of Abnormal Child Psychology,* **12**, 261–76.

Milich, R. and Kramer, J. (1984). Reflections on impulsivity: an empirical investigation of impulsivity as a construct. In *Advances in Learning and Behavioural Disabilities,* vol. 3, K. Gadow and I. Bialer, eds, pp. 57–94. Greenwich, CT: JAI Press.

Milich, R., Landau, S., Kilby, G. and Whitten, P. (1982). Preschool peer perceptions of the behavior of hyperactive and aggressive children. *Journal of Abnormal Child Psychology,* **10**, 497–510.

Mischel, W., Shoda, Y. and Rodriguez, M. (1989). Delay of gratification in children. *Science*, **244**, 933–8.

Moffitt, T. (1990). Juvenile delinquency and attention deficit disorder: boys' developmental trajectories from age 3 to age 15. *Child Development*, **61**, 893–910.

O'Leary, S.G., Slep, A.M.S. and Reid, M.J. (1999). A longitudinal study of mothers' overreactive discipline and toddlers' externalizing behavior. *Journal of Abnormal Child Psychology*, **27**, 331–41.

Olson, S.L. (1989). Assessment of impulsivity in preschoolers: cross-measure convergences, longitudinal stability, and relevance to social competence. *Journal of Clinical Child Psychology*, **18**, 176–83.

Olson, S.L. (1992). Development of conduct problems and peer rejection in preschool children: a social systems analysis. *Journal of Abnormal Child Psychology*, **20**, 27–35.

Olson, S.L. and Brodfeld, P. (1991). Assessment of peer rejection and externalizing behavior problems in preschool boys: a short-term longitudinal study. *Journal of Abnormal Child Psychology*, **19**, 493–503.

Olson, S.L. and Hoza, B. (1993). Preschool developmental antecedents of conduct problems in children beginning school. *Journal of Abnormal Child Psychology*, **22**, 60–7.

Olson, S.L., Bates, J.E. and Bayles, K. (1984). Mothers–infant interaction and the development of individual differences in children's cognitive competence. *Developmental Psychology*, **20**, 166–79.

Olson, S.L., Bayles, K. and Bates, J.E. (1986). Mother–child interaction and children's speech progress: a longitudinal study of the first two years. *Merrill-Palmer Quarterly*, **32**, 1–20.

Olson, S.L. Bates, J.E. and Bayles, K. (1990). Early antecedents of childhood impulsivity: the role of parent–child interacton, cognitive competence, and temperament. *Journal of Abnormal Child Psychology*, **18**, 317–34.

Olson, S.L., Schilling, E.M. and Bates, J.E. (1999). Measurement of impulsivity: construct coherence, longitudinal stability, and relationship with externalizing problems in middle childhood and adolescence. *Journal of Abnormal Child Psychology*, **27**, 151–65.

Patterson, G.R. (1982). *Coercive Family Process*. Eugene, OR: Castalia.

Patterson, G.R., DeBaryshe, B.D. and Ramsey, E. (1989). A developmental perspective on antisocial behavior. *American Psychologist*, **44**, 329–35.

Pennington, B.F. and Ozonoff, S. (1996). Executive functions and developmental psychopathology. *Journal of Child Psychology and Psychiatry*, **37**, 51–87.

Pennington, B.F., Groisser, D. and Welsh, M.C. (1993). Contrasting cognitive deficits in attention defict hyperactivity disorder versus reading disability. *Developmental Psychology*, **29**, 511–23.

Pettit, G.A. and Bates, J.E. (1984). Continuity of individual differences in the mother–infant relationship from six to thirteen months. *Child Development*, **55**, 729–39.

Pianta, R.C. and Caldwell, C.B. (1990). Stability of externalizing symptoms from kindergarten to first grade and factors related to instability. *Development and Psychopathology*, **2**, 247–58.

Porrino, L.J., Rapaport, J.L., Behar, D. et al. (1983). A naturalistic assessment of the motor activity of hyperactive boys. *Archives of General Psychiatry*, **40**, 681–7.

Posner, M.I. and Petersen, S.E. (1990). The attention system of the human brain. *Annual Review of Neuroscience*, **13**, 25–42.

Posner, M.I. and Raichle, M.E. (1994). *Images of Mind*. New York: Scientific American Library.

Posner, M.I. and Rothbart, M.K. (1994). Constructing neuronal theories of mind. In *High Level Neuronal Theories of the Brain*, C. Koch and J. Davis, eds, pp. 183–99. Cambridge, MA: MIT Press.

Prior, M. and Sanson, A. (1986). Attention deficit disorder with hyperactivity: a critique. *Journal of Child Psychology and Psychiatry*, **27**, 307–19.

Quay, H.C. (1997). Inhibition and attention deficit hyperactivity disorder. *Journal of Abnormal Child Psychology*, **25**, 7–13.

Reed, M.A., Pien, D.P. and Rothbart, M.K. (1984). Inhibitory self-control in preschool children. *Merrill-Palmer Quarterly*, **30**, 131–47.

Renken, B., Egeland, B., Marvinney, D., Mangelsdorf, S. and Sroufe, L.A. (1989). Early childhood antecedents of aggression and passive-withdrawal in early elementary school. *Journal of Personality*, **57**, 257–81.

Richman, N., Stevenson, J.S. and Graham, P.J. (1982). *Preschool to School – A Behavioural Study*. London: Academic.

Rose, S.L., Rose, S.A. and Feldman, J.F. (1989). Stability of behaviour problems in very young children. *Development and Psychopathology*, **1**, 5–20.

Ross, D.M. and Ross, S.A. (1982). *Hyperactivity: Current Issues, Research, and Theory*, 2nd edn. New York: Wiley.

Rothbart, M.K. (1988). Temperament and the development of inhibited approach. *Child Development*, **59**, 1241–50.

Rothbart, M.K. (1989). Temperament and development. In *Temperament in Childhood*, G. Kohnstamm, J. Bates and M.K. Rothbart, eds, pp. 187–248. Chichester, UK: Wiley.

Rothbart, M.K. and Bates, J.E. (1998). Temperament. In *Handbook of Child Psychology, Social, Emotional, and Personality Development*, vol. 3, W. Damon and N. Eisenberg, eds, 5th edn, pp. 105–76. New York: Wiley.

Rothbart, M.K., Ahadi, S.A. and Evans, D.E. (1994). Temperament and social behavior in childhood. *Merrill-Palmer Quarterly*, **40**, 21–39.

Routh, D.K., Schroeder, C.S. and O'Tuama, L. (1974). Development of activity level in children. *Developmental Psychology*, **10**, 163–8.

Ruff, H.A. and Rothbart, M.K. (1996). *Attention in Early Development: Themes and Variations*. New York: Oxford University Press.

Rutter, M. (1987). Psychosocial resilience and protective mechanisms. *American Journal of Orthopsychiatry*, **57**, 316–3l.

Sameroff, A.J. (1995). General systems theories and developmental psychopathology. In *Manual of Developmental Psychopathology*, vol. 1, D. Cicchetti and D. Cohen, eds, pp. 659–95. New York: Wiley.

Sameroff, A.J. (2000). Dialectical processes in developmental psychopathology. In *Handbook of Developmental Psychopathology*, 2nd edn, A.J. Sameroff, M. Lewis and S.M. Miller, eds, New York: Wiley.

Sameroff, A.J. and Chandler, M.J. (1975). Reproductive risk and the continuum of caretaking casualty. In *Review of Child Development Research, V.4*, F.D. Horowitz, ed. Chicago: University of Chicago Press.

Sander, L. (1975). Infant and caretaking environment. In *Explorations in Child Psychiatry*, E.J. Anthony, ed., pp. 129–66. New York: Basic Books.

Satterfield, J., Hoppe, C.M. and Schell, A.M. (1982). A prospective study of delinquency in 110 adolescent boys with attention deficit disorder and 88 normal adolescent boys. *American Journal of Psychiatry*, **139**, 797–8.

Satterfield, J., Swanson, J., Schell, A. and Lee, F. (1994). Prediction of antisocial behavior in atention-deficit hyperactivity disorder boys from aggression/defiance scores. *Journal of the American Academy for Child and Adolescent Psychiatry*, **33**, 185–90.

Schachar, R. (1991). Childhood hyperactivity. *Journal of Child Psychology and Psychiatry*, **32**, 155–91.

Schachar, R. and Logan, G.D. (1990). Impulsivity and inhibitory control in normal development and childhood psychopathology. *Developmental Psychology*, **26**, 710–20.

Schachar, R.J., Tannock, R. and Logan, G.D. (1993). Inhibitory control, impulsiveness, and attention deficit disorder. *Clinical Psychology Review*, **13**, 721–39.

Schachar, R., Mota, V., Logan, G.D., Tannock, R. and Klim, P. (2000). Confirmation of an inhibitory control deficit in attention deficit hyperactivity disorder. *Journal of Abnormal Child Psychology*, **28**, 227–36.

Schaffer, H.R. (1984). *The Child's Entry into a Social World*. London: Academic Press.

Schliefer, M., Weiss, G., Cohen, N.J. et al. (1975). Hyperactivity in preschoolers and the effect of methylphenidate. *American Journal of Orthopsychiatry*, **45**, 38–50.

Seifer, R. and Schiller, M. (1999). The role of parenting sensitivity, infant temperament, and dyadic interaction in attachment theory and assessment. *Monographs of the Society for Research in Child Development*, **60**, 146–76.

Semrud-Clikeman, M., Biederman, J., Sprich-Buckminster, S. et al. (1992). Co-morbidity between ADDH and learning disability: a review and report in a clinically referred sample. *Journal of the American Academy of Child and Adolescent Psychiatry*, **31**, 439–48.

Shaw, D.S., Vondra, J.I., Hommerding, K.D., Keenan, K. and Dunn, M. (1994). Chronic family adversity and early child behavior problems: a longitudinal study of low-income families. *Journal of Child Psychology and Psychiatry*, **35**, 1109–22.

Shaw, D.S., Winslow, E.B., Owens, E.B. et al. (1998). The development of early externalizing problems among children from low-income families: a transformational perspective. *Journal of Abnormal Child Psychology*, **26**, 95–107.

Shaywitz, S.E. and Shaywitz, B.A. (1988). Attention deficit disorder: current perspectives. In *Learning Disabilities: Proceedings of the National Conference*, J.L. Kavanagh and T.J. Truss, eds. Parkton, MD: York Press.

Shue, K.L. and Douglas, V.I. (1992). Attention deficit hyperactivity disorder and the frontal lobe syndrome. *Brain and Cognition*, **20**, 104–24.

Silverman, I.W. and Ragusa, D.M. (1992). A short-term longitudinal study of the early development of self-regulation. *Journal of Abnormal Child Psychology*, **20**, 415–35.

Sonuga-Barke, E.J.S., Williams, E., Hall, M. and Saxton, T. (1996). Hyperactivity and delay aversion: III. The effect on cognitive style of imposing delay after errors. *Journal of Child Psychology and Psychiatry*, **37**, 189–94.

Sonuga-Barke, E.J.S. (1995). Disambiguating inhibitory dysfunction in childhood hyperactivity.

In Eunethdis: European Approaches to Hyperkinetic Disorder, J. Sargeant, ed., pp. 209–23. Amsterdam: Sonuga-Barke.

Sroufe, L.A. (1979). The coherence of individual development. *American Psychologist*, **34**, 834–41.

Sroufe, L.A. (1983). Infant–caregiver attachment and patterns of adaptation in preschool: the roots of maladaptation and competence. In *Minnesota Symposia on Child Psychology*, vol. 16, M. Perlmutter, ed., pp. 41–81. Hillsdale, NJ: Erlbaum.

Sroufe, L.A. (1991). Considering normal and abnormal together: the essence of developmental psychopathology. *Development and Psychopathology*, **2**, 335–47.

Sroufe, L.A. (1996). *Emotional Development: The Organization of Emotional Life in the Early Years.* Cambridge: Cambridge University Press.

Sroufe, L.A. and Rutter, M. (1984). The domain of developmental psychopathology. *Child Development*, **55**, 17–29.

Sroufe, L.A., Duggal, S., Weinfeld, N. and Carlson, E. (2000). Relationships, development, and psychopathology. In *Handbook of Developmental Psychopathology*, 2nd edn, A.J. Sameroff, M. Lewis and S.M. Miller, eds, pp. 75–92. New York: Wiley.

Stern, D.N. (1983). *The Interpersonal World of the Infant: A View of Psychoanalysis and Developmental Psychology.* New York: Basic.

Szatmari, P., Boyle, M. and Offord, D.R. (1989). ADDH and conduct disorder: Degree of diagnostic overlap and differences among correlates. *Journal of the American Academy of Child and Adolescent Psychiatry*, **28**, 865–72.

Taylor, E. (1999). Developmental neuropsychopathology of attention deficit and impulsiveness. *Development and Psychopathology*, **11**, 607–28.

Taylor, E., Chadwick, O., Heptinstall, E. and Danckaerts, M. (1996). Hyperactivity and conduct problems as risk factors for adolescent development. *Journal of the American Academy of Child and Adolescent Psychiatry*, **35**, 1213–26.

Teglasi, H. and MacMahon, B.H. (1990). Temperament and common behavior problems of children. *Journal of Applied Developmental Psychology*, **11**, 331–49.

Thomas, A., Chess, S. and Birch, H. (1968). *Temperament and Behavior Disorders in Children.* New York: New York University Press.

Thompson, R. (1994). Emotion regulation: a theme in search of a definition. In *Monographs of the Society for Research in Child Development*, **59**, no. 240.

Thompson, R.A. and Calkins, S.D. (1996). The double-edged sword: emotional regulation for children at risk. *Development and Psychopathology*, **8**, 163–82.

Thorley, G. (1984). Review of follow-up and follow-back studies of childhood hyperactivity. *Psychological Bulletin*, **96**, 116–32.

Tronick, E.Z. (1989). Emotions and emotional communication in infants. *American Psychologist*, **44**, 112–19.

Urban, J., Carlson, E., Egeland, B. and Sroufe, L.A. (1991). Patterns of individual adaptation across childhood. *Development and Psychopathology*, **3**, 445–60.

Vondra, J.I. and Barnett, D. (1999). Atypical patterns of early attachment: theory, research, and current directions. In *Monographs of the Society for Research in Child Development*, **64**, no. 258, pp. 1–24.

Vondra, J.I., Hommerding, K.D. and Shaw, D.S. (1999). Stability and change in infant attachment in a low-income sample. *Monographs of the Society for Research in Child Development*, **64**, 119–44.

Vygotsky, L.S. (1962). *Thought and Language*. Cambridge, MA: MIT Press.

Wakschlag, L. and Hans, S. (1999). Relation of maternal responsiveness during infancy to the development of behavior problems in high-risk youths. *Developmental Psychology*, **35**, 569–79.

Waters, E. and Sroufe, L.A. (1983). Social competence as a developmental construct. *Developmental Review*, **3**, 79–97.

Waters, E., Vaughn, B., Posada, G. and Kondo-Ikemura, K. (eds) (1999). Caregiving, cultural, and cognitive perspectives on secure-base behavior and working models: new growing points of attachment theory and research. *Monographs of the Society for Research in Child Development*, **60**, 244.

Weiss, G. and Hechtman, L.T. (1993). *Hyperactive Children Grown Up*. New York: Guilford Press.

Werner, E.E. and Smith, R.S. (1992). *Overcoming the Odds*. Ithaca: Cornell University Press.

Whalen, C.K. (1989). Attention deficit and hyperactivity disorders. In *Handbook of Child Psychopathology*, T.H. Ollendick and M. Hersen, eds, pp. 131–69. New York: Plenum.

Whalen, C.K., Henker, B. and Granger, D.A. (1990). Social judgement process in hyperactive boys: effects of methylphenidate and comparisons with normal peers. *Journal of Abnormal Child Psychology*, **18**, 297–316.

Zeanah, C.H., Boris, N.W. and Scheeringa, M.S. (1997). Psychopathology infancy. *Journal of Child Psychology and Psychiatry*, **38**, 81–99.

9

Behavioural and molecular genetic studies

Irwin D. Waldman and Soo Hyun Rhee

Department of Psychology, Emory University, Atlanta, GA, USA

Considerable developments have occurred in the research on and conceptualization of attention deficit hyperactivity disorder (ADHD) over the past 15 years. The classification of the disorder has shifted repeatedly in both the USA and Europe, manifested by major changes to both the *International Classification of Disease* (ICD: World Health Organization, 1992) and *Diagnostic and Statistical Manual of Mental Disorders* (American Psychiatric Association, 1994) classifications. A number of studies (Weiss and Hechtman, 1986; Lilienfeld and Waldman, 1990; Manuzza et al., 1993) have increased our understanding of the long-term course and outcome of ADHD, suggesting that ADHD children have lower educational attainment, lower income and underemployment as well as higher rates of school drop-out, adult criminality and substance abuse than children without the disorder. Research on the overlap of ADHD with other conditions (Lilienfeld and Waldman, 1990; Biederman et al., 1991) has shed light on the extensive and varied nature of the psychopathology experienced by many ADHD children, including rates of oppositional defiant disorder (ODD) and conduct disorder (CD) and anxiety and depressive disorders that are much higher than population base rates.

Perhaps the most dramatic increase in the research literature over the last 15 years has been the increase in our knowledge of the aetiology of ADHD. In this chapter we review research that examines the aetiology of ADHD by investigating its underlying genetic and environmental influences. We begin by considering behaviour genetic studies – studies using family, adoption and twin designs – which attempt to disentangle and estimate the magnitude of genetic and environmental influences on ADHD. We then review the burgeoning literature on molecular genetic studies of ADHD, with a primary focus on studies of the relation of ADHD with genes in the dopaminergic system. Towards the end of each section we suggest a number of future research directions that in our view would be especially fruitful for advancing our knowledge of the aetiology of ADHD and related conditions.

The classification of ADHD

ADHD is a childhood disorder characterized by inattention, hyperactivity and impulsivity. According to DSM-IV (American Psychiatric Association, 1994), the prevalence of ADHD is 3–5% in school-age children, with male-to-female ratios ranging from 4:1 to 9:1. ADHD has been known previously as hyperkinetic reaction of childhood, hyperkinetic syndrome, hyperactive child syndrome, minimal brain damage, minimal brain dysfunction, minimal cerebral dysfunction, minor cerebral dysfunction and attention deficit disorder with or without hyperactivity (ADDH or ADD-wo/H, respectively). The DSM (American Psychiatric Association, 1968), which is used more commonly in North America, and the ICD (World Health Organization, 1967–1969), which is used more commonly in Europe, have recognized ADHD as a disorder since the 1960s. Since then, several revisions in the criteria for the diagnosis of ADHD have been made in both the DSM and the ICD. Although the criteria for ADHD in the DSM and ICD have differed in the past, the 18 symptoms listed in the diagnostic criteria for ADHD in the latest versions of the DSM (American Psychiatric Association, 1994) and the ICD (World Health Organization, 1992) are nearly identical (Chapter 5).

DSM-IV recognizes three subtypes of ADHD: the predominantly inattentive type, the predominantly hyperactive-impulsive type and the combined type. The symptom criteria for the predominantly inattentive type are six or more inattention symptoms and fewer than six hyperactivity-impulsivity symptoms, whereas the symptom criteria for the predominantly hyperactive-impulsive type are six or more hyperactivity-impulsivity symptoms and fewer than six inattention symptoms. The symptom criteria for the combined type are six or more inattention symptoms and six or more hyperactivity-impulsivity symptoms. In DSM-IV, ADHD is not excluded in the presence of other disorders. The symptom criteria for ICD-10 hyperkinetic disorder (HKD) are six or more inattention symptoms, three or more hyperactivity symptoms and one or more impulsivity symptoms. No subtypes are recognized. HKD is not diagnosed in the presence of other disruptive disorders and the HKD diagnosis is not recommended in the presence of internalizing disorders such as anxiety or depression. A separate disorder (hyperkinetic conduct disorder) is diagnosed if a CD is also present. Swanson et al.'s (1998) review demonstrated that when diagnostic criteria for DSM ADHD and ICD HKD are used, prevalence differences between countries are small, with the prevalence for DSM ADHD ranging from 5 to 10% and the prevalence for ICD HKD ranging from 1 to 2%.

Behavioural genetic studies of ADHD

Research designs for investigating genetic and environmental influences include family studies, adoption studies and twin studies. The studies reviewed below have examined ADHD as defined by the DSM criteria (Pauls et al., 1983) or using other measures of inattentive, hyperactive or impulsive symptoms (e.g. the Child Behavior Checklist (CBCL); Edelbrock et al., 1995). Unfortunately, no behaviour genetic studies of HKD as defined by ICD or comparing the DSM and ICD criteria have been conducted.

Family studies

Early family studies examined the relation between ADHD in children and psychopathology in their biological parents by employing two major methods for the assessment of parental psychopathology: studying current parental sociopathy (antisocial personality disorder or ASPD), alcoholism and hysteria (Briquet's syndrome or somatization disorder), or retrospectively diagnosing parents for ADHD. Morrison and Stewart (1971) and Cantwell (1972) found that biological parents of hyperactive children had higher rates of sociopathy, hysteria and alcoholism compared with parents of nonhyperactive control children. Stewart et al. (1980) suggested that an association between parental psychopathology and childhood hyperactivity might have been found in these earlier studies because normal children (rather than children with psychiatric disorders) were used as controls, and because hyperactivity was defined very broadly, with antisocial behaviours included in the criteria for diagnosis. They attempted to address these issues by using psychiatric controls and studying hyperactive children with and without antisocial behaviour separately, and failed to find any association between pure childhood hyperactivity and parental psychopathology (alcoholism, antisocial personality and somatization disorder). Lahey et al. (1988b) obtained similar results, finding no association between ADDH (without CD) and parental substance abuse, antisocial personality or somatization disorder.

Morrison (1980) tried to address the criticisms of the earlier studies by using psychiatric instead of normal controls, and found that parents of hyperactive children were more likely to have antisocial personality and Briquet's syndrome (somatization disorder) than parents of control children (11% vs. 2%). He failed, however, to address Stewart et al.'s other important criticism and did not examine a separate group of hyperactive children without antisocial behaviour. Hyperactivity may be related to antisocial personality and Briquet's

syndrome because of its association with CD and because ADHD and CD overlap substantially. Lilienfeld and Waldman (1990) suggested that ADHD in children may not be related to later ASPD unless those children also have conduct problems or aggression. Hence, Morrison should also have examined whether antisocial personality or Briquet's syndrome is more common in the parents of hyperactive children with antisocial symptoms than in the parents of hyperactive children without antisocial symptoms, as well as in both of these groups as compared with the parents of control children.

Morrison and Stewart (1971) used the retrospective method and found that 20% of hyperactive children had a parent who reported childhood hyperactivity, compared with only 5% of medical controls – a statistically unreliable difference. The difference between hyperactive and control children was significant when aunts and uncles were included in the comparison. Thirty-four per cent of hyperactive children had a parent, aunt or uncle formerly diagnosed as hyperactive compared with only 5% of medical controls ($P < 0.001$).

Pauls et al. (1983) also used the retrospective method. They examined 72 children who met DSM-III criteria for ADD with or without hyperactivity and the family history of their first-degree relatives. The risk to the siblings of ADD patients was 0.11 (5 out of 46 siblings) if neither parent was affected, but 0.34 (26 out of 76) if at least one parent was affected, suggesting that ADD is familial and vertically transmitted (i.e. from parents to children).

Sibling studies have also been used to examine the aetiology of ADHD. Safer (1973) studied 17 children with minimal brain dysfunction (hyperactivity) and their 19 full siblings and 22 half siblings. Ten out of 19 full sibling pairs were concordant for minimal brain dysfunction, compared with two out of 22 half sibling pairs. Welner et al. (1977) studied 53 hyperactive children and their siblings and 38 nonhyperactive controls and their siblings. Twenty-six per cent of the brothers of hyperactive children were hyperactive vs. 9% of the brothers of control children. Borland and Heckman (1976) used a slightly different sibling method, studying the children of retrospectively diagnosed hyperactive men and their nondiagnosed brothers. Hyperactivity and behaviour problems were more frequent in children of the probands (i.e. people who are affected by the disorder) than in the children of the probands' brothers, although this difference was not statistically reliable. Borland and Heckman did not report how many children of the probands or the probands' brothers had hyperactivity and behaviour problems.

The most recent family studies come from Biederman and his colleagues at Massachusetts General Hospital. Biederman et al. (1986) studied 22 boys with DSM-III ADD and their 74 first-degree relatives and 20 control boys and their 70 first-degree relatives. ADD was assessed contemporaneously in the subjects and their siblings, and childhood ADD was assessed retrospectively in their parents. The morbidity risk in the first-degree relatives of ADD children was 31.5%, compared with 5.7% in the first-degree relatives of normal control children. Biederman et al. (1990) studied 73 male ADD probands and their 264 first-degree relatives, 26 psychiatric control males and their 101 first-degree relatives, and 26 paediatric control males and their 92 first-degree relatives. The morbidity risks for the relatives of the probands, psychiatric controls and paediatric controls were 25.1%, 5.3% and 4.6%, respectively. Biederman et al. (1992) studied 140 male probands and their 454 first-degree relatives and 120 normal male controls and their 368 first-degree relatives. The relatives of the ADHD probands had a morbidity risk of 25% vs. 8% in the relatives of the controls. Faraone et al. (1991) replicated these results in a sample of 21 ADD girls and their 69 first-degree relatives and 20 control girls and their 71 first-degree relatives. The relatives of ADD girls had a morbidity risk of 19.5% vs. 4.3% in the relatives of the controls.

The degree to which one can learn about the aetiology of ADHD from family studies is severely limited by two methodological obstacles. First, given that ADHD is a childhood disorder, comparisons of hyperactivity in parents and children must involve either retrospective diagnoses of parents for ADHD or contemporaneous diagnoses of adult disorders that are thought to be related to ADHD (e.g. ASPD, somatization disorder or alcoholism). Although sibling comparisons do not have this problem, they are limited by the second insurmountable obstacle, namely that studies of intact families cannot disentangle genetic and environmental influences. Although family studies can elucidate that ADHD is transmitted familially, they cannot demonstrate to what extent the familiality is due to genes or shared environment.

Adoption studies

Morrison and Stewart (1973) compared biological parents of hyperactive children to adoptive parents of hyperactive children and to parents of normal control children. The biological parents of hyperactive children were more likely to have been hyperactive themselves as children and to have associated disorders in adulthood (sociopathy, hysteria and alcoholism) than the other two groups of parents. Cantwell (1975) found similar results, in that biological parents of hyperactive children living with their natural families were more likely to have been hyperactive as children themselves compared with adoptive parents of hyperactive children. Cunningham et al. (1975) used a different adoption study method and compared the adopted-away offspring of psychiatrically disturbed biological parents and psychiatrically normal biological parents. Eight out of 59 (13.6%) adoptees with psychiatrically disturbed biological parents vs. only one out of 55 (1.8%) adoptees with psychiatrically normal biological parents were diagnosed with hyperactivity.

Alberts-Corush et al. (1986) studied 43 hyperactive children (25 children living with their natural families and 18 children living with adoptive families) and 45 normal control children (25 children living with their natural families and 20 children living with their adoptive families). Biological relatives of hyperactive children had more attentional problems, slower mean reaction times and fewer correct recognitions on standardized measures of attention than adoptive parents of hyperactive children or parents of normal children. Also, Cadoret and Stewart (1991) studied the contributions of several variables in predicting increased rates of ADHD in adoptees. These variables included an adoption agency record that mentions psychiatric problems or behavioural disturbance in the biological parents, socioeconomic status of the adoptive home and psychiatric disturbance in the adoptive home (i.e. alcohol problems, antisocial behaviour or psychiatric problems in adoptive parents, siblings or more distant relatives) assessed via adoptive parent interviews. Log linear modelling was used to analyse the relation of these variables to ADHD in adoptees, and only delinquency or adult criminal conviction in the biological parents and socioeconomic status (SES) in the adoptive home predicted increased rates of ADHD in the adoptees.

These results supplement the information that family studies provide by suggesting that the familiality in ADHD can be attributed largely to genetic influences. None the less, some of the same criticisms of family studies apply to these adoption studies. In adoption studies, as in family studies, parents cannot be assessed contemporaneously for ADHD because ADHD is a childhood disorder. Instead, retrospective diagnoses of ADHD or contemporaneous diagnoses of disorders that are thought to be associated with ADHD (e.g. ASPD, somatization disorder or alcoholism) are used. All of the adoption studies cited here used these methods, except that of Alberts-Corush et al. (1986), who used standardized measures of attention. Adoption studies are also limited because the information that would be most useful, the direct comparison of psychopathology in the biological and adoptive families of the same ADHD adoptees, is usually impossible to obtain because of practical obstacles. Cadoret and Stewart's (1991) study was the only adoption study mentioned above that gathered information about both the biological and adoptive families of the same adoptees. Unfortunately, they made no direct comparisons between the biological and adoptive families. Most likely, direct comparisons were not made because they used different criteria for 'psychiatric disturbance' in the biological and adoptive families. An adoption record mentioning psychiatric problems or behavioural disturbance met the criterion for 'psychiatric disturbance' in the biological families, whereas interview-assessed alcohol problems, antisocial behaviour, or psychiatric problems in the adoptive parents, siblings or more distant relatives met the criterion for 'psychiatric disturbance' in the adoptive families.

Twin studies

Twin study designs have certain advantages over both family and adoption studies in that they are more generalizable, more powerful and better able to provide accurate estimates of the magnitude of genetic and environmental influences. Twin studies examine the aetiology of a trait by taking advantage of the fact that monozygotic (MZ) twin pairs share 100% of their genes identical by descent, whereas dizygotic (DZ) twin pairs share 50% of their genes on average. By using this information and comparing the correlations of the trait in MZ and DZ twin pairs, three types of influences on the trait are estimated. Heritability (h^2), or the magnitude of additive genetic influences, is the proportion of individual differences (i.e. variance) in the liability for the trait that is due to genetic differences among individuals. Shared environmental influence (c^2) is the proportion of variance in the liability for the trait that is due to environmental influences that family members experience in common which make them similar to one another. Nonshared environmental influence (e^2) is the proportion of variance in liability that is due to environmental influences that family members experience uniquely that make them different from one another. In addition to these influences, there may be a path leading from one twin's or sibling's trait to their cotwin's or cosibling's trait. This path represents sibling interaction or rater contrast effects that also may influence the phenotype. The sibling interaction may be positive, respresenting cooperation effects, or negative, representing competition.

Additive genetic influences (a^2) refer to alleles from different genetic loci acting independently and 'adding up' to influence the liability for a trait. When genetic influences are nonadditive, however, alleles interact with each other, either at a single locus (dominance) or at different loci (epistasis), to influence the liability for a trait. The magnitude of nonadditive genetic influences (d^2) can also be estimated using a twin design, but c^2 and d^2 cannot be estimated simultaneously because they rely on the same information to infer their effects (Figure 9.1).

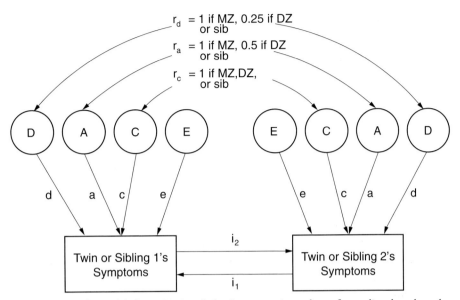

Figure 9.1   Path model for univariate behaviour genetic analyses for a disorder. d, path representing nonadditive genetic influences; a, path representing additive genetic influences; c, path representing shared environmental influences; e, path representing nonshared environmental influences; i, paths representing the influence of one twin or sibling's symptom level on the cotwin or cosibling's symptom level (representing sibling interaction or rater contrast effects); r_d, coefficient of relationship for nonadditive genetic influences; r_a, coefficient of relationship for additive genetic influences; r_c, coefficient of relationship for shared environmental influences.

Twin studies rely on several assumptions in order to disentangle and estimate genetic and environmental influences. These assumptions include the equal environments assumption, no assortative mating and unbiased sampling from the population of twins. Violation of these assumptions can lead to biased estimates of the magnitude of genetic and environmental influences. In twin studies, one makes the equal environments assumption, or the assumption that the shared environmental influences on the trait being examined are no more similar for MZ twins than for DZ twins. It is possible that the environmental influences on MZ twins are more similar because they are treated more similarly. This bias could result in the over-estimation of the magnitude of genetic influences. On the other hand, MZ twin pairs may be less similar in their prenatal influences because sharing the same chorion leads to more prenatal competition. If there are prenatal influences on the trait being examined, the violation of the equal environments assumption could result in the underestimation of the magnitude of genetic influences. A second assumption of the twin study design is absence of assortative, or nonrandom, mating. A correlation between the phenotypes of parents is evidence of assortative mating. Positive assortative mating leads h^2 estimates to be biased downward and c^2 estimates to be biased upward in twin studies because the genetic resemblance between DZ twins is increased due to their receiving more similar genes from both parents than would be expected under conditions of random mating. A third issue to consider when interpreting the results of twin studies is the generalizability of the findings, which may be compromised in several ways. For example, pre- and perinatal complications are more common in twin pairs than in singletons. Twins are born 3–4 weeks premature, are 30% lighter at birth and tend to have delayed language development (Plomin et al., 1997). If these variables are related to the trait being examined, the generalizability of the findings from twin studies to the general population is decreased.

The earliest twin studies of hyperactivity and related characteristics used very small samples. Rutter et al. (1963) examined parents' accounts of activity in 3 MZ twin pairs, 5 DZ (same-sex) twin pairs and 26 pairs of siblings who were at least 2 years old. The within-pair mean rank difference was smaller for the MZ pairs than for the DZ pairs or the sibling pairs. Lopez (1965) studied the hyperkinesis syndrome in four pairs of MZ twins and six pairs of DZ twins (four opposite-sex pairs, two same-sex pairs), age 5–12. All four MZ pairs were concordant, whereas only one DZ pair was concordant.

Willerman (1973) studied 93 twin pairs (aged 11 months to 156 months: 54 MZ pairs and 39 same-sex DZ pairs) recruited from Mothers of Twins Clubs. Heritability, estimated by $(r_{MZ} - r_{DZ})/(1 - r_{DZ})$, was 0.77 for hyperactivity assessed using the Activity Level Questionnaire (Werry, 1970). Torgersen and Kringlen (1978) assessed infant temperament (age 2–9 months) from parent interviews in 34 MZ twin pairs and 16 same-sex DZ twin pairs born at an obstetrical department in Norway. The difference between MZ and DZ within-pair variances was tested by a variance ratio test, which examines the significance of the difference between sample variances. By the age of 9 months, significant differences between MZ and DZ twin pairs in within-pair variance were found for all temperamental characteristics assessed (i.e. rhythmicity, threshold, approach, intensity, activity, persistence, distractibility, mood and adaptability), including activity and distractibility, which are most centrally related to ADHD.

Goodman and Stevenson (1989) conducted the first large twin study (102 MZ and 111 same-sex DZ twin pairs) of ADHD symptoms and reported heritability estimates ranging from 32% to 42% ($c^2 = 12$–28%; $e^2 = 40$–46%) for measures of inattention and 42–100% ($c^2 = 0$–27%; $e^2 = 0$–58%) for measures of hyperactivity. Gilger et al. (1992) assessed DSM-III ADHD in 81 MZ and 52 DZ twin pairs from a reading disability sample using the Diagnostic Interview for Children and Adolescents and found that the proband-wise concordance rates were significantly different for MZ (81%) and DZ (29%) twin pairs. Waldman et al. (1998) examined DSM-III-R ADHD symptoms in a large population-based twin sample (1034 MZ pairs, 1009 DZ pairs and 345 sibling pairs) and found that ADHD was influenced predominantly by genetic influences ($h^2 = 0.90$, $e^2 = 0.10$), with no evidence of shared environmental influences.

A number of studies have examined genetic and environmental influences on the CBCL attentional problems scale. Edelbrock et al. (1995) examined CBCL attentional problems in 99 MZ and 82 DZ twin pairs and found evidence for significant genetic influences and no shared environmental influences ($h^2 = 0.66$, $e^2 = 0.34$). Schmitz et al. (1995) and Gjone et al. (1996) also examined CBCL attentional problems in larger samples and found similar results (Schmitz et al., 1995: $h^2 = 0.65$, $e^2 = 0.35$ in 66 MZ and 137 DZ twin pairs; Gjone et al., 1996: $h^2 = 0.73$–0.79, $e^2 = 0.21$–0.27 in 526 MZ and 389 DZ pairs).

Several studies have examined heritability for extreme levels of activity and inattention (labeled h_g^2, following DeFries and Fulker, 1988). Stevenson (1992) examined several measures of inattention and hyperactivity and reported varying levels of h_g^2 for inattention (0.25–0.76) and for hyperactivity (0.16–0.75). Gillis et al. (1992) and Rhee et al. (1999) reported higher h_g^2 levels for ADHD symptoms ($h_g^2 = 0.98$ and 0.99, respectively). Gjone et al. (1996) reported h_g^2 for attention problems by symptom severity, and found that h_g^2 did not increase as severity increased ($h_g^2 = 0.82$ at the mean level of symptoms, $h_g^2 = 0.88$ for ≥ 0.5 SD above the mean, $h_g^2 = 0.86$ for ≥ 1.0 SD above the mean, and $h_g^2 = 0.77$ for ≥ 1.5 SD above the mean).

If the MZ correlation is more than twice the DZ correlation, the presence of nonadditive genetic influences and/or contrast effects is a possibility. In some twin studies of ADHD, the DZ correlation was very low or even negative (Thapar et al., 1995; Silberg et al., 1996; Nadder et al., 1998). One explanation for extremely low DZ correlations (near-zero or slightly negative) is a contrast effect, i.e. raters exaggerating the difference between DZ twin pairs. Another explanation is sibling interaction, where one twin's ADHD level has a direct negative or inhibiting effect on the other twin's ADHD level. When data from only one rater are used, it is not possible to distinguish between a rater contrast effect and sibling interaction. Several researchers have examined alternative models testing for the presence of sibling interaction/contrast effects.

Thapar et al. (1995) compared a model positing that hyperactivity is caused by additive genetic influences and nonshared environmental influences (an AE model) to a model which also included a sibling interaction/contrast effect (an

AE-B model). The AE-B model ($h^2 = 0.88$, $b = -0.24$) fit significantly better than the AE model, and Thapar et al. interpreted these results as evidence for competitive or inhibitory sibling interaction. Silberg et al. (1996) examined hyperactivity in four groups of children (older boys, older girls, younger boys, younger girls), and also found that an AE-B model was the best-fitting model in all four groups ($h^2 = 0.67$–0.70, $e^2 = 0.25$–0.32, $b = -0.22$ to -0.08). Nadder et al. (1998) compared models including and excluding the sibling interaction/contrast effect for ADHD symptoms. The AE-B model was the best-fitting model, with a heritability estimate of 58–61%, nonshared environment estimate of 39–42%, and a sibling interaction/contrast effect of -0.13 to -0.18, but this model did not fit significantly better than an ADE-B model (i.e. a model that also included nonadditive genetic influences).

Eaves et al. (1997) examined the issue of possible rater bias by testing for the presence of sibling interaction/contrast effects and by comparing the results for parent and teacher reports of ADHD symptoms. For parent reports, the AE-B model fit better than a model that included nonadditive genetic influences but excluded the contrast (the ADE model). Heritability estimates after removing contrast effects ranged from 0.55 to 0.82, the magnitude of nonshared environmental influences ranged from 0.18 to 0.45 and the magnitude of rater contrast effects ranged from -0.09 to -0.24. For teacher reports, the AE model was the best-fitting model ($h^2 = 0.54$–0.62, $e^2 = 0.38$–0.46), and there was no evidence of significant contrast effects. Given that contrast effects were present in parent reports but not teacher reports, Eaves et al's results suggest that the very low DZ correlations are caused by rater contrast effects rather than competitive or inhibitory sibling interaction. In another paper examining hyperactivity in this sample, Simonoff et al. (1998) were also able to show that such findings seem to be due to rater contrast effects rather than direct sibling interaction, given that mother ratings show a contrast effect while teacher ratings show a different form of bias that can be due to either twin confusion (i.e. difficulty attributing behaviour to the correct child) or correlated errors.

As mentioned above, in the most recent version of the DSM (DSM-IV; American Psychiatric Association, 1994), there are three subtypes of ADHD: predominantly inattentive type, predominantly hyperactive-impulsive type and the combined type. These three subtypes are based on surpassing the diagnostic thresholds on one or both of the inattention and hyperactivity-impulsivity symptom dimensions underlying DSM-IV ADHD. This is a significant change from DSM-III-R (American Psychiatric Association, 1987), where ADHD symptoms were viewed as one dimension and a diagnosis of ADHD was given if eight or more of 14 symptoms (of inattention, hyperactivity or impulsivity) were present. This change was based in part on factor analytic evidence that the symptoms of ADHD load on two separate dimensions (inattention-disorganization and hyperactivity-impulsivity; Lahey et al., 1988a; Pelham et al., 1992), as well as on evidence that there are important differences between children with symptoms of inattention only (e.g. greater academic difficulty; Edelbrock et al., 1984) and children with symptoms of both inattention and hyperactivity (e.g. poor peer relations; Lahey et al., 1984).

Given the evidence supporting the distinctiveness of two separate ADHD symptom dimensions, it is important to examine potential heterogeneity in the aetiology of inattentive and hyperactive-impulsive symptoms. Goodman and Stevenson (1989) calculated separate heritability estimates for inattention and hyperactivity and found lower heritabilities for inattention (32–42%) than for hyperactivity (42–100%). Unfortunately, inattention and hyperactivity were assessed using different methods (i.e. laboratory measures for inattention and parent or teacher ratings for hyperactivity), making these results difficult to interpret.

More recently, Sherman et al. (1997) conducted a behaviour genetic study examining inattentive and hyperactive-impulsive symptoms separately. A different pattern of results was found for teacher and mother reports. For teachers, the best-fitting model for inattention was the ACE model ($h^2 = 0.39$, $c^2 = 0.39$ and $e^2 = 0.22$), whereas for hyperactivity-impulsivity the AE model provided the best fit ($h^2 = 0.69$, $e^2 = 0.31$). For mother reports, the AE model was the best-fitting model for both inattention ($h^2 = 0.69$, $e^2 = 0.31$) and for hyperactivity-impulsivity ($h^2 = 0.91$, $e^2 = 0.09$). Sherman et al. also conducted bivariate genetic analyses to examine the aetiology of the covariation between inattentive and hyperactive-impulsive symptoms. The covariation between inattentive and hyperactive-impulsive symptoms was due to genetic influences, shared environmental influences and nonshared environmental influences ($h^2 = 0.33$, $c^2 = 0.45$, $e^2 = 0.22$) for teacher reports, but there was no evidence of shared environmental influences for mother reports ($h^2 = 0.86$, $e^2 = 0.14$). Heath et al. (1996) also examined in other reports of inattention and hyperactivity-impulsivity separately, but reported very similar heritability estimates for inattention ($h^2 = 0.88$, $e^2 = 0.12$) and for hyperactivity-impulsivity ($h^2 = 0.89$, $e^2 = 0.11$) and found a moderate genetic correlation ($r_g = 0.52$) between inattention and hyperactivity-impulsivity. Waldman et al. (1996) reported slightly higher heritability for hyperactivity-impulsivity ($h^2 = 0.88$–0.92, $e^2 = 0.08$–0.12) than for inattention ($h^2 = 0.81$–0.83, $e^2 = 0.17$–0.19), and a higher genetic correlation ($r_g = 0.80$) between inattention and hyperactivity-impulsivity.

Conclusions

The family, adoption and twin studies reviewed above differ on many important characteristics, including the definition of attention/hyperactivity problems, the source of participants, the age range of the subjects, sample size and statistical methods used. Despite these differences, several general conclusions about the aetiology of ADHD can be drawn from these studies. First, both ADHD symptoms in the general population and extreme levels of ADHD in selected populations are highly heritable, with little evidence of shared environmental influences. Several researchers have found near-zero or slightly negative DZ correlations, which suggest the presence of competitive or inhibitory sibling interaction (siblings influencing each other's traits in an opposite direction) or contrast effects (raters exaggerating the difference between twins), rather than nonadditive genetic influences (Thapar et al., 1995; Silberg et al., 1996; Eaves et al., 1997; Nadder et al., 1998; Simonoff et al., 1998). In their comparison of results across multiple informants, Eaves et al. (1997) and Simonoff et al. (1998) provided evidence that the very low DZ correlations for ADHD are most likely the result of rater contrast effects rather than sibling interaction. Most researchers who have conducted behaviour genetic studies of ADHD have examined ADHD symptoms as a single dimension rather than examining inattention and hyperactive-impulsive symptoms separately. Given the evidence regarding the classification of ADHD symptoms, more behaviour genetic studies examining the aetiology of inattention and hyperactivity-impulsivity as two separate dimensions need to be conducted. In addition, behaviour genetic studies of the aetiology of the covariation between the inattentive and hyperactive-impulsive symptom dimensions, and of the covariation of these with symptom dimensions representing overlapping disorders (e.g. ODD, CD, anxiety and affective disorders) will contribute greatly to our understanding of comorbidity.

Molecular genetic studies of ADHD

Association and linkage

In contrast to behavioural genetic studies, which estimate broad, abstract components of genetic and environmental variance that contribute to the liability underlying a disorder, molecular genetic studies examine the role of specific genes or genomic regions that may contribute to the aetiology of a given disorder. Molecular genetic studies of disorders test for association and/or linkage between a given disorder and particular candidate genes or genomic regions. In association studies, the frequency of high-risk and low-risk forms of a candidate gene (i.e. high- and low-risk alleles) are typically contrasted in cases and controls (viz. individuals ascertained based on the presence of the target disorder versus a sample selected based on the absence of the disorder who are matched on a variety of background characteristics), with the expectation that cases will show higher frequencies of the high-risk allele than controls. Several variations on the classic case-control association design have been developed (e.g. a comparison of symptom levels in individuals who have 0, 1 or 2 copies of the high-risk allele of a particular gene in a nonreferred sample, or in siblings that differ in the number of high-risk alleles). One very important variation is family-based association methods, such as the haplotype-based haplotype relative risk (HHRR; Falk and Rubenstein, 1987; Terwilliger and Ott, 1992), which contrast the alleles that are transmitted with those that are not transmitted by parents to their affected children. In this design, the nontransmitted alleles serve as controls for the transmitted alleles, which are expected to be disproportionately transmitted to the affected children if there is indeed an association between the disorder and the gene. Family-based association designs were developed to avoid the problem of population stratification that can often plague conventional case-control association studies, leading to false-positive results. This problem occurs when case and control samples differ in both the frequency of high- and low-risk alleles and rates (or symptom levels) of the disorder. This mixture of subsamples which differ in both allele frequencies and symptom levels/diagnostic rates induces an association in the overall sample which may occur even in the absence of any true relation between the gene and the disorder in either of the subsamples. The most common source of population stratification is thought to be ethnic group differences, wherein ethnic groups differ in both allele frequencies and rates of disorder, although in principle stratification effects may be due to any form of population structure (e.g. SES differences) which varies between cases and controls. Within-family association methods are thought to avoid the biasing effects of population stratification because the transmitted and nontransmitted alleles come from the same individuals within the sample of cases.

In linkage studies, typically the correlation of a disorder and anonymous DNA markers is examined within family members (e.g. sibling pairs, parents and their children). In classical linkage studies, this involves examining the cosegregation of the presence or absence of the disorder with sharing particular allele(s) of a DNA marker through large family pedigrees. Note that in linkage analysis it is commonly assumed that the anonymous DNA markers are not themselves the genes contributing to the aetiology of the disorder, but may be 'linked' with them due to their close contiguity on the chromosome, which results in their frequent coinheritance during meiosis. In the case of strong linkage, there is a strong cooccurrence among relatives of the presence or absence of the disorder with sharing the same DNA marker allele identical by descent (IBD), which means that the shared allele is not merely of the same type (identical by state, or IBS), but is indeed the identical allele transmitted by a common ancestor. Classical linkage analyses are commonly model-based, meaning that the researcher must specify a number of parameters a priori, including the base rate of the disorder, the allele frequencies and the penetrances of the genotypes. (The investigator can also examine genetic heterogeneity by modelling the proportion of families in which the disorder is linked to the genomic region.) Needless to say, in most instances the values of most, if not all, of these parameters would be unknown. This led statistical geneticists to develop model-free linkage analytic methods, which require the specification of few or no parameters a priori. Model-free analyses are typically both more flexible and less powerful than model-based linkage analyses in which values of the parameters are correctly specified. A common form of model-free linkage analysis involves estimating the proportion of alleles shared IBD among affected sibling pairs for each DNA marker examined. A departure of the proportion of alleles shared IBD from the expected Mendelian proportions (0.25, 0.50, 0.25 for 0, 1 and 2 alleles shared IBD, respectively) suggests that the genomic region in which that DNA marker resides is linked with the disorder.

Like association analyses, linkage analyses have undergone many important refinements. First, there has been a shift in contemporary linkage studies toward the use of many smaller family pedigrees, or large numbers of affected sibling pairs, rather than a reliance on a few very large family pedigrees. Second, linkage analyses of specific targeted candidate genes, rather than of large numbers of anonymous DNA markers, are becoming more common. One statistical genetic tool that has become quite popular for such studies is the Transmission Disequlibrium Test (TDT; Spielman et al., 1993). The TDT is similar to the afore-mentioned HHRR, in that both statistics contrast the transmitted and nontransmitted alleles from parents to their affected children. The only methodological difference between the analytic methods is that the TDT contrasts the transmitted and nontransmitted alleles from heterozygous parents only, as opposed to contrasting the alleles transmitted by all parents, as in the HHRR. None the less, the TDT possesses a number of important statistical properties that distinguish it from the HHRR, including being a test of linkage as well as association, being robust to population stratification and enabling one to include multiple affected offspring from a given family in a test of linkage. In contrast, the HHRR is a test of association only, is not completely robust to the biasing effects of population stratification and cannot accommodate data from multiple affected offspring from the same family due to the violation of the assumption of observational independence. Given its favourable characteristics, it is little wonder that the TDT has received so much use and attention regarding its statistical properties as compared with alternative statistical genetic methods in the recent genetics literature. In addition, the TDT has recently been extended by a number of researchers (e.g. Rabinowitz, 1997; Waldman et al., 1999) to enable the examination of linkage between a candidate gene or DNA marker and multiple continuous as well as categorical variables (e.g. symptom levels of a disorder instead of, or in addition to, a diagnosis).

The genetics of complex traits

A number of geneticists (Lander and Schork, 1994; Risch and Merikangas, 1996; Chakravarti, 1999; Risch, 2000) have recently highlighted important differences between the genetics of simple Mendelian diseases and of complex traits or disorders, and have focused on the special challenges posed by the search for genes that underlie the latter. These geneticists define a 'complex trait' as any phenotype that does not exhibit classic Mendelian recessive or dominant inheritance attributable to a single gene locus (Lander and Schork, 1994). Complex traits and disorders have a number of features that distinguish them from Mendelian diseases. First, complex traits are thought to result from the effects of multiple genetic and environmental influences. Second, each of the multiple genes thought to underlie complex disorders probably confers only a relatively small risk for the disorder. Third, these genes are likely to have fairly low penetrance (i.e. the probability of developing the disorder given the presence of the high-risk allele or genotype) and have a relatively high allele frequency in the population. Fourth, there is likely to be genetic heterogeneity for complex traits, such that the same genotype can result in different phenotypes and different genotypes can result in the same phenotype. Fifth, there is likely to be the presence of phenocopies (i.e. disorders caused by environmental influences that have the same symptom presentation as the inherited disorder) for complex disorders. Sixth, specific environmental influences are more likely to be important risk factors for complex disorders, and there may be the presence of gene– or genotype-by-environment interaction. Suffice to say, for complex traits and disorders it is most likely that the aetiology and risk to relatives comprise a multitude of susceptibility genes, each contributing only a small magnitude of the overall risk for the disorder. Indeed, most researchers consider the underlying causes of ADHD to be polygenic (i.e. influenced by many genes and environmental factors), although evidence for a major gene has been found in a segregation analysis (Faraone et al., 1992).

Candidate genes for ADHD

Broadly speaking, there are two general strategies for finding genes that contribute to the aetiology of a disorder. The first is a genome scan, in which linkage is examined between a disorder and a large number of DNA markers scattered at approximately equal distances across the genome. Genome scans may be thought of as exploratory searches for putative genes that contribute to the aetiology of a disorder. What makes genome scans exploratory is that neither the location of the relevant genes nor their function or aetiological relevance is known a priori. On the other hand, the fact that major genes have been found for many medical diseases via genome scans is testament to the usefulness of this method. Unfortunately, the power of linkage analyses in genome scans is typically quite low, making it very difficult, if not impossible, to detect genes that account for less than ~15% of the variance in a disorder. Given this, the promise for genome scans of complex traits (e.g. disorders in which multiple genes and environmental influences contribute to their aetiology) remains largely unknown.

In many ways, candidate gene studies are polar opposites of genome scans. In contrast to the exploratory nature of genome scans, well-conducted candidate gene studies represent a targeted test of the role of specific genes in the aetiology of a disorder. In addition, the location, function and aetiological relevance of candidate genes are most often known or strongly hypothesized a priori, although the specific polymorphism chosen for study in the candidate gene may itself not be functional and the functional mutation(s) in the candidate gene may be as yet unidentified. A big advantage of well-conducted candidate gene studies in comparison with genome scans is that positive findings are easily interpretable because one already knows the gene's location, function and aetiological relevance. Some disadvantages of candidate gene studies are that one cannot find genes that one has not looked for, and that there are still not that many strong candidate genes for psychiatric disorders and the same candidate genes tend to be examined for almost all psychiatric disorders, regardless of how disparate the disorders may be in terms of their symptomatology or conjectured pathophysiology. In well-designed studies, however, candidate genes are selected based on the known or strongly hypothesized role of their gene product in the aetiology of the disorder (i.e., its pathophysiological function and aetiological relevance). Thus, with respect to ADHD, most of the candidate genes heretofore examined underlie various aspects of the dopaminergic neurotransmitter pathway. (Candidate genes underlying the noradrenergic and serotonergic neurotransmitter pathways have also been studied, albeit to a much lesser extent.) This is a result of the strongly conjectured role of the dopaminergic (and, to a lesser extent, noradrenergic) system in the aetiology and pathophysiology of ADHD (Levy, 1991; Pliszka et al., 1996; Biederman and Spencer, 1999), as well as the observation that stimulant medications, the most common and effective treatment for ADHD, appear to act primarily by regulating dopamine levels in the brain (Solanto, 1984; Seeman and Madras, 1998). Another justification for the selection of candidate genes within the dopaminergic system involves the results of 'knockout' gene studies in mice, in which the behavioural effect of the deactivation of these genes is examined. Results of such studies have markedly strengthened the consideration of genes within the dopaminergic system as candidate genes for ADHD, including the dopamine transporter gene (*DAT1*; Giros et al., 1996), and the dopamine receptor D3 and D4 genes (*DRD3* and *DRD4*; Accili et al., 1996; Rubinstein et al., 1997; Dulawa et al., 1999).

In this section of the chapter, we review studies of association and linkage between ADHD and candidate genes within the dopaminergic neurotransmission pathway. Candidate genes for neurotransmitter systems may include:

(1) precursor genes that affect the rate at which neurotransmitters are produced from precursor amino acids (e.g. tyrosine hydroxylase for dopamine)
(2) receptor genes that are involved in receiving neurotransmitter signals (e.g. genes corresponding to the five dopamine receptors, *DRD1*, *D2*, *D3*, *D4* and *D5*)
(3) transporter genes that are involved in the reuptake of neurotransmitters back into the presynaptic terminal (e.g. the dopamine transporter gene, *DAT1*)
(4) metabolite genes that are involved in the metabolism or degradation of these neurotransmitters (e.g. the gene for catechol *O*-methyltransferase, COMT)
(5) genes that are responsible for the conversion of one neurotransmitter into another (e.g. dopamine *β*-hydroxylase, or *DβH*, which converts dopamine into noradrenaline (norepinephrine)).

Studies of association and linkage between ADHD and dopamine candidate genes are appearing in the literature at an accelerating rate, thus this review will necessarily be somewhat incomplete. In addition, several reviews have recently been published on the association between ADHD and *DRD4* (Thapar et al., 1999; Swanson et al., 2000), the most recent being a metaanalysis of case-control and within-family association studies (Faraone et al., 2001). Rather than duplicate these reviews of the *DRD4*-ADHD studies, I will briefly summarize their conclusions. Given these considerations, the following review will be representative but not exhaustive, and is meant to give the reader a sense of the methods and findings of studies of association and linkage between ADHD and dopamine candidate genes. Studies are presented for each candidate gene, starting with those genes for which there are relatively many studies and ending with those for which there are relatively few.

Dopamine receptor D4 (*DRD4*)

The dopamine receptor D4 gene (*DRD4*) is an interesting candidate gene for ADHD given its expression in areas of the brain that are likely to underlie ADHD (Paterson et al., 1999), as well as findings from knockout studies in mice relating the gene to novelty seeking (Dulawa et al., 1999) and to heightened effects of alcohol, cocaine and amfetamine on locomotor activity (Rubinstein et al., 1997). In addition, several studies (e.g. Ashgari et al., 1995) have suggested that the 7-repeat of a 48-base pair (bp) VNTR (i.e. variable number of tandem repeats) in exon 3 of the gene differs, albeit slightly, from the 2- and 4-repeats in secondary messenger (i.e. cyclic adenosine monophosphate) activity and possibly also in response to the antipsychotic medication clozapine.

The *DRD4* gene first garnered attention within the personality and psychopathology domains based on reports of its association with the personality trait of novelty seeking in adults (Benjamin et al., 1996; Ebstein et al., 1996). An association of *DRD4* with ADHD in children was reported soon after (LaHoste et al., 1996) in a small case-control sample ($n = 39$ cases and 39 ethnically matched controls), which reported a greater percentage of the 7-repeat allele and genotype in cases (29% and 49%, respectively) than controls (12% and 21%, respectively). This study was followed by a number of replication studies (seven case-control and 14 within-family studies), the findings and methods of which have been described in a number of previous reviews (Thapar et al., 1999; Swanson et al., 2000). As would be expected for molecular genetic studies of any complex trait or disorder, especially given studies with relatively small sample sizes, the findings of association between ADHD and *DRD4* were replicated in some of these studies but not in others. Thus it is noteworthy that there is a recent metaanalysis of these case-control and within-family association studies (Faraone et al., 2001), which demonstrated a significant *DRD4*-ADHD association for both types of studies (case-control: $P = 0.00000008$; relative risk = 1.9, 95% confidence interval: 1.4–2.2; within-family: $P = 0.02$; relative risk = 1.4, 95% confidence interval: 1.1–1.6). Thus, both designs yielded significant evidence for the association between ADHD and *DRD4*, although the evidence was notably stronger for the case-control studies. This may reflect the possible biasing effects of population stratification or some other systematic difference, such as greater power for case-control than within-family designs.

Dopamine transporter gene (*DAT1*)

The dopamine transporter is involved in the reuptake of dopamine from the synaptic cleft back into the presynaptic cell, and thus plays a major role in regulating functional dopamine levels in the brain. There are several justifications for *DAT1* as a strong candidate gene for ADHD. First, stimulant medications such as methylphenidate, which are the most popular and possibly also the most effective treatments for ADHD, exert their therapeutic effects primarily by inhibiting the dopamine transporter, thus increasing functionally active levels of dopamine at the synapse. Second, a study of *DAT1* 'knockout' mice showed extreme levels of hyperactivity and greatly increased synaptic levels of dopamine in mice who were homozygous for *DAT1* deactivation (Giros et al., 1996). Third, a number of recent brain-scanning studies using single-photon emission computed tomography (SPECT) have found differences in dopamine transporter binding (Jacobsen et al., 2000) and availability (Heinz et al., 2000) as a function of *DAT1* genotype.

The first study to examine the association between *DAT1* and ADHD was by Cook et al. (1995) in a clinic sample of 49 DSM-III-R ADHD and eight undifferentiated attention deficit disorder (UADD) probands (average age = 9.4 years, range 4–17) and their parents. The authors used a within-family design to guard against the potentially biasing effects of population stratification that can lead to spurious association in population-based (case-control) studies. Most of the sample was Caucasian (47 families), with nine African-American and one Hispanic family. Two-thirds of the sample met criteria for a DSM-III-R diagnosis in addition to ADHD/UADD, with 33% of the sample meeting criteria for ODD, 10% for CD, 9% for an anxiety disorder, 7% for an elimination disorder and 2% each for major depressive disorder and dysthymia. A substantial proportion of the sample also met criteria for axis II developmental disorders pertaining to expressive writing (31%), receptive language (14%), articulation (7%), reading (10%) or arithmetic (5%). Diagnoses of ADHD and other disorders were made via a multidisciplinary team consensus based on a 6-h evaluation battery that included semistructured diagnostic interviews, physical and neurological examinations, and review of the parent and teacher questionnaires used in the study (the CBCL and Teacher Report Form (TRF), the Conners' scales, and the ADD-H: Comprehensive Teacher's Rating Scale

(ACTeRS)) by at least three experienced clinicians (Cook et al., 1995). The authors examined a 40 bp VNTR in the $3'$ untranslated region of the gene. Using the HHRR, the authors found evidence for association between the 10-repeat (480 bp) *DAT1* allele and ADHD ($\chi^2 = 7.51$, $P = 0.006$, relative risk = 2.84); this finding was later extended using the TDT to provide a test of linkage in the presence of association and yielded very similar results ($\chi^2 = 7.54$, $P < 0.01$, relative risk = 3.33). Similar associations were also found when the sample was restricted to only the Caucasian probands and only the ADHD probands. Further analyses of the data from this sample (unpublished observations) using analytic methods designed to test for mode of inheritance (dominance and recessivity; Schaid and Sommer, 1994) suggested that *DAT1* may be related to ADHD in a recessive rather than a dominant fashion ($\chi^2 = 6.70$, $P < 0.01$ vs. $\chi^2 = 1.67$, $P > 0.25$, respectively).

The findings of Cook et al. (1995) were first replicated by Waldman et al. (1996, 1998), who also extended these findings to examine the roles of DSM-IV ADHD diagnostic subtype and symptom severity on linkage disequilibrium between *DAT1* and ADHD. This sample included 122 children referred to psychiatric clinics primarily for ADHD and related behavioural and learning problems (average age = 9.3 years, SD = 2.75), their siblings and their parents. Approximately three-quarters of the probands were male, two-thirds were of full Caucasian ethnicity, 12% were African-American, 4% were Hispanic and 16% were of mixed ethnic background. Because the intention was to sample broadly with respect to psychopathology, probands were excluded only if there was clear evidence of mental retardation or pervasive developmental disorder/ autism. All but one of the probands met DSM-IV criteria for an ADHD diagnosis (the remaining proband met criteria for ODD), and the most common ADHD diagnostic subtype in this sample was the combined type (79%), with 16% having inattentive type and only 3% having hyperactive/ impulsive type (all percentages correspond to the low level of severity). As might be expected given the relatively broad selection criteria, there was considerable overlap with other conditions in this sample. For example, 88% of probands also met low-severity-level diagnostic criteria for ODD and 38% for CD (the corresponding percentages for medium-severity-level diagnostic criteria are 69% and 22%, respectively), and symptom levels for depression/ dysthymia were substantially higher for probands than for their siblings and for a nonreferred population of twins. Symptoms were rated by parents on a questionnaire developed by the authors to assess symptoms of the common DSM-IV axis-I disorders pertinent to children.

Waldman et al. (1998) used a number of analytic methods to examine association and linkage between *DAT1* and ADHD. First, they conducted between-family analyses of association in which symptom scores for the hyperactive-impulsive and inattentive ADHD symptom dimensions were regressed on the number of *DAT1* high-risk alleles (0, 1 or 2). Following Cook et al. (1995), the authors hypothesized that the 10-repeat (480-bp) allele would be the 'high-risk' allele. Waldman et al. found that the number of *DAT1* high-risk alleles was significantly related to the number of hyperactive-impulsive but not the number of inattentive symptoms in the predicted direction ($t = 1.87$, $P = 0.032$, $R^2 = 3.6\%$ and $t = 1.10$, $P = 0.137$, $R^2 = 1.1\%$, respectively). These results were unchanged when ethnic background was statistically controlled in an effort to eliminate the possible effects of population stratification. Second, the authors conducted within-family analyses of association in which scores for hyperactive-impulsive and inattentive symptoms were contrasted between siblings who differed in the number of *DAT1* high-risk alleles. Siblings with greater numbers of *DAT1* high-risk alleles than their cosibling also had higher scores on both symptom dimensions (hyperactivity-impulsivity: paired samples $t = 3.42$, $P = 0.003$, effect size = 0.99 SD; inattention: paired samples $t = 2.75$, $P = 0.009$, effect size = 0.79 SD). Third, the authors conducted within-family analyses of linkage disequilibrium using the TDT across both diagnostic subtype and level of symptom severity. These analyses indicated linkage between *DAT1* and ADHD (across all subtypes), which was stronger with increasing symptom severity (low severity: $\chi^2 = 3.57$, $P < 0.10$, relative risk = 1.63; medium severity: $\chi^2 = 4.45$, $P < 0.05$, relative risk = 1.93; high severity: $\chi^2 = 6.53$, $P < 0.025$, relative risk = 2.75). At all levels of symptom severity, linkage was found between *DAT1* and ADHD for the combined subtype (low severity: $\chi^2 = 4.33$, $P < 0.05$, relative risk = 2.00; medium severity: $\chi^2 = 5.76$, $P < 0.025$, relative risk = 3.20; high severity: $\chi^2 = 4.57$, $P < 0.05$, relative risk = 3.67) but not the inattentive subtype (low severity: $\chi^2 = 0.05$, $P < 0.75$, relative risk = 1.10; medium severity: $\chi^2 = 0.25$, $P < 0.50$, relative risk = 1.29; high severity: $\chi^2 = 0.33$, $P < 0.50$, relative risk = 1.40). (There were too few children with the hyperactive-impulsive subtype to include in separate subtype analyses.) Thus, these results replicate those of Cook et al. (1995) for the association (and linkage) between *DAT1* and ADHD, and extend them by suggesting that this relation is stronger with increasing symptom severity and may be stronger with the combined vs. the inattentive subtype (or with the hyperactive-impulsive vs. the inattentive symptoms). In addition, although evidence was mixed for mode of inheritance, the results tended to support a recessive model for the association between *DAT1* and ADHD at higher levels of symptom severity, similar to the findings from Cook et al. (1995).

These findings of association and linkage between *DAT1* and ADHD have also replicated in two separate Irish samples. Gill et al. (1997) used a within-family design in a sample of 40 clinically referred ADHD probands and 68 parents. Consensus diagnoses of ADHD were made by two clinicians using a set of parent and teacher questionnaires which included the CBCL, the Conners' Parent Rating scale and the ACTeRS. The authors found an association between *DAT1* and ADHD using the HHRR ($\chi^2 = 6.07$, $P = 0.014$, relative risk = 2.86). Association and linkage between *DAT1* and ADHD was also examined by this same research group (Daly et al., 1999) in a subsequent study using an independent sample of 118 ADHD probands (86% male, age range 4–14 years old) and 200 of their parents from 111 families. The procedures used to assess and diagnose ADHD and related disorders were identical to those in Gill et al. (1997). By far the most common ADHD diagnostic subtype in this sample was the combined type (90%), with only 7.6% having inattentive type and 2.5% having hyperactive/impulsive type (1.7% also had UADD). There was considerable overlap of ADHD with other disorders in this sample, such that 90% of the ADHD probands also had ODD and CD, and approximately 20% of the probands also had mood or anxiety disorders or specific learning disabilities. With the exception of two families in which the fathers were Arabian and Croatian, the sample was ethnically Irish. The authors again used a within-family design and replicated the association between *DAT1* and ADHD in this independent sample (HHRR: $P = 0.039$, relative risk = 1.88 from the combined Irish samples). In the combined Irish sample, linkage was also demonstrated using the TDT ($P < 0.05$, relative risk = 1.2) and the relative risk was slightly higher for probands with a positive rather than a negative family history of ADHD (relative risks = 1.29 vs. 1.20, respectively).

Association and linkage between *DAT1* and ADHD has also been replicated in a multisite UK sample of 66 ADHD children, 59 with the combined subtype, 6 with the hyperactive-impulsive subtype, and 1 with the inattentive subtype (Curran et al., 2001). Diagnoses of ADHD and related disorders were made on the basis of a parent semistructured interview using a modified version of the Child and Adolescent Psychiatric Assessment (CAPA) and teacher ratings on the Conners' Rating Scale. Participants were described as Caucasian, but no additional information was provided on ethnicity, nor on the age of the sample, the male-to-female ratio, or the rates of overlapping disorders. Linkage disequilibrium between *DAT1* and ADHD was supported using the TDT ($\chi^2 = 6.12$, one-tailed $P = 0.01$, relative risk = 1.95). The authors (Curran et al., 2001) also presented analyses of linkage disequilibrium between *DAT1* and ADHD from a Turkish sample of 111 children with a DSM-IV diagnosis of ADHD combined subtype and their parents (further information on the characteristics of this sample are provided in the section on COMT, below). In contrast to the results for the multisite UK sample, analyses using the TDT failed to support linkage and association between *DAT1* and ADHD ($\chi^2 = 0.93$, one-tailed $P = 0.832$, relative risk = 0.81).

There have been three additional published failures to replicate the association and linkage between *DAT1* and ADHD. In the first of these, Palmer et al. (1999) studied a mixed sample of 209 singly- and multiply-affected ADHD probands (75% male, average age = 11 years, SD = 3.6) in 124 families recruited by a combination of clinic referral and advertisements. Eighty per cent of the sample was Caucasian (the ethnic background of the remaining families was not specified). Over 70% of the sample met criteria for a DSM-IV diagnosis in addition to ADHD, with 44% of the sample meeting criteria for ODD, 20% for CD, 21% for an anxiety disorder, 20% for major depressive disorder, 4% for dysthymia and 2% for bipolar disorder. Lifetime diagnoses of ADHD (DSM-IV and DSM-III-R) and other disorders were made via a best-estimate procedure based on a battery that included semistructured diagnostic interviews (i.e. the KSADS-E or -PL) and parent and teacher questionnaires reviewed by several experienced clinicians (Palmer et al., 1999). IQ was assessed using the age-appropriate Wechsler scale and the IQ of children in the sample was in the average range (average IQ = 105 ± 15). The authors examined linkage between *DAT1* and ADHD using analyses of IBD allele sharing in affected sib pairs, as well as linkage disequilibrium using the TDT. Results were nonsignificant for both analytic methods under a wide variety of diagnostic subtypings and groupings with overlapping disorders (for the TDT, all *P*-values ≥ 0.59 and all relative risks < 1.0, for IBD allele sharing, all *P*-values ≥ 0.33) despite adequate statistical power for most of these tests.

In a second failure to replicate, Swanson et al. (2000) used a within-family design in a sample of 80 parent–proband trios. This sample is quite different from the others reviewed in that probands were selected for a 'refined' ADHD phenotype, which was based on meeting both the DSM-IV criteria for ADHD and the ICD-10 criteria for HKD (essentially DSM-IV ADHD combined type with no serious overlapping disorders), and for showing positive response to methylphenidate. The authors conducted both HHRR analyses of association and TDT analyses of linkage in the presence of association (linkage disequilibrium), although the latter analysis examined only a small number of transmissions (26) from heterozygous parents. There was no evidence for association between *DAT1* and ADHD using the HHRR ($\chi^2 = 1.34$, one-tailed $P = 0.877$, relative risk = 0.64) nor for linkage disequilibrium using the TDT

($\chi^2 = 1.38$, one-tailed $P = 0.879$, relative risk $= 0.62$), and in fact there was a trend for the high-risk allele (the 480-bp allele) to be preferentially nontransmitted in these analyses.

In a third failure to replicate, Holmes et al. (2000) used both a case-control and within-family design to examine association and linkage between *DAT1* and ADHD in a sample of 137 British caucasian children from 133 families (92% male; average age $= 9.3$ years, $SD = 1.8$, age range $= 6$–12 years). Probands were recruited from child and adolescent psychiatry clinics in the northern UK, and were included if they had an IQ > 70, no evidence of a major medical or neurological condition, and the absence of Tourette's syndrome, pervasive developmental disorder (PDD) and fragile X syndrome. The authors used a semistructured interview of mothers (on the Child and Adolescent Psychiatric Assessment (CAPA)) and teachers to assess and diagnose ADHD, HKD and related disorders. The most common ADHD diagnostic subtype in this sample was the combined type (72%), with 7% having inattentive type and 11% having hyperactive-impulsive type (95% also met DSM-III-R criteria for ADHD and 65% met ICD-10 criteria for HKD). There was also considerable overlap of ADHD with other disorders in this sample, such that 58% of the probands also met criteria for ODD, 12% for CD, 13% for tic disorders, and approximately 4.5% of the probands also had mood or anxiety disorders. The control sample was selected at random from general practice registers. No further demographic or diagnostic information was available for them, aside from being described as healthy blood donors and healthy individuals. The frequency of the high-risk (480-bp) allele did not differ between cases and controls (73% vs. 74%, respectively), providing no evidence for association between *DAT1* and ADHD. There was also no evidence for linkage disequilibrium between *DAT1* and ADHD in the TDT ($\chi^2 = 0.56$, $P = 0.75$, relative risk $= 0.89$), as the 480-bp allele was actually preferentially nontransmitted.

The results of these studies of association and linkage between *DAT1* and ADHD raise a number of issues. First, additional studies, especially with larger sample sizes, are needed to resolve the inconsistencies in the above findings, preferably by investigating and providing good explanations for the heterogeneity in effects across studies. Second, a metaanalysis of these studies of association and linkage should facilitate a clearer picture of the relation between *DAT1* and ADHD than that provided by any single study. Third, studies geared toward finding the functional regions of *DAT1* that are of aetiological relevance for ADHD, and establishing whether the VNTR in the 3′ untranslated region of the gene is indeed functional, should be among the highest priority.

Catechol *O*-methyltransferase

COMT is an enzyme that is responsible for the degradation of catecholamines such as dopamine and noradrenaline and thus plays an important role in regulating dopamine levels at the synapse. A number of studies have recently been published examining association and linkage between ADHD and COMT. Researchers have examined an amino acid substitution (valine → methionine) in exon IV that is functional and has been shown to affect substantially COMT enzyme activity, such that homozygosity for valine shows three to four times greater activity than homozygosity for methionine. Given the higher activity of valine, which would lead to less synaptic availability of dopamine than would methionine, it is reasonable to consider valine the high-risk allele. Eisenberg et al. (1999) used a within-family design and the HHRR statistic to test for association between ADHD and COMT in an Israeli sample of 48 ADHD children (40 males, eight females; average age = 9.4 years, range 5–17) and their parents. Although the authors excluded children with primary diagnoses of a number of other conditions (Tourette's syndrome, PDD, mental retardation, psychosis), approximately 40% of the sample met criteria for diagnoses of ODD or CD and 18% showed transient tics. The authors assessed ADHD using a number of measures, including a structured interview of the probands' mothers, the Conners' Teacher Rating Scale and the Continuous Performance Test. A variety of ADHD-related indices were derived from these measures and related to COMT. The most common ADHD diagnostic subtype among probands was ADHD combined type (57%), followed by inattentive type (33%) and hyperactive-impulsive type (10%). As suggested above, the authors considered valine to be the high-risk allele in their analyses. A significant association was found between COMT (valine) and diagnoses of ADHD ($\chi^2 = 4.72$, $P = 0.030$, relative risk = 1.89) which was stronger when the diagnoses were restricted to the hyperactive-impulsive and combined subtypes ($\chi^2 = 8.34$, $P = 0.004$, relative risk = 2.91). There was also some evidence that the association of these diagnostic subtypes was particularly strong with the valine/valine genotype ($\chi^2 = 5.98$, degrees of freedom = 2, $P = 0.050$), as there was excess transmission vs. non-transmission of this genotype (36% vs. 10%) to children diagnosed with the hyperactive-impulsive and combined subtypes. Similar associations were also found with the Conners' Teacher Rating Scale hyperactivity scores and errors of commission on the Continuous Performance Test. No association was observed with the inattentive subtype of ADHD ($\chi^2 = 0.00$, $P = 1.00$) or with the Conners' Teacher Rating Scale inattention scores and errors of omission on the Continuous Performance Test. Although these results are based on a small sample ($n = 48$ parent–offspring trios for all ADHD diagnoses and 31 trios for the hyperactive-impulsive and combined subtypes) and thus need to be replicated in larger samples, this study suggests an association of ADHD with the high-activity (valine) COMT allele and genotype that may be specific to the hyperactive-impulsive symptoms of the disorder.

Three recent failures to replicate the association and linkage between ADHD and COMT have been published, all of which used within-family designs. Hawi et al. (2000) examined this association in an Irish sample of 94 4–14-year-old ADHD probands, 86% of whom were male, and their parents using a within-family design. The 94 probands were sampled from 91 families, 80 of which were parent–offspring trios and 14 of which were mother–offspring duos. This sample was a subsample of that used by Daly et al. (1999) above and thus has the same characteristics. No preferential transmission of valine was observed in the HHRR ($\chi^2 = 0.18$, $P = 0.67$, relative risk $= 0.91$). Similar results were also observed using the TDT. The authors also failed to find any evidence for heterogeneity by children's sex or family history.

Barr et al. (1999) also examined linkage between COMT and ADHD using a within-family design and the TDT in a Canadian sample of 77 probands and 19 affected siblings, ranging in age from 7 to 16 years. Of the 77 families sampled, 59 included a proband and available DNA from both parents, whereas 18 included a proband and available DNA from only one parent. The sample included 77 boys and 19 girls (80% male). Diagnoses of ADHD were based on a multifaceted assessment battery that included semistructured interviews of, and symptom questionnaire ratings by, parents and teachers. Children were included in the sample if they met diagnostic criteria for one of the three ADHD subtypes (diagnostic rates not reported), and excluded if they scored less than 80 on both the verbal and performance scales of the Wechsler Intelligence Scale for Children – Third Edition (WISC-III) or showed evidence of a neurological or relevant medical condition, Tourette syndrome or chronic multiple tics, bipolar disorder, psychotic symptoms or if they had an anxiety or depressive disorder that could better account for their symptoms (Barr et al., 1999). Almost all (96%) of the families were of European ethnic background, with the remaining families being of African-Canadian or native Canadian ethnicity. Of the 136 parents in the sample, 59 were heterozygous for COMT, which led to 65 informative transmissions for the test of linkage via the TDT. There was no evidence for linkage between COMT and ADHD, nor for the preferential transmission of valine, given that the TDT was nonsignificant ($\chi^2 = 1.25$, $P = 0.264$, relative risk $= 0.76$).

Tahir et al. (2000) examined association and linkage between COMT and ADHD using a within-family design in a Turkish sample of 72 proband–parent trios. Probands were 9.4 years old on average (SD = 2.4 years), 86% were male and 79% showed positive response to methylphenidate (90% of the probands were being treated). Children and their families were assessed using a comprehensive battery consisting of a semistructured interview of the parents and child, as well as parent and teacher ratings on a DSM-IV ADHD symptom scale, the Conners' scales, and the CBCL and TRF. All children met criteria for the DSM-IV combined subtype of ADHD, as well as for pervasiveness of ADHD across home and school settings. In addition, 34% of the sample met criteria for Tourette's syndrome or tics, 25% for ODD or CD and 8% for depression (Tahir et al., 2000). Children were excluded from the study if they showed a major neurological disorder (e.g. head injury, epilepsy or fragile X syndrome), had experienced perinatal complications (e.g. premature birth, eclampsia, neonatal seizures), had an IQ score less than 80, or had a personal or family history of psychopathology other than ADHD, tics or Tourette's syndrome, ODD, CD or anxiety disorders (Tahir et al., 2000). The authors conducted analyses of association using the HHRR and of linkage and association using the TDT. Of the 144 parents in the sample, 87 were heterozygous and thus yielded informative transmissions for the TDT. Despite a slight preferential transmission of the valine compared to the methionine allele (48 vs. 39 transmissions), there was no evidence for linkage between COMT and ADHD, given that the TDT was nonsignificant ($\chi^2 = 0.93$, $P = 0.168$, relative risk = 1.23). A test of differential transmission vs. nontransmission of the three COMT genotypes was nonsignificant ($\chi^2 = 2.2$, df = 2, $P = 0.140$). Further analyses of linkage between COMT and symptom severity, comorbid conditions and medication response also yielded nonsignificant findings.

In a recent study, Waldman et al. (unpublished paper) examined association and linkage between COMT and four continuous symptom scales representing the childhood disruptive disorders (the inattention and hyperactive-impulsive symptom dimensions of ADHD, and the ODD and CD symptom dimensions). These analyses were conducted in an extension of the same sample (described above) used previously to examine association and linkage between *DAT1* and ADHD (Waldman et al., 1998). This extended sample included 156 families of clinic-referred children. Similar to that study, we used a combination of between- and within-family association analyses, as well as within-family analyses of linkage disequilibrium. The latter were conducted using an extension of the TDT (Waldman et al., 1999) to continuous traits (e.g. symptom levels) and moderation (e.g. sex differences in linkage). In the association analyses, the hyperactivity-impulsivity symptoms and ODD and CD symptoms were related to COMT such that symptom levels were highest for the valine/valine genotype (i.e. for hyperactivity-impulsivity and CD) or for homozygous relative to the heterozygous genotype (i.e. for ODD). Within-family analyses of linkage disequilibrium using the continuous variable TDT showed no evidence for linkage or association with the valine allele, unless the other allele that was transmitted (i.e. the mode of inheritance) was also considered. When the mode of inheritance was included in the analysis, for all of the symptom dimensions excepting CD there was preferential transmission of the valine allele when accompanied by another valine allele (similar to the findings of Eisenberg et al., 1999, above), as well as preferential transmission of the methionine allele when accompanied by another methionine allele. In addition, there was evidence for sex differences for all four symptom dimensions, as valine was preferentially transmitted with higher symptom levels in girls, and methionine was preferentially transmitted with higher symptom levels in boys.

Dopamine receptor D5 (*DRD5*)

There have been three published studies of association and linkage between ADHD and *DRD5*. The first was in the same study of the Irish sample reported above for *DAT1* (Daly et al., 1999). In this study, a highly polymorphic microsatellite marker was examined in *DRD5* which yielded 12 alleles in this sample. The authors reported preferential transmission of a 148-bp allele using the HHRR ($\chi^2 = 16.36$, $P = 0.0005$, relative risk $= 2.52$), as well as the TDT ($P < 0.01$, relative risk $= 1.67$). The HHRR results were considerably stronger for probands with a negative rather than a positive family history of ADHD (positive: $\chi^2 = 5.00$, $P = 0.025$, relative risk $= 1.59$; negative: $\chi^2 = 11.77$, $P = 0.0006$, relative risk $= 1.72$). The second study was in the same Turkish sample described above that was used to examine association and linkage between ADHD and COMT. In this study, the authors (Tahir et al., 2000) used a multiallelic version of the TDT to examine linkage disequilibrium between ADHD and *DRD5*, and found preferential transmission of a 151-bp allele ($\chi^2 = 2.38$, $P = 0.061$, relative risk $= 1.28$). There was also evidence that linkage disequilibrium between ADHD and *DRD5* was stronger for children with positive response to methylphenidate than for nonresponders ($\chi^2 = 4.90$, one-tailed $P = 0.013$, relative risk $= 1.47$ for methylphenidate responders only). Similarly, stronger linkage findings between ADHD and *DRD4* for methylphenidate responders than for nonresponders were also found in this sample.

The third study was in the Canadian sample described above that was used to examine association and linkage between ADHD and COMT. In this study, the authors (Barr et al., 2000a) also used a multiallelic version of the TDT to examine linkage disequilibrium between ADHD and *DRD5*, and found only a nonsignificant trend for preferential transmission of the 148-bp allele ($\chi^2 = 1.16$, one-tailed $P = 0.140$, relative risk = 1.26). The authors also found preferential transmission of a 134-bp allele ($\chi^2 = 3.60$, $P = 0.058$, relative risk = 4.00), as well as preferential nontransmission of a 136-bp allele ($\chi^2 = 4.46$, $P = 0.035$, relative risk = 4.50) and of a 146-bp allele ($\chi^2 = 5.83$, $P = 0.016$, relative risk = 2.62). Although these studies are consistent in finding linkage between ADHD and *DRD5*, these results are puzzling with respect to linkage disequilibrium or allelic association, as it is not clear that the same specific alleles are being preferentially transmitted across studies. Further research is needed to clarify the linkage disequilibrium between *DRD5* and ADHD, as well as the role that this gene may play in contributing to risk for the disorder.

Dopamine receptor D3 (*DRD3*)

The dopamine receptor D3 gene (*DRD3*) is a good candidate gene for ADHD based on the regions in which it is expressed in the brain (e.g. the nucleus accumbens and striatum; Meador-Woodruff et al., 1996), as well as on the results of a knockout gene study in which mice homozygous for *DRD3* deactivation showed greater locomotor activity and rearing behaviour than heterozygous and wild-type mice (Accili et al., 1996). There are only two published studies of association and linkage between *DRD3* and ADHD, one in the Canadian sample mentioned above for COMT and *DRD5*, the other in the US sample (Waldman et al., unpublished paper) mentioned above for *DAT1* and COMT. In a sample of 100 families, Barr et al. (2000b) examined linkage disequilibrium between ADHD and two polymorphisms in *DRD3*, a functional polymorphism in exon I that results in an amino acid change (serine → glycine) and a polymorphism in intron 5. The results of the TDT did not support linkage disequilibrium between ADHD and either polymorphism (exon I: $\chi^2 = 0.98$, $P = 0.322$, relative risk = 1.22; intron 5: $\chi^2 = 0.09$, $P = 0.769$, relative risk = 1.06). Negative results were also obtained for haplotypes formed from both of these markers. Waldman et al. (unpublished paper) also examined linkage disequilibrium between the exon I polymorphism and disruptive disorder symptoms using an extension of the TDT that can include continuous variables and tests of moderation (e.g. tests of sex differences in linkage disequilibrium). Analyses of the whole sample yielded no evidence for association and linkage between *DRD3* and the hyperactive-impulsive and inattentive symptoms of ADHD. Analyses of sex as a moderator using the extension of the TDT suggested linkage disequilibrium between *DRD3* (serine) and the hyperactive-impulsive and inattentive symptoms of ADHD for girls but not boys, whereas the glycine allele showed a trend for linkage disequilibrium with inattentive symptoms in boys. Interestingly, linkage disequilibrium between DRD3 (serine) was also found for symptoms of ODD and CD for girls but not boys. While these findings are suggestive, they need to be replicated in future studies of association and linkage between DRD3 and childhood disruptive disorders.

Dopamine receptor D2 (*DRD2*)

There are only a few published studies of association and linkage between DRD2 and ADHD, one in the sample (Rowe et al., 1999; Waldman et al., 1999) mentioned above for DAT1, DRD3 and COMT, the other being a series of studies by Comings et al. (1991, 1996) of the association of ADHD with DRD2 (and of many other disorders and traits with many other genes) in a sample selected for Tourette's syndrome. The DRD2 gene first came to the attention of psychopathology researchers based on a reported association with alcoholism. Despite the fact that it has been a decade since the first report of association between the TaqIA 'long' allele of DRD2 and alcoholism, whether this association represents a true relation or an artefact is still a matter of strong disagreement, due in part to the use of case-control designs that do not deal adequately with the potentially biasing effects of population stratification.

Shortly after the report of association between DRD2 and alcoholism, associations of this gene were reported with many other disorders, including ADHD (Comings et al., 1991, 1996). Unfortunately, these studies have a number of limitations that make interpretation of their findings difficult. First, given that they are case-control studies, their findings of association between DRD2 and ADHD may be due (at least in part) to the biasing effects of population stratification. Second, the probands in these studies were selected not on the basis of ADHD, but because they met diagnostic criteria for Tourette's syndrome and tic disorders. Although it is common and even desirable to examine association and linkage of a candidate gene with overlapping disorders, the selection of a sample on the basis of Tourette's syndrome represents very strong selection for a very severe disorder. As such, it is difficult to know how findings from this sample on the association between DRD2 and ADHD generalize to the general ADHD population and compare to the findings from other, more representative samples. Third, it is common in these studies for the association between DRD2 and ADHD to be reported among the results of a multitude of other statistical tests of association between this (and other) candidate gene(s) and other psychiatric disorders and traits. This problem of determining an appropriate P-value in the face of multiple tests is only compounded by the fact that the tests are nonindependent due to the correlation among the disorders and traits. In our opinion, the safest interpretation of the findings from these studies is that they are suggestive but need to be replicated in samples that are not characterized by these limitations.

Association and linkage disequilibrium between *DRD2* and ADHD were also examined in a separate sample in which probands were explicitly selected on the basis of meeting diagnostic criteria for ADHD (Rowe et al., 1999; Waldman et al., 1999). Although evidence for association and linkage was found, this association was between the TaqIA 'short' *DRD2* allele and ADHD symptoms. Thus, even though both sets of studies found evidence for a relation between *DRD2* and ADHD, it is hard to think of these findings replicating those of Comings et al. (1991, 1996) given that the opposite allele was associated. Future studies need to be conducted to elucidate the true relation, if any, between *DRD2* and ADHD. These studies should be conducted in large, representative samples that avoid the limitations mentioned above.

Dopamine β-hydroxylase

DβH converts dopamine to noradrenaline and is thus interesting as a candidate gene for ADHD, given the suggestion by a number of researchers that the underlying pathophysiology of ADHD involves noradrenaline as well as dopamine (Pliszka et al., 1996; Biederman and Spencer, 1999). There is only one published study of association between ADHD and DβH, which was conducted in the afore-mentioned Irish sample (Daly et al., 1999). The authors used a within-family design and found an association between a biallelic marker in intron 5 of DβH and ADHD (HHRR: $\chi^2 = 9.00$, $P = 0.003$, relative risk = 1.87). Linkage was also demonstrated using the TDT ($P < 0.005$, relative risk = 1.31). The HHRR results were considerably stronger for probands with a positive rather than a negative family history of ADHD (positive: $\chi^2 = 7.18$, $P = 0.007$, relative risk = 1.49; negative: $\chi^2 = 2.73$, $P = 0.098$, relative risk = 1.20). Given both the potential role of noradrenaline as well as dopamine in ADHD, and the positive results of association between ADHD and DβH in this study, these findings need to be replicated in independent samples.

Candidate genes outside the dopaminergic system

Molecular genetic studies of ADHD have also begun to examine candidate genes outside the dopaminergic system. A number of researchers have investigated linkage and association between ADHD and genes in the serotonin system. For example, in the Canadian sample above, association and linkage were examined between ADHD and the serotonin receptor 2A gene (*HTR2A*; Quist et al., 2000). Analyses using the TDT revealed linkage disequilibrium between ADHD and one of two markers in *HTR2A* ($\chi^2 = 4.67$, two-tailed $P = 0.03$, relative risk = 2.00; Quist et al., 2000). Association and linkage between ADHD and two serotonergic receptor genes, *HTR2A* and *HTR1B*, were also examined in a multisite study in the UK and Ireland. In the total sample, association and linkage were found for the 861G allele of *HTR1B* (TDT $\chi^2 = 6.7$, two-tailed $P = 0.01$, relative risk = 1.46), whereas linkage with *HTR2A* was marginally significant in the Irish sample ($\chi^2 = 4.5$, two-tailed $P = 0.052$, relative risk = 2.67), but not for the full multisite sample ($\chi^2 = 0.01$, two-tailed $P = 1.00$, relative risk = 0.98). It is worth noting that the associated allele in the Irish sample is opposite from the one found in the Canadian study, thus raising questions regarding the validity and replicability of these findings.

Researchers have also examined association and linkage of candidate genes outside the major neurotransmitter systems. These genes were selected as candidates based on the plausibility of their putative aetiological role for ADHD and/or their location in genomic regions found to be linked with related disorders (e.g. the short arm of chromosome 6, which has been linked with reading disability). A number of such genes have been examined for association and linkage with ADHD in the afore-mentioned Canadian sample. The relation between ADHD and *SNAP-25*, a gene involved in axonal growth and synaptic plasticity, has been examined in this Canadian sample (Barr et al., 2000c). Further motivation for examining *SNAP-25* as a candidate gene for ADHD arose from the observation that a mouse strain with a hemizygous deletion of this gene exhibited hyperactivity that responded to stimulant medication (Barr et al., 2000c). Analyses using the TDT revealed linkage disequilibrium between ADHD and two two-marker haplotypes at *SNAP-25* ($\chi^2 = 3.66$, two-tailed $P = 0.056$, relative risk = 0.65 and $\chi^2 = 4.74$, two-tailed $P = 0.030$, relative risk = 1.77, respectively; Barr et al., 2000c). Pending replication, these findings suggest the potential importance of *SNAP-25* as a gene underlying ADHD. This research group also examined linkage disequilibrium between ADHD and myelin oligodendrocyte glycoprotein gene (*MOG*), which is located on the short arm of chromosome 6, given the replicated findings of linkage of that chromosomal region with reading disability, and the considerable overlap between reading disability and ADHD. Further rationale for *MOG* as a candidate gene for ADHD follows from the suggestion that it may be involved in the completion and maintenance of the myelin sheath (Linnington et al., 1984; Scolding et al., 1989; both cited in Barr et al., 2001a), and its potential role in cognitive and neurophysiological disorders such as ADHD. Analyses of association and linkage between ADHD and two polymorphisms in this gene using the TDT were both nonsignificant, suggesting that *MOG* may not be a risk factor for ADHD (Barr et al., 2001a).

Linkage disequilibrium between ADHD and the nicotinic acetylcholine α4 receptor (*CHRNA4*) was examined in a multisite sample from Ireland and the UK (Kent et al., 2001). This was chosen as a candidate gene for ADHD given the evidence that ADHD is a risk factor for early use of nicotine, maternal cigarette smoking appears to be a risk factor for ADHD, nicotine promotes the release of dopamine and improves attentional performance and may be involved in locomotor activity, and nicotine agonists appear to improve attention in monkeys and adults with ADHD (Kent et al., 2001). Despite this strong rationale for *CHRNA4* as a candidate gene for ADHD, analyses using the TDT demonstrated no evidence for association or linkage ($\chi^2 = 0.89$, two-tailed $P = 0.35$, relative risk $= 1.25$), suggesting that *CHRNA4* may not be a risk factor for the development of ADHD (Kent et al., 2001).

These studies represent the leading edge of research on association and linkage between ADHD and candidate genes outside the dopamine system which are sure to proliferate over the next few years.

Future directions

Examining multiple markers within candidate genes

Molecular genetic studies of ADHD have also begun to examine multiple markers and create haplotypes in candidate genes within the dopaminergic system. The Canadian research team mentioned above has also been at the forefront of this development, as they have investigated linkage disequilibrium between ADHD and multimarker haplotypes for both *DRD4* and *DAT1* in their sample (Barr et al., 2000d, 2001b). The authors found linkage disequilibrium between ADHD and a three-marker haplotype at *DRD4* (Barr et al., 2000a), but failed to find linkage disequilibrium between ADHD and a polymorphism in the tyrosine hydroxylase gene (*TH*). The authors also found linkage disequilibrium between ADHD and two three-marker haplotypes at *DAT1* (Barr et al., 2001b). The evidence for linkage with these haplotypes was stronger than that for any of the individual markers ($\chi^2 = 9.14$, one-tailed $P = 0.02$, relative risk $= 2.08$ and $\chi^2 = 3.90$, one-tailed $P = 0.024$, relative risk $= 0.48$, respectively), although there were also statistical trends in the TDT for the preferential transmission of the 480-bp allele in the 3′ VNTR ($\chi^2 = 2.56$, one-tailed $P = 0.055$, relative risk $= 1.38$) and for the preferential nontransmission of the 440-bp allele ($\chi^2 = 2.32$, one-tailed $P = 0.064$, relative risk $= 1.37$). It remains for further research to determine the incremental value of multiple markers for establishing linkage over those previously associated and linked (e.g. the 3′ VNTR in *DAT1*, the exon 3 48-bp repeat in *DRD4*), as well as for finding the functional region(s) of relevant candidate genes.

Genetic considerations in molecular genetic studies of ADHD

It may sound odd to some, but it is our contention that there is relatively little genetics in molecular genetic studies of ADHD. What we mean by this is that most such studies have been limited to the examination of association (and, at times, linkage) between ADHD and a particular candidate gene, and there are many ways in which these studies could tell us more about the genetics of ADHD. An initial step along these lines are the emerging studies of multi-marker haplotypes mentioned above. Let us offer some additional examples to illustrate our point. First, very few studies have considered the mode of inheritance (cf. the afore-mentioned findings on ADHD and *DAT1* from Cook et al., 1995 and Waldman et al., 1998), examining whether a particular candidate gene acts in an additive, multiplicative, dominant or recessive manner with respect to ADHD. Similarly, few studies have tested for excess homo- or heterozygosity of a candidate gene in relation to ADHD. Second, very few studies have tested for differences in association and/or linkage due to trans-mitting parent, which might indicate the possibility of imprinting. This is especially surprising for *DRD4*, given that it is in a genomic region for which imprinting has already been found. Third, we know very little about allelic heterogeneity, the phenomenon in which there are multiple high-risk alleles for a particular candidate gene. To take the example of the 48-bp repeat in exon III that is the most frequently examined marker in *DRD4*, we do not know if it is the 7-repeat allele per se, or alleles of greater length, that are most strongly related to risk for ADHD. Fourth, an emerging issue in molecular genetic studies of ADHD is that of epistasis, or the interaction between genes as they are related to ADHD. Considering *DAT1* and *DRD4*, for example, we do not know whether these genes simply add together in the risk they confer for ADHD, whether they have a synergistic effect such that having high-risk alleles for both genes increases the risk for ADHD much more strongly than the combination of their individual risks, or whether *DAT1* is a risk factor in the absence of *DRD4* and vice versa. Each of these three models is plausible for the joint effects of these genes on ADHD, and at this point we know very little about how candidate genes may interact in their effects on ADHD. A further elaboration of epistasis involves examining systems of genes (e.g. genes within the dopaminergic system) simultaneously, rather than investigating them singly in a piecemeal fashion. This makes conceptual sense, given that the products of such genes work together in a system, and given that knockout studies of particular candidate genes in mice (e.g. *DAT1*) have shown profound effects that ripple throughout various aspects of the dopaminergic system (Jones et al., 1998).

Examining diagnostic specificity and heterogeneity

Two profitable future directions for molecular genetic studies of ADHD are to examine the specificity of association and linkage between candidate genes and ADHD diagnostic subtypes and/or symptom dimensions, as well as heterogeneity in these relations due to sex, age of onset, age, environmental variables and other moderators that may affect gene–disorder relations. One beginning at addressing issues of diagnostic specificity was in a set of studies of association and linkage between ADHD and *DAT1* and *DRD4* by Rowe and Waldman (Rowe et al., 1998; Waldman et al., 1998). In one study (Rowe et al., 1998), linkage disequilibrium with *DRD4* was observed for inattentive but not hyper-active-impulsive ADHD symptoms, whereas in the other study (Waldman et al., 1998), linkage disequilibrium with *DAT1* was observed for the combined but not the inattentive diagnostic subtype. We have recently extended these analyses to demonstrate that *DAT1* is also associated and linked with ODD and CD symptoms, whereas *DRD4* appears to be associated and linked with only inattentive symptoms (Waldman et al., unpublished paper). One of the more interesting applications along these lines will be to examine the similarity of association and linkage with candidate genes of the DSM-IV diagnostic subtypes and the ICD-10 diagnosis of HKD, as this may help build bridges across the major diagnostic schemes. Unfortunately, at present the closest that studies have come to this goal is to examine the ADHD 'refined phenotype' (Swanson et al., 1998). Another interesting application involves developments in the taxonomy of ADHD using latent class analysis (Hudziak et al., 1998; Neumann et al., 1999), which have suggested that ADHD may best be conceptualized as a set of distinct underlying classes, rather than as two moderately-to-highly correlated underlying symptom dimensions à la DSM-IV. While the jury is still out on whether a latent class approach is superior to a dimensional approach and to the extent DSM-IV diagnostic scheme for understanding both the taxonomy and aetiology of ADHD, future research along these lines will be very profitable for understanding the classification and causes of ADHD and related disorders.

Very little research has been conducted examining the heterogeneity of association and linkage between ADHD and candidate genes. Such analyses can be very important for finding gene–disorder relations, as was demonstrated in the initial linkage analyses of breast cancer and *BRCA1*, where the linkage relationship became clear only when age of onset was considered in the analyses (Hall et al., 1990). We have recently attempted a preliminary foray into this domain by conducting analyses to examine how association and linkage between ADHD symptoms and *DAT1* and *DRD4* may vary by sex and age. In these analyses, we found that association and linkage between hyperactive-impulsive symptoms and *DAT1* was stronger for boys than girls and for older rather than younger children, whereas association and linkage between inattentive symptoms and *DRD4* was stronger for girls than boys and for younger rather than older children (Waldman et al., unpublished paper). Needless to say, much future research needs to address issues of diagnostic specificity and heterogeneity, as it is highly implausible that the candidate genes studied will all be related to the diagnosis of ADHD per se in children who vary in many characteristics such as sex, age and environmental circumstance.

Refining the ADHD phenotype and the use of 'endophenotypes'

Another related arena for future research involves refining and broadening the ADHD phenotype to include laboratory measures of related constructs, such as the executive functions. These may include measures of various forms of attention, impulse control, organization and planning, among other constructs. Incorporating these lab measures into molecular genetic studies of ADHD can have a number of potential advantages for finding association and linkage between ADHD and candidate genes. For example, lab measures of executive functions can be used to refine the ADHD phenotype in order to help find linkage with candidate genes. In addition, lab measures of executive functions may represent endophenotypes, phenotypes that are thought to be more proximal to the products and influence of the gene, and thus may provide an explanatory mechanism for relations between ADHD and candidate genes.

To date, there has been little research on the relation between candidate genes and lab measures related to ADHD. A preliminary report of such an investigation (Swanson et al., 2000) showed somewhat paradoxical findings, such that ADHD children with a copy of the *DRD4* exon III 7-repeat allele appeared to perform better on a number of attentional measures than ADHD children without the 7-repeat. We also have recently investigated the relation between this *DRD4* polymorphism and several measures of executive functions (Hadeishi et al., 1999), which included a Continuous Performance Test, Trails A and B, Word Fluency measures, and the Rey–Osterrieth complex figure. Consistent with a priori hypotheses, we found that performance on the majority of these measures decreased as a function of increasing numbers of the *DRD4* 7-repeat allele. Needless to say, this research is in its infancy and many future studies in this area will be necessary to judge the incremental advantages conferred by lab measures over and above diagnostic symptom ratings in finding association and linkage between ADHD and candidate genes.

Considerations for genome scans of ADHD

To date, molecular genetic studies of ADHD have consisted entirely of candidate gene studies of association and, at times, linkage. No genome scans for ADHD have yet been published, though this will change in the next few years as the first genome scans that are currently underway reach fruition. As more genome scans are planned and implemented for ADHD, a number of important considerations will be raised. These include issues of sample selection, study design and data analysis. With regard to sample selection, is it best to sample randomly from the population, to sample multigenerational pedigrees with multiple affected family members, to sample affected sib pairs only, or to sample extremely discordant and extremely concordant sib pairs? With respect to study design, is it best to examine linkage via highly polymorphic multisatellite markers, newly developed single nucleotide polymorphisms, or association via pooled DNA samples? Finally, with regard to data analysis, there is a panoply of statistical genetic methods available for complex traits, rendering analytic decision making a formidable problem.

Conclusions

Molecular genetic studies of ADHD have to date concentrated mainly on studies of association between ADHD and candidate genes in the dopaminergic system. Although some studies have reported positive associations and some negative findings, the published studies have shown a surprising degree of consistency and replication relative to molecular genetic studies of other psychiatric disorders. It may be the case that over the next few years a preponderance of negative reports will follow the predominance of positive findings that have been published thus far. Further studies examining the majority of the candidate genes reviewed above, as well as metaanalyses of these findings, will be necessary for evaluating the true nature and magnitude of the findings, as well as possible explanations for the heterogeneity in findings across studies. In addition, the above review should be considered a brief exposure to the first wave of studies, rather than an exhaustive review of the literature in this domain, especially given the increasing rate at which new studies are appearing. Thus it will take at least several years before the literature on the molecular genetics of ADHD becomes well established and fully comprehensible.

Although it is hard to predict the future directions of a research literature, a number of roads seem especially promising and likely to be well travelled in the years to come. First, many studies are beginning to incorporate within-family designs and to examine linkage as well as association using the TDT, a step that will be particularly useful to guard against the very real possibility that association findings are due to population stratification artefacts rather than to the causal effects of the gene. Second, many studies are beginning to examine association and linkage with distinct ADHD diagnostic phenotypes and symptom dimensions (rather than with the overall diagnosis only), as well as related disorders. Such research will illuminate both the aetiology and classification of ADHD and its comorbid conditions. Third, the first wave of ADHD genome scans should be appearing before long, and we will see whether the success of candidate gene studies of ADHD relative to other psychiatric disorders will also hold true for genome scans. Needless to say, research on the genetics of ADHD has had a very promising beginning and it will be of great interest to watch its development in the years to come.

REFERENCES

Accili, D., Fishburn, C.S., Drago, J. et al. (1996). A targeted mutation of the D3 dopamine receptor gene is associated with hyperactivity in mice. *Proceedings of the National Academy of Science of the United States of America*, **93**, 1945–9.

Alberts-Corush, J., Firestone, P. and Goodman, J.T. (1986). Attention and impulsivity characteristics of the biological and adoptive parents of hyperactive and normal control children. *American Journal of Orthopsychiatry*, **56**, 413–23.

American Psychiatric Association. (1968). *Diagnostic and Statistical Manual of Mental Disorders*, 2nd edn. Washington, DC: American Psychiatric Association.

American Psychiatric Association. (1987). *Diagnostic and Statistical Manual of Mental Disorders*, 3rd edn, revised. Washington, DC: American Psychiatric Association.

American Psychiatric Association. (1994). *Diagnostic and Statistical Manual of Mental Disorders*, 4th edn. Washington, DC: American Psychiatric Association.

Ashgari, V., Sanyal, S., Buchwaldt, S. et al. (1995). Modulation of intracellular cyclic AMP levels by different human dopamine D4 receptor variants. *Journal of Neurochemistry*, **65**, 1157–65.

Barr, C.L., Wigg, K., Malone, M. et al. (1999). Linkage study of catechnol-O-methyltransferase and attention-deficit hyperactivity disorder. *American Journal of Medical Genetics*, **88**, 710–13.

Barr, C.L., Wigg, K.G., Feng, Y. et al. (2000a). Attention-deficit hyperactivity disorder and the gene for the dopamine D5 receptor. *Molecular Psychiatry*, **5**, 548–51.

Barr, C.L., Wigg, K.G., Wu, J. et al. (2000b). Linkage study of two polymorphisms at the dopamine D3 receptor gene and attention-deficit hyperactivity disorder. *American Journal of Medical Genetics*, **96**, 114–17.

Barr, C.L., Feng, Y., Wigg, K. et al. (2000c). Identification of DNA variants in the SNAP-25 gene and linkage study of these polymorphisms and attention-deficit hyperactivity disorder. *Molecular Psychiatry*, **5**, 405–9.

Barr, C.L., Wigg, K.G., Bloom, S. et al. (2000d). Further evidence from haplotype analysis for linkage of the dopamine D4 receptor gene and attention-deficit hyperactivity disorder. *American Journal of Medical Genetics*, **96**, 262–7.

Barr, C.L., Shulman, R., Wigg, K.G. et al. (2001a). Linkage study of polymorphisms in the gene for myelin oligodendrocyte glycoprotein located on chromosome 6p and attention-deficit hyperactivity disorder. *American Journal of Medical Genetics*, **105**, 250–4.

Barr, C.L., Xu, C., Kroft, J. et al. (2001b). Haplotype study of three polymorphisms at the dopamine transporter locus confirm linkage to attention-deficit/hyperactivity disorder. *Biological Psychiatry*, **49**, 333–9.

Benjamin, J., Li, L., Patterson, C. et al. (1996). Population and familial association between the D4 dopamine receptor gene and measures of novelty seeking. *Nature Genetics*, **12**, 81–4.

Biederman, J. and Spencer T. (1999). Attention-deficit/hyperactivity disorder (ADHD) as a noradrenergic disorder. *Biological Psychiatry*, **46**, 1234–42.

Biederman, J., Newcorn, J. and Sprich, S. (1991). Comorbidity of attention deficit hyperactivity disorder with conduct, depressive, anxiety, and other disorders. *American Journal of Psychiatry*, **148**, 564–77.

Biederman, J., Munir, K., Knee, D. et al. (1986). A family study of patients with attention deficit disorder and normal controls. *Journal of Psychiatry Research*, **20**, 263–74.

Biederman, J., Faraone, S.V., Keenan, K., Knee, D. and Tsuang, M.T. (1990). Family genetic and psychosocial risk factors in DSM-III attention deficit disorder. *Journal of the American Academy of Child and Adolescent Psychiatry*, **29**, 526–33.

Biederman, J., Faraone, S.V., Keenan, K. et al. (1992). Further evidence for family-genetic risk factors in attention deficit hyperactivity disorder: patterns of comorbidity in probands and relatives in psychiatrically and pediatrically referred samples. *Archives of General Psychiatry*, **49**, 728–38.

Borland, B.L. and Heckman, H.K. (1976). Hyperactive boys and their brothers. *Archives of General Psychiatry*, **33**, 669–75.

Cadoret, R.J. and Stewart, M.A. (1991). An adoption study of attention deficit/hyperactivity/

aggression and their relationship to adult antisocial personality. *Comprehensive Psychiatry*, **32**, 73–82.

Cantwell, D. (1972). Psychiatric illness in families of hyperactive children. *Archives of General Psychiatry*, **27**, 414–17.

Cantwell, D. (1975). Genetic studies of hyperactive children: psychiatric illness in biologic and adopting parents. In *Genetic Research in Psychiatry*, R. Fieve, D. Rosenthal and H. Brill, eds, pp. 273–80. Baltimore: Johns Hopkins University Press.

Chakravarti, A. (1999). Population genetics – making sense out of sequence. *Nature Genetics*, **21**, 56–60.

Comings, D.E., Comings, B.G., Muhleman, D. et al. (1991). The dopamine D2 receptor locus as a modifying gene in neuropsychiatric disorders. *Journal of the American Medical Association*, **266**, 1793–800.

Comings, D.E., Wu, S., Chiu, C. et al. (1996). Polygenic inheritance of Tourette syndrome, stuttering, attention deficit hyperactivity, conduct, and oppositional defiant disorder: the additive and subtractive effect of the three dopaminergic genes – DRD2, D beta H, and DAT1. *American Journal of Medical Genetics*, **67**, 264–88.

Cook, E.H. Jr, Stein, M.A., Krasowski, M.D. et al. (1995). Association of attention-deficit disorder and the dopamine transporter gene. *American Journal of Human Genetics*, **56**, 993–8.

Cunningham, L., Cadoret, R.J., Loftus, R. and Edwards, J.E. (1975). Studies of adoptees from psychiatrically disturbed biological parents: psychiatric conditions in childhood and adolescence. *British Journal of Psychiatry*, **126**, 534–49.

Curran, S., Mill, J., Tahir, E. et al. (2001). Association study of a dopamine transporter polymorphism and attention deficit hyperactivity disorder in UK and Turkish samples. *Molecular Psychiatry*, **6**, 425–8.

Daly, G., Hawi, Z., Fitzgerald, M. and Gill, M. (1999). Mapping susceptibility loci in attention deficit hyperactivity disorder: preferential transmission of parental alleles at DAT1, DBH, and DRD5 to affected children. *Molecular Psychiatry*, **4**, 192–6.

DeFries, J.C. and Fulker, D.W. (1988). Multiple regression analysis of twin data: etiology of deviant scores versus individual differences. *Acta Geneticae Medicae et Gemellologiae*, **37**, 205–16.

Dulawa, S.C., Grandy, D.K., Low, M.J., Paulus, M.P. and Geyer, M.A. (1999). Dopamine D4 receptor-knock-out mice exhibit reduced exploration of novel stimuli. *Journal of Neuroscience*, **19**, 9550–6.

Eaves, L.J., Silberg, J.L., Meyer, J.M. et al. (1997). Genetics and developmental psychopathology: 2. The main effects of genes and environment on behavioral problems in the Virginia Twin Study of adolescent behavioral development. *Journal of Child Psychology and Psychiatry*, **38**, 965–80.

Ebstein, R.P., Novick, O., Umansky, R. et al. (1996). Dopamine D4 receptor (D4DR) exon III polymorphism associated with the human personality trait of novelty seeking. *Nature Genetics*, **12**, 78–80.

Edelbrock, C., Costello, A.J. and Kessler, M.D. (1984). Empirical corroboration of the attention deficit disorder. *Journal of the American Academy of Child Psychiatry*, **23**, 285–90.

Edelbrock, C., Rende, R., Plomin, R. and Thompson, L.A. (1995). A twin study of competence and problem behavior in childhood and early adolescence. *Journal of Child Psychology and Psychiatry*, **36**, 775–85.

Eisenberg, J., Mei-Tal, G., Steinberg, A. et al. (1999). Haplotype relative risk study of catechol-*O*-methyltransferase (COMT) and attention deficit hyperactivity disorder (ADHD): association of the high-enzyme activity Val allele with ADHD impulsive-hyperactive phenotype. *American Journal of Medical Genetics*, **88**, 497–502.

Falk, C.T. and Rubenstein, P. (1987). Haplotype relative risk: an easy reliable way to construct a proper control sample for risk calculations. *Annals of Human Genetics*, **51**, 227–33.

Faraone, S.V., Biederman, J., Keenan, K. and Tsuang, M.T. (1991). A family-genetic study of girls with DSM-III attention deficit disorder. *American Journal of Psychiatry*, **148**, 112–17.

Faraone, S.V., Biederman, J., Chen, W.J. et al. (1992). Segregation analysis of attention deficit hyperactivity disorder: evidence for single gene transmission. *Psychiatric Genetics*, **2**, 257–75.

Faraone, S.V., Doyle, A.E., Mick, E. and Biederman, J. (2001). Meta-analysis of the association between the 7-repeat allele of the dopamine D(4) receptor gene and attention deficit hyperactivity disorder. *American Journal of Psychiatry*, **158**, 1052–7.

Gilger, J.W., Pennington, B.F. and DeFries, J.C. (1992). A twin study of the etiology of comorbidity: attention deficit hyperactivity disorder and dyslexia. *Journal of the American Academy of Child and Adolescent Psychiatry*, **31**, 343–8.

Gill, M., Daly, G., Heron, S., Hawi, Z. and Fitzgerald, M. (1997). Confirmation of association between attention deficit hyperactivity disorder and a dopamine transporter polymorphism. *Molecular Psychiatry*, **2**, 311–13.

Gillis, J.J., Gilger, J.W., Pennington, B.F. and DeFries, J.C. (1992). Attention deficit disorder in reading-disabled twins: evidence for a genetic etiology. *Journal of Abnormal Child Psychology*, **20**, 303–15.

Giros, B., Jaber, M., Jones, S.R., Wightman, R.M. and Caron, M.G. (1996). Hyperlocomotion and indifference to cocaine and amphetamine in mice lacking the dopamine transporter. *Nature*, **379**, 606–12.

Gjone, H., Stevenson, J. and Sundet, J.M. (1996). Genetic influence on parent-reported attention-related problems in a Norwegian general population twin sample. *Journal of the American Academy of Child and Adolescent Psychiatry*, **35**, 588–96.

Goodman, R. and Stevenson, J. (1989). A twin study of hyperactivity – II. The aetiological role of genes, family relationships and perinatal adversity. *Journal of Child Psychology and Psychiatry*, **30**, 691–709.

Hadeishi, Y., Waldman, I.D., Mohr, J. and Rowe, D. (1999). Association of DRD4 and measures of executive function relevant to ADHA. Poster presented at the 1999 World Congress on Psychiatric Genetics, Monterey, CA, October 11–14, 1999.

Hall, J.M., Lee, M.K., Newman, B. et al. (1990). Linkage of early-onset familial breast cancer to chromosome 17q21. *Science*, **250**, 1684–9.

Hawi, Z., Millar, N., Daly, G., Fitzgerald, M. and Gill, M. (2000). No association between catechol-*O*-methyltransferase (COMT) gene polymorphism and attention deficit hyperactivity disorder (ADHD) in an Irish sample. *American Journal of Medical Genetics*, **96**, 282–4.

Heath, A.C., Hudziak, J., Reich, W. et al. (1996). The inheritance of hyperactivity and inattention in girls: results from the Missouri Twin Study. *Behavior Genetics*, **26**, 587–8.

Heinz, A., Goldman, D., Jones, D.W. et al. (2000). Genotype influences in vivo dopamine transporter availability in human striatum. *Neuropsychopharmacology*, **22**, 133–9.

Holmes, J., Payton, A., Barrett, J. H. et al. (2000). A family-based and case-control association study of the dopamine D4 receptor gene and dopamine transporter gene in attention deficit hyperactivity disorder. *Molecular Psychiatry*, **5**, 523–30.

Hudziak, J.J., Heath, A.C., Madden, P.F. et al. (1998). Latent class and factor analysis of DSM-IV ADHD: a twin study of female adolescents. *Journal of the American Academy of Child and Adolescent Psychiatry*, **37**, 848–57.

Jacobsen, L.K., Staley, J.K., Zoghbi, S.S. et al. (2000). Prediction of dopamine transporter binding availability by genotype: a preliminary report. *American Journal of Psychiatry*, **157**, 1700–3.

Jones, S.R., Gainetdinov, R.R., Jaber, M. et al. (1998). Profound neuronal plasticity in response to inactivation of the dopamine transporter. *Proceedings of the National Academy of Sciences of the United States of America*, **95**, 4029–34.

Kent, L., Middle, F., Hawi, Z. et al. (2001). Nicotinic acetyoline receptor D4 subunit polymorphism and attention deficit hyperactivity disorder. *Psychiatric Genetics*, **11**, 37–40.

Lahey, B.B., Schaughency, E.A., Strauss, C.C. and Frame, C.L. (1984). Are attention deficit disorders with and without hyperactivity similar or dissimilar disorders? *Journal of the American Academy of Child Psychiatry*, **23**, 302–9.

Lahey, B.B., Pelham, W.E., Schaughency, E.A. et al. (1988a). Dimensions and types of attention deficit disorder. *Journal of the American Academy of Child and Adolescent Psychiatry*, **27**, 330–5.

Lahey, B.B., Piacentini, J.C., McBurnett, K. et al. (1988b). Psychopathology in the parents of children with conduct disorder and hyperactivity. *Journal of the American Academy of Child and Adolescent Psychiatry*, **27**, 163–70.

LaHoste, G.J., Swanson, J.M., Wigal, S.B., et al. (1996). Dopamine D4 receptor gene polymorphism is associated with attention deficit hyperactivity disorder. *Molecular Psychiatry*, **1**, 121–4.

Lander, E.S. and Schork, N.S. (1994). Genetic dissection of complex traits. *Science*, **265**, 2037–48.

Levy, F. (1991). The dopamine theory of attention deficit hyperactivity disorder (ADHD). *Australian and New Zealand Journal of Psychiatry*, **25**, 277–83.

Lilienfeld, S.O. and Waldman, I.D. (1990). The relation between childhood attention-deficit hyperactivity disorder and adult antisocial behavior reexamined: the problem of heterogeneity. *Clinical Psychology Review*, **10**, 699–725.

Lopez, R.E. (1965). Hyperactivity in twins. *Canadian Psychiatric Association Journal*, **10**, 421–6.

Mannuzza, S., Klein, R., Bessler, A., Malloy, P. and LaPadula, M. (1993). Adult outcome of hyperactive boys: educational achievement, occupational rank, and psychiatric status. *Archives of General Psychiatry*, **50**, 565–76.

Meador-Woodruff, J.H., Damask, S.P., Wang, J. et al. (1996). Dopamine receptor mRNA expression in human striatum and neocortex. *Neuropsychopharmacology*, **15**, 17–29.

Morrison, J. (1980). Adult psychiatric disorders in parents of hyperactive children. *American Journal of Psychiatry*, **137**, 825–7.

Morrison, J.R. and Stewart, M.A. (1971). A family study of the hyperactive child syndrome. *Biological Psychiatry*, **3**, 189–95.

Morrison, J.R. and Stewart, M.A. (1973). The psychiatric status of legal families of adopted hyperactive children. *Archives of General Psychiatry*, **28**, 888–91.

Nadder, T.S., Silberg, J.L., Eaves, L.J., Maes, H.H. and Meyer, J.M. (1998). Genetic effects on ADHD symptomatology: results from a telephone survey. *Behavior Genetics*, **28**, 83–99.

Neuman, R.J., Todd, R.D., Heath, A.C. et al. (1999). Evaluation of ADHD typology in three contrasting samples: a latent class approach. *Journal of the American Academy of Child and Adolescent Psychiatry*, **38**, 25–33.

Palmer, C.G., Bailey, J.N., Ramsey, C. et al. (1999). No evidence of linkage or linkage disequilibrium between DAT1 and attention deficit hyperactivity disorder in a large sample. *Psychiatric Genetics*, **9**, 157–60.

Paterson, A.D., Sunohara, G.A. and Kennedy, J.L. (1999). Dopamine D4 receptor gene: novelty or nonsense? *Neuropsychopharmacology*, **21**, 3–16.

Pauls, D.L., Shaywitz, S.E., Kramer, P.L., Shaywitz, B.A. and Cohen, D.J. (1983). Demonstration of vertical transmission of attention deficit disorder. *Annals of Neurology*, **14**, 363.

Pelham, W.E., Gnagy, E.M., Greenslade, K.E. and Milich, R. (1992). Teacher ratings of DSM-III-R symptoms of the disruptive behavior disorders. *Journal of the American Academy of Child and Adolescent Psychiatry*, **31**, 210–18.

Pliszka, S.R., McCracken, J.T. and Maas, J.W. (1996). Catecholamines in attention-deficit hyperactivity disorder: current perspectives. *Journal of the American Academy of Child and Adolescent Psychiatry*, **35**, 264–72.

Plomin, R., DeFries, J.C., McClearn, G.E. and Rutter, M. (1997). *Behavioral Genetics*, 3rd edn. New York: W.H. Freeman.

Quist, J.F., Barr, C.L., Schachar, R. et al. (2000). Evidence for the serotonin HTR2A receptor gene as a susceptibility factor in attention deficit hyperactivity disorder (ADHD). *Molecular Psychiatry*, **5**, 537–41.

Rabinowitz, D. (1997). A transmission/disequilibrium test for quantitative trait loci. *Human Heredity*, **47**, 342–50.

Rhee, S.H., Waldman, I.D., Hay, D. and Levy, F. (1999). Sex differences in genetic and environmental influences on DSM-III-R attention-deficit hyperactivity disorder (ADHD). *Journal of Abnormal Psychology*, **108**, 24–41.

Risch, N.J. (2000). Searching for genetic determinants in the new millennium. *Nature*, **405**, 847–56.

Risch, N. and Merikangas, K. (1996). The future of genetic studies of complex human diseases. *Science*, **273**, 1516–17.

Rowe, D.C., Stever, C., Giedinghagen, L.N. et al. (1998). Dopamine DRD4 receptor polymorphism and attention deficit hyperactivity disorder. *Molecular Psychiatry*, **3**, 419–26.

Rowe, D.C., Van den Oord, E.J.C.G., Stever, C. et al. (1999). The DRD2 TaqI-A2 allele and symptoms of attention deficit hyperactivity disorder. *Molecular Psychiatry*, **4**, 580–6.

Rubinstein, M., Phillips, T.J., Bunzow, J.R. et al. (1997). Mice lacking dopamine D4 receptors are supersensitive to ethanol, cocaine, and methylphenidate. *Cell*, **90**, 991–1001.

Rutter, M., Korn, S. and Birch, H.G. (1963). Genetic and environmental factors in the development of 'primary reaction patterns'. *British Journal of Social and Clinical Psychology*, **2**, 162–73.

Safer, D.J. (1973). A familial factor in minimal brain dysfunction. *Behavior Genetics*, **3**, 175–86.

Schaid, D. and Sommer, S. (1994). Comparison of statistics for candidate-gene association studies using cases and parents. *American Journal of Human Genetics*, **55**, 402–9.

Schmitz, S., Fulker, D.W. and Mrazek, D.A. (1995). Problem behavior in early and middle childhood: an initial behavior genetic analysis. *Journal of Child Psychology and Psychiatry*, **36**, 1443–58.

Seeman, P. and Madras, B.K. (1998). Anti-hyperactivity medication: methylphenidate and amphetamine. *Molecular Psychiatry*, **3**, 386–96.

Sherman, D.K., Iacono, W.G. and McGue, M.K. (1997). Attention-deficit hyperactivity disorder dimensions: a twin study of inattention and impulsivity-hyperactivity. *Journal of the American Academy of Child and Adolescent Psychiatry*, **36**, 745–53.

Silberg, J., Rutter, M., Meyer, J. et al. (1996). Genetic and environmental influences on the covariation between hyperactivity and conduct disturbance in juvenile twins. *Journal of Child Psychology and Psychiatry*, **37**, 803–16.

Simonoff, E., Pickles, A., Hervas, A. et al. (1998). Genetic influences on childhood hyperactivity: contrast effects imply parental rating bias, not sibling interaction. *Psychologcal Medicine*, **28**, 825–37.

Solanto, M.V. (1984). Neuropharmacological basis of stimulant drug action in attention deficit disorder with hyperactivity: a review and synthesis. *Psychological Bulletin*, **95**, 387–409.

Spielman, R., McGinnis, J. and Ewens, W. (1993). Transmission test for linkage disequilibrium: the insulin gene region and insulin-dependent diabetes mellitus (IDDM). *American Journal of Human Genetics*, **52**, 506–16.

Stevenson, J. (1992). Evidence for a genetic etiology in hyperactivity in children. *Behavior Genetics*, **22**, 337–44.

Stewart, M.A., deBlois, C.S. and Cummings, C. (1980). Psychiatric disorder in the parents of hyperactive boys and those with conduct disorder. *Journal of Child Psychology and Psychiatry*, **21**, 283–92.

Swanson, J.M., Sergeant, J.A., Taylor, E. et al. (1998). Attention-deficit hyperactivity disorder and hyperkinetic disorder. *Lancet*, **351**, 429–33.

Swanson, J.M., Flodman, P., Kennedy, J. et al. (2000). Dopamine genes and ADHD. *Neuroscience and Biobehavioral Reviews*, **24**, 21–5.

Tahir, E., Yazgan, Y., Cirakoglu, B. et al. (2000). Association and linkage of DRD4 and DRD5 with attention deficit hyperactivity disorder (ADHD) in a sample of Turkish children. *Molecular Psychiatry*, **5**, 396–404.

Terwilliger, J.D. and Ott, J. (1992). A haplotype-based haplotype relative risk statistic. *Human Heredity*, **42**, 337–46.

Thapar, A., Hervas, A. and McGuffin, P. (1995). Childhood hyperactivity scores are highly heritable and show sibling competition effects: twin study evidence. *Behavior Genetics*, **25**, 537–44.

Thapar, A., Holmes, J., Poulton, K. and Harrington, R. (1999). Genetic basis of attention deficit and hyperactivity. *British Journal of Psychiatry*, **174**, 105–11.

Torgersen, A.M. and Kringlen, E. (1978). Genetic aspects of temperamental differences in infants. *Journal of the American Academy of Child Psychiatry*, **17**, 433–44.

Waldman, I.D., Elder, R.W., Levy, F. and Hay, D.A. (1996). Competing models for the underlying structure of the attention deficit disorders: confirmatory factor analyses and multivariate genetic analyses in an Australian twin sample. *Behavior Genetics*, **26**, 602.

Waldman, I.D., Rowe, D.C., Abramowitz, A. et al. (1998). Association and linkage of the dopamine transporter gene (DAT1) and attention deficit hyperactivity disorder in children. *American Journal of Human Genetics*, **63**, 1767–76.

Waldman, I.D., Robinson, B.F. and Rowe, D.C. (1999). A logistic regression based extension of the TDT for continuous and categorical traits. *Annals of Human Genetics*, **63**, 329–40.

Weiss, G. and Hechtman, L.T. (1986). *Hyperactive Children Grown Up*. New York: Guilford Press.

Welner, Z., Welner, A., Stewart, M., Palkes, H. and Wish, E. (1977). A controlled study of siblings of hyperactive children. *Journal of Nervous and Mental Disease*, **165**, 110–17.

Werry, J.S. (1970). Hyperactivity. In *Symptoms of Psychopathology*, C.G. Costello, ed., pp. 397–417. New York: Wiley.

Willerman, L. (1973). Activity level and hyperactivity in twins. *Child Development*, **44**, 288–93.

World Health Organization. (1967–69). *Manual of the International Statistical Classification of Diseases, Injuries, and Causes of Death*. Geneva: World Health Organization.

World Health Organization. (1992). *The ICD-10 Classification of Mental and Behavioral Disorders: Clinical Descriptions and Diagnostic Guidelines*. Geneva: World Health Organization.

10

Biological underpinnings of ADHD

F. Xavier Castellanos and James Swanson

ADHD Research Unit, National Institute of Mental Health, Bethesda, MD, USA

The clinical diagnosis of *International Classification of Disease* (ICD-10) hyperkinetic disorder (HKD: World Health Organization, 1992, 1993) is a restricted subset of *Diagnostic and Statistical Manual of Mental Disorders* (DSM-IV) attention deficit hyperactivity disorder (ADHD: American Psychiatric Association, 1994), due to more rigorous inclusion and exclusion criteria (Swanson et al., 1998a; Chapter 5). Given the high degree of comorbidity in ADHD (Jensen et al., 1997), it has generally been agreed that neurobiological studies of ADHD should begin by focusing on the 'refined' phenotype of combined-type ADHD. For simplicity, we will refer to this refined phenotype as ADHD unless otherwise specified.

A fully delineated testable neurobiological formulation of ADHD is not yet at hand. However, advances in neuropsychology (Chapters 6 and 7) and molecular genetics (Chapter 9), along with recent pivotal studies from clinical and basic neurosciences, to be reviewed below, suggest that a reasonable 'circuit diagram' can now be delineated. We previously presented preliminary formulations (Castellanos, 1997; Swanson and Castellanos, 1998) that are developed here in greater detail.

There is as yet no general agreement on the psychological deficit or deficits that underlie ADHD. Explanatory concepts such as inhibition, impulsivity and attention are generally evoked, although they have not been sufficiently well defined to test their applicability to ADHD definitively. For heuristics reasons, we will take as our starting point Van der Meere's proposal (Chapter 6) that ADHD represents primarily a disorder of state regulation and will grapple with one basic question. What are the likely anatomical, neurophysiological, and neurochemical substrates that may underlie such disruption of state regulation?

Neuroanatomy of ADHD

The quantitative study of brain development during childhood and adolescence became feasible when magnetic resonance imaging (MRI) became available in the late 1980s (Jernigan and Tallal, 1990; Jernigan et al., 1991). Subsequent cross-sectional (Giedd et al., 1996; Reiss et al., 1996; Sowell et al., 1999a,b) and mixed longitudinal/cross-sectional studies (Giedd et al., 1999a) have confirmed that, although total brain volume changes between ages 5 and 18 years are negligible, there are robust and complex changes in white and grey matter compartments. White matter volume (Reiss et al., 1996) and MRI white matter signal intensity (Paus et al., 1999) increase linearly during this age range, reflecting increasing myelination, and grey matter volume increases until early to mid adolescence before decreasing during late adolescence (Giedd et al., 1999a), presumably from synaptic pruning and reduction of neuropil (Huttenlocher, 1979; Huttenlocher and Dabholkar, 1997). Though there continues to be a gap in the ages studied between the first and fourth years of life, the available data demonstrate that grey matter volumes reach their peak at about age 12 in frontal and parietal lobes, preceding a similar pattern in the temporal lobe by about 4 years. In parallel, anterior regions of corpus callosum reach adult size before posterior regions (Giedd et al., 1999a,b).

Quantitative studies have also shown that even normal individuals who are closely matched for age, sex, height and weight can differ in total brain volume by as much as a factor of 2 (Lange et al., 1997). Thus, analyses of regional brain abnormalities should control statistically for differences among individuals in total brain volume, preferably using analyses of covariance instead of simple ratios or proportions (Arndt et al., 1991).

Prefrontal brain

Anatomical hypotheses of the substrates of ADHD have focused on the role of the prefrontal brain. Normally, the right anterior brain is slightly but consistently larger than the left (Weinberger et al., 1982). Significant decreases of this asymmetry in ADHD have been reported using computed tomography (Shaywitz et al., 1983) and MRI (Hynd et al., 1990; Castellanos et al., 1996a; Reiss et al., 1996; Filipek et al., 1997). Volumetric measures have also detected smaller right-sided prefrontal brain regions measured en bloc (Castellanos et al., 1996a; Filipek et al., 1997) in boys with ADHD which were correlated with neuropsychological performance on tasks that required response inhibition (Casey et al., 1997; Yeo et al., 2000). In the only published study to date to report grey–white segmentation, right anterior white matter was also reduced in ADHD boys (Filipek et al., 1997).

Basal ganglia

Along with the prefrontal cortex, the caudate nucleus and its associated circuits have long been suspected to play a pivotal role in ADHD (Pontius, 1973). Abnormalities of caudate nucleus volume (Castellanos et al., 1996a; Filipek et al., 1997) or asymmetry (Hynd et al., 1993; Castellanos et al., 1996a; Mataró et al., 1997) have been reported, although the studies differ in whether the normal caudate is asymmetric, and whether this asymmetry normally favours the right (Castellanos et al., 1996a) or the left caudate (Hynd et al., 1993; Filipek et al., 1997; Mataró et al., 1997; Giedd et al., 1999a; Castellanos et al., 2001). These inconsistencies may reflect differences in methodology, comorbidity and statistical power. In girls with ADHD, differences in asymmetry relative to controls were not found, although ADHD girls had smaller left and total caudate volumes, which remained significant after covariate adjustment for total cerebral volume and Wechsler Intelligence Scale for Children – Revised (WISC-R) vocabulary subscale score (Castellanos et al., 2001).

Neither of the anatomical MRI studies that evaluated putamen volumes detected significant diagnostic group differences (Aylward et al., 1996; Castellanos et al., 1996a). It is worth noting that anatomical neuroimaging findings in Tourette syndrome have centred on the putamen (Peterson et al., 1993; Singer et al., 1993), the striatal region associated with primary and supplementary motor areas. However, as noted below, a recent preliminary functional imaging study detected decreased blood flow in the putamen of objectively hyperactive boys with ADHD, but not in those boys whose activity levels did not differ from that of controls (Teicher et al., 2000). If confirmed in larger samples, this finding suggests that the putamen may be particularly related to motoric symptoms. Severe closed head injury can produce secondary ADHD (Max et al., 1998). In a study of 76 children with severe closed head injury, those who developed secondary ADHD were significantly more likely to demonstrate lesions in the right putamen (Herskovits et al., 1999).

The caudate, putamen and nucleus accumbens (collectively termed corpus striatum because of their striated appearance on gross examination) receive efferents from essentially the entire cerebral cortex. This impressive convergence of information is then processed and emerges from the output nuclei of the basal ganglia, which in primates are the internal segment of the globus pallidus and the substantia nigra pars reticulata. However, the volume of the latter cannot be reliably measured with current MRI parameters, and the size of the globus pallidus can only be measured as a unit (internal and external segments together), and then only with difficulty. Still, this region was found to be significantly reduced in size in boys with ADHD (Aylward et al., 1996; Castellanos et al., 1996a), although these two studies differed in finding the larger difference on the left and right sides, respectively. Globus pallidus volume differences in girls with ADHD did not survive adjustment for the covariates total cerebral volume and IQ (Castellanos et al., 2001).

Cerebellum

An early computed tomography study found a trend towards greater cerebellar atrophy in adults with a prior history of hyperkinetic minimal brain dysfunction (Nasrallah et al., 1986). In a quantitative MRI study of 112 subjects, the volumes of the cerebellar hemispheres were found to be significantly smaller in ADHD boys (Castellanos et al., 1996a). In a follow-up study within the same sample, the cerebellar vermis as a whole, and particularly the posterior inferior lobules (lobules VIII–X) were found to be significantly smaller in ADHD (Berquin et al., 1998). Smaller lobules VIII–X were independently replicated in boys with ADHD (Mostofsky et al., 1998), and in girls with ADHD (Castellanos et al., 2001), where the posterior inferior cerebellar vermis was the only structure that was rigorously replicated, with a comparable standardized effect size, d ($d = 0.66$ in boys, $d = 0.53$ in girls).

The posterior inferior vermis has also been found to be abnormal in childhood-onset schizophrenia (Jacobsen et al., 1997) and in multiple-episode adult affective disorder patients (DelBello et al., 1999). The potential relevance of the posterior inferior vermis for dopaminergically related psychiatric disorders such as ADHD and schizophrenia has been highlighted by the selective finding of dopamine transporter (DAT) immunoreactivity in ventral cerebellar vermis, particularly in lobules VIII–X, and to a lesser extent in lobules I–II, in nonhuman primate (Melchitzky and Lewis, 2000). DAT immunoreactivity was not present in cerebellar hemispheres. The function and origin of these dopaminergic fibres are not known, but they may form the afferent portion of a cerebellar circuit that influences the ventral tegmental area and the locus coeruleus (Snider et al., 1976a,b; Dempesy et al., 1983). Human functional brain imaging studies, discussed below, have documented the sensitivity of the cerebellum, and particularly the vermis, to the effects of psychostimulants (Ernst et al., 1997a; Volkow et al., 1997; Schweitzer et al., 1998; Anderson et al., 1999).

Summary of anatomical studies

Although most studies have used small samples and quantitative methodology is still evolving, anatomical MRI studies support the notion that a distributed circuit underlies some of the manifestations of ADHD. At least in boys, this circuit appears to include right prefrontal brain regions, the caudate nucleus, globus pallidus and a subregion of the cerebellar vermis. With one exception (Mataró et al., 1997), all groups have reported reduced volumes (or areas), and this is consistent with the broad notion that the relevant brain regions are hypofunctioning. It is generally accepted, as a first approximation, that cortico-striatal-thalamocortical circuits (Alexander et al., 1986) select, initiate and execute complex motor and cognitive responses (Graybiel, 1998), and that cerebellar circuits provide online guidance of these functions (Jueptner and Weiller, 1998). The remarkable selectivity of the result within the cerebellar vermis, i.e. that the region involved is limited to the posterior inferior lobules, together with the finding that this is the only region in the cerebellum that receives a dense dopaminergic innervation (Melchitzky and Lewis, 2000), support the speculation that the vermis exerts important regulatory influences on prefrontal-striatal circuitry via the ventral tegmental area and locus ceruleus (LC). Such effects may go beyond known cerebellar vermal influencing of cardiovascular physiology (Bradley et al., 1991) and heart rate conditioning (Ghelarducci and Sebastiani, 1997), which have been implicated in the state dysregulation hypothesis of ADHD (Chapter 6). More specifically, it is possible that findings described in detail by van der Meere, such as smaller anticipatory cardiac deceleration (Jennings et al., 1997) and greater low-frequency heart rate variability (Börger and Van der Meere, 2000), which are associated with poor motor activation state and greater difficulty in allocating effort, respectively, may be anatomically linked to dysfunction in the vermis outputs to midbrain monoaminergic nuclei.

Functional brain imaging studies of ADHD

At first glance, it would seem that functional imaging studies should be ideal to investigate ADHD. Instead, it has been even more difficult to obtain a consistent picture from the various functional imaging studies, perhaps because of interactions between imaging technology and the disorder itself. For example, performance differences between hyperactive and control children are minimized when testing is performed in the presence of an experimenter as opposed to when testing is performed in the experimenter's absence (Draeger et al., 1986; Chapter 6). Conducting a functional imaging study requires the presence of multiple individuals, all of whom are monitoring a number of parameters with varying degrees of urgency. Also, the time windows for functional studies are strictly determined by technical demands, and rarely represent a good fit with the time frames most useful for highlighting cognitive and/or behavioural impairments.

Despite these limitations, positron emission tomography (PET) with [18F]-fluoro-2-deoxy-D-glucose was used to demonstrate decreased frontal cerebral metabolism in adults with ADHD, although results were confounded with differences in sex distribution between patient and control groups (Zametkin et al., 1990). Inconsistent results in adolescents (Zametkin et al., 1993; Ernst et al., 1994, 1997b) led the authors to use an alternative technique to probe the catecholaminergic system, as discussed further below (Ernst et al., 1998, 1999). Other investigators have measured local cerebral blood flow, which is linked to neuronal activity and tissue metabolism, with a variety of techniques, including 133xenon inhalation and single photon emission computed tomography (SPECT). Decreased blood flow has been reported in ADHD subjects in the striatum (Lou et al., 1990) and in prefrontal regions (Amen et al., 1993). However, these results remain tentative because ethical constraints make it difficult to obtain truly independent observations from normal control children. By contrast, functional magnetic resonance imaging (fMRI) obviates the need to use ionizing radiation.

Nearly all fMRI studies use the blood oxygenation level-dependent (BOLD) method which is dependent on increases in local cerebral perfusion several seconds after increases in local neuronal activity (Bandettini et al., 1997). The BOLD fMRI technique was used in a study of 10 boys with ADHD and six controls, all of whom were scanned on and off methylphenidate while they performed two go–no-go tasks (Vaidya et al., 1998). As expected, methylphenidate improved the performance of normal children and of the patients with ADHD (Rapoport et al., 1978). In caudate and putamen, Vaidya and colleagues found a striking group difference. In the task with the faster stimulus presentation rate, methylphenidate increased the number of activated pixels in striatum in ADHD subjects, but it had the opposite effect in controls. In both caudate and putamen, controls activated significantly fewer pixels when scanned while on methylphenidate compared to drug-free scans. Patients as well as controls activated significantly larger numbers of pixels in prefrontal cortex during this task when on drug compared to placebo. This regional dissociation between prefrontal cortex and striatum supports the notion that even though mesocortical (prefrontal) and nigrostriatal (basal ganglia) circuits are both dopaminergic, they differ in the density of dopaminergic fibres (much higher in the striatum), in the absence or presence, respectively, of terminal autoreceptors (Meador-Woodruff et al., 1994), and in the kinetics of synaptic and extrasynaptic dopamine levels (Frazer et al., 1999). This pattern of results was not confirmed in the companion task, in which the rate of presentation of go and no-go stimuli differed. Furthermore, in this 'response-controlled task', ADHD subjects had greater activation than controls in both basal ganglia and in prefrontal cortex, whether off or on methylphenidate. These results are difficult to interpret, not only because of the complexity of the design and small number of subjects, but also because all the patients had been medicated with methylphenidate until 36 h prior to their scans. Since the normal controls had by definition never been previously exposed to stimulants, the possibility that these findings reflect medication withdrawal, first-dose effects (Volkow et al., 1998a) or type I error must be excluded.

Utilizing a sample of seven adolescent boys with ADHD who were un-medicated or medication-free for at least 1 week before scanning and nine controls, frontal-striatal circuits were targeted in another fMRI study (Rubia et al., 1999). Subjects were scanned while performing the Stop Task (Schachar and Tannock, 1993) and a delay task that required synchronization of a motor response to an intermittently appearing visual stimulus. The hyperactive sub-jects showed less brain activity, predominantly in the right medial frontal cortex during both tasks, and in the right inferior prefrontal cortex and left caudate nucleus during the Stop Task. The authors concluded: 'the right inferior frontal lobe – and its projections to the caudate – has been related to response inhibition . . . It thus seems that the brake system of the brain is localized to the right prefrontal lobe, and its underactivation in ADHD seems to be the neural correlate of a less efficient inhibitory motor control' (Rubia et al., 1999).

The principal limitation of fMRI explorations of ADHD is the exquisite sensitivity of the technique to even minimal movement during scanning. Vaidya and colleagues (1998) required that subjects use a bite-bar. Rubia et al. (1999) included only adolescents who were able to remain sufficiently immo-bile in the scanner. Because physical restlessness decreases with age (Levy, 1980), Bush and colleagues (1999) studied eight adults who had a history of childhood onset and persistence into adulthood of ADHD and eight matched controls. The Counting Stroop was used to avoid verbal responses; rather than colour words, subjects were shown words that were repeated one to four times per presentation. Subjects were required to press the button corresponding to the number of words, and interference was provided by presenting number words that did not match the number of presented words (Bush et al., 1998). Although both groups of subjects showed the expected slowing of response times in the interference condition, significant activation of bilateral anterior cingulate was only found in the normal controls. In contrast, ADHD subjects significantly activated right and left inferior frontal gyrus, right and left insula, left caudate, right putamen, right thalamus and left pulvinar. Thus, the absence of cingulate activation could not be ascribed to a simple failure to activate a neural network, although the authors noted that possible anatomical differences in cingulate volume and stimulant medication history could have confounded their results. Also, the cognitive task did not result in sufficiently robust activations to allow for single-subject analyses, which is a strength of fMRI studies. Thus, absence of averaged activation could simply reflect greater anatomical variability in the subjects with ADHD. Nevertheless, further exploration with this task and technique in younger subjects appears warranted.

BOLD fMRI activation studies typically use a 'subtraction design' in which the blood flow pattern obtained during one cognitive or motor task is subtracted from the blood flow pattern obtained during a control task. An alternative approach involves measuring 'T2 relaxometry' by varying the fMRI scanning parameters so as to obtain the maximum T2 relaxation times for regions of interest. This novel approach has been validated by comparison to gadolinium-based cerebral blood volume estimates (Anderson et al., 2000a), and was used to investigate steady-state blood flow in 11 boys with ADHD compared to six healthy controls (Teicher et al., 2000). Significantly higher T2 relaxation times, which suggest lower steady-state perfusion, were found in the ADHD children in the putamen bilaterally. Treatment with methylphenidate significantly affected the putamen T2 relaxation times, although the magnitude and direction of the normalizing changes depended on the child's unmedicated activity level (Teicher et al., 2000). On methylphenidate, the five patients who were least active during cognitive testing all exhibited increased T2 relaxation times (implying decreased putamen blood flow), whereas four of the six children with greatest activity exhibited decreases in T2 relaxation times, indicating an increase in putamen blood flow. Unlike the Vaidya study, the normal control children were not treated with methylphenidate, but the two studies converge in suggesting that methylphenidate may have differential striatal effects depending on baseline characteristics, whether they be categorical, such as diagnosis, or dimensional, such as motoric activity level.

In a subsequent examination of the same sample, the authors noted that within the 'objectively hyperactive' (at least 25% more active than controls) subset of six subjects, treatment with methylphenidate produced a significant dose-dependent decrease in resting blood flow in the vermis, whereas there was no significant change in vermis blood flow in the five primarily inattentive subjects (Anderson et al., 2000b). This preliminary analysis was limited to four axial slices of the cerebellum, which did not span the entire vermis, and in particular excluded the posterior inferior lobules. Nevertheless, the authors noted an inverse relationship between changes in blood flow in vermis and striatum, and concluded that their data support the notion that one important function of the cerebellar vermis may be to influence and regulate central dopaminergic modulation via fastigial nuclei projections to the ventral tegmental area (VTA: Snider and Maiti, 1976; Heath et al., 1978, 1980; Albert et al., 1985; Supple and Kapp, 1994; Ghelarducci and Sebastiani, 1997; Schmahmann and Sherman, 1998; Melchitzky and Lewis, 2000).

Despite the many advantages of magnetic resonance (lack of ionizing radiation, repeated measures, excellent spatial resolution and sufficient power for individual subject designs), imaging with radiotracers offers the only practical way of assaying the neurochemistry of the human brain in vivo. For example, [^{18}F] fluorodopa ([^{18}F]F-DOPA) was used to label catecholamine terminals in 17 unmedicated adults with ADHD (Ernst et al., 1998). [^{18}F]F-DOPA uptake was significantly diminished in the left and medial prefrontal cortex (relative to occipital uptake) of the ADHD adults compared to the 23 controls, with no differences in striatum or midbrain regions. By contrast, in 10 adolescents with ADHD, [^{18}F]F-DOPA uptake in right midbrain was significantly elevated compared to 10 controls ($P = 0.04$, uncorrected for multiple comparisons; Ernst et al., 1999). However, as the authors acknowledge, the fluorodopa uptake ratio is noisy in regions of low dopaminergic neural density such as the medial prefrontal cortex, where the signal magnitude in ADHD adults was less than 10% that in striatum (Ernst et al., 1998). If replicated, these preliminary results support the notion that catecholamine dysregulation is central to the pathophysiology of ADHD, and not just to its treatment. They also highlight the proposition that dopaminergic and noradrenergic systems cannot be understood without taking developmental effects into account (Castellanos, 1997).

The utility of SPECT, which is more widely available and less expensive than PET, was highlighted in a preliminary report (Dougherty et al., 1999). The highly selective dopamine transporter ligand [^{123}I]-altropane was used in six adults with ADHD who were compared to a database of 30 healthy controls. Striatal binding potential (Bi_{max}/K_d) was elevated in all six ADHD patients, with each patient exceeding the mean values of the corresponding age-matched controls by at least two standard deviations. This report was questioned because four of the six patients had been previously treated with stimulants (Baughman, 2000), even though they were all medication-free for at least 1 month.

A recent manuscript enhanced the credibility of the Dougherty report. Ten previously untreated adults with ADHD were studied before and after 4 weeks of daily treatment with methylphenidate by SPECT with [Tc-99m]-TRODAT-1, a SPECT ligand that binds to the dopamine transporter. Specific binding of

[Tc-99m]-TRODAT-1 to the dopamine transporter was significantly elevated in the patients as compared with age- and sex-matched controls (Krause et al., 2000). Treatment with three doses per day of 5 mg methylphenidate for 1 month significantly decreased specific [Tc-99m]-TRODAT-1 binding in all patients by a mean of 29%. This study forecloses the possibility that the elevated levels of dopamine transporter in ADHD adults might be secondary to prior medication exposure. Furthermore, it shows that even modest therapeutic doses of methylphenidate have robust effects on dopamine transporter availability.

Summary of functional imaging studies

Conducting functional imaging studies in children requires heroic efforts and a willingness to accept numerous compromises, many of which limit the generalizability of the findings. Nevertheless, the studies point to functional differences in prefrontal cortex (Zametkin et al., 1990; Ernst et al., 1998; Rubia et al., 1999), and in striatum between patients and controls (Lou et al., 1998; Dougherty et al., 1999; Rubia et al., 1999; Bush et al., 1999; Krause et al., 2000; Teicher et al., 2000).

Despite the apparent convergence, it has been difficult to integrate these myriad results until now. The recent SPECT results (Dougherty et al., 1999; Krause et al., 2000) appear to offer a straightforward model of pathogenesis, at least in adults who continue to manifest ADHD. Increased binding capacity of the dopamine transporter implies that synaptic dopamine is cleared more rapidly in ADHD individuals in the striatum where reuptake via dopamine transporters is the most important means of removing dopamine from the synapse (relative to prefrontal cortex, where synaptic dopamine activity is primarily decreased by diffusion and uptake by noradrenaline (norepinephrine) transporters; Cass and Gerhardt, 1995; Frazer et al., 1999). When administered therapeutically, methylphenidate appears to return the system towards an optimal equilibrium (Krause et al., 2000). Since treatment was not blind, and controls were only imaged once, placebo-controlled replication will be needed to ensure that nonspecific effects, such as decreased anxiety, did not mediate the reduction in dopamine transporter. Now the pressing question is whether increases in striatal dopamine transporter density represent the primary neurochemical deficit or a secondary overcompensation. This cannot be answered by studying adults with ADHD and will be difficult or impossible to test directly in unmedicated children.

Thus, indirect methods may be required. Using one such method, robust striatal dopamine release was observed in adult normal volunteers playing a video game (Koepp et al., 1998). Tracer doses of radiolabelled raclopride, a dopamine-2 receptor antagonist, were used to measure indirectly endogenous dopamine release. The relevance of this approach to ADHD should be clear, though ethical and regulatory obstacles will still impede such a study in children.

A new technique that will only be mentioned briefly here is transcranial magnetic stimulation. An initial report has found evidence of motor cortical inhibitory deficits in children with ADHD that were reversed by methylphenidate (Moll et al., 2000). Replication and extension will be eagerly awaited.

Electrophysiological studies of ADHD

Spatial techniques such as MRI or positron emission tomography provide images with spatial resolution ranging from excellent to moderate, but both techniques are expensive and have limited temporal resolution. Electrophysiological approaches have the complementary strength of excellent temporal resolution, down into the millisecond range, but with fundamental limits on spatial resolution deriving from the inverse problem. The inverse problem refers to the mathematical impossibility of arriving at a single solution for any given configuration of electrical or magnetic activity recorded at the scalp.

Despite this unavoidable limitation, electrophysiological techniques are noninvasive, potentially quantitative and relatively inexpensive. Two main types of electrophysiological studies are used: those that record continuous electroencephalograms (EEGs), and studies of event-related potentials (ERP).

Clinical EEGs in ADHD children often report nonspecific abnormal slowing, but these qualitative observations have not been clinically or diagnostically useful (Nogueira de Melo and Niedermeyer, 1999). The development of quantitative EEG (QEEG) was an attempt to harness the potential power of this noninvasive technique. In QEEG, EEG is recorded digitally and short artefact-free segments (2 s or so) are selected and then processed by Fourier analyses to obtain spectral information. Spectral gradients can then be displayed topographically, giving rise to the term 'brain mapping', although concerns have been raised regarding excessive false positives and variable training of practitioners (Levy and Ward, 1995; Nuwer, 1997, 1998). Despite protestations (Hoffman et al., 1999), some papers continue to exhibit fundamental statistical flaws (Lubar et al., 1999).

Fortunately, methodological rigor is improving, as demonstrated by a study of 482 individuals, including 85 controls, conducted in order to validate an index of cortical slowing (Monastra et al., 1999). The authors conclude that the θ/β power ratio is strongly related to age and to the diagnosis of ADHD. They also report highly accurate rates of classifying subjects, with a spectacular positive predictive power of 99%. Subsequent reliability and validity studies with independent samples (Monastra et al., 2000) confirm a statistically robust diagnostic difference in the ratio of θ/β power averaged across four brief behavioural conditions. Test–retest correlation in 55 children with ADHD tested 1 month apart was 0.96. Positive predictive power of the θ/β power ratio was 98%, and negative predictive power was 76%.

One reason why it is unlikely that any single technique will yield nearly perfect positive and negative predictive power is that there are so many possible confounders that need to be taken into account, such as sex. For example, in one study decreased right-lateralized frontal activation was detected in boys with ADHD on power spectral analysis of baseline EEG, but girls with ADHD exhibited the opposite pattern (they were more right-lateralized than the comparison normal girls; Baving et al., 1999). This study was conducted in two age ranges, preschoolers (age $4\frac{1}{2}$ years) and 8-year-old children, and results were independent of age. Unfortunately, even though a total of 117 subjects were studied, there were few girls with ADHD per group (eight preschool, seven school-age).

The conclusion that EEG-associated abnormalities in ADHD are not eliminated by chronological maturation was supported by a well-conducted study of 54 adolescent males with ADHD and an equal number of matched controls (Lazzaro et al., 1999). ADHD adolescents had significantly increased absolute θ activity throughout, and not just in anterior regions. ADHD subjects also showed significantly fewer simultaneously recorded skin conductance responses. The two findings were interpreted as supporting the decreased central nervous system arousal hypothesis of ADHD (Satterfield et al., 1974).

The EEG studies discussed to this point all attempted to capture a baseline or resting state by the selection of brief artefact-free intervals. There are two fundamental problems with this process. First, it relies on the operator's decision regarding appropriate sampling intervals, and second, as functional imaging studies have increasingly shown, a neutral resting state does not exist in the brain. These difficulties are avoided by time-locking the recording period to the presentation of stimuli, so that the recorded intervals can elucidate central processing during specific phases of well-defined tasks.

ERP are averaged over multiple trials, with each 'tracing' typically anchored to a time point, such as stimulus presentation. ERP can be performed in any sensory modality, but visual or auditory stimuli are predominantly used.

Individual ERP trials have exceedingly low signal/noise ratios. Thus, large numbers of trials (typically hundreds, and sometimes thousands) are averaged to obtain the best estimate of the electrophysiological signature for a given subject and task. Extensive reviews of ERP studies in ADHD (Klorman, 1991; Tannock, 1998) have concluded, despite a familiarly unfortunate multiplicity of methods, that ADHD children demonstrate 'problems in central arousal patterns and under-reactivity to stimulation . . . likely related to subcortical activation' (Klorman (1991), cited in Tannock, 1998).

Although averaging hundreds of trials provides information about central tendencies, trial-by-trial variance is eliminated, which is regrettable because variability of responses is a hallmark of ADHD cognitive and motor performance. Fortunately, investigators are now attending to this issue. For example, single-sweep ERP can be analysed by extracting simpler mathematically defined 'wavelets' (Heinrich et al., 1999). This approach captured diagnostic differences between 25 boys with ADHD and 25 age-, IQ- and sex-matched controls, whereas traditional ERP analytical methods did not distinguish the groups. As the authors indicate, additional studies are required to validate this novel technique further and establish its potential diagnostic utility. A complementary approach of measuring the variability of single-trial ERP relative to their average demonstrated significantly increased ERP variability within the P300 window in unmedicated ADHD adolescents that was significantly improved by methylphenidate (Lazzaro et al., 1997). As in the prior example, there had been no between-group differences in P300 mean amplitude or latency.

An alternative technique that also enhances signal/noise makes use of steady-state visually evoked potentials (SSVEP; Morgan et al., 1996; Silberstein et al., 1998). A spatially diffuse 13-Hz visual flicker is used, in which are embedded the stimuli for the cognitive task, which in this case was the A–X variation of the Continuous Performance Task. In this task subjects should respond to an X only if it follows an A. Normal subjects exhibited changes in SSVEP latency and amplitude in right frontal lobe suggestive of enhanced speed of processing. Subjects with ADHD did not demonstrate this rapid temporal shift, and also committed significantly more commission errors.

Summary of electrophysiological studies

As noted, these techniques do not provide precise spatial localization and they cannot interrogate subcortical structures, particularly basal ganglia or cerebellum. At the same time, several studies (Silberstein et al., 1998; Baving et al.,

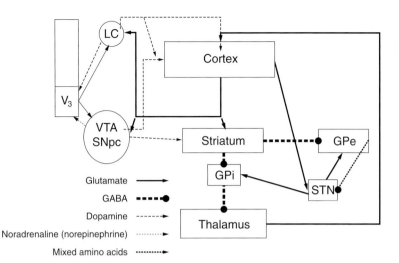

Figure 10.1   Crude diagram demonstrating the known neurochemical linkages among cerebellar, brainstem and cortico-striatal-thalamo-cortical circuits. V_3, posterior inferior cerebellar vermis; LC, locus ceruleus; VTA, ventral tegmental area; SNpc, substantia nigra, pars compacta; Striatum stands for caudate, putamen or nucleus accumbens; GPi, globus pallidus, internal segment; GPe, globus pallidus, external segment; STN, subthalamic nucleus; GABA, γ-aminobutyric acid.

1999; Pliszka et al., 2000) are strongly supportive of other neuroimaging findings of abnormal right prefrontal anatomy (Castellanos et al., 1996a; Filipek et al., 1997; Yeo et al., 2000) and function (Rubia et al., 1999) in ADHD. ERP techniques that capture trial-by-trial variability (Lazzaro et al., 1997; Heinrich et al., 1999) or that enhance signal/noise (Silberstein et al., 1998) are likely to be most useful in ADHD. QEEG approaches are also continuing to be explored with greater methodological rigor (Cox et al., 1998; Monastra et al., 1999, 2000). All of these results are loosely consistent with the notion that ADHD represents a state regulation disorder, as discussed in detail in Chapter 6.

Neurochemistry of ADHD

The delineation of neuroanatomical networks associated with ADHD (Figure 10.1) has renewed the search for specific biochemical abnormalities that may be linked to this neuroanatomy. Since the 1970s (Wender, 1973), the preeminent biochemical theory of ADHD has been based on a catecholamine hypothesis (for historical review, see Pliszka et al., 1996), but even after a quarter-century of investigation its status remains unclear. Recent refinements of this theory have emphasized primary roles of dopamine (Castellanos, 1997) and noradrenaline (Roth and Elsworth, 1995). Castellanos (1997) extended the unitary dopamine theory of ADHD, based on a proposal that different abnormalities might exist in two dopamine regions: underactivity in a cortical region (anterior cingulate) that results in cognitive deficits and overactivity in a subcortical region (caudate nucleus) that results in motor excesses. Arnsten et al. (1996) modified the noradrenergic theory of ADHD in a similar fashion, postulating that different abnormalities may exist in two noradrenergic regions: underactivity in cortex (dorsolateral prefrontal) resulting in primary memory deficits, and overactivity in a subcortical system (LC), resulting in overarousal.

The role of the LC in attention has recently been reviewed (Aston-Jones et al., 1999). Noradrenergic LC neurons have two functional modes, characterized as tonic and phasic. Tonic activity is relatively low-frequency, sustained and closely linked to changes in wakefulness. During waking periods, LC neurons also display phasic fluctuations in response to salient environmental stimuli (Berridge, 2000). At moderate levels of tonic LC activity, phasic LC firing predicts and appears to influence vigilance performance (Rajkowski et al., 1994). If tonic activity is too low, drowsiness and sleep eventually emerge. If LC tonic activity is excessive, the rate of false alarms in vigilance tasks increases in a manner suggestive of ADHD (Usher et al., 1999).

In both of these recent extensions of the catecholamine theory of ADHD (Arnsten et al., 1996; Castellanos, 1997), activity in networks is modulated by subcortical input from midbrain neurons that have receptors strategically located in specialized neuroanatomical networks. For example, the neuroanatomic differentiation of the nigrostriatal dopamine system (cell bodies in the substantia nigra; synaptic connections to receptors primarily in the striatum) and the mesocorticolimbic dopamine system (cell bodies in the ventral tegmental area; synaptic connections to receptors in cortex as well as ventral striatum) is well known and is related to function (sensorimotor vs. emotional control; Roth and Elsworth, 1995), and this knowledge both emerged from and directed pharmacological interventions for motor dysfunctions (parkinsonism) and psychotic disorders (schizophrenia; Sunahara et al., 1993; Civelli, 1995).

As we have also emphasized elsewhere (Swanson et al., 1998b), additional levels of complexity of these neuroanatomical–neurochemical connections are related to the site (Roth and Elsworth, 1995) and type (Civelli, 1995) of dopamine receptors. The site of dopamine receptors (presynaptic on dopaminergic neurons or postsynaptic on dopaminoceptive neurons) can determine whether the net effect of synaptic dopamine is that of an agonist or antagonist (Roth and Elsworth, 1995). Also relevant is the type of dopamine receptors, which are classified as D1-like (D1 and D5 receptors) and D2-like (D2, D3 and D4 receptors). Furthermore, each receptor type has genetic variants (polymorphisms) that potentially introduce further complexity within dopamine pathways (Seeman, 1995).

The two principal central dopaminergic pathways are also differentially regulated. In humans and nonhuman primates, dopamine cells in the VTA, which primarily represent the mesocorticolimbic system, lack autoreceptors, whereas nearby dopamine cells in the substantia nigra, which mostly innervate the striatum, have them in abundance (Meador-Woodruff et al., 1994). Investigations of the neuroanatomic distribution of receptor types have begun (Meador-Woodruff et al., 1996; Lidow et al., 1998), and in situ hybridization studies have shown that relative to D1 and D2 receptors, D3 and D4 receptors are sparse but are localized in the mesocorticolimbic dopamine pathway (Civelli, 1995).

D4 dopamine receptors are located on inhibitory GABAergic interneurons in the cortex, basal ganglia and thalamus (Mrzljak et al., 1996) as well as in the cerebellar vermis (Ariano et al., 1997). Thus, if D4 receptor variations (polymorphisms) are important in the pathophysiology of ADHD (see Swanson et al., 2000b for review and Chapter 9), they are located in the relevant circuits.

Summary of neurochemistry of ADHD

Accumulating evidence continues to point to the catecholamines, dopamine and noradrenaline as key neurotransmitters in the pathophysiology of ADHD. However, we must guard against the conclusion that other substances, such as neuropeptides, are not also involved. Dopaminoceptive neurons contain a bewildering number of other neuropeptide receptors, and the role of substances such as neuropeptide Y (Ault et al., 1998; Zukowska-Grojec, 1998), dynorphin (Gerfen et al., 1998) or substance P (Caille et al., 1995; Tokuno et al., 1996; van der Kooy, 1996) in striatal development and function remains largely undefined.

Neuropharmacology of ADHD

The regions of neuroanatomical abnormalities associated with ADHD and the modulation of neural networks by neurotransmitter systems (Figure 10.1) provide the theoretical basis for neuropharmacological treatment of this disorder. The primary treatment of ADHD is with stimulant medication (methylphenidate and amfetamines; Spencer et al., 1996; Jensen et al., 1999). After a dramatic increase over the past several years (Swanson et al., 1995), it is estimated that over 6% of boys and 2% of girls in the USA are now receiving this pharmacological treatment.

The neuropharmacology of stimulant medications has been investigated extensively in preclinical studies (Kuczenski and Segal, 1975, 1977; Pechnick et al., 1979; Nielsen et al., 1983; Segal and Kuczenski, 1999). However, much of this work has failed to address the efficacy of the stimulants for ADHD for several reasons. First, most preclinical investigations were carried out before the elucidation of multiple receptor subtypes (Civelli, 1995). Second, a large body of preclinical work addressed stimulant-induced psychosis as model for schizophrenia (Robinson et al., 1985) or self-administration of stimulants as a model of substance abuse (Robinson and Kolb, 1997), and the doses investigated have typically been much higher than those used for the treatment of ADHD and have been administered parenterally. Also, most basic studies have been performed in anaesthetized animals, in which neuronal responses are dramatically different from those observed in the conscious behaving animal (Haracz et al., 1993). Finally, while there are undeniable advantages to conducting preclinical studies in rodents, there are also substantial limitations to extrapolating from organisms in whom the ratio of prefrontal brain to striatum is much lower than in nonhuman primates or in humans.

Early neuropharmacological investigations of ADHD were based on the guiding assumption that the primary neurotransmitter system affected by neuroleptic and stimulant medications was the same (dopamine), but the site of action was different (blocking of dopamine receptors by neuroleptics vs. stimulating release and blocking reuptake of dopamine by stimulants). Recent investigations have clearly identified the molecular sites of action of methylphenidate, which blocks the dopamine and noradrenaline transporters (Sonders et al., 1997) and thus increases the temporal and spatial presence of dopamine at the synapse where it is released. It is one of the enduring paradoxes of stimulant psychopharmacology that, while methylphenidate and the amfetamines are clinically very comparable in most children with ADHD, they differ in their specific mechanisms. Methylphenidate is a pure catecholamine reuptake inhibitor, and only has effects on synaptic catecholamine levels if neurotransmitter has been released physiologically. By contrast, the amfetamines, and particularly dextroamfetamine, exert multiple effects, in at least three sites. Unlike methylphenidate, amfetamine releases monoamines (not just dopamine, but also noradrenaline and serotonin) from synaptic vesicles, it inhibits monoamine oxidase and, most importantly, it can convert catecholamine transporters into channels, thereby allowing a massive efflux of dopamine and noradrenaline into synapses (Galli et al., 1996; Frazer et al., 1999).

The recent development of new techniques such as rapid chrono-amperometric measurement of dopamine fluxes (Zahniser et al., 1998; Gerhardt et al., 1999) makes it possible to examine the precise biochemical effects of the stimulants in vivo. However, such studies have yet to be conducted. In the meantime, positron emission tomography has been used to examine the dopaminergic system response to minute traces of radiolabelled methylphenidate in humans and nonhuman primates. Unfortunately, appropriate noradrenergic radioligands have not yet been developed, so that effects on that system in primates remain unknown.

Intravenously administered C^{11}-methylphenidate in normal adults was localized in basal ganglia (putamen, caudate and ventral striatum) and cortex (temporal insula and cingulate gyri; Wang et al., 1995). In a provocatively titled paper, intravenously administered methylphenidate was found to bind to the same sites occupied by radiolabelled cocaine (Volkow et al., 1995). However, clearance of methylphenidate from striatum was more than four times longer (90 min) than that of cocaine (< 20 min), which may underlie some of the differences in abuse liability between the two psychostimulants. Oral dosing also affects pharmacokinetics, and probably accounts for methylphenidate's relatively lower abuse potential. By using orogastric intubation in a baboon, Volkow and colleagues found that peak brain levels are reached 60 min after ingestion. Usual therapeutic doses were found to block upwards of 50% of dopamine transporter in striatum, and clearance from striatum was found to approximate the postpeak length of action following oral administration (2–3 h; Volkow et al., 1998b). Using SPECT, Krause et al. documented even greater decreases in dopamine transporter availability after chronic treatment with 5 mg TID of methylphenidate (Krause et al., 2000).

Using more traditional pharmacodynamic and pharmacokinetic methods in children with ADHD dosed at 30-min intervals, robust tachyphylaxis has been found for methylphenidate (Swanson et al., 1999). This newly described phenomenon was used to design a new delivery system for methylphenidate that would prevent the 40% loss of efficacy produced by constant blood levels (Swanson et al., 2000a).

Additional indirect support for the notion that the primary site of action of stimulants is through the dopamine system was provided by two studies of cerebrospinal fluid (CSF). The baseline level of the primary dopamine metabolite (homovanillic acid, HVA) correlated positively with teacher ratings of hyperactivity (Castellanos et al., 1994) in 29 boys with ADHD. In other words, children with higher baseline HVA levels were more severely hyperactive. A subsequent study confirmed this initially unexpected finding in a new group of

20 ADHD boys, and also found that the behavioural response to multiple stimulant medications in the combined sample (methylphenidate, amfetamine and pemoline) correlated significantly and positively with CSF HVA levels, but not with the noradrenaline or serotonin metabolites (Castellanos et al., 1996b). Unfortunately, the absence of a normal control group or of postdrug CSF made it impossible to interpret these results unambiguously. One possible explanation is that clinical doses of stimulants might act primarily on presynaptic receptors and thus produce a net decrease in dopamine at the synapse (Solanto, 1986, 1998; Solanto et al., 2000). Castellanos speculated that presynaptic effects might predominate in subcortical regions (producing decreased synaptic dopamine) but postsynaptic effects would predominate in cortical regions (producing increased synaptic dopamine; Castellanos, 1997).

The hypothesis that low doses of stimulants have greater presynaptic than postsynaptic effects has been tested and rejected in the rat (Ruskin et al., 2001). Ruskin et al. found that the dose–response curves for individually recorded neurons in the substantia nigra pars compacta (presynaptic dopamine neurons) and the globus pallidus (postsynaptic GABAergic neurons) did not differ for methylphenidate, whereas d-amfetamine was even more potent postsynaptically. Furthermore, the authors noted that both drugs had profound effects on postsynaptic multisecond oscillations, shifting the firing-rate oscillations from periods of ~30 s down to periods of 5–10 s. Dopamine antagonists blocked these remarkably robust effects, which were most pronounced with doses that approximate those used clinically. This unexpected finding raises the possibility that multisecond oscillations may link distributed circuits that include prefrontal cortex (Hudetz et al., 1992, 1998), basal ganglia (Ruskin et al., 1999a,b), VTA (Snider et al., 1976a), substantia nigra (Ruskin et al., 2001), LC (Snider, 1975; Vankov et al., 1995; Aston-Jones et al., 2000) and possibly the cerebellar vermis (Hartmann and Bower, 1998).

Summary of neuropsychopharmacology of ADHD

Neuroscientists have once again become interested in understanding the therapeutic mechanisms of action of the stimulants in ADHD. These drugs enhance synaptic levels of dopamine, noradrenaline and, to a lesser extent, serotonin, but whether these are the primary relevant effects is still unclear. The hypothesis that stimulants preferentially activate release-inhibiting autoreceptors (Solanto, 1986; Castellanos et al., 1996b; Solanto et al., 2000) has been refuted, at least in the rat (Ruskin et al., 2001). At the same time, a novel potential mechanism has been uncovered. At therapeutic doses, stimulants have remarkably robust effects on multisecond oscillations that appear to reflect the properties of a distributed circuit, rather than of a single set of synaptic connections. In our conclusion, we turn to such a possible circuit.

Conclusions: a tentative model of ADHD pathophysiology

A refined phenotype of ADHD has emerged from over a half-century of clinical practice, and recent investigations provide converging evidence that this phenotype is characterized by neuropsychological deficits in executive functions and reduced size in neuroanatomical regions in the frontal lobes, basal ganglia and posterior inferior cerebellar vermis. The convergence of two complementary studies using different SPECT ligands firmly establishes that dopamine transporter density in striatum is elevated in adults with ADHD (Dougherty et al., 1999; Krause et al., 2000), and is decreased by subchronic treatment with low-dose methylphenidate (Krause et al., 2000). It now remains to be seen whether increased dopamine transporter density represents a primary aetiological defect in ADHD, or alternatively, a secondary overcompensation.

Figure 10.1 depicts our speculative model that attempts to link the observations reviewed in this chapter in a parsimonious hypothesis. We propose that primary genetic factors (Swanson et al., 2000b) have their strongest direct effects on the development and function of the cerebellar vermis (Berquin et al., 1998), which has been considered the 'head afferent ganglion of the catecholamine systems' (Snider et al., 1976a). Inadequate vermal efferents would thus lead to excessive and/or dysregulated catecholaminergic neurotransmission in childhood (Castellanos et al., 1996b) and adolescence (Ernst et al., 1999), and deficient prefrontal (Ernst et al., 1998) and striatal (Dougherty et al., 1999; Krause et al., 2000) catecholamine innervation in adulthood. Such dysregulated systems, resulting in the behavioural deficits described elsewhere in this volume (Chapter 6), are temporarily improved by medications that enhance synaptic catecholamine levels (Vaidya et al., 1998; Krause et al., 2000; Teicher et al., 2000), i.e. stimulants. Elaborating this crude model into a series of testable specific hypotheses and determining its applicability across the life span will lead us closer to an understanding of the biological underpinnings of ADHD.

REFERENCES

Albert, T.J., Dempesy, C.W. and Sorenson, C.A. (1985). Anterior cerebellar vermal stimulation: effect on behavior and basal forebrain neurochemistry in rat. *Biological Psychiatry*, **20**, 1267–76.

Alexander, G.E., DeLong, M.R. and Strick, P.L. (1986). Parallel organization of functionally segregated circuits linking basal ganglia and cortex. *Annual Review of Neuroscience*, **9**, 357–81.

Amen, D.G., Paldi, J.H. and Thisted, R.A. (1993). Brain SPECT imaging. *Journal of the American Academy of Child and Adolescent Psychiatry*, **32**, 1080–1.

American Psychiatric Association (1994). *Diagnostic and Statistical Manual of Mental Disorders,* 4th edn. Washington, DC: American Psychiatric Association.

Anderson, C.M., Polcari, A.M., McGreenery, C.E. et al. (1999). Cerebellar vermis blood flow: associations with psychiatric symptoms in child abuse and ADHD. *Society for Neuroscience Abstracts*, **25**, 1637.

Anderson, C.M., Maas, L.C., Renshaw, P.F. and Teicher, M.H. (2000a). Non-invasive T2-relaxation time measures correlate with gadolinium-based cerebral blood volume estimates in the putamen and cerebellar vermis of young adults. *Society for Neuroscience Abstracts*, **27**, 1730.

Anderson, C.M., Polcari, A.M., McGreenery, C.E. et al. (2000b). Methylphenidate dose-dependently alters blood flow in the vermis but not basal ganglia of ADHD boys. *Biological Psychiatry*, **47**, 106S–7S.

Ariano, M.A., Wang, J., Noblett, K.L., Larson, E.R. and Sibley, D.R. (1997). Cellular distribution of the rat D4 dopamine receptor protein in the CNS using anti-receptor antisera. *Brain Research*, **752**, 26–34.

Arndt, S., Cohen, G., Alliger, R.J., Swayze, V.W.2. and Andreasen, N.C. (1991). Problems with ratio and proportion measures of imaged cerebral structures. *Psychiatry Research*, **40**, 79–89.

Arnsten, A.F., Steere, J.C. and Hunt, R.D. (1996). The contribution of alpha 2-noradrenergic mechanisms of prefrontal cortical cognitive function. Potential significance for attention-deficit hyperactivity disorder. *Archives of General Psychiatry*, **53**, 448–55.

Aston-Jones, G., Rajkowski, J. and Cohen, J. (1999). Role of locus coeruleus in attention and behavioral flexibility. *Biological Psychiatry*, **46**, 1309–20.

Aston-Jones, G., Rajkowski, J. and Cohen, J. (2000). Locus coeruleus and regulation of behavioral flexibility and attention. *Progress in Brain Research*, **126**, 165–82.

Ault, D.T., Radeff, J.M. and Werling, L.L. (1998). Modulation of [3H]dopamine release from rat nucleus accumbens by neuropeptide Y may involve a sigma 1-like receptor. *Journal of Pharmacology and Experimental Therapeutics*, **284**, 553–60.

Aylward, E.H., Reiss, A.L., Reader, M.J. et al. (1996). Basal ganglia volumes in children with attention-deficit hyperactivity disorder. *Journal of Child Neurology*, **11**, 112–15.

Bandettini, P.A., Kwong, K.K., Davis, T.L. et al. (1997). Characterization of cerebral blood oxygenation and flow changes during prolonged brain activation. *Human Brain Mapping*, **5**, 93–109.

Baughman, F.A. (2000). Dopamine-transporter density in patients with ADHD. *Lancet*, **355**, 1460–1.

Baving, L., Laucht, M. and Schmidt, M.H. (1999). Atypical frontal brain activation in ADHD: preschool and elementary school boys and girls. *Journal of the American Academy of Child and Adolescent Psychiatry*, **38**, 1363–71.

Berquin, P.C., Giedd, J.N., Jacobsen, L.K. et al. (1998). The cerebellum in attention-deficit/hyperactivity disorder: a morphometric study. *Neurology*, **50**, 1087–93.

Berridge, C.W. (2000). Arousal- and attention-related actions of the locus coeruleus-noradrenergic system: potential target in the therapeutic actions of amphetamine-like stimulants. In *Stimulant Drugs and ADHD: Basic and Clinical Neuroscience*. M.V. Solanto, A.F.T. Arnsten and F.X. Castellanos, eds, pp. 158–84. New York: Oxford University Press.

Börger, N. and Van der Meere, J. (2000). Motor control and state regulation in children with ADHD: a cardiac response study. *Biological Psychology*, **51**, 247–67.

Bradley, D.J., Ghelarducci, B. and Spyer, K.M. (1991). The role of the posterior cerebellar vermis in cardiovascular control. *Neuroscience Research*, **12**, 45–56.

Bush, G., Whalen, P.J., Rosen, B.R. et al. (1998). The counting Stroop: an interference task specialized for functional neuroimaging – validation study with functional MRI. *Human Brain Mapping*, **6**, 270–82.

Bush, G., Frazier, J.A., Rauch, S.L. et al. (1999). Anterior cingulate cortex dysfunction in attention-deficit/hyperactivity disorder revealed by fMRI and the counting Stroop. *Biological Psychiatry*, **45**, 1542–52.

Caille, I., Dumartin, B., Le Moine, C., Begueret, J. and Bloch, B. (1995). Ontogeny of the D1 dopamine receptor in the rat striatonigral system: an immunohistochemical study. *European Journal of Neuroscience*, **7**, 714–22.

Casey, B.J., Castellanos, F.X., Giedd, J.N. et al. (1997). Implication of right frontostriatal circuitry in response inhibition and attention-deficit/hyperactivity disorder. *Journal of the American Academy of Child and Adolescent Psychiatry*, **36**, 374–83.

Cass, W.A. and Gerhardt, G.A. (1995). In vivo assessment of dopamine uptake in rat medial prefrontal cortex: comparison with dorsal striatum and nucleus accumbens. *Journal of Neurochemistry*, **65**, 201–7.

Castellanos, F.X. (1997). Toward a pathophysiology of attention-deficit/hyperactivity disorder. *Clinical Pediatrics*, **36**, 381–93.

Castellanos, F.X., Elia, J., Kruesi, M.J.P. et al. (1994). Cerebrospinal fluid monoamine metabolites in boys with attention-deficit hyperactivity disorder. *Psychiatry Research*, **52**, 305–16.

Castellanos, F.X., Giedd, J.N., Marsh, W.L. et al. (1996a). Quantitative brain magnetic resonance imaging in attention-deficit/hyperactivity disorder. *Archives of General Psychiatry*, **53**, 607–16.

Castellanos, F.X., Elia, J., Kruesi, M.J.P. et al. (1996b). Cerebrospinal homovanillic acid predicts behavioral response to stimulants in 45 boys with attention-deficit/hyperactivity disorder. *Neuropsychopharmacology*, **14**, 125–37.

Castellanos, F.X., Giedd, J.N., Berquin, P.C. et al. (2001). Quantitative brain magnetic resonance imaging in girls with attention-deficit/hyperactivity disorder. *Archives of General Psychiatry*, **58**, 289–95.

Civelli, O. (1995). Molecular biology of the dopamine receptor subtypes. In *Psychopharmacology: The Fourth Generation of Progress*, F.E. Bloom and D.J. Kupfer, eds, pp. 155–61. New York: Raven Press.

Cox, D.J., Kovatchev, B.P., Morris, J.B. Jr. et al. (1998). Electroencephalographic and psychometric differences between boys with and without attention-deficit/hyperactivity disorder (ADHD): a pilot study. *Applied Psychophysiology and Biofeedback*, **23**, 179–88.

DelBello, M.P., Strakowski, S.M., Zimmerman, M.E., Hawkins, J.M. and Sax, K.W. (1999). MRI analysis of the cerebellum in bipolar disorder: a pilot study. *Neuropsychopharmacology*, **21**, 63–8.

Dempesy, C.W., Tootle, D.M., Fontana, C.J. et al. (1983). Stimulation of the paleocerebellar cortex of the cat: increased rate of synthesis and release of catecholamines at limbic sites. *Biological Psychiatry*, **18**, 127–32.

Dougherty, D.D., Bonab, A.A., Spencer, T.J. et al. (1999). Dopamine transporter density is elevated in patients with attention deficit hyperactivity disorder. *Lancet*, **354**, 2132–3.

Draeger, S., Prior, M. and Sanson, A. (1986). Visual and auditory attention performance in hyperactive children: competence or compliance. *Journal of Abnormal Child Psychology*, **14**, 411–24.

Ernst, M., Liebenauer, L.L., King, A.C. et al. (1994). Reduced brain metabolism in hyperactive girls. *Journal of the American Academy of Child and Adolescent Psychiatry*, **33**, 858–68.

Ernst, M., Zametkin, A.J., Matochik, J.A. et al. (1997a). Intravenous dextroamphetamine and brain glucose metabolism. *Neuropsychopharmacology*, **17**, 391–401.

Ernst, M., Cohen, R.M., Liebenauer, L.L., Jons, P.H. and Zametkin, A.J. (1997b). Cerebral glucose metabolism in adolescent girls with attention-deficit/hyperactivity disorder. *Journal of the American Academy of Child and Adolescent Psychiatry*, **36**, 1399–406.

Ernst, M., Zametkin, A.J., Matochik, J.A., Jons, P.H. and Cohen, R.M. (1998). DOPA decarboxylase activity in attention deficit hyperactivity disorder adults. A [fluorine-18]fluorodopa positron emission tomographic study. *Journal of Neuroscience*, **18**, 5901–7.

Ernst, M., Zametkin, A.J., Matochik, J.A. et al. (1999). High midbrain 18F-DOPA accumulation in children with ADHD. *American Journal of Psychiatry*, **156**, 1209–15.

Filipek, P.A., Semrud-Clikeman, M., Steingard, R.J. et al. (1997). Volumetric MRI analysis comparing attention-deficit hyperactivity disorder and normal controls. *Neurology*, **48**, 589–601.

Frazer, A., Gerhardt, G.A. and Daws, L.C. (1999). New views of biogenic amine transporter function: implications for neuropsychopharmacology. *International Journal of Neuropsychopharmacology*, **2**, 305–20.

Galli, A., Blakely, R.D. and DeFelice, L.J. (1996). Norepinephrine transporters have channel modes of conduction. *Proceedings of the National Academy of Sciences of the United States of America*, **93**, 8671–6.

Gerfen, C.R., Keefe, K.A. and Steiner, H. (1998). Dopamine-mediated gene regulation in the striatum. *Advances in Pharmacology*, **42**, 670–3.

Gerhardt, G.A., Ksir, C., Pivik, C. et al. (1999). Methodology for coupling local application of dopamine and other chemicals with rapid in vivo electrochemical recordings in freely-moving rats. *Journal of Neuroscience Methods*, **87**, 67–76.

Ghelarducci, B. and Sebastiani, L. (1997). Classical heart rate conditioning and affective behavior: the role of the cerebellar vermis. *Archives Italiennes de Biologie*, **135**, 369–84.

Giedd, J.N., Snell, J.W., Lange, N. et al. (1996). Quantitative magnetic resonance imaging of human brain development: ages 4–18. *Cerebral Cortex*, **6**, 551–60.

Giedd, J.N., Blumenthal, J., Jeffries, N.O. et al. (1999a). Cerebral cortical gray matter changes during childhood and adolescence: a longitudinal MRI study. *Nature Neuroscience*, **2**, 861–3.

Giedd, J.N., Blumenthal, J., Jeffries, N.O. et al. (1999b). Development of the human corpus callosum during childhood and adolescence: a longitudinal MRI study. *Progress in Neuropsychopharmacology and Biological Psychiatry*, **23**, 571–88.

Graybiel, A.M. (1998). The basal ganglia and chunking of action repertoires. *Neurobiology Learning and Memory*, **70**, 119–36.

Haracz, J.L., Tschanz, J.T., Wang, Z., White, I.M. and Rebec, G.V. (1993). Striatal single-unit responses to amphetamine and neuroleptics in freely moving rats. *Neuroscience and Biobehavioral Reviews*, **17**, 1–12.

Hartmann, M.J. and Bower, J.M. (1998). Oscillatory activity in the cerebellar hemispheres of unrestrained rats. *Journal of Neurophysiology*, **80**, 1598–604.

Heath, R.G., Dempesy, C.W., Fontana, C.J. and Myers, W.A. (1978). Cerebellar stimulation: effects on septal region, hippocampus, and amygdala of cats and rats. *Biological Psychiatry*, **13**, 501–29.

Heath, R.G., Dempesy, C.W., Fontana, C.J. and Fitzjarrell, A.T. (1980). Feedback loop between cerebellum and septal-hippocampal sites: its role in emotion and epilepsy. *Biological Psychiatry*, **15**, 541–56.

Heinrich, H., Dickhaus, H., Rothenberger, A., Heinrich, V. and Moll, G.H. (1999). Single-sweep analysis of event-related potentials by wavelet networks – methodological basis and clinical application. *IEEE Transactions in Biomedical Engineering*, **46**, 867–79.

Herskovits, E.H., Megalooikonomou, V., Davatzikos, C. et al. (1999). Is the spatial distribution of brain lesions associated with closed-head injury predictive of subsequent development of attention-deficit/hyperactivity disorder? Analysis with brain-image database. *Radiology*, **213**, 389–94.

Hoffman, D.A., Lubar, J.F., Thatcher, R.W. et al. (1999). Limitations of the American Academy of Neurology and American Clinical Neurophysiology Society paper on QEEG. *Journal of Neuropsychiatry and Clinical Neurosciences*, **11**, 401–7.

Hudetz, A.G., Roman, R.J. and Harder, D.R. (1992). Spontaneous flow oscillations in the cerebral cortex during acute changes in mean arterial pressure. *Journal of Cerebral Blood Flow and Metabolism*, **12**, 491–9.

Hudetz, A.G., Biswal, B.B., Shen, H., Lauer, K.K. and Kampine, J.P. (1998). Spontaneous fluctuations in cerebral oxygen supply. In *Oxygen Transport to Tissue XX*, A.G. Hudetz and D.F. Bruley, eds, pp. 551–9. New York: Plenum Press.

Huttenlocher, P.R. (1979). Synaptic density in human frontal cortex – developmental changes and effects of aging. *Brain Research*, **163**, 195–205.

Huttenlocher, P.R. and Dabholkar, A.S. (1997). Regional differences in synaptogenesis in human cerebral cortex. *Journal of Comparative Neurology*, **387**, 167–78.

Hynd, G.W., Semrud-Clikeman, M., Lorys, A.R., Novey, E.S. and Eliopulos, D. (1990). Brain morphology in developmental dyslexia and attention deficit disorder/hyperactivity. *Archives of Neurology*, **47**, 919–26.

Hynd, G.W., Hern, K.L., Novey, E.S. et al. (1993). Attention deficit hyperactivity disorder and asymmetry of the caudate nucleus. *Journal of Child Neurology*, **8**, 339–47.

Jacobsen, L.K., Giedd, J.N., Berquin, P.C. et al. (1997). Quantitative morphology of the cerebellum and fourth ventricle in childhood-onset schizophrenia. *American Journal of Psychiatry*, **154**, 1663–9.

Jennings, J.R., van der Molen, M.W., Pelham, W., Debski, K.B. and Hoza, B. (1997). Inhibition in boys with attention deficit hyperactivity disorder as indexed by heart rate change. *Developmental Psychology*, **33**, 308–18.

Jensen, P.S., Martin, D. and Cantwell, D.P. (1997). Comorbidity in ADHD: implications for research, practice, and DSM-V. *Journal of the American Academy of Child and Adolescent Psychiatry*, **36**, 1065–79.

Jensen, P.S., Arnold, L.E., Richters, J.E. et al. (1999). A 14-month randomized clinical trial of treatment strategies for attention-deficit/hyperactivity disorder. *Archives of General Psychiatry*, **56**, 1073–86.

Jernigan, T.L. and Tallal, P. (1990). Late childhood changes in brain morphology observable with MRI. *Developmental Medicine and Child Neurology*, **32**, 379–85.

Jernigan, T.L., Trauner, D.A., Hesselink, J.R. and Tallal, P.A. (1991). Maturation of human cerebrum observed in vivo during adolescence. *Brain*, **114**, 2037–49.

Jueptner, M. and Weiller, C. (1998). A review of differences between basal ganglia and cerebellar control of movements as revealed by functional imaging studies. *Brain*, **121**, 1437–49.

Klorman, R. (1991). Cognitive event-related potentials in attention deficit disorder. *Journal of Learning Disabilities*, **24**, 130–40.

Koepp, M.J., Gunn, R.N., Lawrence, A.D. et al. (1998). Evidence for striatal dopamine release during a video game. *Nature*, **393**, 266–8.

Krause, K.H., Dresel, S.H., Krause, J., Kung, H.F. and Tatsch, K. (2000). Increased striatal dopamine transporter in adult patients with attention deficit hyperactivity disorder: effects of methylphenidate as measured by single photon emission computed tomography. *Neuroscience Letters*, **285**, 107–10.

Kuczenski, R. and Segal, D.S. (1975). Differential effects of D- and L-amphetamine and methylphenidate on rat striatal dopamine biosynthesis. *European Journal of Pharmacology*, **30**, 244–51.

Kuczenski, R. and Segal, D.S. (1997). Effects of methylphenidate on extracellular dopamine, serotonin, and norepinephrine: comparison with amphetamine. *Journal of Neurochemistry*, **68**, 2032–7.

Lange, N., Giedd, J.N., Castellanos, F.X., Vaituzis, A.C. and Rapoport, J.L. (1997). Variability of human brain structure size: ages 4 to 20. *Psychiatry Research: Neuroimaging*, **74**, 1–12.

Lazzaro, I., Anderson, J., Gordon, E. et al. (1997). Single trial variability within the P300 (250–500 ms) processing window in adolescents with attention deficit hyperactivity disorder. *Psychiatry Research*, **73**, 91–101.

Lazzaro, I., Gordon, E., Li, W. et al. (1999). Simultaneous EEG and EDA measures in adolescent attention deficit hyperactivity disorder. *International Journal of Psychophysiology*, **34**, 123–34.

Levy, F. (1980). The development of sustained attention (vigilance) and inhibition in children: some normative data. *Journal of Child Psychology and Psychiatry*, **21**, 77–84.

Levy, F. and Ward, P.B. (1995). Neurometrics, dynamic brain imaging and attention deficit hyperactivity disorder. *Journal of Paediatrics and Child Health*, **31**, 279–83.

Lidow, M.S., Wang, F., Cao, Y. and Goldman-Rakic, P.S. (1998). Layer V neurons bear the majority of mRNAs encoding the five distinct dopamine receptor subtypes in the primate prefrontal cortex. *Synapse*, **28**, 10–20.

Lou, H.C., Henriksen, L. and Bruhn, P. (1990). Focal cerebral dysfunction in developmental learning disabilities. *Lancet*, **335**, 8–11.

Lou, H.C., Andresen, J., Steinberg, B., McLaughlin, T. and Friberg, L. (1998). The striatum in a putative cerebral network activated by verbal awareness in normals and in ADHD children. *European Journal of Neurology*, **5**, 67–74.

Lubar, J.F., White, J.N., Swartwood, M.O. and Swartwood, J.N. (1999). Methylphenidate effects on global and complex measures of EEG. *Pediatric Neurology*, **21**, 633–7.

Mataró, M., García-Sánchez, C., Junqué, C., Estévez-González, A. and Pujol, J. (1997). Magnetic resonance imaging measurement of the caudate nucleus in adolescents with attention-deficit hyperactivity disorder and its relationship with neuropsychological and behavioral measures. *Archives of Neurology*, **54**, 963–8.

Max, J.E., Arndt, S., Castillo, C.S. et al. (1998). Attention-deficit hyperactivity symptomatology after traumatic brain injury: a prospective study. *Journal of the American Academy of Child and Adolescent Psychiatry*, **37**, 841–7.

Meador-Woodruff, J.H., Damask, S.P. and Watson, S.J. Jr. (1994). Differential expression of autoreceptors in the ascending dopamine systems of the human brain. *Proceedings of the National Academy of Sciences of the United States of America*, **91**, 8297–301.

Meador-Woodruff, J.H., Damask, S.P., Wang, J. et al. (1996). Dopamine receptor mRNA expression in human striatum and neocortex. *Neuropsychopharmacology*, **15**, 17–29.

Melchitzky, D.S. and Lewis, D.A. (2000). Tyrosine hydroxylase- and dopamine transporter-immunoreactive axons in the primate cerebellum. Evidence for a lobular- and laminar-specific dopamine innervation. *Neuropsychopharmacology*, **22**, 466–72.

Moll, G.H., Heinrich, H., Trott, G., Wirth, S. and Rothenberger, A. (2000). Deficient intracortical inhibition in drug-naive children with attention-deficit hyperactivity disorder is enhanced by methylphenidate. *Neuroscience Letters*, **284**, 121–5.

Monastra, V.J., Lubar, J.F., Linden, M. et al. (1999). Assessing attention deficit hyperactivity disorder via quantitative electroencephalography: an initial validation study. *Neuropsychology*, **13**, 424–33.

Monastra, V.J., Lubar, J.F. and Linden, M. (2000). The development of a QEEG scanning process for ADHD: reliability and validity studies. *Neuropsychology*, **15**, 136–44.

Morgan, S.T., Hansen, J.C. and Hillyard, S.A. (1996). Selective attention to stimulus location modulates the steady-state visual evoked potential. *Proceedings of the National Academy of Sciences of the United States of America*, **93**, 4770–4.

Mostofsky, S.H., Reiss, A.L., Lockhart, P. and Denckla, M.B. (1998). Evaluation of cerebellar size in attention-deficit hyperactivity disorder. *Journal of Child Neurology*, **13**, 434–9.

Mrzljak, L., Bergson, C., Pappy, M. et al. (1996). Localization of dopamine D4 receptors in GABAergic neurons of the primate brain. *Nature*, **381**, 245–8.

Nasrallah, H.A., Loney, J., Olson, S.C. et al. (1986). Cortical atrophy in young adults with a history of hyperactivity in childhood. *Psychiatry Research*, **17**, 241–6.

Nielsen, J.A., Chapin, D.S. and Moore, K.E. (1983). Differential effects of d-amphetamine, beta-phenylethylamine, cocaine and methylphenidate on the rate of dopamine synthesis in terminals of nigrostriatal and mesolimbic neurons and on the efflux of dopamine metabolites into cerebroventricular perfusates of rats. *Life Sciences*, **33**, 1899–907.

Nogueira de Melo, A. and Niedermeyer, E. (1999). The EEG in infantile brain damage, cerebral palsy, and minor cerebral dysfunctions of childhood. In *Electroencephalography: Basic Principles, Clinical Applications, and Related Fields*, 4th edn, E. Niedermeyer and F.H. Lopes da Silva, eds, pp. 383–92. Baltimore: Williams and Wilkins.

Nuwer, M. (1997). Assessment of digital EEG, quantitative EEG, and EEG brain mapping: report of the American Academy of Neurology and the American Clinical Neurophysiology Society. *Neurology*, **49**, 277–92.

Nuwer, M.R. (1998). Assessing digital and quantitative EEG in clinical settings. *Journal of Clinical Neurophysiology*, **15**, 458–63.

Paus, T., Zijdenbos, A., Worsley, K. et al. (1999). Structural maturation of neural pathways in children and adolescents: in vivo study. *Science*, **283**, 1908–11.

Pechnick, R., Janowsky, D.S. and Judd, L. (1979). Differential effects of methylphenidate and d-amphetamine on stereotyped behavior in the rat. *Psychopharmacology*, **65**, 311–15.

Peterson, B., Riddle, M.A., Cohen, D.J. et al. (1993). Reduced basal ganglia volumes in Tourette's syndrome using three-dimensional reconstruction techniques from magnetic resonance images. *Neurology*, **43**, 941–9.

Pliszka, S.R., McCracken, J.T. and Maas, J.W. (1996). Catecholamines in attention-deficit hyperactivity disorder: current perspectives. *Journal of the American Academy of Child and Adolescent Psychiatry*, **35**, 264–72.

Pliszka, S.R., Liotti, M. and Woldorff, M.G. (2000). Inhibitory control in children with attention-deficit/hyperactivity disorder: event-related potentials identify the processing component and timing of an impaired right-frontal response-inhibition mechanism. *Biological Psychiatry*, **48**, 238–46.

Pontius, A.A. (1973). Dysfunction patterns analogous to frontal lobe system and caudate nucleus syndromes in some groups of minimal brain dysfunction. *Journal of the American Medical Women's Association*, **28**, 285–92.

Rajkowski, J., Kubiak, P. and Aston-Jones, G. (1994). Locus coeruleus activity in monkey: phasic and tonic changes are associated with altered vigilance. *Brain Research Bulletin*, **35**, 607–16.

Rapoport, J.L., Buchsbaum, M.S., Zahn, T.P. et al. (1978). Dextroamphetamine: cognitive and behavioral effects in normal prepubertal boys. *Science*, **199**, 560–3.

Reiss, A.L., Abrams, M.T., Singer, H.S., Ross, J.L. and Denckla, M.B. (1996). Brain development, gender and IQ in children. A volumetric imaging study. *Brain*, **119**, 1763–74.

Robinson, T.E. and Kolb, B. (1997). Persistent structural modifications in nucleus accumbens and prefrontal cortex neurons produced by previous experience with amphetamine. *Journal of Neuroscience*, **17**, 8491–7.

Robinson, T.E., Becker, J.B., Moore, C.J., Castaneda, E. and Mittleman, G. (1985). Enduring enhancement in frontal cortex dopamine utilization in an animal model of amphetamine psychosis. *Brain Research*, **343**, 374–7.

Roth, R.H. and Elsworth, J.D. (1995). Biochemical pharmacology of midbrain dopamine neurons. In *Psychopharmacology: The Fourth Generation of Progress*, F.E. Bloom and D.J. Kupfer, eds, pp. 227–43. New York: Raven Press.

Rubia, K., Overmeyer, S., Taylor, E. et al. (1999). Hypofrontality in attention deficit hyperactivity disorder during higher-order motor control: a study with functional MRI. *American Journal of Psychiatry*, **156**, 891–6.

Ruskin, D.N., Bergstrom, D.A., Kaneoke, Y. et al. (1999a). Multisecond oscillations in firing rate in the basal ganglia: robust modulation by dopamine receptor activation and anesthesia. *Journal of Neurophysiology*, **81**, 2046–55.

Ruskin, D.N., Bergstrom, D.A. and Walters, J.R. (1999b). Multisecond oscillations in firing rate in the globus pallidus: synergistic modulation by D_1 and D_2 dopamine receptors. *Journal of Pharmacology and Experimental Therapeutics*, **290**, 1493–501.

Ruskin, D.N., Bergstrom, D.A., Shenker, A. et al. (2001). Drugs used in the treatment of attention deficit/hyperactivity disorder affect postsynaptic firing rate and oscillation without preferential autoreceptor action. *Biological Psychiatry*, **49**, 340–50.

Satterfield, J.H., Cantwell, D.P. and Satterfield, B.T. (1974). Pathophysiology of the hyperactive child syndrome. *Archives of General Psychiatry*, **31**, 839–44.

Schachar, R.J. and Tannock, R. (1993). Inhibitory control, impulsiveness, and attention deficit hyperactivity disorder. *Clinical Psychology Review*, **13**, 721–39.

Schmahmann, J.D. and Sherman, J.C. (1998). The cerebellar cognitive affective syndrome. *Brain*, **121**, 561–79.

Schweitzer, J.B., Lee, D.O., Ely, T.D. et al. (1998). The effects of methylphenidate on the functional neuroanatomy of working memory in ADHD. *Society for Neuroscience Abstracts*, **24**, 958.

Seeman, P. (1995). Dopamine receptors. Clinical correlates. In *Psychopharmacology: The Fourth Generation of Progress*, F.E. Bloom and D.J. Kupfer, eds, pp. 295–302. New York: Raven Press.

Segal, D.S. and Kuczenski, R. (1999). Escalating dose–binge treatment with methylphenidate: role of serotonin in the emergent behavioral profile. *Journal of Pharmacology and Experimental Therapeutics*, **291**, 19–30.

Shaywitz, B.A., Shaywitz, S.E., Byrne, T., Cohen, D.J. and Rothman, S. (1983). Attention deficit disorder: quantitative analysis of CT. *Neurology*, **33**, 1500–3.

Silberstein, R.B., Farrow, M., Levy, F. et al. (1998). Functional brain electrical activity mapping in boys with attention-deficit/hyperactivity disorder. *Archives of General Psychiatry*, **55**, 1105–12.

Singer, H.S., Reiss, A.L., Brown, J.E. et al. (1993). Volumetric MRI changes in basal ganglia of children with Tourette's syndrome. *Neurology*, **43**, 950–6.

Snider, R.S. (1975). A cerebellar–ceruleus pathway. *Brain Research*, **88**, 59–63.

Snider, R.S. and Maiti, A. (1976). Cerebellar contributions to the Papez circuit. *Journal of Neuroscience Research*, **2**, 133–46.

Snider, R.S., Maiti, A. and Snider, S.R. (1976a). Cerebellar connections to catecholamine systems: anatomical and biochemical studies. *Transactions of the American Neurological Association*, **101**, 295–7.

Snider, R.S., Maiti, A. and Snider, S.R. (1976b). Cerebellar pathways to ventral midbrain and nigra. *Experimental Neurology*, **53**, 714–28.

Solanto, M.V. (1986). Behavioral effects of low-dose methylphenidate in childhood attention deficit disorder: implications for a mechanism of stimulant drug action. *Journal of the American Academy of Child Psychiatry*, **25**, 96–101.

Solanto, M.V. (1998). Neuropsychopharmacological mechanisms of stimulant drug action in attention-deficit/hyperactivity disorder: a review and integration. *Behavioral Brain Research*, **94**, 127–52.

Solanto, M.V., Arnsten, A.F.T. and Castellanos, F.X. (2000). The neuroscience of stimulant drug action in ADHD. In *Stimulant Drugs and ADHD: Basic and Clinical Neuroscience*, M.V. Solanto, A.F.T. Arnsten and F.X. Castellanos, eds, pp. 355–79. New York: Oxford University Press.

Sonders, M.S., Zhu, S.J., Zahniser, N.R., Kavanaugh, M.P. and Amara, S.G. (1997). Multiple ionic conductances of the human dopamine transporter: the actions of dopamine and psychostimulants. *Journal of Neuroscience*, **17**, 960–74.

Sowell, E.R., Thompson, P.M., Holmes, C.J., Jernigan, T.L. and Toga, A.W. (1999a). *In vivo* evidence for post-adolescent brain maturation in frontal and striatal regions. *Nature Neuroscience*, **2**, 859–61.

Sowell, E.R., Thompson, P.M., Holmes, C.J. et al. (1999b). Localizing age-related changes in brain structure between childhood and adolescence using statistical parametric mapping. *Neuroimage*, **9**, 587–97.

Spencer, T., Biederman, J., Wilens, T.E. et al. (1996). Pharmacotherapy of attention-deficit hyperactivity disorder across the life cycle. *Journal of the American Academy of Child and Adolescent Psychiatry*, **35**, 409–32.

Sunahara, R.K., Seeman, P., Van Tol, H.H. and Niznik, H.B. (1993). Dopamine receptors and antipsychotic drug response. *British Journal of Psychiatry Supplement*, **163**, (suppl. 22), 31–8.

Supple, W.F. Jr. and Kapp, B.S. (1994). Anatomical and physiological relationships between the anterior cerebellar vermis and the pontine parabrachial nucleus in the rabbit. *Brain Research Bulletin*, **33**, 561–74.

Swanson, J.M. and Castellanos, F.X. (1998) Biological bases of ADHD: neuroanatomy, genetics, and pathophysiology. In *NIH Consensus Development Conference – Diagnosis and Treatment of Attention Deficit Hyperactivity Disorder*, pp. 37–42. Bethesda, MD: National Institutes of Health.

Swanson, J.M., Lerner, M. and Williams, L. (1995). More frequent diagnosis of attention deficit-hyperactivity disorder. *New England Journal of Medicine*, **333**, 944.

Swanson, J., Castellanos, F.X., Murias, M., LaHoste, G.J. and Kennedy, J. (1998b). Cognitive neuroscience of attention deficit hyperactivity disorder and hyperkinetic disorder. *Current Opinion in Neurobiology*, **8**, 263–71.

Swanson, J., Gupta, S., Guinta, D. et al. (1999). Acute tolerance to methylphenidate in the treatment of attention deficit/hyperactivity disorder in children. *Clinical Pharmacology and Therapeutics*, **66**, 295–305.

Swanson, J., Greenhill, L., Pelham, W. et al. (2000a). Initiating Concerta™ (OROS® methylphenidate HCl) qd in children with attention-deficit hyperactivity disorder. *Journal of Clinical Research*, **3**, 59–76.

Swanson, J.M., Flodman, P., Kennedy, J. et al. (2000b). Dopamine genes and ADHD. *Neuroscience Biobehavioral Reviews*, **24**, 21–5.

Swanson, J.M., Sergeant, J.A., Taylor, E. et al. (1998a). Seminar: attention-deficit hyperactivity disorder and hyperkinetic disorder. *Lancet*, **351**, 429–33.

Tannock, R. (1998). Attention deficit hyperactivity disorder: advances in cognitive, neurobiological, and genetic research. *Journal of Child Psychology and Psychiatry*, **39**, 65–99.

Teicher, M.H., Anderson, C.M., Polcari, A. et al. (2000). Functional deficits in basal ganglia of children with attention-deficit/hyperactivity disorder shown with functional magnetic resonance imaging relaxometry. *Nature Medicine*, **6**, 470–3.

Tokuno, H., Takada, M., Kaneko, T., Shigemoto, R. and Mizuno, N. (1996). Patchy distribution of substance P receptor immunoreactivity in the developing rat striatum. *Brain Research: Developmental Brain Research*, **95**, 107–17.

Usher, M., Cohen, J.D., Servan-Schreiber, D., Rajkowski, J. and Aston-Jones, G. (1999). The role of locus coeruleus in the regulation of cognitive performance. *Science*, **283**, 549–54.

Vaidya, C.J., Austin, G., Kirkorian, G. et al. (1998). Selective effects of methylphenidate in attention deficit hyperactivity disorder: a functional magnetic resonance imaging study. *Proceedings of the National Academy of Sciences of the United States of America*, **95**, 14 494–9.

van der Kooy, K.D. (1996). Early postnatal lesions of the substantia nigra produce massive shrinkage of the rat striatum, disruption of patch neuron distribution, but no loss of patch neurons. *Brain Research: Developmental Brain Research*, **94**, 242–5.

Vankov, A., Herve-Minvielle, A. and Sara, S.J. (1995). Response to novelty and its rapid habituation in locus coeruleus neurons of the freely exploring rat. *European Journal of Neuroscience*, **7**, 1180–7.

Volkow, N.D., Ding, Y.S., Fowler, J.S. et al. (1995). Is methylphenidate like cocaine? Studies on their pharmacokinetics and distribution in human brain. *Archives of General Psychiatry*, **52**, 456–63.

Volkow, N.D., Wang, G.J., Fowler, J.S. et al. (1997). Effects of methylphenidate on regional brain glucose metabolism in humans: relationship to dopamine D2 receptors. *American Journal of Psychiatry*, **154**, 50–5.

Volkow, N.D., Wang, G.J., Fowler, J.S. et al. (1998a). Differences in regional brain metabolic responses between single and repeated doses of methylphenidate. *Psychiatry Research*, **83**, 29–36.

Volkow, N.D., Wang, G.J., Fowler, J.S. et al. (1998b). Dopamine transporter occupancies in the human brain induced by therapeutic doses of oral methylphenidate. *American Journal of Psychiatry*, **155**, 1325–31.

Wang, G.J., Volkow, N.D., Fowler, J.S. et al. (1995). Comparison of two PET radioligands for imaging extrastriatal dopamine transporters in human brain. *Life Sciences*, **57**, PL-187–PL-191.

Weinberger, D.R., Luchins, D.J., Morihisa, J. and Wyatt, R.J. (1982). Asymmetrical volumes of the right and left frontal and occipital regions of the human brain. *Neurology*, **11**, 97–100.

Wender, P.H. (1973). Some speculations concerning a possible biochemical basis of minimal brain dysfunction. *Annals of the New York Academy of Sciences*, **205**, 18–28.

World Health Organization. (1992). *The ICD-10 Classification of Mental and Behavioural Disorders: Clinical Descriptions and Diagnostic Guidelines.* Geneva, Switzerland: WHO.

World Health Organization. (1993). *The ICD-10 Classification of Mental and Behavioural Disorders: Diagnostic Criteria for Research.* Geneva, Switzerland: WHO.

Yeo, R.A., Hill, D., Campbell, R., Brooks, W.M. and Zamora, L. (2000). A proton magnetic resonance spectroscopy investigation of the right frontal lobe in children with attention deficit hyperactivity disorder. *Journal of Cognitive Neuroscience*, (suppl., 64).

Zahniser, N.R., Dickinson, S.D. and Gerhardt, G.A. (1998). High-speed chronoamperometric electrochemical measurements of dopamine clearance. *Methods in Enzymology*, **296**, 708–19.

Zametkin, A.J., Nordahl, T.E., Gross, M. et al. (1990). Cerebral glucose metabolism in adults with hyperactivity of childhood onset. *New England Journal of Medicine*, **323**, 1361–6.

Zametkin, A.J., Liebenauer, L.L., Fitzgerald, G.A. et al. (1993). Brain metabolism in teenagers with attention-deficit hyperactivity disorder. *Archives of General Psychiatry*, **50**, 333–40.

Zukowska-Grojec, Z. (1998). Neuropeptide Y: an adrenergic cotransmitter, vasoconstrictor, and a nerve-derived vascular growth factor. *Advances in Pharmacology*, **42**, 125–8.

11

Psychosocial contributions

Seija Sandberg

Department of Psychiatry and Behavioural Sciences, Royal Free and University College Medical School, London, UK

Introduction

Environmental and psychosocial factors such as socioeconomic deprivation, family discord and dysfunctional parent–child relationships are well acknowledged as risk factors for disruptive behaviour disorders in childhood. Whether the same adversities also contribute to the causal processes of particular subtypes of childhood behaviour disorder, namely hyperactivity and attention deficit disorders, remains less clear. There are two principal reasons for this. First, compared with biological and especially genetically mediated influences, psychosocial factors have tended to be viewed as peripheral to the aetiology of hyperactivity and attention disorders (Schachar, 1991; Cantwell, 1996; Tannock, 1998). Second, a majority of the evidence available so far concerns disruptive behaviour in general, rather than being specific to hyperactivity and attention disorders. Given the high degree of symptom overlap and diagnostic comorbidity between the two groups of disorders it is often unclear whether the reported associations apply to hyperactivity, conduct disorder, or both. Therefore, the presumed psychosocial correlates of hyperactivity may in fact be those of conduct disorder, or even nonspecific correlates of psychiatric disturbance in general.

There is one possible exception regarding the specificity of psychosocial risk for hyperactivity: this concerns the role that may be played by severely disrupted early attachments, occurring in the contexts of institutional rearing and maternal depression, for example, in contributing to the cause of attention deficit and hyperactivity disorders (Haddad and Garralda, 1992; Sroufe 1997; Sroufe et al., 1999; Chapters 8 and 12).

The aim of this chapter is to review the evidence, predominantly made available in the last decade, for psychosocial contributions to childhood hyperactivity and attention disorders (for earlier studies, the reader is referred to Sandberg and Garralda, 1996). As far as it is reasonably possible, the discussion of environmental correlates will be separated from those with causal or maintaining influence. This is important in order to disentangle the possible mechanisms involved. Second, the likely differential associations and contributions in terms of psychosocial background factors to the development of pure hyperactivity attention deficit disorder on the one hand, and to hyperactivity associated with a significant component of conduct and oppositional disorder, on the other, will be delineated. A further main topic of the chapter will be the evidence for the situational nature of hyperactivity, and the implications this has on the possible role of psychosocial causation.

It is the last-mentioned issue, i.e. situational nature of hyperactivity, that will be discussed first as it highlights the possible psychosocial contributions in a useful way. The second section will deal with the nature of the associated psychosocial factors, and consider the differential contributions to pure hyperactivity and to mixed hyperactivity conduct disorder. The third section will examine possible mechanisms by which psychosocial factors may contribute to the development of hyperactivity and attention disorders. For the sake of readability, the term ADHD used to refer both to hyperkinetic disorder and attention deficit hyperactivity disorder, as understood within the World Health Organization *International Classification of Diseases* (ICD-9 and ICD-10: World Health Organization, 1978, 1992), and the American Psychiatric Association's *Diagnostic and Statistical Manual* (DSM-III-R and DSM-IV: American Psychiatric Association 1987, 1994) classification schemes.

Situational nature of hyperactivity

Scores of studies clearly suggest that a child may be hyperactive at home but not at school, or vice versa; or even hyperactive at home and school, but not in some third situation, on a summer camp or in a clinic testing room, or even in one kind of testing situation but not in another (Taylor et al., 1991; Altepeter and Breen, 1992; Ho et al., 1996; Leung et al., 1996; Breton et al., 1999; Gomez et al., 1999). It is possible that a good deal of the reported difference is more apparent than real, the result of idiosyncratic concepts of what constitutes 'a little' or 'a lot' of hyperactive behaviour as measured by questionnaires, for example, or just different degrees of tolerance of overactive and inattentive behaviour on the part of particular parents and teachers acting as informants. Such low levels of agreement have indeed forced the possibility to be considered that a child's 'hyperactivity' may in fact vary a great deal from situation to situation, and therefore in some cases be 'socially caused', as suggested by Conrad (1976). In this respect, ADHD is by no means unique – rather, 'contextual variation, across time as well as situations, is a hallmark of most childhood problems' (Sroufe, 1997).

Whether or not situational factors are the cause of individual differences in hyperactive behaviour, they are nevertheless likely to play a role in determining how such individual differences are manifested. Furthermore, evidence of strong situational variation in hyperactive behaviour does suggest that environmental factors play a significant role in determining the expression of the disorder. But again, ADHD does not form a particular exception. Apart from autism, the manifestations of most childhood disturbances are greatly influenced by social context (Plomin, 1994, 1995; Sroufe, 1997).

The contextual malleability taken to its extreme could, however, well suggest that any given child placed in a particular environment will be labelled hyperactive, whereas were the same child placed in another environment, he or she may not be called hyperactive. Most people would be reluctant to accept such an extreme position, because we believe that there exists an unknown number, however small, of children who will almost certainly be identified as hyperactive regardless of the way they are treated at home or school. However, what we may wish to learn, or indeed should learn, from such apparently exaggerated propositions is that any examination of the possible associations between the environmental dimensions and hyperactive behaviour must take into account factors potentially contributing to the disorder. These may be to do with basic aetiological mechanisms or, as in most cases, affect the severity or persistence of the problems.

There are also further explanations: hyperactive behaviour may in some cases represent an adaptation to the situation (a hypervigilant child raised in an abusive or violent environment); a conflict within the situation (a toddler living with a severely depressed parent); or a 'comment' on the particular social system (classroom behaviour of a child from a chaotic home). By focusing on 'situational hyperactivity' it may be possible to develop a perspective that returns some meaning to the child's behaviour, in contrast to the one of hyperactivity as purely personal pathology, discounting the situation in which it occurs.

Psychosocial correlates

Social and demographic factors

General population-based surveys have provided conflicting evidence for the extent to which children suffering from ADHD differ from their peers on the basis of fairly straightforward indices of psychosocial background such as social class, family size, intactness of the family unit, etc. For example, large population-based studies of primary school-age boys by Leung et al. (1996) in Hong

Kong, and by Taylor et al. (1991) in London failed to find significant associations between hyperactivity (present both at home and at school) and the usual indices of the children's social and demographic background such as social class, family size and parental unemployment. In contrast, children whose problems are of the pure inattentive type have been shown to differ from community controls by having fathers with low occupational status (Taylor et al., 1991; Warner-Rogers et al., 2000). Some epidemiological studies (Scahill et al., 1999) have, however, reported low social class, often combined with associated high score on a combined index of social disadvantage, to be associated with the diagnosis of ADHD.

In this context it is important to note that factors such as social class and family size can at best be regarded as risk indices that as such don't take us far in trying to understand the mechanisms involved in bringing about particular disorder. Furthermore, it is hardly sufficient to examine selective correlates of an already manifest disorder. Findings based on a mere statistical associations between low social class and attention problems, for example, at best only point to certain likely explanations. Some variables may have stronger differential links with onset of problems, while others may be more related to their persistence (Brooks-Gunn et al., 1995; August et al., 1996a; Conger et al., 1997). Sadly, however, this has frequently been the extent to which a cross-sectional enquiry has been limited. Moreover, these associations are just as likely to have their origins in wider societal influences as in interpersonal interaction patterns between the child and family. These intrafamiliar factors as possible risk mechanisms for the maintenance, even if not causation, of hyperactivity disorder will be the next topic.

Intrafamiliar factors

The stability of the family, the quality of parental relationship, illness in a family member and other chronic intrafamilial stress are all factors that influence the functioning of the family unit. This, in turn, is likely to affect child-rearing conditions, with consequences for the physical and emotional well-being of the children growing up in that particular family. It is therefore plausible that such intrafamilial processes exert their influence on the development of hyperactivity disorder, among other effects. The latest evidence regarding each of these factors will now be examined.

Family stability

When compared with 'normal', nonhyperactive controls, according to some studies hyperactive children have suffered more family instability. Carlson et al.

(1995) followed up a sample of socially disadvantaged families and found that marital disruption (along with intrusive caregiving) best distinguished children suffering from ADHD in middle childhood. Similarly, in a study by Schachar and Wachsmuth (1991) an increased rate of family break-up among hyperactive children was detected. This finding was not, however, endorsed by a community-based survey of primary school-aged boys by Taylor et al. (1991).

Marital discord

Conflictful relationship between the parents has been shown in some studies to be associated with childhood hyperactivity (Jenkins and Smith, 1991). Two caveats, however, are important here. First, the methods of sample selection in most studies do not allow for specific associations between childhood hyperactivity and parental marital problems to be unequivocally demonstrated even if they existed: few studies have differentiated between children suffering from hyperactivity, conduct disorder and the common group with features of the two (Schachar, 1991). In studies where this distinction has been made, no differences have been found in the proportions of children from maritally discordant homes (Marshall et al., 1990), with one exception (Taylor et al., 1991). Even here the association was in a direction opposite to what might have been expected: the children suffering from hyperkinetic disorder (as defined by ICD-9 criteria) significantly less often came from homes characterized by marital problems as compared with a matched group of children diagnosed as conduct-disordered.

Furthermore, rather than involving a direct cause, parents' discordant relationship is likely to exert its negative influence on children's emotional development via a qualitatively altered parent–child interaction. This issue will be discussed more fully in the section on child-specific family environment, below.

Psychiatric disorder in a parent

Mental disorder in a parent represents a definite risk factor for psychiatric disturbance in children (Jensen et al., 1991; Cummings and Davies, 1994; Murray and Cooper, 1997; Rutter et al., 1997a). Nevertheless, rather than increasing the risk of one particular type of childhood disorder, the effect is largely nonspecific. Similarly, when the risks associated with parental mental disorder and the risks stemming from other forms of psychosocial adversity are compared, few differences are found with respect to the common types of emotional and conduct problems in childhood. The implication therefore is that the risk stems from some aspects of family disturbance associated with parental mental disorder rather than from the psychiatric condition in the parent as such.

However, like the studies looking at psychosocial causes in general for childhood hyperactivity, with few exceptions (Schachar and Wachsmuth, 1990; Taylor et al., 1991), most of those aimed at examining the specific role of parental psychiatric illness have been methodologically inadequate. This is because the studies have either relied on clinical samples or failed to provide independent assessments of child behaviour and parental psychiatric state. The main problem with studies relying on clinical samples is that, given the diversity of factors influencing referral to a specialist service, it is likely that the presence of parental psychiatric disorder in itself increases the chances of a child with an existing problem behaviour, such as hyperactivity, being referred. This means that the correlations between hyperactivity and parental disorder are probably artificially high in clinic-based studies.

The issue of nonindependence of measurement of child behaviour and parents' psychiatric problems is pertinent to all studies relying on information obtained by questionnaires completed by parents of child hyperactivity. However, an equally plausible explanation for the high correlation would be that the distressed mothers perceived more hyperactivity in their children's behaviour than did the nondistressed mothers, i.e. the child behaviour in fact has been very similar. Therefore, when interpreting research findings we should be alerted to the possibility that depressed mothers will have a tendency to rate their children's behaviour as more deviant than objective assessments of behaviour warrant – an issue which is pertinent to interpreting questionnaire-based research of child behaviour (Murray et al., 1999). This parental quality is likely to be at least partly rooted in a disturbed perception and cognitive distortion due to depressed affect, and also to reduced tolerance for child misconduct in a depressed parent (Bendell et al., 1994).

Conclusions regarding psychosocial correlates

Psychosocial correlates such as family stability, marital discord or parents' mental health are primarily features characterizing the overall family environment. Therefore, as such they are likely to influence the general child-rearing conditions of the family unit in question. When assessed in terms of being 'present' or 'absent' they have to be viewed as factors exerting a 'shared' environmental influence on all children growing up in that particular family, and it would be hard to claim that they impinge on one child any more than on another. To argue the latter, these factors need to be specifically defined and measured in relation to a particular child.

Maintaining psychosocial factors

Child-specific family environment

The role of intrafamilial factors as likely contributors to the maintenance of children's hyperactive behaviour has been extensively reviewed by Barkley (Barkley, 1990a; Barkley et al., 1992). In his account, Barkley noted the many problems hyperactive children have in their relationships with their families, but also quite clearly argued that the negative interactions in the first place stem from the hyperactive child, rather than it being the case that the behaviour of other family members brings about hyperactivity in the child. This evidence predominantly rests on studies that have examined the interactions between hyperactive children and their mothers, often in the context of stimulant medication trials (Hinshaw and McHale, 1991). The interactions of hyperactive children and their fathers, as well as siblings, also show similar patterns of conflict, although to a lesser degree (Taylor et al., 1991). There is also evidence from several studies suggesting that hyperactive children elicit similar negative, controlling and generally directive behaviours from adults, such as teachers, outside the family (Barkley, 1990a; Hinshaw and McHale, 1991).

Parent–child interactions

The conclusions on the nature of the parent–child relationship in hyperactivity have traditionally been based on observational studies of mother–child interaction, and it is only relatively recently that the role of fathers and siblings has been considered. Accordingly, this review will first deal with qualities of the relationship between hyperactive children and their mothers in home-based observations of mother–child interaction. The results show that the key differences between hyperactive and nonhyperactive children appear less to do with the amount of parent–child interaction than with the patterns of the interaction. Parents of ADHD children tend to make specific, rather than general, remarks and seldom offer the child positive encouragement. The mothers of non-ADHD children make an equal number of remarks, but they contain fewer specific suggestions. These mothers also encouraged persistence and provided answers only when the child requested them (see Danforth et al. (1991) for a review; Chapter 8).

The issue of child-specific interactions within the context of the social and family factors discussed above will now be examined more closely. The following topics will be specifically dealt with:

(1)   affective content of parent–child relationship

(2)   styles of parenting

(3)   parental psychiatric illness

(4)   marital discord

(5)   the effect of drug therapy on the relationship between hyperactive children and their parents.

Affective content of parent–child relationship

Research in the area of parenting and child hyperactivity has tended to focus on child compliance with parental commands and directives. However, there exists clear evidence for the need to broaden our conceptualization of parenting in relation to child hyperactivity (Marshall et al., 1990; Dix, 1991; Feldman et al., 1999). Thus, in their two-stage epidemiological study Taylor et al. (1991), for example, showed that mothers of pervasively hyperactive boys were more often rated as lacking warmth but expressing high levels of criticism towards the child than the mothers of any of the comparison group children (i.e. boys showing conduct problems without hyperactivity, or inattentiveness without hyperactivity, or the random community controls). The higher levels of criticism also held for the fathers. In addition, mothers' coping skills with the child's challenging behaviour and 'emotional upsets' were significantly poorer in the pervasively hyperactive groups (regardless of whether hyperactivity occurred on its own or in combination with other behaviour problems). Critical expressed emotion from parents was also a predictor of worse long-term outcome in an untreated group of children with hyperactivity (Rutter et al., 1997b).

These findings were largely replicated in a subsequent study (Woodward et al., 1998) involving 28 pervasively hyperactive boys, aged 7–10, and their 30 classroom controls from two outer London boroughs. Poor parent coping, disciplinary aggression, negative affect, lower parental sensitivity to child needs and authoritative parenting style were significantly associated with hyperactivity. Furthermore, the results suggest that negative affect and parental insensitivity may be attributable to their respective associations with parent mental health and child conduct problems. Children whose parents were coping less well with child challenging behaviour were 3.3 times more likely to be hyperactive, and 2.5 times more likely to be hyperactive if their parents used harsh and aggressive discipline methods. However, given the correlational nature of the associations, the direction of the effect between parent coping and disciplinary aggression and hyperactivity cannot be determined.

Styles of parenting

Findings common to two epidemiological studies, one carried out in Hong Kong (Leung et al., 1996) and one in East London (Taylor et al., 1991), indicate a significant association between inconsistent parenting styles and childhood hyperactivity. The characteristic highlighted by both surveys is parental disagreement in how to handle challenging child behaviour, and in some cases a near-complete laissez faire attitude of the parents. Further characteristics of parenting that have been shown to correlate with child hyperactive behaviour are lowered parental aspirations regarding the child's academic achievement, less parental involvement and interest in the child's early learning, and less opportunities and encouragement offered to the child.

Another indicator of severe child-specific psychosocial stress of possible relevance has been highlighted by a study by Famularo et al. (1992), which draws attention to excessively punitive child-rearing practices as a possible contributor to hyperactivity. A group of 61 maltreated children, aged 5–10 years and drawn from attenders to a juvenile court, were compared with 35 control children. The two groups were compared on diagnoses based on a structured psychiatric interview, carried out separately with the child and the parent. The children who had suffered maltreatment significantly more often received the diagnosis of ADHD (as well as conduct disorder and posttraumatic stress disorder) than controls. Whether physical child maltreatment was a characteristic of parenting even before the children showed signs of hyperactivity, or whether it resulted from an inappropriate style of parental control brought about by the child's difficult behaviour in the first place cannot be ascertained on the basis of data provided. However, there is evidence to suggest that the parents of hyperactive children are inclined to use more discipline, and particularly resort to physical methods of disciplining the child, even when compared with behaviour problem controls (Marshall et al., 1990; Barkley et al., 1991).

Maternal depression

The relationship between psychiatric illness in a parent and behavioural difficulties in the offspring is well established. It is especially depression in the mother as a contributory factor to difficult parent–child interactions that has received most attention (Downey and Coyne, 1990; Hibbs et al., 1991; Cummings and Davies, 1994). In the East London study by Taylor et al. (1991), maternal depression was associated with both teacher and parent interview assessment of the children's hyperactive behaviour. Furthermore, the presence of depressive illness in the mother during the previous year correlated significantly with persistence of such a pervasive form of child hyperactivity.

Depressed mothers have been shown to be more critical, disapproving, aversive and less positive in their interactions with their children than mothers who are not depressed (Field, 1992; Murray and Cooper, 1997). More specifically, depressed mothers are also more likely to initiate hostile behaviours towards their children in an indiscriminative manner rather than this being contingent on the immediately preceding child behaviour. However, certain characteristics of the child are also more likely to predict unsatisfactory 'linking' of mother–child responses when the mother is depressed; these are existing emotional or behavioural disturbance and poor expressive language skills. Both of these factors are relevant here: hyperactive children, when younger, frequently have less well-developed language skills and show difficult temperamental characteristics, which are easily perceived as 'bad behaviour' (Taylor et al., 1991).

On the other hand, it has been observed that, with depressed mothers, the child has to get attention by high intensity of demand. Furthermore, there is also a matching unfavourable response from the child: even if the depressed mother succeeds in picking up the child's 'cue', though possibly in a less finely tuned manner, the child response in turn is less likely to be contingent, either in tone or content, on the mother's response (Murray et al., 1993, 1996b; Campbell et al., 1995). The endresult of this interactional pattern is a poorer 'meshing' of parent–child responses, with both parties frequently failing to sustain interaction and effectively meet each other's approaches.

Thus, it appears that associations between maternal depression and child behaviour stem from a mixture of factors. Depressed mothers have altered perceptions on child misconduct and perhaps less tolerance of child behaviour in general. In addition, they also use excessive disapproval, irritability and aversiveness, and less approval and less positive behaviour in their interactions with their children than nondepressed mothers would to the same behaviours. However, the children of depressed mothers also display more aversion in their interactions with their mothers, as well as behaving more aggressively towards them (Campbell et al., 1996).

Given the considerable hereditary evidence for hyperactivity, the issue also needing to be raised here relates to the fact that, because the parents who are providing the parenting experiences are also passing on genes, there is the possibility that the risks from adverse experiences are, at least partially, genetically mediated, either in relation to hyperactivity in particular (Frick and Jackson, 1993) or psychiatric disturbance in general (Plomin and Bergeman, 1991; Plomin, 1995). This has even been suggested by adoption studies showing that psychopathology in the biological parents is associated with more negative parenting by the adoptive parents (Ge et al., 1996; O'Connor et al., 1998); the children's genetically influenced disruptive behaviour thus has an effect on the parents. The same research has also shown effects on the children of the parents' behaviour, thus supporting the existence of a two-way interactive process.

In summary, the findings referred to above quite clearly suggest that the effects of parental depression or other forms of psychiatric disturbance on child behaviour are likely to be via the interactions between the parent and child. Furthermore, when allowing for a psychiatric disorder in a parent, the qualities of the child are important in determining which child, and to what extent, becomes the recipient of negative parental behaviour and attitudes: a temperamentally difficult or demanding child, or one who has a problem in communicating, is more likely to become the target of parental anger and irritation than a more placid child with a more 'easy-going' disposition.

Marital discord

Marital discord may function in a similar manner to depression in altering parental perceptions and styles of management of child behaviour (Jenkins and Smith, 1991). The combination of maternal depression and marital discord results in even higher rates of perceived child deviance and actual parent–child conflict, as well as child aggression, than the presence of these two factors in isolation (Campbell et al., 1996; Murray et al., 1996a). Furthermore, there tends to be a high correlation between maternal depression and marital discord in any given family. Aversive mother–child interactions tend also to be further increased in families where depressed mothers themselves experience a greater degree of negative interaction with other adults, such as spouses or relatives.

It is therefore highly likely that marital discord, maternal depression, paternal antisocial behaviour and marital aggression are significantly interrelated in the families of some hyperactive children (Barkley et al., 1992). It is this subgroup of hyperactive children with multiple features of family dysfunction who in turn are at a particular risk for developing additional conduct disorder (Taylor et al., 1991). The psychosocial risk factors for hyperactivity associated with the significant component of conduct disorder will be examined in more detail in the next section.

Effect of medication on parent–child relationship

A number of studies have demonstrated that methylphenidate given to hyperactive children results in significant reductions in child negative and off-task behaviour, as well as in an increase in both contingent and sustained compliance (Barkley, 1990a; Hinshaw and McHale, 1991). Furthermore, a child being placed on methylphenidate has been shown to increase expressed maternal warmth and decrease maternal criticism (Schachar et al., 1987), whereas, family cohesion, efficiency of parental coping and the pattern of interpersonal family interaction remained unchanged.

Caution is, however, needed against interpreting the results of methylphenidate studies in an unduly optimistic light. On the surface, the early mother–child interaction studies by Barkley and his colleagues (summarized in Barkley, 1990a), have showed a significant increase in child compliance and decrease in mother directiveness and intrusiveness when the hyperactive child is placed on psychostimulant medication. However, at the same time other changes have also been noted taking place: while on the active drug the children tend to become less sociable, which means that they initiate fewer interactions with the mother and generally become less responsive. Drugs like methylphenidate make children less sociable. As a result, instead of actively interacting with their environment, the children tend to engage in solitary play. Because in most studies maternal responses have been rated as 'conditional' to child behaviour, it is possible that the apparent increase in maternal positive attitudes, as displayed in the mothers' interactions with their children, is at least partly a reflection of the children simply demanding or requiring less attention and interaction when placed on methylphenidate. One might also argue, albeit somewhat speculatively, that in a situation analogous to that involving depressed mothers and their children, the child 'keeping to himself' is welcomed by the mother because it 'leaves her alone'. Thus, negative interaction could largely be replaced by lack of interaction – a fact that might easily be overlooked when interpreting findings of similar studies. Such a conclusion would also receive support from the recent MTA study (The MTA Cooperative Group, 1999; Chapter 13). Among the socioeconomically disadvantaged group a decrease in parent-reported closeness and positive interactions with their children on medication was noted.

It therefore appears legitimate to ask whether the controlling and intrusive behaviour on the part of the mothers is, besides a response to the child's overactive behaviour, also contributing to the child's behavioural difficulties in the first place. This possibility is highlighted by the lack of a balancing positive response on the part of the mother to child compliance, as succinctly demonstrated by Gardner (1994) in an observation study of preschool-age children with teacher-identified behaviour problems. The study showed the mothers of problem children to be particularly ready to respond with criticism and intrusiveness when the child did something wrong, but at the same time slow to offer positive comments and praise when the child behaved well.

Psychosocial causes of hyperactivity

Sroufe (1997) has poignantly noted that 'pathology is not something a child "has", it is a pattern of adaptation reflecting the totality of the developmental context to that point' (p. 258). Along with others he has also stressed the need to abandon the search for single pathogens, conceptualized as linear causes for a particular outcome, and search for complex influences initiating developmental pathways (Cicchetti and Tucker, 1994; Rutter, 1996; Seifer et al., 1996; Sroufe, 1997). Furthermore, the aetiology of disturbance is best conceptualized in terms of a combination of risk factors and protective factors of diverse sorts, and the way these arise, evolve, combine and recombine over time. Besides, such influences are only probabilistically associated with disturbed behaviour.

This also applies to the relationship between parental behaviour and child problems of inattention and hyperactivity. As is well acknowledged (Barkley, 1990a), managing a child with ADHD problems is very difficult. Therefore, it would seem quite natural for parents to be controlling and even critical of such a child. If then with intervention the child's problems decrease, one would also expect controllingness to decline. Such a finding in no way removes the relevance of care-giving factors to aetiology. How child factors interact with parenting variables has, however, been little explored so far.

Disrupted attachments

More than two decades ago Tizard and Hodges (1978) presented powerful evidence that disruptive early experiences, such as institutional rearing and parenting breakdown, are associated with overactivity and attentional problems in a school-aged child. The association between disrupted parenting and hyperactivity appears to apply especially when disrupted parenting occurs before the age of 3 years, suggesting that there is a sensitive attachment period when certain cognitive as well as social skills are acquired (Hersov, 1990; Greenberg et al., 1993; Speltz et al., 1999). Disrupting this developmentally vital process would lead to continuing parallel problems of overactivity and poor social relationships.

Subsequently, Haddad and Garralda (1992) described school-age children presenting to child psychiatric clinics with a combination of hyperkinetic syndrome and severely disrupted early experiences. In children with such life histories hyperactivity was unaccompanied by biological indicators; the problem behaviour had an onset in early childhood and had persisted in spite of children having lived for years in stable substitute families. Furthermore, hyperactivity in these children was associated with other features of attachment disorders such as attention-seeking behaviour, indiscriminate friendliness, poorly modulated peer interactions, and in some cases hoarding of food. The authors argued that early deprivation would have resulted in difficulties by the children in developing enduring attachments and an inner sense of emotional security, and led to problems in controlling and regulating attention and activity levels. It is, however, unclear whether the emotional insecurity and poor sense of safety and consequent disrupted attachments are the crucial factor leading to hyperactivity in children who have experienced major early disruptions (Chapter 12).

The period involving the first 3 years of life is seen as important, not just for social and emotional development, but also for the development of the regulation of motor and attentional behaviours (Chapter 8). Lack of adequate availability for the child of the mother, or the main caretaker, at this crucial time, would result in persisting dysfunction in the child's ability to regulate attention and motor activity. This is likely to be due to the failure to experience the required sense of security drawn from the predictability of the mother's presence. There is also evidence that a history of patterned responsive care is central in tuning and balancing excitatory and inhibitory systems in the central nervous system itself (Schore, 1994). This would in turn support emotional regulation and behavioural flexibility. In accord with the developmental model, avoidant and disorganized patterns of attachment may be thought of as initial developmental variations, probabilistically associated with later disturbance (Sroufe, 1997; Sroufe et al., 1999). Also, a good deal of evidence suggests that the attachment pattern with each parent/caregiver is different (Fox et al., 1991), and changes as a function of that parent's changing life stress. The quality of a particular attachment relationship, whether secure or anxious, is based on the history of interaction within the pair. (See the section on experience dependent brain development, below.)

Patterns, as evolving in a given attachment relationship, are taken forward at the behavioural level as well. The child has been entrained into particular patterns of reciprocity and affective sharing, as well as having evolved a sense of curiosity and a skill in exploration, supported by the secure attachment. Supporting the behavioural level are patterns of arousal regulation, which will allow the full range of emotional expression with sufficient modulation, such that organized behaviour can be maintained. Such patterns are readily established in the context of responsive care, because responsiveness entails appropriate affective stimulation and interventions to keep arousal within reasonable bounds.

Olson (Chapter 8) has reviewed the evidence regarding attachment anomalies and overactivity. Although not entirely unequivocal, the available studies offer evidence that the security of the mother–child attachment is related to a toddler's willingness to comply with the mother's request and engage in constructive problem solving, as well as 'on-task' behaviour. Thus, securely attached children are on the whole more compliant, enthusiastic and attentive to maternal suggestions than insecurely attached children. Security of mother–infant attachments has also been found to predict cognitive nonimpulsivity and ability to delay gratification at the time the child enters school (Olson et al., 1990). Conversely, insecurity of early mother–child attachments has been shown to be related to teacher ratings of behavioural impulsivity and interpersonal hostility in preschool age.

The disorganized subtype of attachment is one of the atypical patterns that does not fit previously defined categories (Main and Solomon, 1990; Barnett and Vondra, 1999). Infants with this attachment type lack a consistent strategy for organizing security seeking following the stress of maternal separation. The pattern is most prevalent in high-risk samples, where it has in turn been linked to lack of maternal responsiveness. Several studies now indicate that infants with disorganized attachment are at elevated risk for later disruptive behaviour problems (Lyons-Ruth, 1996), often with high levels of aggression in preschool years (Greenberg et al., 1991; Speltz et al., 1999).

Parental psychopathology

The role of parental psychiatric disorder as a causal influence on childhood hyperactivity has been the focus of several studies. The findings, though somewhat inconsistent, have pointed towards maternal depression possibly contributing to the cause of hyperactivity in the younger age group. Various routes for this effect to come about have been postulated, all of them primarily operating via the disordered interaction between mother and child, and through this adversely influencing the child's ability to achieve cognitive competence or ability to modulate his or her activity level. These results can be interpreted as showing that young children's attention is affected by their mother's illness. The most likely mechanism by which this happens is via an impaired mother–child relationship – the attachment relationship possibly being the crucial one (Seifer et al., 1996) – engendered by psychiatric disorder, especially major depression.

At the same time, it needs to be noted that maternal depression involves a specific condition of biological and environmental stress. Infants of depressed mothers have been shown to differ from infants whose mothers are not depressed by having more frequent negative facial expressions, more irregular sleep and by being less active and crying less (Field, 1995; Field et al., 1995; Jones et al., 1997). The infants of depressed mothers also exhibit greater right frontal asymmetry (due to reduced left frontal activation). The explanations offered for this have included biological or genetic predisposition, prenatal influences caused by elevated stress hormone levels and learned depressive pattern of interaction. These features suggest greater physiological disequilibrium, which is reflected, for example, in the electroencephalogram.

In this respect the findings of the work by Murray and her colleagues (1993, 1996a,b, 1999) examining the influence of postnatal depression on later child adjustment are particularly relevant. The results, based on a low-risk community sample, indicated that several aspects of child behaviour at the age of 5 years were related to the occurrence of maternal depression in the early postpartum months. This applied, independently of the child's gender and family social class, even when account was taken of current circumstances such as marked conflict between parents or a recent episode of depression in the mother. Furthermore, none of the effects of postnatal depression was explained by the child's earlier impairments in cognitive functioning.

At 5 years of age the children displayed diminished responsiveness in their interactions with the mother, even in cases where the mother's behaviour had shown some recovery. The children also manifested more disturbed behaviour at home, as compared with school. However, the child's home behaviour was not related to the early attachment patterns. This the authors attributed to two possible reasons: either a child's attachment system may not be specifically challenged in the home environment or many avenues are open to the child for the expression of insecurity, particularly of the avoidant type, in behaviours that bear no relation to the symptoms of disturbance assessed in maternal questionnaire reports, as they may be adaptive in that particular context. At school, instead, the children's play appeared to lack planning and structure, and there was little social contact with peers.

Early mother–infant relationship in the context of postnatal depression is characterized by reduced quality of interaction (Stein et al., 1991), raised levels of maternal hostility and failure to acknowledge infant autonomy (Field, 1992), even in low-risk samples (Murray et al., 1993). It therefore seems possible that, despite the mother's subsequent recovery from depression, these initial attitudes to the infant may set up a cycle of marked difficulties that come to influence the child's subsequent behaviour. This is consistent with the findings of Field et al. (1993) and Bendell et al. (1994), who reported that postpartum depressed mothers' early perceptions of their infants were more negative compared with those of independent observers, and showed considerable continuity throughout preschool years.

Concluding remarks

A number of environmental factors have been suggested as playing a causal role in hyperactivity disorders. These include maternal depression and inter-parental discord. Because of their known associations, both these factors may lead to overactivity via any of the mechanisms described above. Thus, maternal depression has been shown to be associated with suboptimal parenting and poor parent–child relationship, with delayed cognitive development in young children, with behavioural and with attachment disorders. Furthermore, parental discord is commonly found in association with maternal depression.

Therefore, it may be concluded that there does seem to exist some theoretical, clinical and empirical support for the possibility that the mechanisms described above mediate the links between family and environmental factors and the causation of childhood hyperactivity. However, much of the evidence is indirect, and the relative validity and specificity of these mechanisms in relation to different types of comorbidity can only be ascertained by future clinical observations and carefully targeted research.

Genes versus experiences

Of the 30 000 or so genes expressed in the human body, possibly as many as one-half may be specifically expressed in the brain. However, while the basic wiring of the central nervous system is genetically preprogrammed, its fine tuning throughout different phases of infancy, childhood and adulthood is highly experience-dependent (Hopkin, 1997; Post and Weiss, 1997). The genetically predetermined sequence of neurodevelopment proceeds from lower to higher brain centres, from the brain stem to the cerebral cortex (Nelson and Bloom, 1997). At the same time there exists the potential for plasticity in both the developing and mature brain (Emerit et al., 1992; Linden, 1994; Abraham and Bear, 1996). Some of this plasticity is mediated through neuronal activity (neurotransmission). For processes such as emotional memory, this neuroplasticity appears to occur at large numbers of synapses, with increasing complexity and self-organization. The higher-order and integrative systems such as cortical association areas and prefrontal cortex further help to integrate emotion and experience, guiding the person's subsequent actions and enabling him or her to plan for the future, for example (Schore, 1994).

Consequently, it is also apparent that the subtleties of individual responsiveness and responses by others can make a major impact on gene expression and on the longlasting sequelae of traumatic and other types of experience, pertinent to emotional and cognitive development (Mack, 1995; Plomin, 1995; Yehuda et al., 1995). Given the strong hereditary influence in hyperactivity as evidenced in family, adoption and twin studies (Chapter 9), it is natural that the focus has recently moved towards directly searching for a candidate gene for the disorder. The focus is on genes within the dopamine system. The potential candidacy of 7-repeat allele is particularly interesting for cross-ethnic studies (Chapter 3). It has, however, been suggested that this particular allele may turn out to be virtually absent in some ethnic groups (such as Asian populations, for example), while hyperactivity occurs there none the less. This would be more proof of the potent role of environment in determining how and where genes express themselves.

Impact of stressful experiences on the brain

There are many possibilities by which the effects of stressful experiences may be carried forward in time. Persistence may come about because the initial adverse experiences led to altered patterns of interpersonal interaction that, in turn, brought about further negative experiences (Rutter and the English and Romanian Adoptees Study Team, 1998). Alternatively, experiences such as physical or emotional abuse may lead to altered styles of emotional and cognitive processing (Dodge et al., 1990, 1995). A further possibility is that stress affects neuroendocrine structure and function, as suggested by findings in both animals (Sapolsky, 1996a,b; Liu et al., 1997) and humans (McEwen and Sapolsky, 1995; Hart et al., 1996). There is also some indication that this may happen with prenatal stressors (Kraemer, 1992; Kraemer and Clarke, 1996; Schneider et al., 1998). The mechanism with respect to severe and lasting early adversities could also lie in the developmental programming of the brain (Stone, 1992; Singer, 1995). It has been well demonstrated through animal studies that sensory input is necessary for the normal development of the visual cortex, and it is likely that there are parallel experience-dependent neural development effects with respect to other experiences (Thoenen, 1995; Pollak et al., 1997).

Animal studies of severe stress have shown that this can result in hippocampal damage (Liu et al., 1997). There is also limited evidence that the neural effects of social privation may differ from those of separation stresses. It remains uncertain whether the similar effects apply in humans, but it is reasonable to suppose that they may (Bremner et al., 1997; Bremner and Narayan, 1998).

Prenatal stress

Primate research has presented strong evidence that chronic unpredictable stress during pregnancy may have longlasting effects on brain activity and behaviour of the offspring (Schneider et al., 1998). The postulated mechanism for this action is that prenatal stress affects the neurobiology of the neonate so that its responses to common events and stimuli are markedly altered. However, its effects on brain mechanisms are likely to be diffuse, rather than specific. As a consequence, the neonate may, for example, be more fussy and difficult, and in turn this affects how the caregiver is able to cope. In this way, prenatal stress may set the infant's neurobiology into a state in which vital attachments are hard to achieve and adverse experiences are more likely (Kraemer, 1992; Kraemer and Clarke, 1996).

Prenatal effects on fetal neurobiological development may be easily confused with genetic predisposition. It therefore remains a challenge to future research to determine how prenatal environmental effects contribute to persisting and trait-like organization of neurobiological systems. This, in turn, would markedly further our understanding of how genetic and post-natal environmental factors play a role in the expression of developmental psychopathology (Schore, 1994; Trevarthen and Aitken, 1994; Sroufe et al., 1999).

Experience-dependent brain development

The recent evidence concerning experience-dependent brain development (Greenough et al., 1987; Kraemer, 1992; Cicchetti and Tucker, 1994; Schore, 1994; Kim et al., 1997; Hockfield and Lombroso, 1998) makes it clear that there are substantial experiential influences on the development of the central nervous system, including the tuning of systems concerned with activation and regulation of affect and behaviour. Inadequate input from the environment not only results in downregulation, but if it is of sufficient proportion, in neuronal and dendritic retraction, and ultimately preprogrammed cell death, perhaps as the extreme result of disuse (Goodman and Shatz, 1993; Katz and Shatz, 1996). Neglect during early developmental periods can have devastating consequences likened to those caused by extreme starvation, as seen for example in Romanian orphanages (Kaler and Freeman, 1994; Carlson and Earls, 1997; Chapter 12).

Mechanisms involved in neuronal learning and memory are used and reused not only in sculpting the brain in its initial establishment, but also in the moulding of behaviour and personality, based on experience (Edelman, 1992; Abraham and Bear, 1996). In the light of this, it is likely that phenomena such as overexcitation or deprivation can profoundly affect the neuronal substrates involved in cognitive and emotional development (Mesulam, 1990; Brown, 1994; Byrne and Kandel, 1996).

Animal studies provide further evidence for the potential longlasting impact of early experience, not only on behaviour and cognitive function, but also on important neural substrates mediating affect on anatomical and biochemical levels (Plotsky and Meaney, 1993; McEwen, 1994). For example, repeated separations from the mother in the immediate postnatal period can lead to lifelong disturbance in the immunological functions, or to dependence on substrates such as cocaine and alcohol (Plotsky, 1997). Likewise, there is animal evidence for the deleterious effects of maternal distress on other endocrine functions in the offspring, a phenomenon closely resembling severe depression in humans (Pihoker et al., 1993; Coplan et al., 1996). Conversely, longlasting consequences for brain anatomy and biochemistry of enriched environments in increasing the number of synapses and dendritic sprouting have been demonstrated (Meaney et al., 1988; Wallace et al., 1992; Liu et al., 1997).

Neglect and traumatic experiences

It has been suggested that there are some important differences between the effects of neglect and traumatic experiences on the maturing brain (Rieder and Cicchetti, 1989; Winslow et al., 1993; Perry, 1996; Pollak et al., 1997; see also review by Glaser, 2000). The absence of crucial experiences such as touch, love or being spoken to can lead to permanent absence of capabilities, reflected by the lack of growth of parts of the brain. In the case of a traumatic experience, it is the abnormal and persisting presence of response which may profoundly alter an existing part of the brain.

There are good reasons to believe that it is easier to treat and mend a part of the brain that has been impaired by trauma than it is to grow a part anew after the critical periods of childhood are over. The situation is particularly bleak for those young children who are forced to undergo repeated episodes of physical or sexual abuse, and the deprivation and neglect associated with such contexts. The neglect might lead to deficient development of neural systems responsible for emotional and cognitive modulation, while at the same time memories of traumatic experiences may be etched into the brain, thereby doubling the set of maldevelopmental lesions (Rieder and Cicchetti, 1989; Pollak et al., 1997).

Of the 30 or so neurotransmitters in the central nervous system, biogenic amines, such as noradrenaline (norepinephrine), adrenaline (epinephrine), dopamine and serotonin, play a central role in mediating an alarm reaction. Short periods of threat result in the mobilization of the alarm reaction and restoration towards normal. Persistence of threat, or an extremely traumatic single event, has the capacity to redefine the baseline level, resulting in a dysfunctional or maladaptive set of brain activities (Giller et al., 1990; see also Rogeness et al., 1992; Rogeness and McClure, 1996). One of the core neuro-transmitter systems in stress response is the noradrenergic nucleus, the locus ceruleus, with its neurons originating in the pons, a more primitive part of the brain, but with projections throughout the brain. The locus ceruleus plays a critical role in arousal, vigilance, regulation of affect, behavioural irritability, locomotion, attention, sleep regulation and startle response (Svensson, 1987; Fillenz, 1990).

In general, the earlier and the more pervasive the trauma, the more brain development will be disrupted with an impact on emotional, cognitive and behavioural functions (Lauder, 1988; LeDoux et al., 1989; Courchesne et al., 1994). Children exposed to neglect or prolonged abuse early in life almost by rule have little cognitive understanding of how the anxiety, impulsivity and social and emotional distress they suffer are related to the memories their brains have created (Perry, 1996).

The brain's record of experiences
Sensory experiences leave their mark on the brain by altering the synapses between neurons (Bear, 1997). However, unless these modifications are con-solidated, the synaptic strengths decay back to their original state and the memory is lost. Research suggests that memories may reside in the very core of a neuronal cell, the nucleus, and be maintained by self-sustaining changes of protein synthesis in gene transcription (Frey and Morris, 1997). The vividness of 'flashbulb' memories may derive in part from this cellular mechanism.

It has been argued that all parts of the brain have capabilities for changing in response to alterations in neuronal activity (Post and Weiss, 1997). This can be taken to mean that all parts of the brain store information and have, in some sense memory (Squire, 1992). The specific nature of the memory, and the kind of information stored and recalled, differs depending on its function. The word 'memory' for most part has come to signify some aspect of cognitive memory, accessible to words and residing in the cortex of the brain. The emotional and history-dependent context of experiences, on the other hand, is largely laid down at the amygdala and hippocampus (LeDoux, 1992, 1994; Rolls, 1992; Xu et al., 1997; Lombroso and Sapolsky, 1998). Such memories commonly mani-fest as 'first impressions'. Activation of the motor vestibular parts of the brain, such as basal ganglia, gives rise to motor memory (Greenwald et al., 1996; Knowlton et al., 1996). The sensitizing, chronic or prolonged activation of state-regulating parts situated in the brain stem and midbrain leads to the development of state memories (Greenwald et al., 1996; Knowlton et al., 1996). These same areas also modulate physiological reactivity, vigilance, anxiety, emotional lability, behavioural impulsivity and sleep. Negative-state memories are created, for example, by domestic violence and other traumatic stress.

Traumatic events disrupt familiar patterns and cause disequilibrium. They do this by influencing and altering brain functioning from the cortex (cognition) to the brain stem (the site of core physiological state regulation; Post et al., 1997). When repeated over time, a thought recalling the trauma may activate limbic, basal ganglia and brain stem areas, resulting in emotional, motor and arousal or state changes that are functional residuals associated with the original event (Perry, 1994). Conversely, a state may lead to activation in the amygdala, resulting in an emotional change, which may or may not be sufficient to activate associated cognitive memories (LeDoux, 1989). The external or internal triggers may not be something the person is aware of. A particular aspect of acute stressors occurring in the neonatal period is that they may become associated with longlasting deficits, based on the formation of long-term memory traces. For this reason, the early acquisition of emotional memory, mediated through amygdala, in the absence of a fully developed cortex, may remain particularly fixed (LeDoux et al., 1989).

Use-dependent learning and state-dependent storage and recall
The brain changes in use-dependent fashion (Mack, 1995; Post and Weiss, 1997). The alterations in brain functioning take place in response to specific repetitive patterns of activation, and result in changes of cognition, emotional and motor functioning and state regulation capacity. Mismatch between the modality of teaching and the receptive portions of a child's brain occurs frequently. This is particularly true with regard to the learning experiences of a traumatized child – sitting in a classroom in a persistent state of arousal, anxiety or dissociated (Perry et al., 1995; Castro-Alamancos and Connors, 1996). In a constantly aroused child the primary areas of the brain which process information are different from those of a child who remains calm (McNally et al., 1990).

Two children may have the same results on an IQ test, but only the one who is relaxed can focus on the words of the teacher, and using his or her cortex, engage in abstract cognition. The child in an alarm state will be less efficient at processing and storing verbal information. The child's cognition will be dominated by subcortical and limbic areas, focusing on nonverbal information – the teacher's facial expressions and hand gestures – and consequently, the child will appear distracted. The fact that the sense of time is altered in alarm states also has implications for understanding the thinking of a traumatized child. With his or her sense of future foreshortened, the child finds it almost impossible to think of the future even days ahead (Perry et al., 1995). Also, immediate reward is most reinforcing, and delayed gratification most improbable.

Developmental consequences

During development, if a stress response is required to be frequently and persistently active, the brain may mirror the environment and the whole system may become overactive and hypersensitive (Perry, 1994, 1996). However, it is highly adaptive for an individual developing in a violent or chaotic environment to be hypervigilant, hypersensitive to external stimuli and remain in a ready state of alarm. It is also possible that many states of distress in children are activated through accessing state or affective memories entirely void of cognitive or narrative associations to a specific trauma or experience (Greenwald et al., 1996; Bremner and Narayan, 1998). This is particularly likely to occur in young or developmentally delayed children who are preverbal or cognitively immature. However, their behaviour or symptoms may never get connected to past experiences by adults around them. Neither is it uncommon for traumatized children to be labelled as having attention deficit disorder or conduct disorder, judged on the basis of their current presenting symptoms. Such diagnostic labels may well be totally accurate concerning the child's behaviour, but as such they hardly offer a clinician any cues to aetiology, prognosis or treatment.

Individuals at various developmental stages respond differently when confronted with threat (Perry et al., 1995; Perry, 1996; Cicchetti and Rogosch, 1997). A sensory overload will often cause an infant to turn away from the overstimulating input and even fall asleep. The capacity to disengage from stressful stimuli, and dissociate, is the psychological equivalent to 'flight'. As children grow older, the capacity to dissociate may persist. In some circumstances, a child who is able to disengage and dissociate can be seen as having an adaptive advantage. Therefore, the ability to modulate arousal and anxiety associated with the stress response for periods of time may well be highly adaptive.

Sometimes a fearful child may simply appear defiant (Perry, 1994; Perry and Pollard, 1998). This is typically interpreted as wilfulness and the child striving to be in control. An adult confronted by such obstinate child behaviour is easily roused to fury. The nonverbal cues of the frustrated and angry adult further increase the child's terror, and he or she is soon ready for combat. Yet, the child's behaviour may merely reflect attempts to adapt and respond to a perceived threat. Many traumatized children also have significant impairments in social and emotional functions. These again may be learned capabilities which have developed in response to experience. Likewise, it is not uncommon for hypervigilant children to possess considerable nonverbal skills compared with their verbal skills. For this reason, they may, for example, overread nonverbal cues: eye contact may only mean threat, while a friendly touch may be interpreted as an antecedent of seduction. Such skills are all appropriate in the world such children come from (McNally et al., 1990; Kim and Fanslow, 1992; Eich, 1995).

Comorbidity and its psychosocial implications

A finding common to several epidemiological and clinic-based studies is that conduct problems and activity or attention problems in school-age children correlate highly (August et al., 1996a,b; Leung et al., 1996; Lynam, 1996). At preschool age the two behavioural dimensions show even stronger overlap (Bennett et al., 1998, 1999; Hughes et al., 2000). Indeed, the most common child psychiatric disorders that are comorbid with ADHD are conduct disorder and oppositional defiant disorder (Biederman et al., 1991; Fergusson et al., 1991; Fergusson and Horwood, 1993; Angold et al., 1999). However, comorbidity is the rule, not the exception, and not just in relation to ADHD but across a range of childhood disturbances (Caron and Rutter, 1991; Biederman et al., 1991; Rutter, 1997a; Angold et al., 1999). Comorbid internalizing disorders (depression more often than anxiety) have increasingly been claimed to be almost as common in children with ADHD as externalizing disorders (Biederman et al., 1991; Bird et al., 1993; Jensen et al., 1993; Costello et al., 1997). There is some suggestion that specific forms of familial transmission operate in connection with this comorbidity: parental internalizing disorders are associated with ADHD comorbidity with anxiety/depression in children, whereas parental externalizing disorders show a stronger association with ADHD comorbidity with conduct disorder or oppositional defiant disorder in children (Pfiffner et al., 1999). Results from the Virginia twin study (Silberg et al., 1996) have also suggested that the covariation between hyperactivity and oppositional or conduct problems is almost entirely attributable to genetic factors. Furthermore, in younger children the same set of genes appears to explain all the variations in both cooccurring disorders.

Psychosocial factors distinguishing hyperactivity and conduct disorder

One important criterion for two disorders forming independent diagnostic entities is whether or not they can be shown to have distinctly separate aetiologies. In relation to hyperactivity, the key questions here have been: is ADHD a valid diagnostic entity, separate from conduct disorder, and can this distinction be made on the basis of the psychosocial correlates which are of likely aetiological importance?

Early studies approached this question by allocating children into two problem groups on the basis of parent and/or teacher questionnaire scores, and more or less assumed that the two forms of behavioural disturbance occurred independent of one another, and in different children. However, subsequent studies based on more adequate diagnostic criteria have clearly demonstrated that this is not the case. Although ADHD without a concomitant conduct disorder does occur at a reasonable rate, the reverse is not true – conduct disorder without hyperactivity is a relatively rare phenomenon (Taylor et al., 1991). Therefore, the question, as set out above, can be further articulated as follows: does the combined ADHD + conduct disorder/oppositional defiant disorder differ from pure ADHD (and from pure conduct disorder/oppositional defiant disorder) in terms of psychosocial factors likely to have causal significance? The findings from less than a handful of relevant studies (based on general population samples and making adequate diagnostic distinctions) published in the last decade suggest that, although the two groups largely resemble each other, the addition of conduct disorder tends to bring greater social disability and more adverse family environments (Taylor et al., 1991; Fletcher et al., 1996; Leung et al., 1996; Carlson et al., 1997). The same applies to clinic-based studies (Luk et al., 1991; Abikoff and Klein, 1992; Schachar and Tannock, 1995; Kuhne et al., 1997). It therefore seems likely that many of the psychosocial adversities attributed in the past to ADHD are particularly associated with ADHD that is comorbid for conduct disorder (Biederman et al., 1996; Fletcher et al., 1996; Satterfield and Schell, 1997).

In clinic-referred samples, a number of psychosocial adversities have been found to characterize more strongly the mixed hyperactive-conduct-disordered group than those children suffering from pure hyperactivity (Luk et al., 1991; Schachar and Tannock, 1995). In population studies, the differences have been less sharp and consistent (Taylor et al., 1991; Leung et al., 1996; Carlson et al., 1997). Examining 61 clinic-referred boys, aged 6–12 years, all meeting DSM-III-R criteria for ADHD, and the ICD-9 criteria for hyperkinetic disorder, and 34 of them comorbid for conduct disorder, Luk et al. (1991) found several differences with regard to intrafamilial distress and discord in relationships. For example, the quality of the father–child relationship was less optimal in the mixed group, with lower levels of parental expressed warmth towards the child and poorer coping with the child's challenging behaviour and emotional upsets. (The differences for the mothers were in the same direction but less substantial.) Also, the parents of the mixed group reported that their marriage was more discordant and generally less satisfactory, and the children themselves had more negative interactions with their siblings compared with the pure hyperactivity group. The results obtained by Schachar and Tannock (1995) were largely similar.

The two general population studies (Taylor et al., 1991; Leung et al., 1996) that also shared rather similar methodologies (questionnaire screening followed by detailed investigations of identified contrast groups) yielded results which were comparable in many ways. In both studies the groups with mixed hyperactivity–conduct disorder generally scored highest on indices of suboptimal parent–child relationship, parental coping and consistency between parents. It also appeared that in the Taylor et al. (1991) study such measures of psychosocial adversity were more clearly associated with hyperactivity than conduct problems, while this pattern was less consistent in the findings of Leung et al. (1996). For example, Taylor et al. (1991) found that a high score on expressed criticism towards the child, as measured separately for mothers and fathers was being significantly more common in the group showing both hyperactivity and conduct disorder. However, the parents of boys with pure hyperactivity were almost as critical as those with the mixed disorder, whereas both the mothers and fathers of the boys selected for conduct problems alone expressed far lower levels of criticism towards the child. In addition, the mother's poor skills in dealing with the child's problem behaviour and emotional upsets were particularly characteristic of the hyperactive groups, regardless of whether conduct disorder featured in the problems or not. The presence of depressive symptoms (not necessarily meeting the criteria for clinical diagnosis of depression) experienced by the mothers over the previous year distinguished the boys with a mixed hyperactivity-conduct disorder from the other two problem groups, i.e. pure hyperactivity or pure conduct disorder. The mixed group also stood out from the rest by a significantly higher composite score of family relationship problems – a finding similar to that reported by Leung et al. (1996).

Strong evidence for differential developmental pathways initiated by the presence or absence of early maternal responsiveness comes from the 10-year follow-up of 77 children born to high-risk mothers (Wakschlag and Hans, 1999). Responsiveness, pertaining to maternal behaviour in terms of timing, pacing, flexibility and emotional engagement, was assessed through videotaped observations at 4, 12 and 24 months. At 10 years of age, a lack of early maternal responsiveness was found to be differentially associated with child disruptive behaviour (both in terms of clinical diagnosis and symptom score), but not with attention problems (diagnosis of ADHD or symptom score). The results further suggested that the effects of early responsiveness may be moderated by the experience of later adversity. Children who experienced responsive parenting during infancy showed low levels of later disruptive behaviour, regardless of later family adversity, whereas those with unresponsive early parenting were at increased risk only if they were living in high-risk conditions at school age.

An issue relevant to clinical decision making and case management has been highlighted by Overmeyer et al. (1999). Their results demonstrated the danger related to the knowledge of diagnosis: psychosocial adversities may be under-detected among hyperactive children because the disorder is commonly as-cribed to biological causes. The parents of 21 children with hyperkinetic disorder and 26 children with conduct disorder were first interviewed by clinicians (who were aware of the diagnosis, as is normal in clinical practice), and then by researchers who were blind to the diagnosis. The clinicians detected significantly higher levels of psychosocial adversity in children with conduct disorder than in children with hyperkinetic disorder. By contrast, the researchers detected equal amounts of adversity in both. Logistic regression confirmed the presence of strong interaction effects between raters, and knowl-edge of diagnosis, especially regarding intrafamilial relationships (lack of warmth in the parent–child relationship, hostility or scapegoating of child, discord between adult family members).

Hyperactivity a risk factor for conduct disorder

There is a strong suggestion, deriving from separate lines of research, that a link exists between childhood hyperactivity, family adversity (stemming from fac-tors such as parental psychopathology or marital discord, for example) and the development of childhood conduct disorder. According to such a model, childhood hyperactivity acts as a vulnerability factor (Campbell, 1995; Hughes et al., 2000), while intrafamilial adversity operates as a mediating factor for the risk of conduct disorder (Moffitt, 1990; Toupin et al., 2000). Furthermore, the different components of intrafamilial adversity seem to mediate the risk in their unique ways (Frick et al., 1992; Wakschlag and Hans, 1999).

Farrington (1991, 1995), Pagani et al. (1999) and Moffitt (1993) have sugges-ted that many aspects of ADHD could significantly contribute to an individual's propensity to antisocial behaviour. These include impulsivity, daring, low intelligence, high activity level and physical strength. Similarly, Lahey et al. (1999) have argued that antisocial behaviour cannot be fully understood without taking individual differences into account, even though situational influences are also very powerful. In an 8–11-year follow-up of children participating in the Bloomington Longitudinal Study (Olson et al., 1999), laboratory measures of impulsivity at 8 years of age significantly predicted parent-rated delinquency in adolescent girls, and impulsivity at both 6 and 8 years of age predicted the young person's own ratings of aggression and delinquency in both sexes. There is also evidence that youths with onset of antisocial behaviour at an earlier age are more likely to meet diagnostic criteria for ADHD during childhood than youths with later ages of onset (Moffitt, 1990; Loeber et al., 1995). Most of the studies have involved only boys, but the more recent evidence suggests that the situation may be different in girls with perhaps both ADHD and oppositional defiant disorder turning out to be independent precursors of conduct disorder (Lahey et al., 1999).

The reviews by Lahey et al. (1999) and Lilienfeld and Waldman (1990) have called for caution when drawing conclusions from existing research findings. The point has been made that in earlier studies ADHD may have been incorrectly identified as a developmental precursor to conduct disorder in boys because it is frequently comorbid with oppositional defiant disorder. The evidence presented in these reviews, instead, seems to suggest that boys comorbid for both ADHD and oppositional defiant disorder in childhood are at increased risk for later antisocial behaviour, but boys with ADHD alone are not. However, there is also evidence that boys with both ADHD and oppositional defiant disorder are more likely to develop antisocial behaviour than boys with oppositional defiant disorder/conduct disorder alone (Hinshaw et al., 1993; Kuhne et al., 1997). Also, antisocial youths who meet the criteria for concurrent ADHD exhibit higher numbers and/or more persistent antisocial behaviours (Moffitt, 1990; Toupin et al., 2000). The findings by Taylor et al. (1996) make a partial exception. Their study of children followed up from ages 6–7 to 16–18 years suggested that hyperactivity was a risk factor for later conduct problems, even after the coexistence of initial conduct problems was taken into account. In this context, it also needs to be noted that AHHD is important because it confers additional risks of its own for poor outcomes. Independent of antisocial behaviour, ADHD is associated with academic underachievement relative to intelligence, early drop-out from school and restricted occupational success (Frick et al., 1991; Mannuzza et al., 1997).

The role of hyperactivity and conduct disorder, separately or jointly predisposing to psychiatric disorder in general rather than acting as risk factors for one another, was investigated by Taylor et al. (1991). In a two-stage epidemiological study, a short-term longitudinal design was employed utilizing the results of the initial screening with parent and teacher questionnaires and subsequent detailed interview measures 9 months later. The presence of pervasive hyperactivity was found to influence the short-term development of overall psychiatric disturbance. At follow-up, hyperactivity, conduct disorder and a mixture of the two were significantly predicted by membership of the screening group. Among the children rated high on the mixed hyperactivity-conduct disorder scale at screening stage, the overall rate of any disorder at follow-up was 81%, compared with 51% in the pure hyperactivity group, 28% in the pure conduct disorder group and 16% in controls. The types of succeeding disorders were also different according to screening group: membership of the conduct disorder group initially was only a risk factor for subsequent conduct disorder; but membership of the hyperactivity group carried risks for both conduct disorder and hyperactivity, as well as the mixture of the two. This suggests that hyperactivity leads to conduct disorder, not the other way round.

To disentangle the relative contribution of the two, analysis of covariance was employed. When conduct disorder symptoms derived from the parent and teacher rating scales at screening were both covaried, adverse family life still remained associated with persistence of hyperactivity. Conversely, when the family relationship index was used as a covariate, the persistence of hyperactivity was still associated with the initial teacher and parent ratings of conduct disorder. The findings of the survey by Taylor et al. (1991) thus indicate that unhappy family life, represented by angry, inconsistent parental reactions and high levels of depressive symptoms in the mothers, is likely to affect negatively the outcome of children with an early onset of hyperactivity. However, the significance of the dysfunctional patterns of family relationships may not be a specific cause of hyperactivity, but rather it is a factor strongly associated with persistence of the disorder. Furthermore, this prediction is considerably strengthened if the early hyperactivity is accompanied by defiant child behaviour.

The following observations regarding the role of maternal depression and parental marital conflict may offer some clues about the possible mechanisms by which early hyperactivity can lead to conduct disorder in the context of psychosocial adversity. A number of studies have indicated that maternal depression or distress gives rise to inconsistent and noncontingent management of fairly 'normal' child noncompliance, which in turn increases the likelihood of further child misbehaviour. This is likely to be even more pronounced in hyperactive children. Such evidence is obviously less convincing if based on studies that have relied on maternal perceptions, rather than objective assessments of child behaviour. However, recent studies have demonstrated evidence of actual observed maternal behaviours, such as expressed criticism or aversiveness, as being characteristic features of interactions between depressed mothers and their young children (Murray et al., 1993; Campbell et al., 1995). Of the other intrafamilial stresses, marital discord has been shown to be associated with episodes of child aggression and defiance during observed parent–child interaction sequences.

A prospective study by Campbell and Ewing (1990) suggested that maternal depression and marital discord interact in unique ways, depending on the measure examined. Each factor occurring separately increased maternal defensive and complaining behaviour during conflict discussions, but when both were present, complaining occurred less than when marital discord existed without depression. These factors also predicted less use of maternal facilitative behaviour towards the child and less use of remarks helping the child to solve specific problems, all of which could contribute to the development of antisocial behaviour, particularly in vulnerable hyperactive children. The relevance of these same intrafamilial adversities throughout childhood was demonstrated by Barkley et al. (1991) in a study of adolescents. This showed that both maternal depression and marital discord were separately associated with the mother's verbal insults and putdowns directed at the adolescent, and with a reduction in the mother's facilitative behaviour. The study by Campbell and Ewing (1990) similarly indicated that maternal perceptions of child misconduct, and actual maternal controlling behaviour in early childhood, are more predictive of conduct problems later in childhood and in adolescence than is actual child behaviour during the earlier years.

The presence of a hostile and unhappy family environment, often accompanied by poor exercising of control for the child's behaviour, seems of special relevance when hyperactivity is associated with defiant and antisocial behaviour (Taylor et al., 1991). Angry, inconsistent parental reactions and high levels of maternal depression contribute to a hostile atmosphere of poor coping, with frequent criticizing of the child. The combination of these factors is also a powerful predictor for the persistence of hyperactivity regardless of whether there is accompanying conduct disorder.

An alternative model, involving two independent routes, one via child aggressiveness and one via negative family climate, to determine the long-term course of hyperactivity was suggested by Marshall et al. (1990), on the basis of a longitudinal study of 29 families with a hyperactive son. Direct observations of parent–child interaction, standardized assessments of expressed emotion and ratings of child aggressiveness were used to determine the relative importance of each one of these factors for the long-term course of ADHD. Parental expressed emotion turned out to predict parental behaviour towards the child in observed interactions, whereas child aggressiveness failed to do so. The child's behaviour towards the parents, however, was highly correlated with observed child aggressiveness, but not with child expressed emotion.

Barkley (1990b) has expressed rather similar views regarding the links between hyperactivity and conduct disorder. While ADHD is a developmental disorder of behavioural disinhibition associated with neuromaturational immaturity and having a strong hereditary predisposition, conduct disorder is likely to arise with, and be maintained by, family characteristics, particularly parental psychiatric problems and social adversity and family discord. Parental beliefs, attitudes, psychological distress, the family's deficient communication and conflict resolution skills also contribute to the development of conduct disorder in hyperactive children. Thus, the progression of hyperactivity into conduct disorder takes place via the mechanisms of intrafamilial adversity. Parental psychiatric symptoms are central in causing a parent's unfavourable mood, which in turn gives rise to an altered perception of child behaviour in terms of exaggerating deviance of behaviour in the hyperactive child. This further increases parental negative behaviour towards the child and decreases positive statements and general social interactions with the child. The child responds with increased negative behaviour and decreased compliance. Mutually coercive exchanges ensue, predicting a further escalation of the child's deviant behaviour through parental negative reinforcement.

In spite of current abundant discussion on the issue of ADHD with and without conduct disorder, the implications for classification are unclear. For example, it is acknowledged that the outcomes for the children so diagnosed are very different. However, next to nothing is known about their respective antecedents, i.e. are the antecedents of conduct disorder alone (or ADHD alone) different from the antecedents of those showing the combined type? Such questions must be approached developmentally. It is not enough to examine selective correlates of already manifest disorders. Some variables may have stronger differential links with onset of problems, while others may be more tied to persistence or desistance (August et al., 1996a). Angold et al. (1999) also call for community-based longitudinal diagnostic studies that are large enough to separate out the specific and nonspecific effects of risk factors across a range of diagnoses. Family genetic approaches and twin studies that focus on comorbidity may also be helpful (Rutter, 1997a,b).

Hyperactivity and anxiety disorder

There does indeed exist evidence from epidemiologically based studies to suggest that in some children hyperactivity is part of an anxiety disorder, though the link is far less strong than with conduct disorder or with cognitive deficits (Taylor et al., 1991; Biederman et al., 1992). Relating to what was postulated above, it is likely that specific underlying psychological and biological factors operate in such cases. Thus, it has been shown that children whose hyperactivity or attention deficit is linked to anxiety disorder exhibit lesser degrees of impulsivity and motor overactivity and fewer antisocial symptoms than hyperactive children without an underlying anxiety disorder (Pliszka, 1992). There is also some controversy about the usefulness of stimulant medication in children whose inattention and hyperactivity are accompanied by anxiety symptoms (DuPaul et al., 1994; Taylor, 1999; The MTA Cooperative Group, 1999; Chapter 13).

Psychosocial theories

An earlier section made an attempt to take on board the demanding task of examining the extent to which there exists evidence to claim that psychosocial factors may be responsible for the cause of hyperactivity and attention problems. It is to be concluded that what evidence there is is largely indirect and based on studies which did not specifically set out to examine the causes of hyperactivity. The aim of this search would be for some theoretical basis for the postulated causal mechanisms, such as disrupted core attachments, parental depression and early traumatic life experiences, in particular. In this respect, the roles of motivation, cognitive and emotional factors and some physiological mechanisms will be considered.

Role of motivation

Most attempts at understanding the underlying deficits in hyperactivity have concentrated on the study of attentional processes. However, in order to explain the way in which social and, more particularly, family and other interactions may contribute to hyperactivity, it also seems important to consider motivational aspects. Furthermore, in striving to understand the central role of motivation, it is essential to deal with the issue of purpose. Hyperactivity may be defined as a behavioural style characterized by persistent marked motor activity which is excessive in relation to what would generally be regarded as necessary for achieving any particular goal. Such surplus activity may serve a purpose which is different from the obvious task at hand, or reflect motivations of which the subject may need not be aware. Overactivity, whether motor, cognitive or emotionally expressed, could be construed as a search for stimulation and exploration, or for a sense of physical and emotional well-being and safety. It may result from a difficulty in integrating psychological functions in the achievement of a special aim. This formulation of over-activity is congruent with that outlined by Olson (Chapter 8), describing hyperactivity as a disorder of self-regulation with problems in flexibly adapting to life situations that call for differing standards of conduct. The general deficit is in rule-governed behaviour which in itself is under the control of immediately occurring contingencies. It is proposed that at crucial stages in development the quality of the caregiver–infant interaction, via its effect on the formation of cognitive/affective schemata, mediates the emergence of basic attentional, motivational and problem-solving skills.

The reasons for emotional unavailability in a parent may stem, for example, from debilitating physical or mental illness, major life stress or constraints placed by the family's inadequate or unsuitable living conditions. Due to these reasons the parents may simply be 'out of touch', or impeded in coping with the high levels of energy characteristic of early childhood. The child's restlessness and inability to concentrate are perceived as troublesome by many parents and this is reflected in these being relatively common complaints among the small group of parents whose children, though referred to psychiatric clinics, eventually fail to qualify for a clinically confirmed psychiatric disorder (Garralda and Bailey, 1988).

According to Bozarth (1991), two main explanatory models can be outlined: one based on drive reduction theory and the other one on incentive motivational theory. The drive reduction theory postulates that organisms are motivated by drives pushing towards the goal object; the behavioural objective is reduction of the drive. The incentive theory in turn stipulates that organisms are motivated by the incentive value of various stimuli pulling towards the goal object; motivation is generated by the expectancy of reward: the primary motivation is not to reduce the drive but to increase and maintain contact with the incentive stimuli. The evidence would suggest that, in the case of hyperactive children, both drive reduction, shown by the combination of delay aversion and sensation seeking, and incentive orientation (reward orientation) operate together.

Bozarth (1991) also proposed that the hypothalamus plays an important role as a possible centre for motivational effects on the grounds that electrical stimulation through electrode placements along the medial forebrain bundle (extending from the lateral hypothalamus to the ventral segmental areas) produces the strongest intrinsically rewarding effects. Dopamine is regarded as the neurotransmitter which is particularly active in relaying the rewarding effects of electrical brain stimulation, with the role of noradrenaline being less well supported. Therefore, changes in dopamine function may underlie some of the incentive-based motivations.

Contributing cognitive factors

A major driving force which is already apparent in a young child is the search for mental and intellectual stimulation and active exploration of the environment. Cognitive limitations, including poor language skills, therefore interfere with the child's ability to engage effectively in activities where intellectual and verbally mediated demands dominate. Such activities will rapidly become devoid of purpose for the child; they will fail to hold the child's interest and attention, and may result in a restless search for more satisfying stimulation through overactivity.

At the same time there is considerable evidence to support the central and primary role of cognitive anomalies for the development of ADHD. Regardless of whether studies have been based on clinical or epidemiological samples, decreased IQ levels and communication problems have consistently been found to be associated with pervasive and severe hyperactivity (Taylor et al., 1991; Chapter 7). Furthermore, this association seems to be of special relevance in situations where overactivity and distractibility are unaccompanied by other clinical features of psychopathology, in other words, in the absence of psychiatric comorbidity.

Though an intrinsic feature of the child, cognitive deficit may well be closely linked to a suboptimal environment during the early years of development. Thus, an impoverished or unsettled environment which fails to provide sufficient and consistent intellectual stimulation may contribute to both cognitive deficits and hyperactivity in the child. It is therefore somewhat surprising that descriptions of the effects of extreme environmental deprivation on children have not singled out overactivity and inattention as main consequences. They may, of course, have been present, but not mentioned because of being regarded as expected consequences of delayed development. Alternatively, it is possible that overactivity is not a consequence when, as appears to be the case, severe deprivation is linked to physical neglect and reduced opportunities for physical activity (see Chapter 12 for further discussion on the subject).

In children growing up in less extreme circumstances, factors such as large family size, changes in family structure, less than optimal quality of the mother–child relationship and institutional rearing have been shown to be related to problems in children's cognitive and language development (Hinde and Stevenson-Hinde, 1987). The study by Taylor et al. (1991) also reported that, among children in the general population inattention was specifically associated with parents' low social class, thus suggesting that an environment lacking in stimulation may contribute both to a slowing of intellectual development and to attention problems.

Contributing emotional factors

The purpose of the child's excessive activity may appear as a fruitless, stereotyped search for experiences to satisfy unmet emotional needs. In such cases the deficiencies in the ability to regulate motor and mental activities may be a result of the child growing up in an environment which repeatedly frustrates his or her wish to have the needs for basic well-being, either physical or psychological, met. This may be through abuse, neglect, or markedly and persistently negative attitudes towards the child. Their effect would be further aggravated by parenting styles which fail to provide sufficient controls and guidance to help the child contain the wish for immediate need gratification. The result could be a behavioural style involving an impulsive and compulsively incessant search for compensatory rewarding experiences which will persist regardless of the likely negative consequences.

A study of physiological arousal responses by Garralda et al. (1991) suggested the possibility that both reward seeking and sensation seeking operate in children whose hyperactive behaviour is part of a conduct disorder. An increased autonomic nervous system reactivity to experiences with positively rewarding connotations was found in children with conduct disorder, many of whom also had significant symptoms of hyperactivity. These children showed a failure to lower their arousal levels during periods of silence, suggesting problems in modulating arousal, which in turn could be underlying the sensation-seeking behaviour. The concept of excessive search for sensation is consistent with findings from experimental work suggesting that the impulsiveness component of hyperactivity is related to 'delay aversion', with the main difficulty being an inability to wait for a delayed reward (Sonuga-Barke et al., 1992); the immediacy rather than the size of reward is important.

Some physiological bases

The development of a positive view of oneself and favourable self-concept are regarded as essential for a person's good psychological adjustment. Persistent negative feedback, whether as a result of the child's overactivity or not, will reduce his or her chances of encountering socially rewarding experiences. If this occurs at a crucial time in development, when he or she is learning to integrate motor and mental activity, it could lead to motor restlessness, overactivity and disruptive behaviour in the futile search for rewarding experiences.

Physiological studies of arousal offer evidence of factors which are of possible relevance in hyperactivity accompanied by anxiety. Children suffering from emotional disorders, a number of whom also exhibit high levels of motor activity, have been shown to differ from children with conduct disorder and from healthy controls, in terms of background arousal levels, as measured by skin conductance and heart rate, as well as in their electrophysiological responses to stimulation. This is, for example, evidenced by their excessive autonomic nervous system responses to the anticipation of potentially stressful or unpleasant experiences (Garralda et al., 1991). Those whose emotional symptoms are particularly severe also exhibit high resting heart rate levels and reduced responses to neutral stimuli (Garralda et al., 1989).

A picture emerges of the hyperactive anxious child as one with increased adrenergic autonomic baseline activity, with decreased general reactivity to overall 'neutral' environmental stimulation, but hypersensitivity to negative and potentially threatening life situations. In children with a proneness to overactive motor behaviour this might well lead to a characteristic tendency to fidgetiness, and in a search for safety, to anxious 'running away' from environmental changes or demands which are perceived as threatening.

Anxiety is linked to overactivity in some children but not in others. It is possible that the presence of temperamental overactivity in the child is a prerequisite. The experience of a sheltered or specially overprotective environment, as is often described in children with anxiety disorder, may reduce the risk of an overactive response. Alternatively, anxious hyperactivity may be a result of especially stressful experiences of loss, or threat of loss, early on in childhood. It may be further compounded by exposure to parental anxiety, since increased rates of anxiety disorder have been noted in the families of children with attention deficit hyperactivity disorder (Biederman et al., 1991). It is therefore possible that children model their behaviour on anxious-restless overactivity in their parents. In such situations overactive behaviour may allow the child to create some physical distance in order to reduce the burden of anxiety fuelled by parental psychiatric disorder.

Constitutional vs. environmental determinants

In one of his salutary reviews, Sroufe (1997) has presented a very elegant synthesis of the interplay between constitutional and environmental factors within a developmental framework. It therefore seems appropriate to conclude this chapter by echoing some of his ideas. One very crucial idea is the need of 'environment' to be broadened to include experiential factors, rather than simply demographic variables and aspects of the physical environment. Regrettably, however, research on developmental psychopathology is still too often guided by the narrow tradition of a medical model, within which environment is defined akin to toxins, precursors seen as pathogens or simply early forms of the disorder, and the course is viewed as linear. Instead, a strong case for the need for longitudinal research – one that begins prior to the onset of disorder – has to be made. The paucity of research on experiential risk factors, early adaptation and processes of change is also to be noted. In addition, because treatment tends to be viewed narrowly as symptom management, few guidelines for early intervention or primary prevention are uncovered by the research.

It is crucial to start by defining early patterns of adaptation, and then follow individuals who show different early patterns to observed outcomes. The notion that children and their caretakers mutually shape each other's behaviour has to form the basis for such research. Sroufe (1997) also stresses that attachment is a relationship construct, not an individual trait construct. Therefore, it needs to be remembered that there are interindividual differences in biologically rooted styles of behaviour, with such differences in turn affecting children's interactions with their environment (Rutter, 1996). Taken in the context of childhood hyperactivity, it is postulated that characteristics such as high activity level, short attention span and impulsivity are 'temperamental' expressions of biological risk which in some environmental conditions will contribute to the development of the clinical syndrome of hyperactivity. Thus, even genetic aetiology is likely to be multifactorial and due to underlying neurochemical factors. The inheritance is polygenic, with the liability being influenced by sex hormonal factors and/or very early social influences, which will both increase the liability of hyperactivity in boys (Plomin and Bergeman, 1991; Plomin, 1995; Rutter, 1997b; Rutter et al., 1997a).

More research is needed on processes of continuity and change, with the emphasis on experiential factors such as changing support and guidance of the child (Sroufe et al., 1990). Likewise, far too little is known about the interaction between prior adaptation and current risks. Ongoing parenting influences on endogenous factors, as well as endogenous influences on parenting, constitute another focus for study. Sroufe (1997) also warns that changes in behaviour in response to stimulant medication do not allow aetiological interpretations, as models of aetiology and models of treatment bear no relation to one another.

REFERENCES

Abikoff, H. and Klein, R.G. (1992). Attention-deficit hyperactivity and conduct disorder: comorbidity and implications for treatment. *Journal of Consulting and Clinical Psychology*, **60**, 881–92.

Abraham, W.C. and Bear, M.F. (1996). Metaplasticity: the plasticity of synaptic plasticity. *Trends in Neuroscience*, **19**, 126–30.

Altepeter, T.S. and Breen, M.J. (1992). Situational variation in problem behaviour at home and school in attention deficit disorder with hyperactivity: a factor analytic study. *Journal of Child Psychology and Psychiatry*, **33**, 741–8.

American Psychiatric Association. (1994). *Diagnostic and Statistical Manual of Mental Disorders*, 4th edn. Washington, DC: APA.

American Psychiatric Association. (1987). *Diagnostic and Statistical Manual of Mental Disorders*, 3rd edn, revised. Washington, DC: APA.

Angold, A., Costello, E.J. and Erkanli, A. (1999). Comorbidity. *Journal of Child Psychology and Psychiatry*, **40**, 57–87.

August, G., MacDonald, A., Realmuto, G. and Skare, S. (1996a). Hyperactive and aggressive pathways: effects of demographic, family, and child characteristics on children's adaptive functioning. *Journal of Clinical Child Psychology*, **25**, 341–51.

August, G.J., Realmuto, G.M., MacDonald, A.W., Nugent, S.M. and Crosby, R. (1996b). Prevalence of ADHD and comorbid disorders among elementary school children screened for disruptive behavior. *Journal of Abnormal Child Psychology*, **24**, 571–95.

Barkley, R.A. (1990a). *Attention Deficit Hyperactivity Disorder: A Handbook for Diagnosis and Treatment*. New York: Guilford Press.

Barkley, R.A. (1990b). The adolescent outcome of hyperactive children diagnosed by research criteria: I. An 8-year prospective follow-up study. *Journal of the American Academy of Child and Adolescent Psychiatry*, **29**, 546–57.

Barkley, R.A., Fischer, M., Edelbrock, C.S. and Smallish, L. (1991). The adolescent outcome of hyperactive children diagnosed by research criteria: III. Mother–child interactions, family conflicts and maternal psychopathology. *Journal of Child Psychology and Psychiatry*, **32**, 233–5.

Barkley, R.A., Anastopoulos, A.D., Guevremont, D.C. and Fletcher, K.E. (1992). Adolescents with attention deficit hyperactivity disorder: mother–child interactions, family beliefs and conflicts, and maternal psychopathology. *Journal of Abnormal Psychology*, **20**, 263–88.

Barnett, D. and Vondra, J. (1999). Atypical patterns of early attachment: theory, research, and current directions. *Monographs of the Society for Research in Child Development*, **64**, 1–24.

Bear, M.F. (1997). How do memories leave their mark? *Nature*, **385**, 481–2.

Bendell, D., Field, T., Yando, R. et al. (1994). 'Depressed' mothers' perceptions of their preschool children's vulnerability. *Child Psychiatry and Human Development*, **24**, 3.

Bennett, K.J., Lipman, E.L., Racine, Y. and Offord, D.R. (1998). Do measures of externalising behaviour in normal populations predict later outcome? Implications for targeted interventions to prevent conduct disorder. *Journal of Child Psychology and Psychiatry*, **39**, 1059–70.

Bennett, K.J., Lipman, E.L., Brown, S. et al. (1999). Predicting conduct problems: can high-risk children be identified in kindergarten and grade I? *Journal of Consulting and Clinical Psychology*, **67**, 470–80.

Biederman, J., Newcorn, J. and Sprich, S. (1991). Comorbidity of attention deficit hyperactivity disorder with conduct, depressive, anxiety, and other disorders. *American Journal of Psychiatry*, **148**, 564–77.

Biederman, J., Faraone, S.V., Keenan, K. et al. (1992). Further evidence for family-genetic risk factors in attention deficit hyperactivity disorder. *Archives of General Psychiatry*, **49**, 728–38.

Biederman, J., Faraone, S.V., Milberger, S. et al. (1996). Is childhood oppositional defiant disorder a precursor to adolescent conduct disorder? Findings from a four-year follow-up study of children with ADHD. *Journal of the American Academy of Child and Adolescent Psychiatry*, **35**, 1193–204.

Bird, H.R., Gould, M.S. and Staghezza, B.M. (1993). Patterns of diagnostic comorbidity in a community sample of children aged 9 through 16 years. *Journal of the American Academy of Child and Adolescent Psychiatry*, **32**, 361–8.

Bozarth, M.A. (1991). The mesolimbic dopamine system as a model reward system. In *The Mesolimbic Dopamine System: From Motivation To Action*, P. Willner and J. Scheel-Kruger, eds, pp. 301–30. New York: John Wiley.

Bremner, J. and Narayan, M. (1998). The effects of stress on memory and the hippocampus throughout the life cycle: implications for childhood development and ageing. *Development and Psychopathology*, **10**, 871–85.

Bremner, J., Randall, P., Vermetten, E. et al. (1997). Magnetic resonance imaging-based measurement of hippocampal volume in post-traumatic stress disorder related to childhood physical and sexual abuse – a preliminary report. *Biological Psychiatry*, **41**, 23–32.

Breton, J.J., Bergeron, L., Valla, J.P. et al. (1999). Quebec child mental health survey: prevalence of DSM-III-R mental health disorders. *Journal of Child Psychology and Psychiatry*, **40**, 375–84.

Brooks-Gunn, J., Klebanov, P.K. and Liaw, F. (1995). The learning, physical, and emotional environment in the home in the context of poverty: the Infant Health and Development Program. *Children and Youth Services Review*, **17**, 251–76.

Brown, J.W. (1994). Morphogenesis and mental process. *Development and Psychopathology*, **6**, 551–63.

Byrne, J.H. and Kandel, E.R. (1996). Presynaptic facilitation revisited: state and time dependence. *Journal of Neuroscience*, **16**, 425–35.

Campbell, S.B. (1995). Behaviour problems in preschool children: a review of recent research. *Journal of Child Psychology and Psychiatry*, **36**, 113–49.

Campbell, S.B. and Ewing, L.J. (1990). Follow-up of hard to manage preschoolers: adjustment at age 9 and predictors of continuing symptoms. *Journal of Child Psychology and Psychiatry*, **31**, 871–89.

Campbell, S.B., Cohn, J.F. and Meyers, T. (1995). Depression in first-time mothers: mother–infant interaction and depression chronicity. *Developmental Psychology*, **31**, 349–57.

Campbell, S.B., Pierce, E.W., Moore, G., Marakovitz, S. and Newby, K. (1996). Boys' externalizing problems at elementary school age: pathways from early behavior problems, maternal control, and family stress. *Development and Psychopathology*, **8**, 701–19.

Cantwell, D.P. (1996). Attention deficit disorder: a review of the past 10 years. *Journal of the American Academy of Child and Adolescent Psychiatry*, **35**, 978–87.

Carlson, M. and Earls, F. (1997). Psychological and neuroendocrinological sequelae of early social deprivation in institutionalized children in Romania. *Annals of the New York Academy of Sciences*, **807**, 419–28.

Carlson, E.A., Jacobvitz, D. and Sroufe, L.A. (1995). A developmental investigation of inattentiveness and hyperactivity. *Child Development*, **66**, 37–54.

Carlson, C.L., Tamm, L. and Gaub, M. (1997). Gender differences in children with ADHD, ODD, and co-occurring ADHD/ODD identified in school population. *Journal of the American Academy of Child and Adolescent Psychiatry*, **36**, 1706–14.

Caron, C. and Rutter, M. (1991). Comorbidity in child psychopathology. Concepts, issues and research strategies. *Journal of Child Psychology and Psychiatry*, **32**, 1063–80.

Castro-Alamancos, M.A. and Connors, B.W. (1996). Short-term plasticity of a thalamocortical pathway dynamically modulated by behavioral state. *Science*, **272**, 274–6.

Cicchetti, D. and Rogosch, F.A. (1997). The role of self-organization in the promotion of resilience in maltreated children. *Development and Psychopathology*, **9**, 797–815.

Cicchetti, D. and Tucker, D. (1994). Development and self regulatory structures of the mind. *Development and Psychopathology*, **6**, 533–49.

Conger, R.D., Conger, K.J. and Elder, G.H. Jr. (1997). Family economic hardship and adolescent adjustment: mediating and moderating processes. In *Consequences of Growing Up Poor*, G.J. Duncan and J. Brooks-Gunn, eds, pp. 288–310. New York: Russell Sage Foundation.

Conrad, P. (1976). *Identifying Hyperactive Children. The Medicalisation of Deviant Behavior*. Massachusetts: Lexington Books.

Coplan, J.D., Andrews, M.W., Rosenblum, L.A. et al. (1996). Persistent elevations of cerebrospinal fluid concentrations of cortioctropin-releasing factor in adult nonhuman primates exposed to early-life stressors. Implications for the pathophysiology of mood and anxiety disorder. *Proceedings of the National Academy of Sciences of the United States of America*, **93**, 1619–23.

Costello, E.J., Farmer, E., Angold, A., Burns, B. and Erkanli, A. (1997). Psychiatric disorders among American Indian and white youth in Appalachia: the Great Smoky Mountains study. *American Journal of Public Health*, **87**, 827–32.

Courchesne, E., Chisum, H. and Townsend, J. (1994). Neural activity-dependent brain changes in development: implications for psychopathology. *Development and Psychopathology*, **6**, 697–722.

Cummings, E.M. and Davies, P.T. (1994). Maternal depression and child development. *Journal of Child Psychology and Psychiatry*, **35**, 73–112.

Danforth, J.S., Barkley, R.A. and Stokes, T.F. (1991). Observations of parent–child interactions with hyperactive children: research and clinical implications. *Clinical Psychology Review*, **11**, 703–27.

Dix, T. (1991). The affective organization of parenting: adaptive and maladaptive processes. *Psychological Bulletin*, **110**, 3–25.

Dodge, K.A., Bates, J.E. and Pettit, G.S. (1990). Mechanisms in the cycle of violence. *Science*, **250**, 1678–83.

Dodge, K.A., Pettit, G.S., Bates, J.E. and Valente, E. (1995). Social information processing patterns partially mediate the effect of early physical abuse on later conduct problems. *Journal of Abnormal Psychology*, **104**, 632–43.

Downey, G. and Coyne, J.C. (1990). Children of depressed parents: an integrative review. *Psychological Bulletin*, **108**, 50–76.

DuPaul, G.J., Barkley, R.A. and McMurray, M.B. (1994). Response of children with ADHD to methylphenidate: interaction with internalizing symptoms. *Journal of the American Academy of Child and Adolescent Psychiatry*, **33**, 894–903.

Edelman, G.H. (1992). *Bright Air, Brilliant Fire: On the Matter of Mind*. New York: Basic Books.

Eich, E. (1995). Searching for mood-dependent memory. *Psychological Science*, **6**, 67–75.

Emerit, M.B., Riad, M. and Hamon, M. (1992). Trophic effects of neurotransmitters during brain maturation. *Biological Neonate*, **62**, 193–201.

Famularo, R., Kinscherff, R. and Fenton, T. (1992). Psychiatric diagnoses of maltreated children: preliminary findings. *Journal of the American Academy of Child and Adolescent Psychiatry*, **31**, 863–7.

Farrington, D.P. (1991). Antisocial personality from childhood to adulthood. *Psychologist*, **4**, 389–94.

Farrington, D.P. (1995). The development of offending and antisocial behaviour from childhood: key findings from the Cambridge Study in Delinquent Development. *Journal of Child Psychology and Psychiatry*, **36**, 929–64.

Feldman, R., Greenbaum, C.W. and Yirmiya, N. (1999). Mother–infant affect synchrony as an antecedent of the emergence of self-control. *Developmental Psychology*, **35**, 223–31.

Fergusson, D.M. and Horwood, L.J. (1993). The structure, stability and correlations of the trait components of conduct disorder, attention deficit and anxiety/withdrawal reports. *Journal of Child Psychology and Psychiatry*, **34**, 749–66.

Fergusson, D.M., Horwood, L.J. and Lloyd, M. (1991). Confirmatory factor models of attention deficit and conduct disorder. *Journal of Child Psychology and Psychiatry*, **32**, 257–74.

Field, T. (1992). Infants of depressed mothers. *Development and Psychopathology*, **4**, 49–66.

Field, T. (1995). Infants of depressed mothers. *Infant Behavior and Development*, **18**, 1–13.

Field, T., Morrow, C. and Adlestein, D. (1993). 'Depressed' mothers' perceptions of infant behaviour. *Infant Behaviour and Development*, **16**, 99–108.

Field, T., Fox, N.A., Pickens, J. and Nawrocki, T. (1995). Relative right frontal EEG activation in 3- to 6-month old infants of depressed mothers. *Developmental Psychology*, **31**, 358–63.

Fillenz, M. (1990). *Noradrenergic Neurons*. Cambridge: Cambridge University Press.

Fletcher, K.E., Fisher, M., Barkley, R.A. and Smallish, L. (1996). A sequential analysis of the mother–adolescent interactions of ADHD, ADHD/ODD, and normal teenagers during neutral and conflict discussions. *Journal of Abnormal Child Psychology*, **24**, 271–97.

Fox, N., Kimmerly, N. and Schafer, W. (1991). Attachment to mother/attachment to father: a meta-analysis. *Child Development*, **62**, 210–25.

Frey, U. and Morris, R.G.M. (1997). Synaptic tagging and long-term potentiation. *Nature*, **385**, 533–6.

Frick, P.J. and Jackson, Y.K. (1993). Family functioning and childhood antisocial behavior: yet another reinterpretation. *Journal of Clinical Child Psychology*, **22**, 410–19.

Frick, P.J., Kamphaus, R.W., Lahey, B.B. et al. (1991). Academic underachievement and the disruptive behavior disorders. *Journal of Consulting and Clinical Psychology*, **59**, 289–94.

Frick, P.J., Lahey, B.B., Loeber, R. et al. (1992). Familial risk factors to oppositional defiant disorder and conduct disorder: parental psychopathology and maternal parenting. *Journal of Consulting and Clinical Psychology*, **60**, 49–55.

Gardner, F.E. (1994). The quality of joint activity between mothers and their children with behaviour problems. *Journal of Child Psychology and Psychiatry*, **35**, 935–48.

Garralda, M.E. and Bailey, D. (1988). Child and parental factors related to the referral of children to child psychiatry. *British Journal of Psychiatry*, **153**, 81–9.

Garralda, M.E., Connell, J. and Taylor, D. (1989). Peripheral psychophysiological changes in children with conduct and emotional disorders: basal levels and reactivity to sounds. *Behavioural Neurology*, **2**, 125–33.

Garralda, M.E., Connell, J. and Taylor, D. (1991). Psychophysiological anomalies in children with conduct and emotional disorders. *Psychological Medicine*, **21**, 947–57.

Ge, X., Conger, R.D., Cadoret, R.J. et al. (1996). The developmental interface between nature and nurture: a mutual influence model of child antisocial behavior and parent behaviors. *Developmental Psychology*, **32**, 574–89.

Giller, E.L., Perry, B.D., Southwick, S. and Mason, J.W. (1990). Psychoneuroendocrinology of post-traumatic stress disorder. In *Post-Traumatic Stress Disorder: Etiology, Phenomenology and Treatment*, M.E. Wolf and A.D. Mosnaim, eds, pp. 158–70. Washington, DC: American Psychiatric Press.

Glaser, D. (2000). Child abuse and neglect and the brain – a review. *Journal of Child Psychology and Psychiatry*, **41**, 97–116.

Gomez, R., Harvey, J, Quick, C., Scharer, I. and Harris, G. (1999). DSM-IV AD/HD: confirmatory factor models, prevalence, and gender and age differences based on parent and teacher ratings of Australian primary school children. *Journal of Child Psychology and Psychiatry*, **40**, 265–74.

Goodman, C.S. and Shatz, C.J. (1993). Developmental mechanisms that generate precise patterns of neuronal connectivity. *Cell*, **72** (suppl.), 77–98.

Greenberg, M.T., Speltz, M.L., DeKlyen, M. and Endriga, M.C. (1991). Attachment security in preschoolers with and without externalizing problems. *Development and Psychopathology*, **3**, 413–30.

Greenberg, M., Speltz, M.L. and DeKlyen, M. (1993). The role of attachment in the early development of disruptive behavior problems. *Development and Psychopathology*, **5**, 191–214.

Greenough, W.T., Black, J.E. and Wallace, C.S. (1987). Experience and brain development. *Child Development*, **58**, 539–59.

Greenwald, A.G., Draine, S.C. and Abrams, R.L. (1996). Three cognitive markers of unconscious semantic activation. *Science*, **273**, 1699–702.

Haddad, P.H. and Garralda, M.E. (1992). Hyperkinetic syndrome and disruptive early experiences. *British Journal of Psychiatry*, **161**, 700–3.

Hart, J., Gunnar, M. and Cicchetti, D. (1996). Altered neuro-endocrine activity in maltreated children related to symptoms of depression. *Development and Psychopathology*, **8**, 201–14.

Hersov, L. (1990). Aspects of adoption: the seventh Jack Tizard memorial lecture. *Journal of Child Psychology and Psychiatry*, **31**, 493–510.

Hibbs, E.D., Hamburger, S.D., Lenane, M. et al. (1991). Determinants of expressed emotion in families of disturbed and normal children. *Journal of Child Psychology and Psychiatry*, **32**, 757–70.

Hinde, R.P. and Stevenson-Hinde, J. (1987). Interpersonal relationships and child development. *Developmental Review*, **7**, 1–21.

Hinshaw, S. and McHale, J. (1991). Stimulant medications and the social interactions of hyperactive children. In *Personality, Social Skills and Psychopathology*, D. Gilbert and J. Connolly, eds, pp. 229–53. New York: Plenum.

Hinshaw, S.P., Lahey, B.B. and Hart, E.L. (1993). Issues of taxonomy and comorbidity in the development of conduct disorder. Special issue: toward a development perspective on conduct disorder. *Development and Psychopathology*, **5**, 31–49.

Ho, T.P., Luk, S.L., Leung, P.W.L. et al. (1996). Situational versus pervasive hyperactivity in a community sample. *Psychological Medicine*, **26**, 309–21.

Hockfield, S. and Lombroso, P.J. (1998). Development of the cerebral cortex: IX. Cortical development and experience: I. *Journal of the American Academy of Child and Adolescent Psychiatry*, **37**, 992–3.

Hopkin, K. (1997). Too much information? Making sense of genome sequencing. *Journal of the Institutes of Health Research*, **9**, 23–7.

Hughes, C., White, A., Sharpen, J. and Dunn, J. (2000). Antisocial, angry, and unsympathetic: 'hard to manage' preschoolers' peer problems and possible cognitive influences. *Journal of Child Psychology and Psychiatry*, **41**, 169–79.

Jenkins, J.M. and Smith, M.A. (1991). Marital disharmony and children's behaviour problems: Aspects of poor marriage that affect children adversely. *Journal of Child Psychology and Psychiatry*, **32,** 793–810.

Jensen, P.S., Richters, J., Ussery, T., Bloedau, L. and Davis, H. (1991). Child psychopathology and environmental influences: discrete life events versus ongoing adversity. *Journal of the American Academy of Child and Adolescent Psychiatry*, **30**, 303–9.

Jensen, P., Salzberg, A., Ricters, J. and Watanabe, H. (1993). Scales, diagnoses, and child psychopathology: I. CBCL and DISC relationships. *Journal of the American Academy of Child and Adolescent Psychiatry*, **32**, 397–406.

Jones, N.A., Field, T., Fox, N.A., Lundy, B. and Davados, M. (1997). EEG-activation in 1-month old infants of depressed mothers. *Development and Psychopathology*, **9**, 491–505.

Kaler, S.R. and Freeman, B.J. (1994). Analysis of environmental deprivation: cognitive and social development in Romanian orphans. *Journal of Child Psychology and Psychiatry*, **35**, 769–81.

Katz, L. and Shatz, C. (1996). Synaptic activity and the construction of cortical circuits. *Science*, **274**, 1133–8.

Kim, J. and Fanslow, M. (1992). Modality specific retrograde amnesia of fear. *Science*, **256**, 675–7.

Kim, K., Relkin, H., Lee, K. and Hirsch, J. (1997). Distinct cortical areas associated with native and second languages. *Nature*, **388**, 171–4.

Knowlton, B., Mangels, J.A. and Squire, L.R. (1996). A neurostriatal habit learning system in humans. *Science*, **273**, 1399–401.

Kraemer, G.W. (1992). Psychobiological attachment theory (PAT) and psychopathology. *Behavioral and Brain Sciences*, **15**, 525–34.

Kraemer, G.W. and Clarke, A.S. (1996). Social attachment, brain function, and aggression. *Annals of the New York Academy of Sciences*, **794**, 121–35.

Kuhne, M., Schachar, R. and Tannock, R. (1997). Impact of comorbid oppositional or conduct problems on attention-deficit hyperactivity disorder. *Journal of the American Academy of Child and Adolescent Psychiatry*, **36**, 1715–25.

Lahey, B.B., Waldman, I.D. and McBurnett, K. (1999). Annotation: the development of antisocial behavior: an integrative causal model. *Journal of Child Psychology and Psychiatry*, **40**, 669–82.

Lauder, J.M. (1988). Neurotransmitters as morphogens. *Progress in Brain Research*, **73**, 365–88.

LeDoux, J.E. (1989). Cognitive-emotional interaction in the brain. *Cognition and Emotion*, **3**, 267–90.

LeDoux, J.E. (1992). Emotion and the amygdala. In *The Amygdala: Neurobiological Aspects of Emotion, Memory and Mental Dysfunction*, J.P. Aggleton, ed., pp. 339–51. New York: Wiley-Liss.

LeDoux, J.E. (1994). Emotion, memory and the brain. *Scientific American*, **270**, 50–7.

LeDoux, J.E., Romanski, L. and Xagoraris, A. (1989). Indelibility of subcortical emotional memories. *Journal of Cognitive Neuroscience*, **1**, 238–43.

Leung, P.W.L., Ho, T.P., Luk, S.L. et al. (1996). Separation and comorbidity of hyperactivity and conduct disturbance in Chinese school-boys. *Journal of Child Psychology and Psychiatry*, **37**, 841–53.

Lilienfeld, S.O. and Waldman, I.D. (1990). The relation between childhood attention-deficit hyperactivity disorder and adult antisocial behavior reexamined: the problem of heterogeneity. *Clinical Psychology Review*, **10**, 699–725.

Linden, R. (1994). The survival of developing neurons: a review of afferent control. *Neuroscience*, **58**, 671–82.

Liu, D., Diorio, J., Tannenbaum, B. et al. (1997). Maternal care, hippocampal glucocorticoid receptors, and hypothalamic–pituitary–adrenal responses to stress. *Science*, **277**, 1659–62.

Loeber, R., Green, S.M., Keenan, K. and Lahey, B. B. (1995). Which boys will fare worse? Early predictors of the onset of conduct disorder in a six-year longitudinal study. *Journal of the American Academy of Child and Adolescent Psychiatry*, **34**, 499–509.

Lombroso, P.J. and Sapolsky, R. (1998). Development of the cerebral cortex: XII. Stress and brain development: I. *Journal of the American Academy of Child and Adolescent Psychiatry*, **37**, 1337–9.

Luk, S.L., Leung, P.W.L. and Yuen, J. (1991). Clinic observations in the assessment of pervasiveness of childhood hyperactivity. *Journal of Child Psychology and Psychiatry*, **32**, 833–50.

Lynam, D.R. (1996). Early identification of chronic offenders: who is the fledgling psychopath? *Psychological Bulletin*, **120**, 209–34.

Lyons-Ruth, K. (1996). Attachment relationships among children with aggressive behavior problems: the role of disorganized early attachment patterns. *Journal of Consulting and Clinical Psychology*, **64**, 64–73.

Mack, K.J. (1995). The effects of neurotransmission on neuronal gene expression. *Mental Retardation and Developmental Disabilities Research Reviews*, **1**, 169–76.

Main, M. and Solomon, J. (1990). Procedures for identifying infants as disorganized/disoriented during the Ainsworth strange situation. In *Attachment in the Preschool Years*, M. Greenberg, D. Cicchetti and E. Cummings, eds, pp. 121–60. Chicago: University of Chicago Press.

Mannuzza, S., Klein, R.G., Bessler, A., Malloy, P. and Hynes, M.E. (1997). Educational and occupational outcome of hyperactive boys grown up. *Journal of the American Academy of Child and Adolescent Psychiatry*, **36**, 1222–7.

Marshall, V.G., Longwell, L., Goldstein, M.J. and Swanson, J.M. (1990). Family factors associated with aggressive symptomatology in boys with attention deficit hyperactivity disorder: a research note. *Journal of Child Psychology and Psychiatry*, **31**, 629–36.

McEwen, B.S. (1994). Corticosteroids and hippocampal plasticity. *Annals of the New York Academy of Sciences*, **746**, 134–42.

McEwen, B. and Sapolsky, R. (1995). Stress and cognitive function. *Current Opinion in Neurobiology*, **5**, 205–16.

McNally, R.J., Kaspi, S.P., Riemann, B.C. and Zeitlin, S.B. (1990). Selective processing of threat cues in post-traumatic stress disorder. *Journal of Abnormal Psychology*, **99**, 398–402.

Meaney, M.J., Aitken, D.H., Van Berkel, C., Bhatnagar, S. and Sapolsky, R.M. (1988). Effect of neonatal handling on age-related impairments associated with the hippocampus. *Science*, **239**, 766–8.

Mesulam, M. (1990). Large-scale neurocognitive networks and distributed processing for attention, language and memory. *Annals of Neurology*, **28**, 597–613.

Moffitt, T.E. (1990). Juvenile delinquency and attention deficit disorder: boys' developmental trajectories from age 3 to 15. *Child Development*, **61**, 893–910.

Moffitt, T.E. (1993). Adolescence-limited and life-course-persistent antisocial behavior: a developmental taxonomy. *Psychological Review*, **100**, 674–701.

Murray, L. and Cooper, P.J. (1997). *Postpartum Depression and Child Development*. New York: Guilford Press.

Murray, L., Kempton, C., Woolgar, M. and Hooper, R. (1993). Depressed mothers' speech to their infants and its relation to infant gender and cognitive development. *Journal of Child Psychology and Psychiatry*, **34**, 1083–101.

Murray, L., Fiori-Cowley, A., Hooper, R. and Cooper, P.J. (1996a). The impact of postnatal depression and associated adversity on early mother–infant interactions and later infant outcome. *Child Development*, **67**, 2512–26.

Murray, L., Hipwell, A., Hooper, R., Stein, A. and Cooper, P.J. (1996b). The cognitive development of 5-year-old children of postnatally depressed mothers. *Journal of Child Psychology and Psychiatry*, **37**, 927–35.

Murray, L., Sinclair, D., Cooper, P. et al. (1999). The socioemotional development of 5-year-old children of postnatally depressed mothers. *Journal of Child Psychology and Psychiatry*, **40**, 1259–71.

Nelson, A. and Bloom, E. (1997). Child development and neuroscience. *Child Development*, **68**, 970–87.

O'Connor, T.G., Deater-Deckard, K., Fulker, D., Rutter, M. and Plomin, R. (1998). Genotype-environment correlations in late childhood and early adolescence: antisocial behavioural problems and coercive parenting. *Developmental Psychology*, **34**, 970–81.

Olson, S.L., Bates, J.E. and Bayles, K. (1990). Early antecedents of childhood impulsivity. The role of parent–child interaction, cognitive competence, and temperament. *Journal of Abnormal Child Psychology*, **18**, 317–34.

Olson, S.L., Schilling, E.M. and Bates, J.E. (1999). Measurement of impulsivity: construct coherence, longitudinal stability, and relationship with externalizing problems in middle childhood and adolescence. *Journal of Abnormal Child Psychology*, **27**, 151–65.

Overmeyer, S., Taylor, E., Blanz, B. and Schmidt, M.H. (1999). Psychosocial adversities underestimated in hyperkinetic children. *Journal of Child Psychology and Psychiatry*, **40**, 259–63.

Pagani, L., Boulerice, B., Vitaro, F. and Tremblay, R.E. (1999). Effects of poverty on academic failure and delinquency in boys: a change and process model approach. *Journal of Child Psychology and Psychiatry*, **40**, 1209–19.

Perry, B.D. (1994). Neurobiological sequelae of childhood trauma: post-traumatic stress disorders in children. In *Catecholamines in Post-Traumatic Stress Disorder: Emerging Concepts*, ed. M. Murberg, ed., pp. 253–76. Washingon, DC: American Psychiatric Press.

Perry, B.D. (1996). *Maltreated Children, Brain Development and the Next Generation*. New York: W.W. Norton.

Perry, B.D. and Pollard, R. (1998). Homeostasis, stress, trauma, and adaptation. A neurodevelopmental view of childhood trauma. *Child and Adolescent Clinics of North America*, **7**, 33–51.

Perry, B.D., Pollard, R., Blakely, T., Baker, W. and Vigilante, D. (1995). Childhood trauma, the neurobiology of adaptation and 'use-dependent' development of the brain: How 'states' become 'traits'. *Infant Mental Health Journal*, **16**, 271–91.

Pfiffner, L.J., McBurnett, K., Lahey, B.B. et al. (1999). Association of parental psychopathology to the comorbid disorders of boys with attention deficit–hyperactivity disorder. *Journal of Consulting and Clinical Psychology*, **67**, 881–93.

Pihoker, C., Owens, M.J., Kuhn, C.M., Schanberg, S.M. and Nemeroff, C.B. (1993). Maternal separation in neonatal rats elicits activation of the hypothalamic–pituitary–adrenocortical axis: a putative role of corticotropin-releasing factor. *Psychoneuroendocrinology*, **18**, 485–93.

Pliszka, S.R. (1992). Comorbidity of attention-deficit hyperactivity disorder and overanxious disorder. *Journal of the American Academy of Child and Adolescent Psychiatry*, **31**, 197–203.

Plomin, R. (1994). Genetic research and identification of environmental influences: Emanuel Miller memorial lecture (1993). *Journal of Child Psychology and Psychiatry*, **35**, 817–34.

Plomin, R. (1995). Genetics and children's experiences in the family. *Journal of Child Psychology and Psychiatry*, **36**, 33–68.

Plomin, R. and Bergeman, C.S. (1991). The nature of nurture: genetic influences on 'environmental' measures. *Behavioral and Brain Sciences*, **14**, 373–427.

Plotsky, P.M. (1997). Long-term consequences of adverse early experience: a rodent model. *Biological Psychiatry*, **41**, 778.

Plotsky, P.M. and Meaney, M.J. (1993). Early post-natal experience alters hypothalamic corticotropin-releasing factor (CRF) mRNA, median eminence CRF content and stress-induced release in adult rats. *Molecular Brain Research*, **18**, 195–200

Pollak, S.D., Cicchetti, D., Klorman, R. and Brumaghim, J.T. (1997). Cognitive brain event-related potentials and emotion processing in maltreated children. *Child Development*, **68**, 773–87.

Post, R.M. and Weiss, S.R.B. (1997). Emergent properties of neural systems: how focal molecular neurobiological alterations can affect behavior. *Development and Psychopathology*, **9**, 907–29.

Post, R.M., Weiss, S.R.B., Smith, M., Li, H. and McCann, U. (1997). Kindling versus quenching: implications for the evolution and treatment of post-traumatic stress disorder. *Annals of the New York Academy of Sciences*, **821**, 285–95.

Rieder, C. and Cicchetti, D. (1989). Organizational perspective on cognitive control functioning and cognitive-effective balance in maltreated childen. *Developmental Psychology*, **25**, 382–93.

Rogeness, G. and McClure, E. (1996). Development and neurotransmitter–environmental inter-actions. *Development and Psychopatholoy*, **8**, 183–99.

Rogeness, G., Javors, M. and Pliszka, S. (1992). Neurochemistry and child and adolescent psychiatry. *Journal of the American Academy of Child and Adolescent Psychiatry*, **31**, 765–81.

Rolls, E.T. (1992). Neurophysiology and functions of the primate amygdala. In *The Amygdala: Neurobiological Aspects of Emotion, Memory, and Mental Dysfunction*, J.P. Aggleton, ed., pp. 143–65. New York: Wiley-Liss.

Rutter, M. (1996). Developmental psychopathology: concepts and prospects. In *Frontiers of Developmental Psychopathology*, M. Lenzenweger and J. Havgaard, eds, pp. 209–37. New York: Oxford University Press.

Rutter, M. (1997a). Comorbidity: concepts, claims and choices. *Criminal Behavior and Mental Health*, **7**, 265–85.

Rutter, M. (1997b). Implications of genetic research for child psychiatry. *Canadian Journal of Psychiatry*, **42**, 569–76.

Rutter, M., Dunn, J., Plomin, R. et al. (1997a). Integrating nature and nurture: implications of person–environment correlations and interactions for developmental psychology. *Development and Psychopathology*, **9**, 335–64.

Rutter, M., Maughan, B., Meyer, J. et al. (1997b). Heterogeneity of antisocial behavior: causes, continuities, and consequences. *Nebraska Symposium on Motivation*, **44**, 45–118.

Rutter, M. and the English and Romanian Adoptees (ERA) Study Team (1998). Developmental catch-up, and deficit, following adoption after severe global early privation. *Journal of Child Psychology and Psychiatry*, **39**, 465–76.

Sandberg, S. and Garralda, M.E. (1996). Psychosocial contributions. In *Hyperactivity Disorders of Childhood*, S. Sandberg, ed., pp. 280–328. Cambridge: Cambridge University Press.

Sapolsky, R. (1996a). Stress, glucocorticoids, and damage to the nervous system: the current state of confusion. *Stress*, **1**, 1–9.

Sapolsky, R. (1996b). Why stress is bad for your brain. *Science*, **273**, 749–50.

Satterfield, J.H. and Schell, A. (1997). A prospective study of hyperactive boys with conduct problems and normal boys: adolescent and adult criminality. *Journal of the American Academy of Child and Adolescent Psychiatry*, **36**, 1726–35.

Scahill, L., Schwab-Stone, M.E., Merikangas, K.R. et al. (1999). Psychosocial and clinical corre-lates of ADHD in a community sample of school-age children. *Journal of the American Academy of Child and Adolescent Psychiatry*, **38**, 976–84.

Schachar, R. (1991). Childhood hyperactivity. *Journal of Child Psychology and Psychiatry*, **32**, 155–91.

Schachar, R. and Tannock, R. (1995). Test of four hypotheses for the comorbidity of attention-deficit hyperactivity disorder and conduct disorder. *Journal of the American Academy of Child and Adolescent Psychiatry*, **34**, 639–48.

Schachar, R. and Wachsmuth, R. (1990). Hyperactivity and parental psychopathology. *Journal of Child Psychology and Psychiatry*, **31**, 381–92.

Schachar, R.J. and Wachsmuth, R. (1991). Family dysfunction and psychosocial adversity: comparison of attention deficit disorder, conduct disorder, normal and clinical controls. *Canadian Journal of Behavioral Science*, **23**, 332–48.

Schachar, R.J., Taylor, E., Wieselberg, M., Thorley, G. and Rutter, M. (1987). Changes in family function and relationships in children who respond to methylphenidate. *Journal of the American Academy of Child and Adolescent Psychiatry*, **26**, 728–32.

Schneider, M.L., Clarke, A.S., Kraemer, G.W. et al. (1998). Prenatal stress alters brain biogenic amine levels in primates. *Development and Psychopathology*, **10**, 427–40.

Schore, A. (1994). *Affect Regulation and the Origin of the Self.* Hillsdale, NJ: Erlbaum.

Seifer, R., Sameroff, A.J., Dickstein, S. et al. (1996). Parental psychopathology, multiple contex-tual risks, and one-year outcomes in children. *Journal of Clinical Child Psychology*, **25**, 423–35.

Silberg, J., Rutter, M., Meyer, J. et al. (1996). Genetic and environmental influences on the covariation between hyperactivity and conduct disturbance in juvenile twins. *Journal of Child Psychology and Psychiatry*, **37**, 803–16.

Singer, W. (1995). Development and plasticity of cortical processing architectures. *Science*, **270**, 758–64.

Sonuga-Barke, E.J., Taylor, E. and Heptinstall, E. (1992). Hyperactivity and delay aversion: II. The effect of self versus externally imposed stimulus presentation periods on memory. *Journal of Child Psychology and Psychiatry*, **33**, 399–409.

Speltz, M.L., DeKlyen, M. and Greenberg, M.T. (1999). Attachment in boys with early onset conduct problems. *Development and Psychopathology*, **11**, 269–85.

Squire, L. (1992). Declarative and non-declarative memory: multiple brain systems supporting learning and memory. *Journal of Cognitive Neuroscience*, **4**, 232–43.

Sroufe, L.A., Egeland, B. and Kreutzer, T. (1990). The fate of early experience following developmental change: longitudinal approaches to individual adaptation in childhood. *Child Development*, **61**, 1363–73.

Sroufe, L.A. (1997). Psychopathology as outcome of development. *Development and Psychopathol-ogy*, **9**, 251–68.

Sroufe, L.A., Carlson, E.A., Levy, A.K. and Egeland, B. (1999). Implications of attachment. *Development and Psychopathology*, **11**, 1–13.

Stein, A., Gath, D.H., Bucher, J. et al. (1991). The relationship between post-natal depression and mother–child interaction. *British Journal of Psychiatry*, **158**, 46–52.

Stone, E. (1992). Stress and brain neurotransmitter receptors. In *Receptors and Ligands in Psychiatry*, A.K. Sen and T. Lee, eds, pp. 400–23. New York: Cambridge University Press.

Svensson, T.H. (1987). Peripheral, autonomic regulation of locus coeruleus noradrenergic neurons in brain: putative implications for psychiatry and psychopharmacology. *Psychopharmacology*, **92**, 1–7.

Tannock, R. (1998). Attention deficit hyperactivity disorder: advances in cognitive, neurobiological, and genetic research. *Journal of Child Psychology and Psychiatry*, **39**, 65–99.

Taylor, E. (1999). Development of clinical services for attention-deficit /hyperactivity disorder. *Archives of General Psychiatry*, **56**, 1097–9.

Taylor, E., Sandberg, S., Thorley, G. and Giles, S. (1991). *The Epidemiology of Childhood Hyperactivity. Maudsley Monographs*, **33**. Oxford: Oxford University Press.

Taylor, E., Chadwick, O., Heptinstall, E. and Danckaerts, M. (1996). Hyperactivity and conduct problems as risk factors for adolescent development. *Journal of the American Academy of Child and Adolescent Psychiatry*, **35**, 1213–26.

The MTA Cooperative Group. (1999). Moderators and mediators of treatment response for children with attention-deficit/hyperactivity disorder: the Multimodal Treatment Study of children with attention-deficit/hyperactivity disorder. *Archives of General Psychiatry*, **56**, 1088–96.

Thoenen, H. (1995). Neurotrophins and neuronal plasticity. *Science*, **270**, 593–8.

Tizard, B. and Hodges, J. (1978). The effect of early institutional rearing on the development of eight-year-old children. *Journal of Child Psychology and Psychiatry*, **19**, 99–118.

Toupin, J., Déry, M., Pauzé, R., Mercier, H. and Fortin, L. (2000). Cognitive and familial contributions to conduct disorder in children. *Journal of Child Psychology and Psychiatry*, **41**, 333–44.

Trevarthen, C. and Aitken, K.J. (1994). Brain development, infant communication, and empathy disorders: Intrinsic factors in child mental health. *Development and Psychopathology*, **6**, 597–633.

Wakschlag, L.S. and Hans, S.L. (1999). Relation of maternal responsiveness during infancy to the development of behavior problems in high-risk youths. *Developmental Psychology*, **35**, 569–79.

Wallace, C.S., Kilman, V.L., Withers, G.S. and Greenough, W.T. (1992). Increases in dendritic length in occipital cortex after 4 days of differential housing in weanling rats. *Behavioural and Neural Biology*, **58**, 64–8.

Warner-Rogers, J., Taylor, A., Taylor, E. and Sandberg, S. (2000). Inattentive behavior in childhood: epidemiology and implications for development. *Journal of Learning Disabilities*, **33**, 520–36.

Winslow, J.T., Hastings, N., Carter, C.S., Harbaugh, C.R. and Insel, T.R. (1993). A role for central vasopressin in pair bonding in monogamous prairie voles. *Nature*, **365**, 545–8.

Woodward, L., Taylor, E. and Dowdney, L. (1998). The parenting and family functioning of children with hyperactivity. *Journal of Child Psychology and Psychiatry*, **39**, 161–9.

World Health Organization (WHO). (1978). *International Classification of Diseases*, 9th edn. Geneva: WHO.

World Health Organization (WHO). (1992). *ICD-10 Classification of Mental and Behavioural Disorders: Clinical Descriptions and Diagnostic Guidelines*. Geneva: World Health Organization.

Xu, L., Anwyl, R. and Rowan, M.J. (1997). Beavioral stress facilitates the induction of long-term depression in the hippocampus. *Nature*, **387**, 497–500.

Yehuda, R., Kahana, B., Schmeidler, J. et al. (1995). Impact of cumulative lifetime trauma and recent stress on current post-traumatic stress disorder symptoms in holocaust survivors. *American Journal of Psychiatry*, **152**, 1815–18.

12

Institutional care as a risk factor for inattention/overactivity

Michael Rutter, Penny Roy and Jana Kreppner

Social, Genetic and Developmental Psychiatry Research Centre, Institute of Psychiatry, London, UK

Numerous clinical and epidemiological studies have shown substantial associations between a range of psychosocial adversities and attention deficit hyperactivity disorder (ADHD: Taylor, 1986; Taylor et al., 1991; Biederman et al., 1995; Scahill et al., 1999; Chapter 11). It is usually assumed that the associations represent the operation of environmentally mediated risk factors. This would seem to be justified on the basis that rigorous research designs have shown significant effects on psychopathology of features such as family negativity and conflict (Rutter, 2000a), and therapeutic interventions designed to reduce coercive family interactions have been shown to bring about worthwhile benefits (Rutter et al., 1998). In recent times, attention has tended to shift away from the role of possible psychosocial influences in aetiology, because of the consistent finding that genetic factors account for a major part of the variation in individual liability to ADHD; that influence is probably greater than that for any other child psychiatric disorder other than autism (Tannock, 1998; Rutter et al., 1999; Thapar et al., 1999), and because of the huge body of evidence showing the benefits stemming from stimulant medication (MTA Cooperative Group, 1999a,b). Nevertheless, the genetic findings show that ADHD is a multifactorial disorder in which environmental as well as genetic factors play a role in aetiology. Also, there is some evidence that the best therapeutic results may come from multimodal interventions that include, but are not restricted to, medication (Taylor, 1999). Several difficulties have bedevilled attempts to identify specific psychosocial risk factors for ADHD.

To begin with, much of the evidence concerns influences on disruptive behaviour generally, rather than specifically on ADHD. A further problem concerns the uncertainty about whether or not the associations reflect environmental risk mediation. Children showing ADHD present many difficulties in management for parents and teachers, and it is necessary to consider the possibility that the family adversities may derive from the *effects* of the children's behaviour, rather than that the adversities serve as causal influences on that behaviour. The reality of this possibility is shown by both genetic and intervention studies. Thus, studies of away-adopted children born to antisocial parents have shown that the disruptive behaviour of the children has elicited raised rates of negative interactions from the adopting parents. Children's behaviour shapes and selects the environments that they experience (Ge et al., 1996; O'Connor et al., 1998). Similarly, treatment studies have shown that, when stimulant medication improves children's behaviour, this may also have secondary beneficial effects on parent behaviour (Schachar et al., 1987; Barkley, 1989). Passive gene–environment correlations may also be important. Because genetic influences on ADHD are quite strong, it may be inferred that the increased rate of parental psychopathology will partially reflect genetic mediation and that this will result in the parents with disorder being more likely to provide adverse rearing environments (Rutter et al., 1997a,b).

An alternative research strategy involves starting with a postulated psychosocial risk factor and determining whether this leads to the increased rate of ADHD. One such risk factor that lends itself to this approach is institutional rearing. Several studies of children with ADHD have noted the high frequency with which this appears in the background of the children. For example, Taylor (1986), in a clinic study, singled out a prolonged period of institutional care as the one psychosocial adversity that seemed to have a specific association with hyperkinetic disorder. Haddad and Garralda (1992) reported five case studies of children with the hyperkinetic syndrome who had had severely disrupted early rearing; this involved residential care in three instances and family foster care in the other two. Several of the children were said to show indiscriminate friendliness, attention seeking and poorly modulated peer interactions, and it was suggested that there may have been an impaired development of selective attachments. Tizard and Hodges (1978), in their follow-up of children initially reared in residential nurseries, also noted that inattention/overactivity (I/O) sometimes accompanied relationship difficulties. Carlson et al. (1995), in their longitudinal study of socially disadvantaged families, found that early marital disruption, along with intrusive caregiving, was the best differentiator of children who showed ADHD in middle childhood. Schachar and Wachsmuth (1991) somewhat similarly commented on the association with parent–child separations.

The findings raise the query of whether institutional care is just serving as an index of multiple psychosocial adversities or whether the experience of rearing in residential group care itself constitutes a specific risk factor. There is also the query of whether institutional care serves as a direct contemporaneous situational influence on I/O or whether this pattern of rearing has some kind of developmental programming effect that persists even if there is later rearing in a harmonious stable family. Finally, there is the query of whether the I/O that sometimes follows institutional care represents a different form of psychopathology than 'ordinary' varieties of ADHD or hyperkinetic disorder. To answer these questions, prospective studies of children initially reared in residential group care are required.

Two key methodological issues need to be addressed when using this research strategy. First, it is crucial to rule out the possibility that the institutional care has been provided because of the children's disruptive behaviour, in which case the association would reflect an effect of the child on the environment, rather than the other way around. The solution to that problem lies in focusing on children admitted to institutional care in early infancy. The second methodological issue concerns the measurement of ADHD as an outcome variable. The problem is that both overactivity and inattention not only serve as defining symptoms for a specific psychiatric disorder, namely ADHD, but are also the nonspecific indicators of a much broader range of psychopathology. The problem is by no means unique to ADHD because exactly the same sort of issue arises in relation to anxiety and to depression. In a real sense, all of these behaviours function rather like fever or fatigue in somatic medical disorders. Psychological malfunction of any type may interfere with concentration, or lead to restlessness. Most obviously, this is the case with anxiety disorders, mania and major depression. Accordingly, if institutional care is found to be associated with overactivity and inattention, it will be necessary to consider whether or not these behaviours are reflecting the specific condition of ADHD or, rather, are indexing psychopathology that has a rather different meaning. In this chapter, we consider two studies that have set out to examine the sequelae of institutional rearing, and in which the outcome measures have included a specific focus on I/O.

Adoptees from Romania

The first investigation concerned children who spent their early life in extremely depriving institutions in Romania and who were subsequently adopted into well-functioning homes in the UK (Rutter and the ERA study team, 1998, 2000; Kreppner et al., 2001). The conditions experienced by most of the children were extremely poor, with a life largely confined to cots without toys, with little in the way of play or conversation with caregivers. Malnutrition was rife and, at the time of coming to the UK, over half the children had weights below the third percentile. The mean developmental quotient was in the mildly retarded range, and some half of the children were severely retarded in their functioning. During the 2 years or so following adoption, there was quite remarkable developmental catch-up, regaining of normal height and weight and major improvements across the whole range of psychological functioning. The outcome for Romanian adoptees who experienced an institutional upbringing was compared with that of nondeprived UK children adopted into UK families in the first 6 months of life. Compared with these within-UK adoptees, the Romanian adoptees as a group were more likely to show various forms of disturbance, although many were functioning normally in all domains (Rutter et al., 2001). An attempt was made to identify those sequelae that seemed to be specifically associated with psychological privation associated with institutional care. Two criteria were laid down to identify specificity. First, there should be a significant difference in the rates of behaviour between the two groups of adoptees; and, second, the pattern of behaviour should show a systematic dose–response relationship for the duration of institutional care within the Romanian adoptee group. In each case, this was considered in relation to the children's behaviour as assessed at the age of 6 years. Hyperactivity/inattention was assessed through the use of the relevant subscale on the Rutter parent and Teacher Questionnaires (Schachar and Wachsmuth, 1991; Elander and Rutter, 1996; Hogg et al., 1997).

At 6 years of age, the adoptees from Romania (both boys and girls) had a mean level of I/O that was higher than that for the within-UK adoptees; the difference was most marked for those who came to the UK over the age of 2 years (Kreppner et al., 2001). On the teacher scale, their I/O score was about a standard deviation higher than that in the UK group; on the parent scale, the difference was about half a standard deviation. Strikingly, there was no increase in I/O in the children from Romania who had been adopted under the age of 6 months. Expressed in categorical terms, just over a third of children from Romania adopted over the age of 2 years showed pervasive I/O (defined in terms of a score in the top decile on the basis of information from either parent or teacher and a score that was at least above the median from the other informant). The comparable figure for the within-UK adoptees was about 10%, as it was too in the children adopted from Romania when they were aged under 6 months.

By contrast, neither oppositional defiant/conduct difficulties nor emotional difficulties were any more frequent in the group of adoptees from Romania, and neither showed any association with duration of privation. The association (a correlation of c. 0.3) between institutional privation and I/O was relatively specific to this particular form of disruptive behaviour.

The findings at age 4 years were closely similar, although the between-group differences were not as marked. Again, no association was found between institutional privation and either oppositional or conduct disorder or emotional disturbance.

At both 4 and 6 years of age, there was a moderately strong correlation between the ratings of parents and teachers for I/O (c. 0.5), and this was higher than those for either conduct problems or emotional difficulties (these ranged between 0.17 and 0.36). Similarly, there was a moderate consistency over time for both parent and teacher ratings of I/O (0.74 for the former and 0.43 for the latter). There was a difference, however, in the longitudinal course of the parent and teacher ratings of I/O between 4 and 6 years of age; the latter tended to remain stable whereas the former tended to decrease. It seems likely that the consistency in I/O on teacher ratings reflects the difficulties experienced by the children in coping with task-oriented group teaching situations, whereas the decrease in parent ratings reflects the extent to which families adapted to the children's behaviour and avoided situations that seemed likely to predispose to I/O. Whatever the explanation, in the children seen clinically by Michael Rutter (MR), it did seem apparent both that entry to school made difficulties more overt and that these tended to be most marked in group situations and least marked in dyadic ones. It was evident that the effect of duration of institutional privation on I/O was as strong on this behaviour at age 6 as it had been at age 4. The implication is that, whatever the mechanism, it represented a relatively persistent effect that continued over the transition to school.

Three main possible confounders needed to be considered. Not surprisingly, given the fact that most of the Romanian children came from very poor families, there was an excess of prematurely born children of low birth weight. It was possible that brain dysfunction stemming from obstetric hazards could have predisposed to I/O, but no association was found. Second, most of the children were severely nutritionally deprived, and it was possible that malnutrition constituted the key causal influence. However, this did not prove to be the case. The children's weight at entry showed no significant association with I/O at 4 years of age; at age 6 years, there was a significant association but more strongly so with teacher reports ($r = -0.27$) than parent reports ($r = -0.18$). When multiple variables were entered into a regression equation, weight at entry continued to have a significant effect ($\beta = 0.25$) on teacher ratings of I/O at 6, but the effect of age of entry was somewhat stronger ($\beta = 0.33$), and there was no significant effect of weight at entry on parent ratings. For children whose weights at the time of entry to the UK were in the top third of the distribution, the correlation between age at entry and I/O were 0.42 and 0.30 for parent and teacher reports respectively. It may be concluded that malnutrition played a contributory predisposing role but that it was not the main causal influence.

The third possible confound is provided by intellectual impairment. At age 6 years, I/O, as assessed by both parent and teacher reports, showed a moderate correlation with the McCarthy General Cognitive Index (GCI: -0.43 and -0.36, respectively). This was to be expected because both the GCI and I/O were associated with duration of privation, and this would result in an intercorrelation between the two outcomes. The question was, however, whether the rating of I/O primarily arose as a consequence of intellectual impairment rather than of institutional privation. This possibility was tested in two different ways. First, a multivariate analysis determined whether the effects of duration on I/O remained after taking cognitive ability into account. The findings showed that they did, although the effects were reduced. Second, using the category of pervasive I/O, we determined whether this was associated with duration of privation within the middle of the IQ range. The findings showed that it was to a significant extent, although the rate of I/O was highest in those with mild cognitive impairment. Excluding the top and bottom 15% of the distribution (thereby focusing on the range of 86–127), the rate of pervasive I/O in the UK adoptees was 11.4%; in the Romanian children adopted before 6 months it was 15.6%; it was 36.8% in the group adopted between 6 and 24 months; and 27.3% in the group adopted after 2 years. It may be concluded that, although there is a meaningful association of moderate strength between I/O and mild cognitive impairment within the normal range, this does not account for the association between I/O and duration of privation.

A necessary further question, however, concerned the meaning of I/O. One way of approaching that question was to determine the extent to which I/O cooccurred with attachment problems. These were assessed on the basis of three items from the interview with the adoptive parents: a definite lack of differentiation between adults, a clear indication that the child would readily go off with a stranger, and a definite lack of checking back with the parent in anxiety-provoking situations. Whereas both conduct problems and emotional difficulties showed some overlap with attachment problems, the associations lacked consistency (they were significant on teacher report but not on parent report), there was a substantial association between attachment problems and I/O on both parent and teacher reports (Kreppner et al., 2001; Rutter et al., 2001). The polychoric correlation between the two, when assessed as categories, was 0.47. Moreover, a cluster analysis showed that the children from Romania who were placed in UK families after the age of 2 years were most likely to show either a combination of I/O and attachment problems or a more complex multiproblem cluster that included both I/O and attachment difficulties but also impaired peer relationships and conduct difficulties.

When the same issue was dealt with dimensionally, the conclusions were essentially the same. The correlation coefficients between I/O and attachment difficulty scales were 0.44 and 0.38 for parent and teacher reports of I/O, respectively, at age 4 years and 0.44 and 0.45 at age 6 years. Multivariate analysis showed that both the GCI and attachment problems had independent effects on I/O, the effects of the two being of roughly similar magnitude (but those of attachment problems were marginally stronger).

The last topic with respect to the I/O shown by these Romanian adoptees is the extent to which the clinical pattern is the same as that associated with ordinary ADHD or hyperkinetic syndrome. No firm answer to that crucial question is yet available but case histories provide some useful pointers.

Peter was noted to be very inattentive from the time of first starting school. He was very friendly with everyone, liked and sought people's attention, was markedly lacking in shyness and even at 6 years would still tend to approach strangers to tell them his life story. Although very talkative, it was difficult to hold a conversation with him because his ideas, like his attention, tended to wander off or jump from topic to topic. Often he talked over other people and also he frequently repeated phrases from videos out of context. He was strikingly fidgety, was 'on the go' all the time, was restless during his sleep and he needed constant supervision because of his tendency to climb everywhere or to go into inappropriate places. There were several unusual circumscribed interests involving frequent caressing of his special objects (such as a particular type of telephone). He seemed not to learn from experience and had been to hospital several times for lacerations to be sutured. There was a lack of awareness of social boundaries so that, for example, he insisted on kissing a doctor whom he was meeting for the first time. At home he was defiant, oppositional and confrontational, but at school he was, if anything, unusually keen to follow rules. His cognitive abilities were found on testing to be towards the lower end of the normal range. Independently of the study, he was prescribed methylphenidate. This was followed by a definite improvement in his behaviour but the general pattern remained much the same, and he continued to present major difficulties in management.

Barbara was seen by her teachers at school as markedly inattentive, restless, fidgety, demanding of attention, and failing to finish tasks. Her behaviour in school was also problematic because she had difficulty accepting authority or criticism, reacted badly to teasing and had difficulty controlling her anger or frustration. Her cognitive skills were well within the normal range but were below average. She was at her best in a one-to-one session and concentrated reasonably well during individual psychological testing. She was much less good in a classroom setting and had difficulty following group instruction. Her parents found her better behaved than her teachers did but they commented on her relative passivity and lack of curiosity. She was strikingly socially naive so that other children found it easy to get her to do silly things that put her into trouble. This was exacerbated by her lack of concern about the effects on others of her behaviour, her lack of appreciation of how situations might turn out, and by a relative lack of awareness of social boundaries. In a one-to-one meeting with a new person she was friendly, lacking shyness and was socially disinhibited, but she was not either overactive or inattentive.

Ralph had an IQ just below average but lagged behind other children in his scholastic achievements. Both at home and at school he had difficulty concentrating and tended to give up easily if faced with a challenging task; he was also fidgety, tending to fiddle with objects and play with things he was not supposed to touch. His general restlessness was irritating to other people but he did not appear pervasively overactive. It was noteworthy that he was somewhat inappropriately friendly with people whom he did not know, he readily talked to strangers in the street or in the shops, he would occasionally ask personally intrusive questions and generally was rather lacking in social modulation and adequate awareness of social boundaries. Compared with Peter and Barbara, however, all these features were much milder, and he was generally getting on much better than had been the case when he was younger.

The behaviour of these three children illustrates well the extent to which inattention and overactivity tended to be bound up with difficulties in social relationships and especially with limitations in their awareness of social cues, social boundaries and the effects of their behaviour on other people. They varied in both the degree and pervasiveness of their inattention and overactivity. Peter had been firmly diagnosed as suffering from a clearcut attention deficit disorder with hyperactivity, and methylphenidate was seen as the solution. The medication brought some worthwhile benefits but it did not alleviate his more widespread problems and the particular nature of his social relationship difficulties had not been highlighted by the clinician he saw. Barbara did not appear particularly inattentive or overactive when seen individually although, evidently, she was both at school. Her social naivety was the most obvious feature both at home and at interview. Ralph's fidgetiness and difficulty sticking with tasks were clearly manifest, although less associated with a broader range of problems than those seen with the other two children. His social disinhibition was more marked when he was younger but still persisted to some extent.

Institutional and family foster care in the UK

The findings from our study of Romanian adoptees provided a strong case for the hypothesis that institutional privation has a relatively specific effect in predisposing to I/O. It has the particular strength of showing that the effect persisted some years after the children left the depriving environment and experienced good-quality rearing in their new adoptive homes. A direct situation-specific effect could be ruled out. On the other hand, it had three important limitations. First, because the conditions in the Romanian institutions were usually so pervasively poor in all respects, it was not possible to differentiate between the effects of, say, gross experiential deprivation (being confined to cots/cribs, no toys, lack of play and conversation, etc.), and a lack of an opportunity to develop selective attachment relationships (as a result of very poor staff–child ratios, lack of individualized care and lack of continuity in the adults providing security and comfort, insofar as anyone did so). Second, because the very poor institutional conditions predisposed to cognitive impairment, it was difficult to determine the extent to which institutional rearing led to I/O in the absence of cognitive impairment. Third, although standardized measures from both parents and teachers were available, there were no direct observations of the children's behaviour in the classroom (even though there were videotaped observations of the children's interactions with parents and with researchers).

The research design for our second study dealt with all three limitations. It took as its starting point the well-established finding that, as a group, children experiencing various forms of alternative or substitute care as a result of a breakdown in parenting in the biological family show rates of emotional/behavioural disturbance (including I/O) well above general population base rates (Rutter, 2000b). The question we tackled was whether the particular form of substitute care contributed to this increased risk and, in particular, whether group residential care constituted a substantial environmentally mediated risk for psychopathology (Roy et al., 2000). In order to focus specifically on the effects of care, the sample was restricted to children removed from their biological parents in the first year of life (in the event, the mean age was 3 months), and the group excluded children known to have handicaps at the time of placement.

Children placed in residential group care were compared with those placed in family foster care. Blind ratings of the social service records showed that both groups came from biological homes with very high rates of parental psychopathology and of adverse family circumstances, but they did not differ in that respect. The family foster homes showed personalized caregiving with high stability but, by contrast, the group homes provided caregiving that was dispersed across a changing range of adults. However, both groups were well looked after, and the children in group homes were both well nourished and had extensive social and other experiences (in marked distinction from those in the Romanian institutions). Both groups were followed up to age 5–7 years and were assessed in the same way through psychometric testing, teacher interview and questionnaire, parental interview and questionnaire, and direct observations in school. Classroom controls were selected for both groups.

Both the group care (institutional) and family foster care groups had a mean Wechsler Intelligence Scale for Children (WISC) IQ of slightly above 100, and there was no difference between the groups in IQ level. Findings throughout were examined both before and after controlling for IQ, with essentially the same results.

The first step in the analysis comprised a comparison of the institution and foster care groups, on the Rutter Teacher Questionnaire (Elander and Rutter, 1996; Hogg et al., 1997), with the further comparison of both these groups with their respective classroom controls. Three items (very restless, squirmy/fidgety, and cannot settle for more than a few moments) were used to assess I/O (Schachar et al., 1981). The findings showed an overall increase in rate of behavioural disturbance in the institutional group that fell just short of statistical significance, but a much greater (and statistically significant) increase in I/O. The mean hyperactivity score was 3.0 in the institutional group, as compared with 1.4 in the foster group – a difference of about two-thirds of a standard deviation. Parent questionnaire scores gave the same picture on the rate of overall disturbance so that the high rate in the institutional group was particularly evident with respect to problems that spanned both home and school settings. This applied to 42% of the children in residential group care as compared with only 5% of the children in family foster care. Observational measures showed that this pervasive disturbance included I/O.

Inevitably, questionnaire ratings are potentially susceptible to rater biases deriving from knowledge (albeit imperfect and sometimes inaccurate) about the children's backgrounds. Accordingly, systematic nonparticipant classroom observations were undertaken and used to derive composite measures of inattention and overactivity (Roy et al., 2000). These showed the same raised rate of inattention in the institutional group; their mean score was well over half a standard deviation higher than that in the foster group. A comparable pattern was found for observed overactivity, although the difference was not as great (and just less than half a standard deviation). Interestingly, however, although the raised rate of I/O in the institutional group applied to both boys and girls on the teacher ratings, it applied only to boys on the observational measures (Roy et al., submitted).

In order to understand better the meaning of the raised rate of I/O in the institutional group, similar between-group comparisons were undertaken for various measures of the children's social relationships at home and at school and these, in turn, were examined for their associations with I/O. Selectivity of attachment to caregivers and peers was assessed from the caregiver interview on the basis of items tapping specificity of affection, seeking of comfort, selectivity of attachment to main carer and overfriendliness to strangers (in the case of caregivers) and specificity of friendships, selective attachment to peers and indiscriminate relationships (in the case of peer attachment).

A marked lack of selective attachment to caregivers was found only in the institutional group (21%), but possible attachment was equally frequent in the two groups, being present in about a third. A marked lack of selective attachment to peers as reported by caregivers was similarly only found in the institutional group (21% vs. 0%). Altogether, over a third of the institutional children (all boys) showed a marked lack of selective attachment to caregivers or peers, but this applied to none of the children in foster families. In short, a marked lack of selective attachments was a feature only of children reared in group care institutions. Other types of social relationship difficulties, however, were found in both groups.

The next question was whether I/O tended to be associated with either a marked lack of selective attachments or with other relationship difficulties. The findings were clearcut in showing significant associations between I/O (as measured by the teacher scale, or by observational measures of inattention or overactivity) and a marked lack of selective attachments. Two important qualifiers, however, need to be added to that finding. First, although the association was very strong, it applied only to a marked lack of selective attachments and not to milder degrees of uncertain selective attachment. Second, the differences between the institutional and foster groups on I/O, and the associations with a marked lack of attachments, did not hold up in girls. It remains uncertain whether the gender specificity in this small sample was a function of small numbers or rather a gender difference in response to group care when it is not accompanied by gross deprivation (as in the Romanian sample).

Conduct problems tended to be more frequent in the institutional group than in either the family foster group or the controls but there was no association with a marked lack of selective attachments in the institutional group.

The findings with respect to associations between I/O and other types of relationship difficulties were both weaker and less consistent. It seems that, although they tended to be more frequent in children reared in institutions, they did not represent the same construct of combined I/O and attachment problems.

It may be concluded that, as in the study of Romanian adoptees, I/O is particularly common in children who have been reared under the conditions of residential group care, and that the behaviours of I/O (unlike other forms of disruptive behaviour) tend to be associated with a marked lack of selective attachments.

Discussion

These two studies, considered in combination, strongly suggest that an institutional rearing during the preschool years predisposes to a pattern of inattention and overactivity that is often associated with a relative lack of specificity in selective attachments and a lack of social boundaries, as reflected in an undue friendliness with strangers. The association with these attachment features seems to be relatively specific to I/O as found in institution-reared children (it was not found in children brought up in family foster care), and it was not found with other forms of disruptive behaviour. There was a weak association with peer relationship problems and other social difficulties, but this was much less specific. In some cases, they may reflect the same underlying construct but in many instances it is likely that they do not.

Three main queries arise out of these findings: do they simply index a more general psychosocial risk for ADHD? Are they truly due to some aspect of experiences that are specific to residential group rearing? What faulty psychological function do they represent? No clearcut answers to any of these three questions are possible in view of the limited database but provisional suggestions may be made.

To begin with, it seems unlikely that institutional care is no more than an index of general psychosocial risks for ADHD or the hyperkinetic syndrome. The most crucial finding in that connection is that, in both studies, there was a substantial overlap between I/O and a particular form of attachment difficulties characterized by weak selective attachments. Because both have closely comparable correlates, the implication is that they may reflect the same underlying construct. Much more detailed clinical and experimental investigation would be required to determine whether the I/O in our two institution-reared groups represents 'ordinary' ADHD that happened to be comorbid with a form of attachment disorder. We suggest that this is not the most likely explanation both because of the closeness of the overlap in phenomena and because in the small subsample of cases seen by MR the quality of the I/O did not seem quite the same as that in ordinary ADHD. The responsiveness to social context seemed more marked, the inattention was much more striking than the overactivity, and in most of the few cases where it was tried the response to stimulant medication was generally unimpressive (although occasionally it seemed helpful). For the time being, it would seem prudent not to assume that the I/O seen in a substantial minority of institution-reared children represents the usual varieties of ADHD, but equally it would be premature to conclude that necessarily it is fundamentally different.

A somewhat firmer answer to the query regarding the specific role of institutional rearing is probably possible. The study of Romanian adoptees left open the possibility that malnutrition played an important contributory role, but this was not a feature of the UK children in the second study and, hence, this does not appear to be a necessary predisposing factor. The same applies to cognitive impairment. It was unassociated with I/O in the institution-reared children in the second study. Accordingly, that cannot be regarded as a necessary predisposing or mediating variable. Both the group care and family foster care groups in the second study came from dysfunctional – often severely dysfunctional – families, and it could be argued that genetic risk played a crucial predisposing role. That is less likely in the Romanian adoptees, for whom family poverty rather than family dysfunction constituted the most prominent background feature. Nevertheless, the data on the biological parents were meagre in the extreme, and that possibility cannot be entirely ruled out. Adverse experiences in the biological family prior to the children's entry into substitute care seem likely to be unimportant in these two studies, if only because the children were admitted to institutions so young (a mean age of a few weeks in the first study and 3 months in the second). The finding that there was no increase in I/O in the Romanian children adopted before 6 months makes it unlikely that experiences in the 3 months of care by biological families in the second study played any major role. Nevertheless, that certainly cannot be ruled out when entry into care takes place at a later age. Vorria et al. (1998a,b) found that there were few adverse effects of institutional rearing when the children had experienced a stable upbringing (albeit in impoverished circumstances) for a few years prior to institutional care.

In summary, we conclude that the crucial risk factor was indeed group rearing in an institutional environment. It seems likely that a lack of continuity in personalized caregiving constituted the key risk variable (because other aspects of care in the second stage were relatively satisfactory), but that hypothesis remains to be tested in a rigorous fashion. Moreover, it cannot be concluded that I/O would develop in normal children as a result of institutional rearing. The Romanian sample were at risk as a result of malnutrition, poor physical care and possibly inappropriate use of medication to control behaviour; and the UK sample were likely to be at risk from presumed genetic risk factors. The risks in the two groups were quite different in type and degree but it may be that some kind of increased vulnerability is needed for I/O to be caused by institutional rearing.

The last question is the most difficult of all to answer on the basis of existing evidence. The second study findings could be compatible with a contemporaneous situation-specific effect whereby I/O represented an adaptive (albeit disadvantageous) response to group situations resulting from patterns learned in the institution. That explanation, however, is implausible in the case of the Romanian adoptees who had left the institutions at least $2\frac{1}{2}$ years earlier, and usually much longer than that. Moreover, the I/O (and associated attachment difficulties: see O'Connor et al., 2000) showed rather strong persistence over the 2-year period between 4 and 6 years, during which time there was also the important transition to school. The findings strongly point to some sort of relatively enduring effect on the organism (although not necessarily an effect that could not be altered through some appropriate form of intervention).

What process might be involved and is it the same process in these two very different samples that nevertheless showed such surprisingly similar problems? The cluster analysis findings in the study of Romanian adoptees suggest that the initial assumption ought to be that the attachment difficulties and the I/O might represent the same basic psychopathological construct. This could arise in at least three different ways. First, it could be a consequence of both stemming from the same mediating risk mechanism. That would have to be some aspect of institutional rearing that did not result in either cognitive impairment or quasiautistic features (because neither was found in the second study and because both these features fell into a different cluster in the study of Romanian adoptees). The lack of personalized caregiving constitutes an obvious contender because that is the feature that most obviously differentiates residential group care from family foster care, and because it constitutes a central feature in attachment theory (Cassidy and Shaver, 1999). However, there are other contenders, such as the lesser opportunities in institutions for exercising individual initiative, autonomy, responsibility and personal control over decisionmaking (Rutter et al., 1979; Quinton and Rutter, 1988). Perhaps these elements are more important for I/O and personalized caregiving for attachment difficulties.

Second, it could be that the I/O is a secondary consequence of impaired selective attachments. The difficulty with that suggestion lies in the uncertainty of what is involved in the attachment difficulties. Traditionally, reactive attachment disorders have been conceptualized in terms of attachment insecurity and of fear in relation to separations and reunions but that is not at all how the difficulties appear in our samples. If anything, anxiety and fear are prominent by their absence. Instead, what was striking was the lack of social boundaries and the relative failure to appreciate social cues and to perceive the results of their actions on other people (O'Connor et al., 2000). Indiscriminate friendliness is the term that has tended to be applied (Chisholm et al., 1995), but to some extent that seems a misnomer. The children do make some distinctions in the ways in which they react to family members, peers and strangers but they fail to pick up social expectations. Thus, they may be more 'touchy-feely' than is culturally acceptable with people whom they do not know; they may be overfamiliar in situations that require respect and reserve; and they intrude into social situations in which they should hold back. That could well lead to behaviours that would be regarded as 'impulsive' but the associations with impulsivity were weaker than with I/O. It is by no means obvious how I/O could be directly conceptualized in attachment feature terms. What stands out clinically is the children's difficulties in attending to group instruction, their difficulty in organizing their approach to assigned tasks, in their sorting out a strategy to prioritize what they do, and in adopting an organized hierarchical approach to learning and to task performance. This could stem from attachment difficulties but, if so, the mechanisms need much better specification than they have received up to now.

The third possibility is that I/O is basic and that the attachment difficulties are secondary. That seems implausible, if only because most cases of I/O (in the absence of institutional rearing) are not accompanied by attachment difficulties. Indeed, it is not obvious how this could come about, particularly as clinically the inattention problem seems more marked than the overactivity.

At present, there is no satisfactory resolution of these dilemmas. The 'take home' message, however, is that clinicians need to be aware of the clinical picture of I/O associated with difficulties or impairments in selective attention. It may or may not prove to constitute a valid, homogeneous, meaningfully distinct syndrome but, in the meanwhile, caution should be exercised before assuming that it constitutes just another variant of ADHD or the hyperkinetic syndrome.

REFERENCES

Barkley, R.A. (1989). Hyperactive girls and boys. Stimulant drug effects on mother–child interactions. *Journal of Child Psychology and Psychiatry*, **30**, 379–90.

Biederman, J., Millberger, S., Faraone, S.V. et al. (1995). Family–environment risk factors for attention-deficit hyperactivity disorder: a test of Rutter's indicators of adversity. *Archives of General Psychiatry*, **52**, 464–70.

Carlson, E.A., Jacobvitz, D. and Sroufe L.A. (1995). A developmental investigation of inattentiveness and hyperactivity. *Child Development*, **66**, 37–54.

Cassidy, J. and Shaver, P.R. (1999). *Handbook of Attachment: Theory, Research, and Clinical Applications.* New York: Guilford Press.

Chisholm, K., Carter, M.C., Ames, E.W. and Morison, S.J. (1995). Attachment security and indiscriminately friendly behavior in children adopted from Romanian orphanages. *Development and Psychopathology*, **7**, 283–94.

Elander J. and Rutter M. (1996). Use and development of the Rutter parents' and teachers' scales. *International Journal of Methods in Psychiatry*, **6**, 63–78.

Ge, X., Conger, R.D., Cadoret, R.J. et al. (1996). The developmental interface between nature and nurture: a mutual influence model of child antisocial behavior and parent behaviors. *Developmental Psychology*, **32**, 574–89.

Haddad, P.M. and Garralda, M.E. (1992). Hyperkinetic syndrome and disruptive early experiences. *British Journal of Psychiatry*, **161**, 700–3.

Hogg, C., Rutter, M. and Richman, N. (1997). Emotional and behavioural problems in children. In *Child Psychology Portfolio*, I. Sclare, ed., pp. 1–13. Windsor: NFEF-Nelson.

Kreppner, J., O'Connor, T., Rutter, M. and the English and Romanian Adoptees (ERA) study team (2001). Can inattention/overactivity be an institutional deprivation syndrome? *Journal of Abnormal Child Psychology*, **29**, 513–28.

MTA Cooperative Group. (1999a). A 14-month randomized clinical trial of treatment strategies for attention-deficit/hyperactivity disorder. *Archives of General Psychiatry*, **56**, 1073–86.

MTA Cooperative Group. (1999b). Moderators and mediators of treatment response for children with attention-deficit/hyperactivity disorder. *Archives of General Psychiatry*, **56**, 1088–96.

O'Connor, T.G., Deater-Deckard, K., Fulker, D., Rutter, M. and Plomin, R. (1998). Genotype–environment correlations in late childhood and early adolescence: antisocial behavioural problems and coercive parenting. *Developmental Psychology*, **34**, 970–81.

O'Connor, T.G., Rutter, M. and the English and Romanian Adoptees (ERA) Study Team (2000). Attachment disorder behavior following early severe deprivation: extension and longitudinal follow-up. *Journal of the American Academy of Child and Adolescent Psychiatry*, **39**, 703–12.

Quinton, D. and Rutter, M. (1988). *Parenting Breakdown: The Making and Breaking of Intergenerational Links.* Aldershot: Avebury.

Roy, P., Rutter, M. and Pickles, A. (2000). Institutional care: risk from family background or pattern of rearing? *Journal of Child Psychology and Psychiatry*, **411**, 139–49.

Roy, P., Rutter, M. and Pickles, A. (submitted). Institutional care: associations between overactivity and lack of selectivity in relationships.

Rutter, M. (2000a). Psychosocial influences: critiques, findings and research needs. *Development and Psychopathology*, **12**, 375–405.

Rutter (2000b). Children in substitute care: some conceptual considerations and research implications. *Children and Youth Services Review*, **22**, 685–703.

Rutter, M., Maughan, B., Mortimore, P., Ouston, J. and Smith, A. (1979). *Fifteen Thousand Hours: Secondary Schools and their Effects on Children*. Cambridge, MA: Harvard University Press.

Rutter, M., Dunn, J., Plomin, R. et al. (1997a). Integrating nature and nurture: implications of person–environment correlations and interactions for developmental psychology. *Development and Psychopathology*, **9**, 335–64.

Rutter, M., Maughan, B., Meyer, J. et al. (1997b). Heterogeneity of antisocial behavior: causes, continuities and consequences. In *Nebraska Symposium on Motivation*, vol. 44: *Motivation and Delinquency*, R. Dienstbier and D.W. Osgood, pp. 45–118. Lincoln, NE: University of Nebraska Press.

Rutter, M. and the ERA study team (1998). Developmental catch-up, and deficit, following adoption after severe global early privation. *Journal of Child Psychology and Psychiatry*, **39**, 465–76.

Rutter, M., Giller, H. and Hagell, A. (1998). *Antisocial Behavior by Young People*. New York: Cambridge University Press.

Rutter, M., Silberg, J., O'Connor, T. and Simonoff, E. (1999). Genetics and child psychiatry: II Empirical research findings. *Journal of Child Psychology and Psychiatry*, **40**, 19–55.

Rutter, M., O'Connor, T., Beckett, C. et al. (2000). Recovery and deficit following profound early deprivation. In *Intercountry Adoption Developments, Trends and Perspectives*, P. Selman, ed., pp. 107–25. London: British Association for Adoption and Fostering.

Rutter, M., Kreppner, J., O'Connor, T. and the English and Romanian Adoptees (ERA) study team (2001). Specificity and heterogeneity in children's responses to profound privation. *British Journal of Psychiatry*, **179**, 97–103.

Scahill, L., Schwab-Stone, M., Merikangas, K.R. et al. (1999). Psychosocial and clinical correlates of ADHD in a community sample of school-age children. *Journal of the American Academy of Child and Adolescent Psychiatry*, **38**, 976–84.

Schachar, R.J. and Wachsmuth, R. (1991). Family dysfunction and psychosocial adversity: Comparison of attention deficit disorder, conduct disorder, normal and clinical controls. *Canadian Journal of Behavioural Science*, **23**, 332–48.

Schachar, R.J., Rutter, M. and Smith, A. (1981). The characteristics of situationally and pervasively hyperactive children: Implications for syndrome definition. *Journal of Child Psychology and Psychiatry*, **22**, 375–92.

Schachar, R.J., Taylor, E., Wieselberg, M., Thorley, G. and Rutter, M. (1987). Changes in family function and relationships with children who respond to methylphenidate. *Journal of the American Academy of Child and Adolescent Psychiatry*, **26**, 728–32.

Tannock, R. (1998). Attention deficit hyperactivity disorder: advances in cognitive, neurobiological, and genetic research. *Journal of Child Psychology and Psychiatry and Allied Disciplines*, **39**, 65–99.

Taylor, E.A. (ed.) (1986). *The Overactive Child*. Clinics in Developmental Medicine no. 97. Oxford: SIMP/Blackwell Scientific.

Taylor, E. (1999). Development of clinical services for attention-deficit/hyperactivity disorder: Commentary. *Archives of General Psychiatry*, **56**, 1097–9.

Taylor, E., Sandberg, S., Thorley, G. and Giles, S. (1991). *The Epidemiology of Childhood Hyperactivity: Maudsley Monographs no. 33*. Oxford: Oxford University Press.

Thapar, A., Holmes, J., Poulton, K. and Harrington, R. (1999). Genetic basis of attention deficit and hyperactivity. *British Journal of Psychiatry*, **174**, 105–11.

Tizard, B. and Hodges, J. (1978). The effect of early institutional rearing on the development of eight-year-old children. *Journal of Child Psychology and Psychiatry*, **19**, 99–118.

Vorria, P., Rutter, M., Pickles, A., Wolkind, S. and Hobsbaum, A. (1998a). A comparative study of Greek children in long-term residential group care and in two-parent families: (I) Social, emotional and behavoural differences. *Journal of Child Psychology and Psychiatry*, **39**, 225–36.

Vorria, P., Rutter, M., Pickles, A., Wolkind, S. and Hobsbaum, A. (1998b). A comparative study of Greek children in long-term residential group care and in two-parent families: (II) Possible mediating mechanisms. *Journal of Child Psychology and Psychiatry*, **39**, 234–45.

13

Treatments: the case of the MTA study

Peter S. Jensen and the MTA Group

Columbia and New York City University, New York, USA

Peter S. Jensen, L. Eugene Arnold, Stephen P. Hinshaw, James M. Swanson, Laurence L. Greenhill, C. Keith Conners, Howard B. Abikoff, Glen Elliott, Lily Hechtman, Betsy Hoza, John S. March, Jeffrey H. Newcorn, William E. Pelham, Joanne B. Severe, Benedetto Vitiello, Karen Wells and Timothy Wigal.

The MTA is a cooperative treatment study performed by six independent research teams in collaboration with the staff of the Division of Clinical and Treatment Research of the National Institute of Mental Health (NIMH), Rockville, Maryland and the Office of Special Education Programs (OSEP) of the US Department of Education (DOE). The NIMH principal collaborators are Peter S. Jensen, MD, L. Eugene Arnold, MEd, MD, John E. Richters, PhD, Joanne B. Severe, MS, Donald Vereen, MD and Benedetto Vitiello, MD. Principal investigators and coinvestigators from the six sites are as follows: University of California at Berkeley/San Francisco (UO1 MH50461): Stephen P. Hinshaw, PhD, Glen R. Elliott, MD, PhD; Duke University (UO1 MH50447): C. Keith Conners, PhD., Karen C. Wells, PhD, John S. March, MD, MPH; University of California at Irvine/Los Angeles (UO1 MH50440): James M. Swanson, PhD; Dennis P. Cantwell, MD; Timothy Wigal, PhD; Long Island Jewish Medical Center/Montreal Children's Hospital (UO1 MH50453): Howard B. Abikoff, PhD, Lily Hechtman, MD; New York State Psychiatric Institute/Columbia University/Mount Sinai Medical Center (UO1 MH50454): Laurence L. Greenhill, MD, Jeffrey H. Newcorn, MD; University of Pittsburgh (UO1 MH50467): William E. Pelham, PhD, Betsy Hoza, PhD. Helena C. Kraemer, PhD (Stanford University) is statistical and design consultant. The OSEP/DOE Principal collaborator is Ellen Schiller, PhD.

Portions of the manuscript were previously published in Jensen, P.S., Hinshaw, S.P., Swanson, J.M., Greenhill, L.L. and the MTA Cooperative Group. (2001). Findings from the NIMH multimodal treatment study of ADHD (MTA): implications and applications for primary care providers. *Journal of Developmental and Behavioral Pediatrics*, **22**, 1–14.

Introduction

Attention deficit hyperactivity disorder (ADHD) occurs in 3–5% of school-aged children (Shaffer et al., 1996) and accounts for as many as 30–50% of child referrals to mental health services (Popper, 1988). Children meeting full (DSM-IV: American Psychiatric Association, 1994) criteria (early onset, 6-month duration and symptoms in more than one setting) have substantial impairment in peer, family and academic functioning (Hinshaw, 1992). Long-term outcome studies indicate that the syndrome persists into adulthood in most cases (Barkley et al., 1990; Mannuzza et al., 1993; Weiss and Hechtman, 1993), with increased risk for substance abuse and delinquency-related outcomes (Satterfield et al., 1987; Mannuzza et al., 1993).

Although a very large literature (Pelham and Murphy, 1986; Swanson, 1993; Spencer et al., 1996; Hinshaw et al., 1998) has documented the beneficial effects of medication (principally stimulants), psychosocial treatments (principally behaviour therapy) and their combination, this body of research has suffered from significant limitations, including the brief duration of treatment (typically days to months), small sample sizes and reliance on a restricted range of outcome measures. Despite nearly 30 years of research on ADHD treatments, few controlled studies have examined the effectiveness of long-term treatments. Two recent exceptions (Hechtman and Abikoff, 1995; Gillberg et al., 1997) were of 1–2 years' duration, and suggested that stimulant effects may persist when the stimulant is taken faithfully. However, the generalizability and interpretability of these and other studies have been constrained by the failure to include ADHD children with the full range of comorbidity and impairment (e.g. conduct disorder (CD)) encountered in 'real-world' practice. Further limitations of past studies result from the fact that none had the necessary ingredients of adequate statistical power, coupled with the analytic and design strategies that have become the de facto standard for state-of-the-art clinical trials (e.g. intent-to-treat analyses, random regression approaches, etc.: Greenhouse et al., 1991a,b; Hedeker et al., 1994; Elkin et al., 1995). Also, long-term (> 4 months) studies have not directly compared optimal medication management with intensive behavioural interventions. Given the public concern about the large numbers of children being treated with stimulants (Safer et al., 1996; Jensen et al., 1999), the severe, chronic nature of the symptoms and the wide variation in nature and quality of ADHD treatment practices (Kwasman et al., 1995; Moser and Kallail, 1995; Sloan et al., 1999), the lack of information about the long-term effectiveness of these two major forms of treatment (alone and in combination) constitutes an urgent public health issue.

To address these urgent public health informational needs, in 1992 the National Institute of Mental Health (NIMH) sponsored the development of a randomized clinical trial, the Multimodal Treatment Study of Children with Attention Deficit/Hyperactivity Disorder (the so-called MTA study). The MTA's rationale (Richters et al., 1995) and methodology (Greenhill et al., 1996; Arnold et al., 1997a,b; Hinshaw et al., 1997; Wells et al., 2000a) have been detailed previously.

Primary study aims and hypotheses

The MTA posed three questions:

(1)   How do long-term medication and behavioural/psychosocial treatments compare in effectiveness? (This was specified as a two-tailed question based on the null hypothesis, because no long-term studies had previously compared the two treatments head-to-head)

(2)   Are there additional benefits when medication and behavioural treatments are used together? (This was specified as a unidirectional hypothesis, with the combined treatment presumed to be superior to single forms of treatment)

(3)   What is the relative effectiveness of systematic, carefully delivered treatments vs. routine treatments typically received in the community? (This was specified as a unidirectional hypothesis, with the three MTA-delivered treatments presumed to be superior to routine community care)

To address these questions, the MTA Cooperative Group designed three treatment strategies:

(a)   a medication management (MedMgt) treatment, composed of initial individualized titration followed by careful monthly monitoring and brief education and support as needed

(b)   a behavioural therapy-only (Beh) treatment, consisting of clinical behaviour therapy (individual and group parent training plus teacher consultation), as well as direct contingency management via an intensive summer treatment programme (STP), followed by 12 weeks of paraprofessional aides in the child's regular classroom in the autumn

(c)   a combined treatment (Comb), amalgamating the strategies in (a) and (b).

A fourth condition (d) was the community comparison (CC) group, in which families found treatments of their own choosing from community providers (not project staff), while also relying upon their own financial resources.

Note that these questions, hypotheses and design were all intended to address the *relative effectiveness* of the treatments (compared to each other), not absolute effectiveness (i.e. compared to no treatment). All of the three MTA-delivered treatments were chosen because they were well documented to be efficacious in the short term. Thus, the MTA study constitutes the first-ever test of the relative effectiveness of these various forms of treatments *in the long term*, vis-à-vis children's course and outcomes through 14 months, using an intent-to-treat (ITT) analytic strategy with random regression techniques (Hedeker and Gibbons, 1996a,b).

Analyses of the MTA study findings have allowed two additional questions to be addressed:

(4)   Why and how did the MTA treatments work?

(5)   What is the overall impact of the various treatments, in terms of proportions of children normalized?

The first reports of study findings have been published (MTA Cooperative Group, 1999a,b), followed by secondary analyses in two special sections in the *Journal of Abnormal Child Psychology* (Hinshaw et al., 2000; Hoza et al., 2000; March et al., 2000; Pelham et al., 2000; Wells et al., 2000b) and the *Journal of the American Academy of Child and Adolescent Psychiatry* (Conners et al., 2001; Greenhill et al., 2001; Jensen et al., 2001; Newcorn et al., 2001; Swanson et al., 2001; Vitiello et al., 2001). These latter publications focus in more depth on how, why and for whom the MTA treatments appear to work (so-called mediators and moderators of treatment effects).

Methods

Recruitment procedures and sample characteristics

Four-step participant selection procedures

A four-step multiple-gating procedure screened potential participants and ascertained caseness (Hinshaw et al., 1997). These recruitment, screening and selection procedures were developed to collect a carefully diagnosed, impaired sample of ADHD children with a wide range of comorbidities and demographic characteristics, representative of patients seen clinically. These four steps involved telephone screening for eligibility, scores above the 83rd percentile on parent- and teacher-completed standardized hyperactivity rating scales (Conners, 1990), face-to-face diagnostic assessment using the Diagnostic Interview Schedule for Children (DISC: version 2.3/3.0; Shaffer et al., 1996) and a comprehensive baseline assessment battery prior to randomization (Hinshaw et al., 1997). Ninety-five per cent of subjects meeting these criteria consented to randomization.

Participants were referred for study entry from multiple sources: almost half were referred by schools, 18% responded to newspaper ads, 9% came from mental health settings, 8% by word of mouth, 6% from paediatricians, and the rest were from other sources. Each site was required to recruit from all sources and not just one 'convenient' source. No attempt was made to stratify on referral source. Subjects entering the fourth and final phase did not differ from initial phone screen subjects on parental education, ethnicity or gender.

Inclusion/exclusion criteria and subject characteristics

In addition to meeting the selection criteria noted above, at the time of randomization children participating in the study were required to be between 7.0 and 9.9 years, in the first to fourth grades, living with primary caretakers for at least 6 months and diagnosed by study staff as ADHD combined type. Exclusion criteria were limited to conditions or situations that would preclude a family's full participation in treatment or that would ethically necessitate conflicting nonstudy treatments (additional details are provided in Arnold et al., 1997a,b, and Hinshaw et al., 1997).

The presence of comorbidities such as oppositional defiant disorder (ODD), CD, internalizing disorders or specific learning disabilities were not exclusionary conditions, because the MTA study team wanted to determine the potential interaction of these factors with treatment outcomes.

Demographic characteristics of the final selected MTA participants were as follows: 80% male and 20% female; 61% Caucasian, 20% Black and 19% Hispanic, racially mixed or of other ethnic origin. Mean age at study entry was 8.5 years. Sixty-nine per cent of the children lived in two-parent families, 30% in one-parent families and 1% lived with other relatives (e.g. grandparents, aunts or long-term foster families). Nineteen per cent of the families were receiving some type of public assistance. In general, the baseline clinical profile (MTA Cooperative Group, 1999a) is typical of a sample of children this age with ADHD (Conners, 1990; Lahey et al., 1993).

In addition to all children meeting criteria for the ADHD combined type using the DISC, the DISC was used to determine the presence of other psychiatric disorders at baseline. Based on the DISC, in terms of cooccurring conditions, 33.5% of children had a comorbid anxiety disorder (not including simple phobia; 38.7% including simple phobia), 14.3% had CD, 39.9% had ODD, 3.8% had affective disorder and 10.9% tic disorder. Only 31.8% of children had pure ADHD, that is, ADHD only with no comorbidities. The robust comorbidity in the sample attests to the similarity of the sample to other clinical as well as epidemiological studies (Szatmari et al., 1989; Biederman et al., 1991, Nottelmann and Jensen, 1995).

Study protocol: treatment conditions

Principles guiding the choice of MTA-delivered treatments were that they had to be:

(1)   state of the art, with research evidence of at least short-term efficacy

(2)   manualized and transportable
(3)   sufficiently intense, integrated and flexible for the treatment to stand on its own credibly
(4)   distinguished sharply enough from each other to support the contrasts and comparisons required by the primary questions

Because of the intensive use of clinical algorithms to guide the implementation of each treatment, the three treatment arms are best viewed as *treatment strategies* (because each was composed of multiple interventions) rather than single specific treatments, as described below.

Medication management (MedMgt)

This condition involved careful initial titration (Greenhill et al., 1996; Arnold et al., 1997b; Greenhill et al., 2001; Vitiello et al., 2001), manualized algorithms guiding dosage adjustments in response to monthly clinical assessments (including reports from parents and teachers), algorithms for systematically testing other drugs (if needed to achieve an adequate response) and brief parent education and support during each monthly visit. The order in which medications were tried was methylphenidate, dextroamfetamine, pemoline, imipramine, then other drugs as determined by a cross-site pharmacology panel. Deviations from the above-described order could only be approved by the cross-site panel. Pharmacotherapists provided encouragement, brief advice (but not behaviour therapy, which was limited to the other two active MTA treatment arms) and when necessary or requested by the parent, 'bibliotherapy' (readings from an approved list). Thus, the services provided in this arm could be readily delivered in a paediatric or psychiatric setting, without extensive behaviour therapy expertise but consistent with pharmacological practice.

Behavioural (Beh) treatment

The Beh treatment strategy included parent training in home behavioural management, school-based intervention and direct treatment of the child. These components were organized and integrated with the timing of the school year, in order to capitalize on the strengths of each treatment. The parent training regimen, based on work by Barkley (1987) and Forehand and McMahon (1980), involved 27 group and eight individual sessions for each family over the study period. Parent training (six families per group) began weekly after randomization (concurrent with biweekly teacher consultation), and both were tapered over time. The same therapist-consultant (TC) conducted both parent training and 10–12 sessions of face-to-face teacher consultation for a given child, with each TC having a case load of 12 families.

The child-focused treatment was provided in a STP developed by Pelham (Pelham and Hoza, 1996). The 8-week, all-day STP employed behavioural interventions including a point system (reward and response cost), time out, social reinforcement, modelling, group problem solving, sports skills and social skills training. STP classrooms provided individualized academic skills practice and reinforcement of appropriate classroom behaviour.

School-based treatment

In addition to teacher consultation in behavioural techniques, this treatment component included 12 weeks of a half-time behaviourally trained paraprofessional aide in the classroom, adapted from the Irvine Paraprofessional Model (Swanson, 1992). The aide was provided in the autumn of the second school year, in order to help generalize previously well-documented STP gains (Pelham and Hoza, 1996) to the new classroom. STP counsellors later became the classroom aides to provide continuity of treatment. By the end of the aide's 12 weeks, parents and teachers were trained to continue the programme the rest of the year and to prepare for the summer and following school year. Across the entire 14 months, parents and teachers used a 'daily report card' (DRC) to enhance children's behavioural and academic functioning. The DRC was completed by the teacher, while the child was rewarded for compliance by the parents at home.

Combined treatment (Comb)

In general, the MTA combined treatment provided all of the treatments outlined above for the MedMgt and Beh arms. However, the Comb arm was structured to take advantage of the potential synergy of both treatments together. For example, data were collected by and shared between the TC and the pharmacotherapist in regular treatment team planning meetings. Also, algorithms guided when and if an adjustment in one treatment should be made, vis-à-vis its potential impact on the other treatment (Arnold et al., 1997b).

Subjects in each of the three MTA-provided treatment arms had a 'bank' of eight additional clinic sessions. These sessions were provided on an 'as needed' basis to respond to emergencies with the child or in the families, or to address instances of possible or imminent attrition from the study.

Community comparison (CC) group

CC participants received no active treatment from the MTA treatment teams, but were instead evaluated and provided with the report of their initial study assessments, along with a list of community mental health resources. They were subsequently reassessed periodically in parallel with participants in the three active treatment arms. At each assessment point, the types of treatments they obtained in the community were documented.

Randomization was done centrally by the NIMH Data Center, stratified by site, in blocks of 16 – four to each group. Sealed ordered envelopes were sent to sites for successive entries. Allocation of subjects to study arms was concealed until the family had agreed to accept randomization, at which point the principal investigator and the family jointly opened the sealed envelope containing the study assignment. Additional details concerning specific treatments and the overall design are detailed in Greenhill et al. (1996); Arnold et al. (1997a,b); Hinshaw et al. (1997); Wells et al. (2000a).

Study variables

Assessment battery

Key assessment domains included:

(1) ADHD symptoms
(2) academic functioning
(3) peer relationships/social skills
(4) aggressive-oppositional behaviours
(5) anxious/depressive symptoms
(6) biological/medical factors (e.g. height, weight, presence of tics, laboratory tests when needed)
(7) competencies/self-esteem
(8) demographics
(9) parental characteristics and family functioning
(10) cognitive ability
(11) general impairment
(12) service use, attitudes and barriers (Hinshaw et al., 1997)

The first five of these domains were selected as the primary study outcome domains, using the procedure described below in the section on data analytic strategy.

Because parent and teacher ratings could be affected by expectancy effects and biases resulting from satisfaction about one's treatment assignment (independently of the effects of the treatment itself), the MTA team also obtained objective measures that could not reasonably be influenced by such factors for several outcome domains:

(1) school-based ADHD symptoms using the Abikoff Classroom Observational System (Abikoff and Gittelman, 1985)
(2) social skills and peer relations, using peer sociometric procedures
(3) academic achievement (Wechsler Individual Achievement Test scores: Wechsler, 1992)

(4)   ratings of videotaped parent–child interactions during standardized laboratory tasks, done by raters blind to treatment condition

Such procedures are not without limitations, however. For example, objective observers potentially lack sensitivity to subtle behaviours which are only discernible by someone who knows the child well or who has many opportunities for observation. Likewise, a videotaped interaction in a university laboratory may not reflect actual behaviours in the home setting. None the less, taken as a group, the study's reliance on a range of measures across different settings, raters and formats made a more complete and valid assessment possible.

Fidelity and compliance

The MTA study achieved a high degree of adherence to protocol by a combination of fidelity and compliance measures. Thus, fidelity to protocol by therapists was achieved by cross-arm emphasis on subject rapport, manualization of all treatments, regular supervision of pharmaco- and psychotherapists by highly skilled clinician investigators, cross-site weekly therapy panels and audiotaping of all sessions to monitor clinician practices. Good compliance by patients to protocol was achieved by monthly pill counts, intermittent saliva levels to monitor taking of methylphenidate and encouragement of families to make up missed visits.

Families' initial acceptance and compliance with their randomly assigned treatment was as follows: beginning immediately after randomization five (3.4%) and 14 (9.7%) subjects from the Comb and MedMgt arms, respectively, refused (and continued to refuse) participation in the medication component of these two arms. Concerning psychosocial treatment components, however, only one (0.7%) and none (0%) of Comb and Beh subjects refused to participate in this treatment for the whole time from randomization forward.

Patterns of families' adherence to protocol and compliance with various treatment components changed over the course of the 14 months of treatment. Thus, despite families' high acceptance of Beh treatment at initial randomization, 38 Beh subjects 'crossed over' to receive ADHD medication, either because the family sought it out on their own (i.e. 'noncompliance') or because MTA clinical staff determined that medication was ethically required due to a child's clinical deterioration. In contrast, only three MedMgt subjects 'crossed over' to receive psychosocial treatments during the study (MTA Cooperative Group, 1999b).

Over the course of the study, 83.5% ($n = 121$) and 81.3% ($n = 117$) of Comb and MedMgt subjects, respectively, participated in their assigned medication treatment for 80% or more of the study's duration. Also, 64.1% ($n = 93$) and 62.5% ($n = 90$) of Comb and Beh subjects, respectively, participated in 80% or more of their assigned psychosocial treatment during the study period. Import-antly, none of these comparisons yielded significant differences between the combined treatment arm and the two single treatment arms (within or across sites) in compliance with specific Beh or MedMgt treatment components. Thus, the degree of psychosocial treatment participation did not differ between Beh and Comb, nor did pharmacotherapy compliance differ between Comb and MedMgt. None the less, these data suggest that a higher level of compli-ance was achieved with the medication component of the Comb and MedMgt treatment arms than was achieved with the psychosocial component of Comb and Beh arms. Despite this difference in compliance in the two forms of treatment, analyses indicated that compliance factors did not affect overall results (see MTA Cooperative Group, 1999b, for complete compliance ana-lyses).

Data analysis

Sample size

The procedure for estimating statistical power needs was based on Cohen (1988) and Kazdin and Bass (1989). Power analyses were based on a between-subjects factorial design with treatment site (six levels) crossed with treatment, either four levels (all treatments) or two (contrasts of averaged MTA treat-ments vs. the community CC condition or contrasts between any two treat-ment arms). Power analyses indicated that 24 subjects per condition per site (for a total 96 at each site) were required in order to estimate a minimum effect size of 0.3–0.4 (for ADHD core symptoms) for comparisons between any two treatment arms (yielding a power of 0.82).

Data analytic strategy

We used random regression (RR) techniques whenever appropriate for our principal ITT analyses (Hedeker and Gibbons, 1996a,b; MTA Cooperative Group, 1999a,b). RR analysis is a powerful technique to analyse longitudinal study data with multiple assessment points, because it offers increased measurement reliability resulting from its ability to model change for each participant over time, without requiring the same adjustment for each member of a group, such as traditional analysis of covariance (Laird and Ware, 1982; Bryk and Raudenbush, 1988; Hedeker et al., 1994; Elkin et al., 1995). Further, data from each participant can be entered into the analysis even if not all follow-up data are obtained, so attrition need not affect the number of partici-pants in the analysis.

For each of the major outcome variables selected (see the section on selection of outcome measures, below), tests for site, time, time × treatment (the treatment effect over time) and site × treatment interactions were examined with ITT RR analyses. When the omnibus RR analyses comparing all four groups were significant, six planned contrasts among the treatment groups were tested for each variable: MedMgt vs. Beh (two-tailed); Comb vs. MedMgt and Comb vs. Beh (with both contrasts one-tailed, assuming the superiority of Comb); and CC vs. MedMgt, CC vs. Beh and CC vs. CC vs. Comb (all contrasts one-tailed, assuming the inferiority of CC to the MTA treatments; MTA Cooperative Group, 1999a,b).

Selection of outcome measures

Outcome measures were prioritized a priori for:

(1) conceptual coherence
(2) simplicity
(3) availability of norms and/or standardization from other studies
(4) ability to tap parallel constructs across different raters
(5) repeated administration over time

Given the number of measures employed in the study, we applied data reduction procedures to those measures that met these criteria, using principal components analyses (PCA) to refine the selection of outcome domains and to eliminate redundant measures. Using this method, five major outcome domains were identified. Measures from each rating source that loaded highest on each of the five factors were selected to represent that domain, while ensuring that two or more informants' ratings were used to assess each domain, whenever possible. The five domains were assessed as follows:

(1) core ADHD symptoms – parents' and teachers' SNAP (Swanson, Nolan and Pelham) inattention and hyperactivity-impulsivity subscales (Swanson, 1992), complemented by the composite score of interference, off-task, and gross motor behaviours from the Abikoff Classroom Observation Rating System (Abikoff and Gittelman, 1985)

(2) oppositional-aggressive symptoms – assessed via parents' and teachers' SNAP ratings and augmented by observers' ratings of classroom-based aggression using the Abikoff System

(3) social skills – assessed via parent- and teacher-completed scales from the Social Skills Rating System (SSRS: Gresham and Elliott, 1989) and augmented by peer sociometric ratings

(4) internalizing symptoms – rated by parents and teachers from SSRS subscales, and augmented by children's self-ratings on the Multidimensional Anxiety Scale for Children (MASC: March et al., 1997)

(5)   academic functioning – assessed via three subscales from the Wechsler Individual Achievement Test (reading, maths, spelling).

Because we obtained multiple informants for each domain whenever possible (the widely accepted standard for measuring childhood functioning and psychopathology), appropriate Bonferonni corrections were applied to *P*-values, based upon the number of measures in that domain. A total of 19 measures was selected for final analyses, representing the five domains.

Results

Below we review the overall 14-month findings, comparing outcomes across the four treatment groups, based on the original five questions outlined above:

(1)   Which treatments work best for which types of outcomes?

(2)   How do optimal (MTA-delivered) treatments compare with community treatments?

(3)   Which treatments work best for which children (treatment moderators with the goal of eventually matching patients to treatments)?

(4)   Why do treatments work (treatment mediators)?

(5)   What proportion of children were normalized by each of the treatment modalities?

Questions 1 and 2: Which treatments work best for which types of outcomes (e.g. MedMgt vs. Beh; and Comb vs. MedMgt or Beh)?

ADHD symptom outcomes

Findings from the initial ITT analyses are outlined in detail in two publications (MTA Cooperative Group, 1999a,b). In general, these analyses indicated that Comb and MedMgt interventions did not differ from each other in any clinically or statistically significant fashion in the degree of improvement in core ADHD symptoms, whether inattention, hyperactivity-impulsivity or overall ADHD symptom ratings. In sharp contrast to the generally equivalent results in comparisons between Comb and MedMgt treatments, Comb and MedMgt were both clinically and statistically superior to Beh and CC *for ADHD outcomes*, with pre–post changes generally 1.0–1.2 standard deviation units in terms of their degree of change from baseline. Beh and CC subjects did not differ from each other on any ADHD outcome measures.

Other functioning outcomes

For outcomes other than ADHD symptoms (oppositional-aggressive symptoms, internalizing symptoms, social skills, parent–child relations and academic functioning) a different pattern of findings emerged. For these analyses, the three active MTA-delivered treatments rarely differed from each other. In addition, only the Comb intervention fairly consistently showed evidence of statistical superiority to the CC condition. In several instances, Comb proved superior to Beh (14-month academic functioning – Wechsler Individual Achievement Test (WIAT) reading scores, parent-reported internalizing (anxiety-depression) ratings, parent-reported oppositional-aggressive symptoms), whereas MedMgt subjects usually scored in between both groups, showing no significant differences from either of the other two MTA treatments. For these functioning outcomes, it is important to note that the relative advantages of the Comb intervention over the other interventions – though adjudged to be real – was small, with overall effect sizes of 0.26–0.28. Thus, statistical testing between Comb and the two other MTA-treated groups often failed to show significant differences, despite the fact that it usually placed first, showing numerical superiority over other modalities for 12 of 19 outcome measures. By way of comparison, MedMgt, Beh and CC each placed first four, two and one times each, respectively. But because the original design and sample sizes selected for the study were based on 80% power to detect effect sizes of 0.4 or greater, smaller effects (e.g. 0.26–0.28, the apparent difference between Comb and MedMgt) would not be discernible by traditional methods, particularly after Bonferonni corrections for multiple comparisons. Thus, caution is warranted to avoid premature and inappropriate conclusions that the Comb intervention did not offer anything over and above MedMgt, or that Comb and MedMgt did not offer anything over and above Beh, *for these non-ADHD functioning outcomes.*

As one means of addressing the issue of overall outcomes (combining both ADHD symptoms and other functioning domains), we conducted secondary analyses to explore the utility of a single, statistically derived composite measure of treatment outcome for the MTA trial (Conners et al., 2001). Total scores from 25 baseline assessment measures were analysed by principal components analysis, and a composite created from the sum of 17 of the standardized scores retained by the Varimax rotated factor analysis. The factor analysis produced two source factors from parents and teachers. A composite of these measures was internally consistent ($\alpha = 0.85$) and reliable (baseline to 3-months test–retest $= 0.86$). Using this approach, Comb was significantly better than all other treatments, with effect sizes ranging from small (0.28 for comparison to MedMgt) to large (0.70 for comparison with CC).

Question 3: What are the benefits of state-of-the-art (MTA-delivered) treatments vs. treatments as delivered in the community?

MTA-delivered treatments vs. community care

These analyses revealed that Comb and MedMgt were generally superior to CC for parent- and teacher-reported ADHD symptoms, whereas Beh was not. In non-ADHD domains, MedMgt and Beh were superior to CC on one domain each (teacher-reported social skills and one measure of parent–child relations, respectively). In contrast, Comb was significantly superior to CC on all five non-ADHD domains of functioning (parent-reported oppositional/aggressive behaviours, internalizing symptoms, teacher-reported social skills, parent–child relations and WIAT reading achievement scores).

Although Comb and MedMgt were generally quite superior to CC, 68% of CC subjects were also treated with medication. However, it is noteworthy that while MTA-treated subjects received medication on a t.i.d. regimen (actual average 2.9 methylphenidate doses/day), CC medication-treated subjects received only twice-daily dosing (averaging 2.1 doses/day) and methylphenidate doses were generally substantially lower (18.7 mg total daily dose, vs. 32.8 mg/day for Comb and MedMgt subjects). In addition, medication visits were of shorter duration (18 vs. 30 min) and much less frequent (2.3 vs. 8.8 visits/year). Other differences included monthly phone contacts made by the pharmacotherapists to the teachers in order to get information and feedback to guide medication adjustments. These components may have enhanced the effectiveness of our medication management over medication treatments as provided in the CC group.

Question 4: For whom do treatments work (moderator analyses)?

Based on theoretical considerations and prior research, a wide range of variables were explored vis-à-vis their potential impact as moderators of treatment outcomes. These variables included age, gender, ethnicity, socioeconomic status and parental education and the presence or absence of specific comorbidities. Moderator variables are those factors that modify the overall ITT random regression analyses described above. In other words, despite these overall findings from these analyses, were there some subjects for whom the overall findings did not apply? For example, though Comb and MedMgt were generally superior to Beh and CC for ADHD symptoms, did these average findings apply equally to boys and girls? These findings are reported in detail elsewhere (MTA Cooperative Group, 1999b), and indicated that only two factors showed evidence of a meaningful impact: first, the presence of a comorbid anxiety disorder (parent-reported) at baseline, and second, family status of being on public assistance or welfare.

For both of these subgroups of families, two major differences emerged. First, Beh appeared more effective than in the primary analyses, such that it diverged from CC subjects and appeared similar in magnitude and direction of effects to MedMgt. Second, Comb diverged from MedMgt, such that substantially greater gains accrued to Comb vs. MedMgt subjects in the moderator subgroups. Outcomes apparently affected by these moderators included parent-reported hyperactivity and inattention, parent–child relations and teacher social skills.

Expressed another way, for subjects with a baseline comorbid anxiety disorder or on public assistance, Comb appeared to offer meaningful advantages over MedMgt for parent-reported ADHD symptoms, teacher-reported social skills and parent–child relations. And in contrast to the primary analyses, Beh appeared quite comparable to MedMgt for these same outcomes for these particular subgroups of subjects (MTA Cooperative Group, 1999b).

Given the multiple comorbid subgroups in the MTA sample, most notably anxiety and disruptive behaviour disorders (ODD or CD together totalled over 54% of the sample), we conducted additional analyses to compare four subgroups of children, based on the presence or absence of an anxiety disorder and the presence or absence of a disruptive behaviour disorder. For these four subgroups (ADHD only, ADHD + anxiety only, ADHD + disruptive only and ADHD + anxiety + disruptive), findings indicated that these comorbid groupings yielded meaningful information that might be used to guide treatment considerations. These analyses indicated that ADHD-only and ADHD + disruptive only subjects achieved meaningful benefits over CC subjects only if they received MedMgt or Comb interventions. For these children, effect sizes for Beh over and above CC were essentially nil. However, ADHD + anxiety only subjects responded well and similarly to all MTA-delivered interventions. Moreover, doubly comorbid (ADHD + anxiety + disruptive) subjects clearly showed the greatest benefits for the Comb intervention (Jensen et al., 2001; see also March et al., 2000).

Because the subgroup of ADHD + anxiety + disruptive subjects constituted only 24.7% of the 579 MTA subjects, and because they showed greater clinical benefits via Comb (vs. MedMgt) interventions, it is possible that a more cost-effective strategy would be to use Comb interventions for this particular needy and severely impaired subgroup. Similarly, in terms of matching patients to treatments, clinicians might consider that ADHD + anxiety only subjects (14.0% of the overall sample) respond equally well to MedMgt and Beh interventions. This finding may provide information to guide them in offering an evidence-based, similarly efficacious option to offer to parents and families who prefer not to use medication.

Why and how did the MTA treatments work (mediator analyses)?

Analyses of factors that mediate treatment outcomes are necessarily post hoc and are not protected by randomization. Thus, factors such as compliance/ attendance, medication dose, relationship with the therapist (therapeutic alliance), parental attitudes/beliefs about the treatment and change in parenting practices over the course of study are all possible explanations of why a given treatment may have worked, either within or across treatment arms. But because such factors all occur after randomization, it cannot be known with certainty that the particular factor has caused the particular effect. To demonstrate causality, additional studies which attempt systematically to vary those factors via random assignment are required.

None the less, mediator (after randomization) analyses of the MTA study data can either tend to support (or not) overall study findings. If analyses suggest the presence of possibly important treatment mediators, additional studies would then be warranted to explore, define and refine the active ingredients of an effective treatment. If, for example, compliance/attendance is related to specific outcomes, that finding would suggest that either failing to get an adequate dose (by not complying) or some other psychological factor externally observed as a noncompliant attitude would be a possible explanatory factor. Finding such effects, future studies might then randomly assign and compare subjects on the basis of different doses, the presence or absence of specific psychological factors, or even to induce experimentally a particular psychological state, in an attempt to control better for these nonrandom factors in the original study design.

With these cautions in mind, MTA investigators have examined a number of possible treatment mediators – overall treatment compliance/session attendance (MTA Cooperative Group, 1999b), characteristics of the medication treatment (Greenhill et al., 2001), cognitive factors in the parent (Hoza et al., 2000), use of behavioural methods at home (Pelham et al., 2000) and changes in parenting practices over the course of the study (Hinshaw et al., 2000; Wells et al., 2000b). Other factors, such as therapeutic alliance, are planned for future analyses as well, but have not begun.

Initial analyses exploring treatment mediators examined the impact of attendance and apparent compliance with the treatment protocol. These analyses indicated that attendance at regular medication visits, where pills were counted and new prescriptions were provided on a monthly basis, was strongly related to treatment outcomes. Those subjects not taking medication or refusing medication treatment altogether show significantly inferior outcomes on many, though not all domains (MTA Cooperative Group, 1999b). Similarly, several MTA investigators (MTA Cooperative Group, 1999b; Greenhill et al., 2001) have explored the impact of medication compliance and optimal use of medication, both within the MedMgt and CC groups. These analyses confirmed original results, namely that high-quality medication practices were likely important factors explaining a substantial portion of the successful outcomes in MTA medication-treated subjects.

To explore potential psychological processes underlying treatment outcomes, Hinshaw and colleagues (2000) conducted mediator analyses to determine whether changes in self-reported parenting practices were correlated with the effects of behavioural, medication or combination treatments on teacher-reported outcomes (disruptive behaviour, social skills, internalizing symptoms). Findings indicated that Comb families showing the greatest reductions in negative/ineffective parenting practices also showed in parallel the greatest teacher-reported benefits of treatment vis-à-vis regular community care. Thus, the success of combination treatment for school-related outcomes appeared to be closely related to reductions in negative and ineffective parenting practices at home. In fact, children in the Comb condition whose parents showed substantial improvement in negative/ineffective discipline were rated by their teachers as normalized in terms of rates of disruptive (ADHD and aggressive) symptomatology at school. Of note, similar reductions in negative parenting practices among Beh-treated children did not yield appreciably different success rates, suggesting that positive changes in parenting practices could result in meaningful school changes, if those same children also had the benefit of medication during the school day. Stated differently, for medication to exert its optimal effect in school, parents had to change home discipline practices.

Question 5: What is the overall impact of the various treatments, in terms of proportions of children normalized?

To supplement our primary analyses, MTA investigators developed and analysed a qualitative outcome measure of success to explore the study's clinical relevance and practical significance (Swanson et al., 2001). Thus, the end-of-treatment status of each subject was evaluated based on a combined overall rating completed by both parents and teachers of DSM-IV symptoms of ADHD and ODD, using the SNAP scale developed by Swanson et al. (2001). This rating scale allowed parents and teacher to score each symptom on a range from 0 (none) through 1 (just a little), 2 (moderate) and 3 (a lot). All items were tallied and then divided by the mean number of items to yield an average item response, and then parents' and teachers' scores were averaged. A low overall symptom severity rating (less than 1, or just a little) was selected as the criterion for successful treatment. Using this threshold, 88% of a sample of comparison children drawn from the children's classrooms fell under this threshold, and was specified as a criterion for successful treatment, i.e. normal. Logistic regression analyses were used to compare success rates for the treatments. Results showed that the success rates for MTA treatments mirrored the primary results, with the following proportions of children being normalized in each of the groups: Comb = 68%, MedMgt = 56%, Beh = 34% and CC = 25%. These findings should be viewed in the context of the symptom scores of children drawn from the same classrooms, 88% of whom were in the normal range, and in view of the fact that none of the MTA children scored in the normal range prior to randomization.

These secondary analyses suggest what clinicians should expect if MTA treatment algorithms are adopted to replace the usual treatment of children with ADHD: first, adopting the MTA MedMgt approaches may as much as double the success rate in most settings and second, adopting Comb treatment interventions may modestly increase the success rate further, matching the small effect size of the Comb vs. MedMgt contrast reported earlier, although the extent of this increase is likely to vary across settings. In contrast, substituting the Beh-only approaches for usual treatment may increase success rates in some settings but decrease it in other settings (Swanson et al., 2001).

Discussion

Overall MTA results indicate that long-term combined and medication-only treatments reduce ADHD, oppositional-aggressive and internalizing symptoms, while enhancing children's peer interactions. These findings are noteworthy, emphasizing that careful medication management approaches can reduce not just the classic ADHD symptoms, but also enhance other areas of functioning which are less well established as salient medication treatment targets (anxiety, peer interactions). In a few areas of functioning (specifically, internalizing symptoms, reading performance), combined approaches may be modestly superior to medication-only approaches. By and large, however, few differences were found between the Comb and MedMgt treatment groups. In addition, Comb and MedMgt approaches are generally significantly superior to community treatments, whereas intensive psychosocial treatment is not. It is noteworthy that the superiority of Comb and MedMgt (and lack of significant difference of P) to CC occurred despite the fact that two-thirds of the community group received medication over the course of the study. Importantly, no meaningful site by treatment interactions were found, thus lending strength, credibility and generalizability to the overall pattern of findings.

The MTA is the largest, most methodologically sophisticated randomized multisite ADHD trial conducted to date, comparing therapeutic strategies that have previously been shown to be effective in briefer, single-site studies. Because of its size and duration, the MTA is able to address key treatment questions which were not fully answered by previous studies. First, it extends the findings of previous studies demonstrating short-term, robust efficacy from medication management approaches out to a period of 14 months, showing that these effects continue during long-term treatment. These effects were realized across diverse settings, patient groups and outcome domains. For example, medication management benefited children's sociometric (peer status and likeability) ratings, demonstrating that the acute effects of medication on negative peer interactions continue with long-term medication use. Given the refractoriness of problems in that domain, such effects are especially note-worthy.

Second, we found positive results on parent ratings of child functioning, in contrast to those long-duration studies that used twice-daily (b.i.d.) dosing (Schachar et al., 1997), and in agreement with other long-duration studies which – like the MTA – used t.i.d. medication (Hechtman and Abikoff, 1995). In contrast to widespread concerns, Comb and MedMgt children tolerated the third medication dose given in the afternoon, confirming findings reported earlier by Kent et al. (1995). By and large, the relative improvements attributed to medication management replicate and extend those reported by other long-duration stimulant trials (Hechtman and Abikoff, 1995; Gillberg et al., 1997; Schachar et al., 1997).

Third, adding psychosocial interventions to stimulant treatments – creating a multimodal intervention, the current 'gold standard' for ADHD treatment – yielded few additional benefits, paralleling earlier findings reported by Hecht-man and Abikoff (1995). Our finding of modest benefits of Comb on reading achievement versus CC appears to 'split the difference' between the 'no-effect' findings of previous, less well-controlled long-term studies, vs. findings from short-term studies that have uniformly shown that medication improves daily classwork. The fact that Comb subjects showed improved reading achievement may have resulted from improved academic productivity during the school year, due either to the Comb intervention itself, or because of the additional academic activity provided in the summer programme that Comb subjects received. Whatever the source, this finding highlights the potential benefits of combined pharmacological and psychoeducational strategies on reading achievement in ADHD children.

Fourth, despite our prediction that extending multidomain, intensive psy-chosocial interventions over a long duration would increase their efficacy, the

MTA's purely behavioural treatment for ADHD did not equal the effects of medication management. Thus, the MTA was not able to replicate the findings of Klein and colleagues that intensive classroom behavioural modification treatments of ADHD using token economies matched methylphenidate in efficacy (Klein and Abikoff, 1997). In part, however, some or all of these differences may have been due to aspects of the MTA's design (see discussion below).

Clinical impact of treatment

The relatively greater clinical benefits for children receiving the intensive medication management strategies appear to be substantial. For example, across parent and teacher ratings of children's ADHD symptoms, Comb and MedMgt subjects' baseline scores improved over treatment by a factor of 1.5–1.8 standard deviations (SD), compared to smaller, though sizeable (0.9–1.2 SD), changes in Beh and CC subjects. Similar findings were noted in oppositional and anxiety symptoms, where Comb and MedMgt subjects generally manifested about 50% more change over time (measured by SD units) than Beh and CC subjects. Such differences are not inconsequential, and are comparable to two different treatments improving a child with symptoms in the 99th percentile (2.5 SD above the mean) to either the 93rd percentile (1.5 SD above the mean) or to the 84th percentile (1.0 SD above the mean).

From a clinician's point of view, what was the impact of the various treatments on the ADHD condition itself? DISC interviews were readministered to all parents at 14 months. These data indicated that, among Comb and MedMgt subjects, only 19 of 127 (15.0%) and 22 of 121 (18.2%) still met full diagnostic criteria for ADHD, compared to 45 of 133 (33.8%) and 40 of 129 (31.0%) of Beh and CC subjects, respectively ($\chi^2 = 18.0$, degrees of freedom (df) = 3, $P < 0.001$). Similar patterns were noted in the proportions of children who met criteria for a disruptive disorder (CD/ODD) at study endpoint: thus, 20 of 125 (16.0%) and 26 of 119 (21.9%) of Comb and MedMgt subjects met criteria for CD/ODD at 14 months, compared to 41 of 129 (31.8%) and 44 of 122 (36.1%) of Beh and CC subjects, respectively ($\chi^2 = 16.0$, df = 3, $P < 0.001$).

In order to make final treatment recommendations to the family as the MTA-delivered treatments concluded, each site developed clinical consensus ratings of children's overall functioning at a final treatment team meeting. These ratings, made after review of the last 3 months of parents', teachers' and clinicians' reports of children's overall functioning, assigned subjects into one of three categories. Category 1 designated children receiving consensus ratings of improved or much improved over the course of the study, and for whom no additional treatments were recommended (other than to continue what they were already receiving). Category 3 ratings denoted just the opposite, namely, subjects judged not to be doing well at all, and whose families were encouraged to seek additional treatments above and beyond what the MTA had provided. Category 2 subjects were intermediate in functioning levels. For these subjects, final clinical recommendations were determined by consensus during a cross-site meeting (with clinicians from all sites participating), after review and discussion of all data. This was done to ensure that sites did not develop dramatically different recommendations at the end-of-treatment debriefing. Notably, 60.6%, 48.4% and 26.3% of Comb, MedMgt and Beh subjects, respectively, were coded to the best outcome group (Category 1), while 13.1%, 14.7% and 30.6% of Comb, MedMgt and Beh subjects, respectively were assigned to the worst outcome group (Category 3). Of course, these data do not represent objective outcome data, because differences among treatment arms could have been influenced by clinicians' biases about the satisfactoriness of the treatments children were receiving. None the less, they do represent consensus judgements made by each site's treatment team (including pharmaco- and psycho-therapists) about the degree of clinical improvement made by each child and family, after careful review of clinical data from parents and teachers over the final 3 months of treatment. In that respect, these data do provide an important clinical perspective of the improvement experienced by participants in each of the three MTA treatments.

Our findings suggest that high-quality treatments may have considerable impact on restoring ADHD children to normal or near-normal functioning at home and in the classroom. Because essentially none of the ADHD children met the normal criteria met by 88% of comparison children drawn from the same classrooms at study outset, the notion that ADHD is just normal behaviour labelled by uninformed parents or overwhelmed teachers appears not only implausible, but preposterous. But even more importantly, substantial proportions of these children could be helped and returned to essentially normal functioning, particularly through the Comb and MedMgt interventions. To deny such children an appropriate diagnosis and high-quality treatments cannot be defended on ethical, scientific or pragmatic grounds. Unfortunately, given the current situation where constraints are often placed on the amount of time available within busy paediatric practices and school classrooms to diagnose, treat, follow-up and coordinate interventions for these children, substantial changes in schools and health systems appear to be necessary. Further studies of the costs and cost-effectiveness of the various interventions, both in terms of short- and long-term outcomes, as well as for specific subgroups of especially impaired ADHD children (such as those doubly comorbid with ADHD, anxiety disorders and CD/ODD) are planned. Coupled with the current long-term follow-up of the MTA sample, such data may be useful to demonstrate the need and pragmatic benefits of intensive high-quality interventions and careful follow-up with these children.

Interpretation of findings: implications of the MTA study design

Notably, Comb and MedMgt were generally superior to CC treatments, even though two-thirds of CC subjects were on medication for some or all of the 14-month period. However, it is not clear exactly what components of the MTA medication interventions rendered them so much more effective than routine community (CC) treatments. Unlike medication treatments as delivered in the community, we used a carefully controlled, manualized medication titration procedure, in order to maximize positive effects while minimizing side-effects (Greenhill et al., 1996). As noted above, we administered t.i.d. medication dosing, versus the common practice of b.i.d. dosing. Moreover, as part of our medication management strategy, we met with parents monthly and obtained systematic feedback both from them and from their children's teachers. In addition, parent guidance and 'bibliotherapy' were provided as needed; this had previously been reported to provide some benefits over simple pill dispensing alone (Long et al., 1993). All these components do not appear to be part of routine paediatric ADHD treatment practices (Sloan et al., 1999), and may have enhanced the relative effectiveness of our medication management. In addition, analyses done by Greenhill et al. (2001) indicate that differences between the MTA-treated and CC-treated groups across a variety of factors (e.g. dose, dosing regimen, visit frequency and length) were the principal factors explaining the sizeable differences between the MTA MedMgt groups and CC subjects who also received medication. Ultimately, however, it may be necessary to undertake some 'dismantling' research on the MTA MedMgt strategy, to determine the relative contributions of the various components.

These findings may have considerable import for primary care providers. Based on our findings of the medication practices used by physicians in the community (CC subjects), they may tend to use lower than optimal doses and twice- rather than three-times-daily dosing. In our experience, providers and parents alike may sometimes be afraid of the medication, and too often settle for a less than a complete response (full normalization).

The monthly medication monitoring and follow-up visits employed by the MTA pharmacotherapists stand in further contrast to the twice-yearly physician visits for medication monitoring provided to families in the CC group.

Given this lack of communication between and general disconnect between physicians and families, as well as the lack of systematic and regular feedback between physicians and teachers – all problems documented in the ADHD Consensus Development Conference (National Institutes of Health Consensus Development Conference Statement, 2000) – it should not be surprising that medication approaches under such conditions do not yield optimal outcomes, perhaps due to very concrete and practical problems such as compliance and under- or overdosing. To the extent that routine ADHD treatment practices could more effectively address such problems, better outcomes seem likely.

Concerning the relative benefits of our Beh treatments (alone or combined with MedMgt), results must be understood within the context of several limitations of our study design. First, our design did not include a no-treatment or placebo group – an ethically unacceptable option for a study of this length. The CC group was treated in the same manner that subjects seek out and receive treatment in many communities (i.e. private practice or clinic-based care, self-pay or insurance options, etc.). Therefore, the fact that Beh subjects' outcomes rarely differed significantly from those of CC subjects does not mean that these treatments were ineffective. To the contrary, substantial improvement occurred over time across all groups, regardless of the rating source or method. In addition, the comparability of Beh and CC outcomes occurred despite the fact that approximately most CC subjects were treated during the study with medication provided by their family physician – arguably a powerful treatment. Post hoc analyses (MTA Cooperative Group, 1999b; Greenhill et al., 2001) indicated that CC children treated with medication over the 14 months fared significantly better than CC subjects not so treated, based on a range of teacher-completed, sociometric and classroom observers' ratings. In all these instances, MTA Beh-treated subjects fared substantially better than un-medicated CC subjects, with their scores closely approximating CC medication-treated subjects (MTA Cooperative Group, 1999b).

These findings suggest that a substantial subset of Beh-assigned children were probably helped by the MTA psychosocial treatment alone, even though this treatment in general was not as effective as the two MTA treatments employing ongoing medication management. Further, our subgroup analyses yielded different treatment effects for specific patient groups than the main ITT analyses (MTA Cooperative Group, 1999b; Jensen et al., 2001), with these analyses indicating that ADHD children with cooccurring anxiety disorders, and especially those with doubly comorbid conditions (ADHD + anxiety + CD/ODD), were most likely to benefit specifically from combined and psychosocial treatments for some outcome domains.

Thus, findings from our ITT moderator analyses (MTA Cooperative Group, 1999b) and further subgroup analyses (March et al., 2000; Jensen et al., 2001) suggest that some children do in fact show a preferential benefit to specific treatments, in a pattern different from the overall pattern of findings. Parent-reported anxiety disorder as a comorbidity with ADHD may have a considerable impact on children's treatment responses, depending upon whether the anxiety occurs with or without a disruptive disorder such as ODD or CD. A simple rule of thumb that summarizes these findings suggests that if a child presents with an ADHD/anxiety only profile, all interventions (other than routine community care) are likely to be effective. If a child presents with ADHD only or ADHD/CD/ODD, treatments with medication appear especially indicated, and Beh alone strategies may be contraindicated. And finally, if a child presents with ADHD/anxiety/CD/ODD, Comb interventions may offer substantial advantages over other treatments, particularly in overall impairment and functioning outcomes.

These findings suggest that more precise matching of patients to treatment using patients' comorbidity profiles may mitigate initial clinical uncertainty, reduce the number of therapeutic trials until a workable treatment is found and yield larger treatment gains for specific patients.

Such considerations highlight the need for careful clinical assessments of children presenting with ADHD, as the ADHD diagnosis alone may not be sufficient to determine optimal treatments for specific children. These findings argue against a 'one size fits all' approach to treatment. Of course, these results cannot necessarily be generalized beyond ADHD combined type; other ADHD subtypes (e.g. inattentive subtype) may warrant somewhat different treatments. Moreover, replication of these findings in new samples is very much needed.

Previous research has shown that the medication benefits may persist only as long as such treatments are being delivered (Firestone et al., 1986; Pelham and Murphy, 1986). Thus, another design issue that may have affected results regarding the relative impact of Beh treatments is that, except for difficulties with compliance and/or side-effects, Comb and MedMgt subjects were maintained on medication throughout the 14 months, including at all assessment points. By contrast, for Beh subjects the frequency of contact with therapists was gradually faded to once-monthly contacts 3–6 months prior to posttreatment assessment. In part, this was done because of the financial constraints set by the total funds made available by NIMH to address the study's questions. In addition, it was unclear how intensive and prolonged our psychosocial treatment could be without losing families due to increasing compliance problems over time. Also, because we wanted to compare treatment strategies that would be feasible and affordable within the constraints of 'real-world' settings, we further concluded that it might be necessary to limit the total amount of psychosocial treatment provided if we were to test a treatment strategy that third-party payers would approve. Last, and perhaps most importantly, previous research had shown that maintenance of acute treatment effects – that is, generalization across settings and over time – has been the Achilles heel (Pelham and Murphy, 1986) of behavioural treatments. Given this combination of logistical constraints, theoretical considerations and practical concerns, we built procedures for maintenance and generalization throughout the Beh treatment components (Wells et al., 2000a), with the goal that benefits would persist as parents and children learned and consolidated their skills. For example, these procedures included several sessions in which parents were taught skills designed to help them interact with their child's teacher in order to maintain the school interventions. However, our Beh procedures, which were increasingly nonintensive during fading, were insufficient to produce overall effects comparable or additive to 14 months of ongoing medication management. Future analyses after the 14-month end-of-treatment period will examine the extent to which treatment effects across all arms persist, at which point all MTA-delivered treatments will have ceased.

As noted above, the actual quality of and compliance with the medication treatments are probably important factors in the effectiveness of the MTA treatment strategies. Yet medication alone is not likely to tell the full story. Behavioural treatments may help families actively cope with their child's disorder and to make the necessary life accommodations to optimize family functioning, even when such treatments are not as effective as medication in reducing children's ADHD symptoms. Indeed, 14-month endpoint analyses indicated that parent satisfaction ratings differed significantly by treatment group, with pairwise contrasts showing that treatment satisfaction scores for Comb and Beh parents were significantly superior to MedMgt parents' ratings (though not differing between themselves), suggesting that the Beh components benefited this area of family-relevant outcomes. Relatedly, our further analyses suggested that actual changes in parents' attitudes and disciplinary practices accompanied evidence of increased benefits of the combined treatments (Hinshaw et al., 2000; Hoza et al., 2000; Wells et al., 2000b), such that the only MTA subgroup identified to date that yielded full normalization of school-based disruptive behaviour patterns included families receiving Comb treatment who significantly improved their negative and ineffective discipline practices during the trial. Such factors must remain active areas of ongoing investigations in refining and improving behavioural and combined treatments.

Thus, unanswered in our study are important questions concerning psychosocial and combined treatments for ADHD. For example, might there be some children for whom medication management is no longer necessary (Gillberg et al., 1997), and if so, how might such children be identified? Can and should psychosocial treatments be faded, and how can that be accomplished while maintaining effects? Is there an optimal length and combination of medication and psychosocial treatments, and how should such treatments be sequenced? Might combined treatments enable medication benefits to be achieved at lower medication doses, a post hoc finding that emerged from our analyses (Vitiello et al., 2001)? Can combined treatments increase the likelihood that children will eventually succeed without medication? Will findings differ as children age and move into critical developmental transitions, such that those who have learned increased skills via a psychosocial intervention eventually function better than those who received only medication? Follow-up study of the MTA subjects past 14 months (which is currently underway) will allow some of these critical questions to be addressed.

Since ADHD is now regarded by most experts as a chronic disorder (Barkley et al., 1990), ongoing treatment appears to be often necessary. As with other chronic conditions like heart disease, diabetes and asthma, however, the need for active treatment may wax and wane, depending upon the course of the disorder and various external circumstances. Just as exercise, diet and pollen load may affect these other chronic illnesses, the nature of persons' learning or work environments and intercurrent stressors may affect the specific need for, type and intensity of ADHD treatments over the life course (Biederman et al., 1995). Under such conditions, psychosocial treatments may help families cope with their child's disorder and to make the necessary life accommodations to optimize family functioning, even when such treatments are not as effective as medication in reducing children's symptoms. In this regard, it is perhaps not surprising that 14-month endpoint analyses indicated that parent satisfaction ratings differed significantly as a function of treatment group, with pairwise contrasts indicating that treatment satisfaction scores for Comb and Beh parents were both significantly superior to MedMgt parents' ratings, but did not differ among themselves.

These findings suggest that the Beh components benefited this area of family-perceived outcomes. Another potential benefit of psychosocial interventions for some families may be improved compliance with medication over the long term due to greater parental satisfaction with treatment, particularly because many medicated children do not continue medication for as long as it is indicated. This issue is explored in depth elsewhere (MTA Cooperative Group, 1999a). Follow-up study of the MTA subjects past 14 months (currently underway) will allow this and other questions to be addressed.

In terms of practicality and feasibility of our various treatments, one 'real-world' limitation consists of the expensive, intensive nature of our Beh, and to a lesser extent, MedMgt treatments. Beh treatments required nearly 30 parent clinic visits and an 8-week daily summer programme. Our MedMgt condition required weekly parent clinic visits during the first month, and monthly parent visits thereafter. Despite the well-documented benefits of psychosocial strategies, for example (Hinshaw et al., 1998), it may be difficult for some families to participate fully and comply with these treatments (MTA Cooperative Group, 1999b), by virtue of their costs, the amount of time required or family characteristics that limit their ability to learn and implement the treatments. Regardless, other clinical considerations, such as medication contraindications for some children, or because many families want to avoid medication strategies altogether, indicate that psychosocial treatments have a necessary role in the therapeutic armamentarium. Similarly, other families may find medication a preferable strategy.

In general, our findings suggest that both our pharmacological and psycho-social treatments could be delivered across six different clinical settings. Of course, whether these treatments are transportable to community settings will ultimately determine their utility. Future research will be required to determine how these treatments might be administered in a more effective and efficient manner, such that families' compliance is maximized, and that these treatments are feasible, transportable and affordable in 'real-world' practice settings.

Conclusion

The MTA study is the largest clinical trial ever conducted by NIMH, and exceeds by several orders of magnitude in size, scope and length other studies of child treatment. Juxtaposed against its several limitations, the strengths of the study are considerable, and include the explicit use of evidence-based treatments; the high degree of compliance across arms and over the course of the study; very low subject attrition; low cross-over rates; a comprehensive range of objective and valid assessments across multiple areas of functioning; measures of therapist competence, treatment alliance and treatment fidelity, collected from various sources; a sample size that well exceeds previous studies in size and diversity; and the absence of any site-by-treatment interactions. For the future, the MTA's multisite, long-duration, parallel randomized controlled trial design using manualized treatments will set an important benchmark for trials testing new treatments for childhood ADHD (Taylor, 1999).

Overall study findings indicate that long-term treatments that employ systematic, frequent (e.g. monthly) medication management with brief parent guidance greatly reduce children's symptoms of ADHD, oppositional-aggressive behaviours and anxiety, while also enhancing other areas of functioning. Given that the MTA findings clearly document various levels of improvement for several different commonly recommended treatment strategies across multiple domains of functioning, results are likely to be relevant for clinicians, as well as valuable for health care planners and policy makers. Despite the ongoing public controversies concerning the use of medication for ADHD children, our data suggest that medication management approaches which are carefully done, monitored and continued over 14 months realize greater benefits across most outcome domains than gradually faded psychosocial-only treatments or routine community care. Moreover, these treatments can be delivered with high success across diverse settings and patient populations. Although our study provides some modest evidence that there may be circumstances where psychosocial treatments (alone or in combination with medication) may help specific children and enhance consumer satisfaction, additional research is needed to define these areas further, as well as to strengthen the overall impact of behavioural interventions, alone and in combination with medications.

REFERENCES

Abikoff, H. and Gittelman, R. (1985). Classroom observation code: a modification of the Stony Brook code. *Psychopharmacology Bulletin*, **21**, 901–9.

American Psychiatric Association. (1994). *Diagnostic and Statistical Manual of Mental Disorders*, 4th edn. Washington, DC: American Psychiatric Association.

Arnold, L., Abikoff, H., Cantwell, D. et al. (1997a). NIMH collaborative multimodal treatment study of children with ADHD (MTA): design challenges and choices. *Archives of General Psychiatry*, **54**, 865–70.

Arnold, L.E., Abikoff, H.B., Cantwell, D.P. et al. (1997b). NIMH collaborative multimodal treatment study of children with ADHD (MTA): design, methodology, and protocol evolution. *Journal of Attention Disorders*, **2**, 141–58.

Barkley, R.A. (1987). *Defiant Children: A Clinician's Manual for Parent Training*. New York: Guilford Press.

Barkley, R.A., Fischer, M., Edelbrock, C.S. and Smallish, L. (1990). The adolescent outcome of hyperactive children diagnosed by research criteria: I. An 8-year prospective follow-up study. *Journal of the American Academy of Child and Adolescent Psychiatry*, **29**, 546–57.

Biederman, J., Newcorn, J. and Sprich, S. (1991). Comorbidity of attention deficit hyperactivity disorder with conduct, depressive, anxiety, and other disorders. *American Journal of Psychiatry*, **148**, 564–77.

Biederman, J., Milberger, S., Faraone, S.V. et al. (1995). Family–environment risk factors for attention-deficit hyperactivity disorder. A test of Rutter's indicators of adversity. *Archives of General Psychiatry*, **52**, 464–70.

Bryk, A.S., Raudenbush, S.W. (1988). Toward a more appropriate conceptualization of research on school effects: a three-level heirarchical linear model. *American Journal of Education*, **97**, 68–108.

Cohen, J. (1988). *Statistical Power Analyses for the Behavioral Sciences*, 2nd edn. Hillsdale, NJ: Lawrence Erlbaum.

Conners, C.K. (1990). *Manual for the Conners' Rating Scales*. Toronto, Canada: Multi-Health Systems.

Conners, C.K., Epstein, J.N., March, J.S. et al. (2001). Multimodal treatment of ADHD (MTA): an alternative outcome analysis. *Journal of the American Academy of Academy Child and Adolescent Psychiatry*, **40**, 159–67.

Elkin, I., Gibbons, R.D., Shea, M.T. et al. (1995). Initial severity and differential treatment outcome in the National Institute of Mental Health treatment of depression collaborative research program. *Journal of Consulting and Clinical Psychology*, **63**, 841–7.

Firestone, P., Crowe, D., Goodman, J.T. and McGrath, P. (1986). Vicissitudes of follow-up studies: differential effects of parent training and stimulant medication with hyperactives. *American Journal of Orthopsychiatry*, **56**, 184–94.

Forehand, R. and McMahon, R. (1980). *Helping the Noncompliant Child: A Clinician's Guide to Parent Training*. New York: Guilford Press.

Gillberg, C., Melander, H., von Knorring, A.L. et al. (1997). Long-term stimulant treatment of children with attention-deficit hyperactivity disorder symptoms. A randomized, double-blind, placebo-controlled trial. *Archives of General Psychiatry*, **54**, 857–64.

Greenhill, L.L., Abikoff, H.B., Arnold, L.E. et al. (1996). Medication treatment strategies in the MTA: relevance to clinicians and researchers. *Journal of the American Academy of Child and Adolescent Psychiatry*, **35**, 1304–13.

Greenhill, L.L., Swanson, J.M., Vitiello, B. et al. (2001). Determining the best dose of methylphenidate under controlled conditions: lessons from the MTA titration. *Journal of the American Academy of Child and Adolescent Psychiatry*, **40**, 180–7.

Greenhouse, J.B., Stangl, D. and Bromberg, J. (1991a). An introduction to survival analysis: statistical methods for the analysis of clinical trials. *Journal of Consulting and Clinical Psychology*, **57**, 536–44.

Greenhouse, J.B., Stangl, D., Kupfer, D.J. and Prien R.P. (1991b). Methodologic issues in maintenance therapy clinical trials. *Archives of General Psychiatry*, **48**, 313–18.

Gresham, F.M. and Elliott, S.N. (1989). *Social Skills Rating System – Parent, Teacher, and Child Forms*. Circle Pines, Minnesota: American Guidance Systems.

Hechtman, L. and Abikoff, H. (1995). Multimodal treatment plus stimulants vs. stimulant treatment in ADHD children: results from a two year comparative treatment study. In *Proceedings of the Annual Meeting of the American Academy of Child and Adolescent Psychiatry*, p. 63. New Orleans: American Academy of Child and Adolescent Psychiatry.

Hedeker, D. and Gibbons, R.D. (1996a). MIXREG: a computer program for mixed-effects regression analysis with autocorrelated errors. *Computer Methods and Programs in Biomedicine*, **49**, 229–52.

Hedeker, D. and Gibbons, R.D. (1996b). MIXOR: a computer program for mixed-effects ordinal regression analysis. *Computer Methods and Programs in Biomed0cine*, **49**, 157–76.

Hedeker, D., Gibbons, R.D. and Flay, B.R. (1994). Random-effects regression models for clustered data with an example from smoking prevention research. *Journal of Consulting and Clinical Psychology*, **62**, 757–65.

Hinshaw, S.P. (1992). Externalizing behavior problems and academic underachievement in childhood and adolescence: causal relationships and underlying mechanisms. *Psychological Bulletin*, **111**, 127–55.

Hinshaw, S.P., March, J.S., Abikoff, H. et al. (1997). Comprehensive assessment of childhood attention-deficit hyperactivity disorder in the context of a multisite, multimodal clinical trial. *Journal of Attention Disorders*, **1**, 217–34.

Hinshaw, S.P., Klein, R.G. and Abikoff, H. (1998). Childhood attention-deficit hyperactivity disorder: nonpharmacologic and combination treatments. In *A Guide to Treatments that Work*, Nathan, P.E. and Gorman, J.M., eds, pp. 26–41. New York: Oxford University Press.

Hinshaw, S.P., Owens, E.B., Wells, K.C. et al. (2000). Family processes and treatment outcome in the MTA: negative/ineffective parenting practices in relation to multimodal treatment. *Journal of Abnormal Child Psychology*, **28**, 555–68.

Hoza, B., Owens, J.S., Pelham, W.E. et al. (2000). Parent cognitions as predictors of child treatment response in attention-deficit/hyperactivity disorder. *Journal of Abnormal Child Psychology*, **28**, 569–83.

Jensen, P.S., Kettle, L., Roper, M.S. et al. (1999). Are stimulants over-prescribed? Treatment of ADHD in four US communities. *Journal of the American Academy of Child and Adolescent Psychiatry*, **38**, 797–804.

Jensen, P.S., Hinshaw, S.P., Kraemer, H.C. et al. (2001). ADHD comorbidity findings from the MTA study: comparing comorbid subgroups. *Journal of the American Academy of Child and Adolescent Psychiatry*, **40**, 147–58.

Kazdin, A.E. and Bass, D. (1989). Power to test differences between alternative treatments in comparative psychotherapy outcome research. *Journal of Consulting and Clinical Psychology*, **57**, 138–47.

Kent, J.D., Blader, J.C., Koplewicz, H.S., Abikoff, H. and Foley, C.A. (1995). Effects of late-afternoon methylphenidate administration on behavior and sleep in attention-deficit hyperactivity disorder. *Pediatrics*, **96**, 320–5.

Klein, R.G. and Abikoff, H. (1997). Behavior therapy and methylphenidate in the treatment of children with ADHD. *Journal of Attention Disorders*, **2**, 89–114.

Kwasman, A., Tinsley, B.J. and Lepper, H.S. (1995). Pediatricians' knowledge and attitude concerning diagnosis and treatment of attention deficit and hyperactivity disorders. *Archivies of Pediatrics Adolescent Medicine*, **149**, 1211–16.

Lahey, B., Applegate, B., McBurnett, K. et al. (1993). DSM IV field trials for attention deficit/hyperactivity disorder in children and adolescents. *American Journal of Psychiatry*, **151**, 1673–85.

Laird, N.M. and Ware, J.H. (1982). Random effect models for longitudinal data. *Biometrics*, **38**, 963–74.

Long, N., Rickert, V.I. and Ashcraft, E.W. (1993). Bibliotherapy as an adjunct to stimulant medication in the treatment of attention-deficit hyperactivity disorder. *Journal of Pediatrics and Health Care*, **7**, 82–8.

Mannuzza, S., Klein, R.G., Bassier, A., Malloy, P. and LaPadula, M. (1993). Adult outcome of hyperactive boys. *Archives of General Psychiatry*, **50**, 565–76.

March, J.S., Parker, J.D., Sullivan, K., Stallings, P. and Conners, C.K. (1997). The Multidimensional Anxiety Scale for Children (MASC): factor structure, reliability, and validity. *Journal of the American Academy of Child Adolescent Psychiatry*, **36**, 554–65.

March, J.S., Swanson, J.M., Arnold, L.E. et al. (2000). Anxiety as a predictor and outcome variable in the multimodal treatment study of children with ADHD. *Journal of Abnnormal Child Psychology*, **28**, 527–41.

Moser, S.E. and Kallail, K.J. (1995). Attention-deficit hyperactivity disorder: management by family physicians. *Archives of Family Medicine*, **4**, 241–4.

MTA Cooperative Group. (1999a). A 14-month randomized clinical trial of treatment strategies for attention-deficit/hyperactivity disorder. *Archives of General Psychiatry*, **56**, 1073–86.

MTA Cooperative Group. (1999b). Moderators and mediators of treatment response for children with attention-deficit/hyperactivity disorder. *Archives of General Psychiatry*, **56**, 1088–96.

National Institutes of Health Consensus Development Conference Statement. (2000). Diagnosis and treatment of attention-deficit/hyperactivity disorder. *Journal of the American Academy of Child and Adolescent Psychiatry*, **39**, 182–93.

Newcorn, J.H., Halperin, J.M., Jensen, P.S. et al. (2001). Symptom profiles in children with ADHD: effects of comorbidity and gender. *Journal of the American Academy of Child and Adolescent Psychiatry*, **40**, 137–46.

Nottelmann, E. and Jensen, P. (1995). Comorbidity of disorders in children and adolescents: developmental perspectives. In *Advances in Clinical Child Psychology*, vol. 17, T. Ollendick and R. Prinz, eds., pp. 109–55. New York: Plenum.

Pelham, W.E. and Hoza, B. (1996). Comprehensive treatment for ADHD: a proposal for intensive summer treatment programs and outpatient follow-up. In *Psychosocial Treatments for Children and Adolescents: Empirically Supported Approaches*, Hibbs, E. and Jensen, P., eds, pp. 311–40. New York: APA Press.

Pelham, W.E. and Murphy, H.A. (1986). Behavioral and pharmacological treatment of hyperactivity and attention-deficit disorders. In *Pharmacological and Behavioral Treatment: An Integrative Approach*, M. Herson and S.E. Breuning, eds, pp. 108–47. New York: Wiley.

Pelham, W.E., Gnagy, E.M., Greiner, A.R. et al. (2000). Behavioral vs. behavioral and pharmacological treatment in ADHD children attending a summer treatment program. *Journal of Abnormal Child Psychology*, **28**, 507–25.

Popper, C.W. (1988). Disorders usually first evident in infancy, childhood, or adolescence. In *Textbook of Psychiatry*, J.A. Talbott, R.E. Hales and S.C. Yudofsky, eds, pp. 649–735. Washington, DC: American Psychiatric Press.

Richters, J., Arnold, L.E.A., Jensen, P.S. et al. (1995). NIMH collaborative multisite, multimodal treatment study of children with ADHD: I. Background and rationale. *Journal of the American Academy of Child and Adolescent Psychiatry*, **34**, 987–1000.

Safer, D.J., Zito, J.M. and Fine, E.M. (1996). Increased methylphenidate usage for attention deficit disorder in the 1990s. *Pediatrics*, **98**, 1084–8.

Satterfield, J.H., Satterfield, B.T. and Schell, A.M. (1987). Therapeutic interventions to prevent delinquency in hyperactive boys. *Journal of the American Academy of Child and Adolescent Psychiatry*, **26**, 56–64.

Schachar, R.J., Tannock, R., Cunningham, C. and Corkum, P.V. (1997). Behavioral, situational, and temporal effects of treatment of ADHD with methylphenidate. *Journal of the American Academy of Child and Adolescent Psychiatry*, **36**, 754–63.

Shaffer, D., Fisher, P., Dulcan, M. et al. (1996). The second version of the NIMH Diagnostic Interview Schedule for Children (DISC-2), *Journal of the American Academy of Child and Adolescent Psychiatry*, **35**, 865–77.

Sloan, M., Jensen, P. and Kettle, L. (1999). Assessing services for children with ADHD: gaps and opportunities. *Journal of Attention Disorders*, **3**, 13–29.

Spencer, T., Biederman, J., Wilens, T. et al. (1996). Pharmacotherapy of attention-deficit hyperactivity disorder across the life cycle. *Journal of the American Academy of Child Adolescent Psychiatry*, **35**, 409–32.

Swanson, J.M. (1992). *School-based Assessments and Interventions for ADD Students*. Irvine, CA: K. C. Publications.

Swanson, J. (1993). Effect of stimulant medication on hyperactive children: a review of reviews. *Exceptional Child*, **60**, 154–62.

Swanson, J.M., Kraemer, H.C., Hinshaw, S.P. et al. (2001). Clinical relevance of the primary findings of the MTA: success rates based on severity of symptoms at the end of treatment. *Journal of the American Academy of Child and Adolescent Psychiatry*, **40**, 168–79.

Szatmari, P., Offord, D.R. and Boyle, M.H. (1989). Correlates, associated impairments, and patterns of services utilization of children with attention deficit disorder: findings from the Ontario Child Health Study. *Journal of Child Psychology and Psychiatry*, **30**, 205–17.

Taylor, E. (1999). Development of clinical services for attention-deficit/hyperactivity disorder. *Archives of General Psychiatry*, **56**, 1097–9.

Vitiello, B., Severe, J.B., Greenhill, L.L. et al. (2001). Methylphenidate dosage for children with ADHD over time under controlled conditions: lessons from the MTA. *Journal of the American Academy of Child and Adolescent Psychiatry*, **40**, 188–96.

Wechsler, D. (1992). *Wechsler Individual Achievement Test – Manual*. San Antonio: Psychological Corporation.

Weiss, G. and Hechtman, L.T. (1993). *Hyperactive Children Grown up. ADHD in Children, Adolescents, and Adults*, 2nd edn. New York: Guilford Press.

Wells, K.C., Pelham, W.E., Kotkin, R.A. et al. (2000a). Psychosocial treatment strategies in the MTA study: rationale, methods, and critical issues in design and implementation. *Journal of Abnormal Child Psychology*, **28**, 483–505.

Wells, C.K., Epstein, J.N., Hinshaw, S.P. et al. (2000b). Parenting and family stress treatment outcomes in attention deficit hyperactivity disorder (ADHD): an empirical analysis in the MTA study. *Journal of Abnormal Child Psychology*, **28**, 543–53.

14

Attention deficit hyperactivity disorder in adults

Brian Toone

Department of Psychological Medicine, King's College Hospital, London, UK

Introduction

This chapter will review the developing concept of adult attention deficit hyperactivity disorder (ADHD) as it has evolved through changes and modifications in the classificatory system. The most convincing evidence of symptom persistence into adult life and of new patterns of adult comorbidity comes from the longitudinal follow-up studies of childhood hyperactivity and these will be considered in some detail. The chapter will conclude with a section on treatment and management. *Diagnostic and Statistical Manual of Mental Disorders*, 4th edition (DSM-IV: American Psychiatric Association, 1994) uses the diagnostic term ADHD; *International Classification of Disease* (ICD-10) (World Health Organization, 1992) uses hyperkinetic disorder (HD). In essence these terms refer to the same disorder, although the differing criteria will identify distinct though overlapping patient populations. In this chapter ADHD rather than ADHD/HD will be used for simplicity; it should not be taken to imply any classificatory preference on the part of the author.

Classification

The central concept of what is now referred to as ADHD (DSM-IV) or HD (ICD-10) has undergone several transformations, in the course of which a recognition that features may persist into adulthood has gradually emerged. Minimal brain damage, an overarching clinical concept, embraced a number of distinct disorders and syndromes that have since been disaggregated; these included 'impairment . . . of attention, impulse, or motor function' (Clements, 1966). DSM-II recognized hyperkinetic reaction of childhood (or adolescence) as a distinct entity characterized by overactivity, restlessness, distractibility and short attention span. Impulsivity was no longer included. The condition was thought to diminish in adolescence (DSM-II, American Psychiatric Association, 1968). In the third edition (DSM-III, American Psychiatric Association, 1980) the replacement term attentional deficit disorder (ADD) emphasized the salience of attentional features. The syndrome was subdivided into ADD with (ADDH) or without hyperactivity. The core features of inattention, impulsivity or hyperactivity were each diagnosed according to whether a threshold number of key symptoms were deemed to be present. For the first time the persistence of symptoms into adult life was clearly recognized. There could be three outcomes. In the first, all of the symptoms would persist into adult life. In the second, the disorder was self-limited and all of the symptoms disappeared completely at puberty. In the third, the hyperactivity resolved, but the impulsivity and inattentiveness continued into adult life. This condition was referred to as the residual type.

In the revised version of the third edition (DSM-III-R, American Psychiatric Association, 1987) the three core features were no longer evaluated separately and inattention and hyperactivity were subsumed within one diagnostic term: ADHD. A persistence of features of the disorder in one-third of adults was acknowledged. In DSM-IV the clinical evaluative structure and subclassificatory systems revert to a model closer to DSM-III than to DSM-III-R. The core features are again evaluated separately, but hyperactivity and impulsivity are subsumed within one subcategory, and inattention forms the other. Criteria are therefore generated to diagnose three ADHD subtypes: a combined subtype; a predominantly inattentive subtype; and a predominantly hyperactive-impulsive subtype. Only a minority of patients were thought to retain the full complement of symptoms into 'mid-adulthood', but others might retain some, thus earning the diagnosis ADHD in partial remission. The diagnosis ADHD not otherwise specified is reserved for those individuals 'with prominent symptoms of inattention and/or hyperactivity/impulsivity' who neither meet criteria for ADHD nor seem ever to have done so. This somewhat loosely defined category may appear to offer licence to the diagnosis of ADHD in any adult presenting for the first time with any psychiatric disorder in which inattention is a prominent feature.

DSM therefore begins with an emphasis on hyperactivity, later shifts to an emphasis on inattention, then incorporates both within a unitary diagnosis, and finally allows for each a separate identity. DSM-IV also recognizes that the pattern may vary with age, with hyperactivity becoming less prominent. ICD-10 takes a similar position as DSM-III-R, recognizing a unitary diagnosis in which hyperactivity and inattention (but not impulsivity, which is considered an associated rather than a diagnostic feature) are each central components. It appears unconvinced of the ADHD concept of a separate inattention subtype. It acknowledges the persistence of symptoms into adult life.

Epidemiology

The ascertainment of prevalence of adult ADHD is beset by difficulties. Criteria for diagnosis and approaches to classification vary, not only between present classificatory systems, but also within classificatory systems across time, a complication that any prospective longitudinal study must face. The diagnosis of ADHD embraces a spectrum of behaviours, symptoms and disabilities that may be conceived as an extreme exaggeration of normal childhood characteristics; consequently they exhibit a dimensional rather than categorical distribution. The point at which a constellation of dimensionally distributed characteristic variables becomes a clinical entity is, to a degree, arbitrary and owes as much to the need for reliability as for validity. In clinical practice the diagnostic threshold may be influenced by the individual family and educational context and by the needs and expectations of patient and family. These uncertainties, which are present during childhood, become even more evident during adolescence and adulthood, at a time when symptoms are fading. This might suggest a need for quantitative rather than qualitative measurement variables, but so far few studies (Taylor et al., 1996) have adopted this approach. A final consideration, and one that has therapeutic as well as epidemiological relevance, concerns the need to distinguish between the persistence of core ADHD features, the presence and functional implications of comorbid disorders such as substance abuse, and a range of disadvantages and disabilities that may be directly related to either ADHD or comorbid disorder or both, or may be a legacy of the effects of a no-longer-extant childhood ADHD.

The prevalence of adult ADHD would best be determined by a prospective community-based longitudinal study of the evolution of ADHD features from childhood into adult years; this has yet to be carried out and would be difficult to achieve. Prospective longitudinal cohort studies have been carried out in a very limited number of centres and it is to these studies that we must turn for such understanding as at present exists about the natural history of ADHD. However, these cohorts were formed from clinic referrals and are unlikely to be representative or unbiased. An alternative approach would be to ascertain the point prevalence of ADHD in an adult community survey. This might complement the prospective longitudinal cohort strategy, though it would be unavoidably subject to the difficulties and limitations of first-time diagnosis during adulthood. Little work of this kind has yet been carried out.

Longitudinal cohorts

There are few prospective studies that have begun in childhood and continued into adulthood and only two centres that have published controlled data based on clinical assessment. The Montreal Group (Weiss et al., 1985) followed up 61 members of an original group of 104 hyperactive children first seen at a children's hospital between the ages of 6 and 12. At 15-year follow-up their average age was 25.1 years. Sixty-one per cent of the probands still reported one or more of the following: restlessness, poor concentration, impulsivity and explosiveness, compared with 7% of a matched normal control group recruited through advertisements. In a little over a third, symptoms were moderate to severe. Forty-four per cent (vs. 9.7% of controls) were observed to be physically restless. DSM-III was not used to make a diagnosis of ADDH. The hyperactive subjects complained of sexual problems, difficulties in interpersonal relationships and neurotic symptoms. Twenty-three per cent received a DSM-III diagnosis of antisocial personality disorder compared with 2.4% of controls. A history of alcohol abuse did not distinguish the groups and nonalcohol substance abuse was not commented on. No excess of schizophrenic subjects was noted. The testimony of a close relative was not sought and most of the assessments were nonblind. A further study based on the same cohort (Hechtman and Weiss, 1986) found a trend towards alcohol abuse and towards drug use and involvement. The researchers also reported increased antisocial behaviour and a trend towards more frequent criminal offending.

A second group of studies is based on two New York cohorts. The first cohort (Gittelman et al., 1985) comprised 101 white male children aged between 6 and 12 years who had been referred to a specialist clinic for disturbed behaviour and who had been deemed hyperactive. Subjects with comorbid conduct disorder were excluded. Most were from middle-class backgrounds. Parents were also interviewed and assessments were carried out blind. At 9-year follow up criteria for a DSM-III diagnosis of attention deficit disorder with hyperactivity (ADDH) was satisfied in 31% of the index group, the salient features of attention deficit, impulsivity and hyperactivity all being present; a further 9% had varying combinations of two of the three features. The diagnosis of ADDH was shared with only 3% of a carefully matched control group. A diagnosis of antisocial personality disorder was made in 27% of the index group compared with 8% of the controls, but among those of the index group who retained a diagnosis of ADDH it was 48%; among those who failed to retain the diagnosis it was 13%, only a little higher than the controls. An increased prevalence of substance abuse in the index group was due to drugs

(16% vs. 3%), not alcohol. Again, the excess substance abuse in the index group was largely accounted for by the ADDH subgroup. Drug abuse was encountered almost exclusively in probands with antisocial personality disorder.

A further study (Mannuzza et al., 1991a), designed to explore the respective genetic and environmental contributions, compared probands, siblings and normal controls. The proportion of subjects with ADD syndrome, partial syndrome or ADD symptoms did not differ between siblings and controls and was low, but the proportion of siblings with antisocial personality disorder and with nonalcoholic substance abuse was in each instance intermediate between probands and controls. A replication study (Mannuzza et al., 1991b) employed a cohort of 94 hyperactive boys and obtained similar results to the first study. In an extension of the first cohort follow-up period to 16 years (Mannuzza et al., 1993), the full ADHD syndrome, now diagnosed according to DSM-III-R, had fallen to 8% compared to 1% of controls and the prevalence of at least one ADHD cardinal feature to 11% vs. 1%. The prevalence of antisocial personality disorder, though still excessive, had fallen, as indeed it had in the controls, but was no longer linked to the retention of the ADHD diagnosis. Antisocial personality disorder would thus seem to emerge from its (possibly confounding) association with ADHD as a disorder in its own right. The prevalence of nonalcoholic substance abuse remained unchanged, i.e. considerably higher in the index group, and remained closely associated with antisocial personality disorder. Probands completed fewer years of schooling and socioeconomic status, which had not differed during adolescence, had by the age of 25 declined relative to the control group.

A British study (Taylor et al., 1996) conducted a community-based prospective study of children aged 6–7 years through to late adolescence. Dimensional measures were used to identify children with hyperactivity, conduct disorder or combined disorders. At 16–18 years respectively 20%, 11% and 29% met DSM-III-R criteria for ADHD. No member of the normal control group achieved the diagnosis. The respective percentages for a diagnosis of hyperkinetic disorder using ICD-10 were 10%, 6% and 14%. These findings demonstrate the effect that initial inclusion criteria may have on outcome: the exclusion of hyperactive children comorbid for conduct disorder would substantially reduce the proportion of adult subjects with persistent features of ADHD. They also give some indication of the effect that the stricter ICD criteria may have on prevalence figures.

Direct comparisons between these studies are limited by classificatory changes and the use of different outcome measures. The Montreal (Weiss et al., 1985) and New York (Mannuzza et al., 1993) cohorts were both reviewed at

25–26 years. In the former the presence of at least one salient feature of hyperactivity was detectable in 60% of the probands; in the latter, one feature of ADHD could be detected in only 11%. Yet proband/control ratios were similar – nine in the first study and 11 in the second – suggesting a considerable difference in symptom detection thresholds rather than a genuine difference in outcome; and indeed, when Weiss et al. considered only 'severe' symptoms, the prevalence fell to 9%. Gittelman et al. (1985) and Taylor et al. (1996) both carried out assessments during late adolescence. In the first study 30% of the probands met criteria for ADDH; in the second 20% met criteria for ADHD. The shortfall in the English study may reflect classificatory differences, but may also be due to the recruitment of less severely affected cases in a community-based study.

Relatively unbiased cross-sectional data have only recently been reported (Murphy and Barkley, 1996). Applicants for driver licence renewal were invited to participate and 720 responded. Diagnosis was based on self-report. Persistent ADHD symptoms were reported in 4.7%; the rate of symptom endorsement declined with increasing age. This is consistent with the data emerging from the longitudinal studies, summarized by Hill and Schoener (1996): the prevalence of ADHD was shown to decline exponentially by approximately 50% every 5 years.

In summary, it is now clear that the symptoms of ADHD do persist beyond childhood, but that the proportion of subjects in which they persist declines steadily throughout adolescence and early adulthood. During late adolescence 20–30% will meet criteria for diagnosis; by the middle of the third decade this will have fallen to 10%. The exact prevalence figure will depend upon adult age at time of assessment, the classificatory system used and cohort selection criteria.

Variables that might predict persistence of symptoms have received surprisingly little attention. In children 4-year follow-up studies (Cantwell and Baker, 1992; Hart et al., 1995) find that hyperactivity and impulsivity, but not inattention, predict symptom persistence. In a follow-up study into early adulthood of children cormorbid for ADHD and conduct disorder, hyperactivity-impulsivity and conduct disorder, independently and jointly, predicted adult criminal activity; inattention did not (Babinsky et al., 1999). Biederman et al. (1995) reported an increased rate of ADHD in the children of parents diagnosed with the disorder and concluded that persistence in to adulthood might represent a more familial form of the disorder.

In childhood ADHD is more prevalent in boys in a ratio of 2.9 : 1 (Bird et al., 1988; Safer and Krager, 1988). This gender difference is no longer apparent in adult pharmacotherapy studies (Wender et al., 1985; Willens et al., 1996). The reasons for this are unclear. Conduct disorder, cognitive difficulties and impaired peer relationships are more marked in girls and the poor long-term outlook relative to boys (Sandberg, 1996) may lead to less gender imbalance among adult ADHD patients.

Comorbidity

High levels of psychiatric comorbidity are as much a feature of ADHD in its adult phase as in its childhood manifestation. However, there is little agreement about the degree of comorbidity, with estimates varying from 77% (Biederman et al., 1993) to less than a third (Mannuzza et al., 1993). Comorbidity has implications for assessment, diagnosis and treatment. Both in adults presenting for the first time and in known ADHD cases undergoing periodic evaluation its presence may mask the underlying features of ADHD, preventing adequate assessment. The presence of comorbidity also makes it difficult to determine the extent to which the penumbra of socioeconomic disadvantage that surrounds ADHD is directly due to the effect of core symptoms rather than to associated disorders. This is of practical consequence as, in the individual case, it may influence the decision whether or not to treat. Views differ on the effect of comorbidity on treatment response. The response of ADHD symptoms to stimulants may be decreased (Spencer et al., 1996) but the same group also reported a robust response to methylphenidate that was independent of comorbidity.

The comorbid disorders identified by the longitudinal studies, most emphatically in the New York cohorts (Mannuzza et al., 1991, 1993), are antisocial personality disorder and nonalcoholic substance abuse. Studies based on adult presentation of ADHD (Biederman et al., 1993; Roy-Byrne et al., 1997; van der Linden et al., 2000) report similar findings. Biederman et al. (1993) have reported a high level of comorbidity principally due to affective disorders (multiple anxiety disorders 52%; major depression 32%). In the New York cohort studies (Mannuzza et al., 1991, 1993) affective disorders of any kind were distinctly uncommon. These differences may, in part, be explained by different cohort characteristics, in particular age (the average age of the Biederman et al. study was 39) and gender distribution.

The relationship between childhood and adult ADHD comorbidity has received little attention. Taylor et al. (1996), in a follow-up study of childhood into late adolescence, found that hyperactivity alone or in combination with conduct disorder, but not conduct disorder alone, predicted the persistence of hyperactivity and the development of antisocial characteristics. Within the spectrum of childhood ADHD, hyperactivity-impulsivity but not inattention predicted later criminal behaviour (Babinski et al., 1999). If, as has been suggested (Taylor et al., 1996), conduct disorder is a consequence of hyperactivity sustained over a period of time, it remains to be seen whether antisocial personality disorder is a continuation of conduct disorder into adult years and the extent to which the spectrum of antisocial behaviour (antisocial personality disorder, nonalcoholic substance abuse, criminal activity) is dependent on the persistence of ADHD symptoms – hyperactivity and impulsivity in particular. In this context a continuation study of ADHD in remission would be rewarding.

Assessment

The full evaluation of ADHD features in an adult comprises a number of components: these include self-report of present and past symptoms and disabilities; a mental state examination; a neuropsychological assessment with an emphasis on tests purporting to measure aspects of attention and impulsivity; and the compilation of information from whatever sources are available (school reports, educational psychology reports, parental testimony) that might provide confirmation of the presence of childhood ADHD. The last section is arguably the most important. ADHD is a disorder of childhood that may persist into adult years. Diagnosis in the adult is conditional on the convincing demonstration of the disorder in the child. The symptoms with which the adult usually presents – poor personal organization, inability to get things done, inattentiveness, impulsivity sometimes bordering on recklessness, and a restlessness that is usually less overt than that seen in hyperactive children – and the consequential disabilities and inadequacies that are claimed – educational and occupational underachievement, interpersonal difficulties – are those that are common to many psychiatric disorders that present for the first time in adult life. This lack of specificity places a burden on the diagnostician to demonstrate a historical continuity of symptomatology and disability from early childhood into adulthood. Finally, in adults and in children, comorbid disorders may not only obscure genuine ADHD symptoms, they may also mimic them. These diagnostic imperatives – the need to demonstrate historical continuity and to distinguish between the material and the comorbid – received emphasis in an influential editorial (Shaffer, 1994). Shaffer also commented anecdotally on the prevalence of self-diagnosis and the use of this diagnosis to justify past and present failures. Others (Silver, 2000) take a different view, welcoming the greater self-awareness of patients and deploring the lack of self-awareness among professional staff, resulting in a failure to refer and to diagnose. Certainly in the UK, a lack of familiarity with not only the assessment procedures, but with the very concept of adult ADHD, leads to a failure of the usual screening processes that precede a referral. In a recent UK study (van der Linden et al., 2000) referral to an adult ADHD clinic was initiated by the patient in 46% of cases, 44% by the parents, and by health professionals in only 10%. Thirty-one per cent received a diagnosis of ADHD. These patients differed from the non-ADHD group in that they were younger (average age 22.4 years), overwhelmingly male and exhibited significantly greater comorbidity (substance abuse; dissocial and impulsive personality disorders according to ICD-10). In these respects they closely resembled the childhood cohorts followed up longitudinally (Mannuzza et al., 1993). Other first assessments during adulthood studies have also reported a low proportion of positive ADHD diagnosis (Roy-Byrne et al., 1997). Asked to comment on the diagnosis, 77% of those diagnosed with ADHD expressed satisfaction; 58% of those who failed to receive that diagnosis expressed dissatisfaction (van der Linden et al., 2000).

DSM-IV criteria are detailed and explicit and can form a framework through which ADHD symptomatology can be elicited. ADHD symptoms are, however, ubiquitous and the issue of symptom overlap has never been satisfactorily resolved (Shaffer, 1994; Milberger et al., 1995; Roy-Byrne et al., 1997). Moreover, the risk of patient rater bias should not be underestimated (van der Linden et al., 2000). DSM-IV does not provide adequate quantification of symptom severity. The ADHD rating scale (Barkley, 1990) is sensitive to drug effects, but has been used mainly in that context. The accurate measure of symptom severity is a particular concern in the assessment of a disorder, the core symptoms of which are likely to attenuate over time. The self-identification of core symptoms is not in itself invariably grounds for initiating treatment; there is still need to demonstrate consequential distress and disability. The evaluation of ADHD symptoms should be supplemented by a more wide-ranging inventory of psychiatric symptomatology using an appropriate instrument, e.g. the Clinical Interview Schedule, revised edition (CIS-R), if DSM-IV is to be used. Ratings of depression, e.g. Beck's Depression Inventory (Beck et al., 1961), and personality, e.g. the Standardized Assessment of Personality (Mann et al., 1981; Pilgrim and Mann, 1990), are also recommended.

Behavioural observations play an important part in the assessment of childhood ADHD. Children exist in a highly structured, closely observed environment. Parent and teacher rating scales have been developed and refined to quantify behaviour and behavioural change in response to treatment in the home and in the school respectively. Such opportunities are rarely available in adult psychiatry. Many patients live alone. Many are unemployed. The observations of a parent, a partner or a close companion may be extremely useful and should always be sought, but such information may lack the detail and pervasiveness available during childhood. Although quantitative psychometric testing is widely used in the assessment of childhood ADHD, its role in the diagnosis of adult ADHD is less clearly established.

The choice of tests varies across studies. Some administer standardized tests of intellectual function, usually the Wechsler Adult Intelligence Scale (WAIS: Wechsler, 1981), and academic performance, such as the Wide Range Achievement Test (WRAT: Jastak and Jastak, 1978). Others use alone or in addition to the above tests that purport to measure sustained attention e.g. the Continuous Performance Test (CPT: Erlenmeyer-Kimling and Cornblatt, 1978) and impulsivity, e.g. the Matching Familiar Figures Test (MFFT: Cairnes and Cammock, 1978). Although the role of executive function in the genesis of ADHD disability is of considerable interest, there is little published work in adults. A few studies include tests such as the Stroop, the Wisconsin Card Sorting Test and the Trail-making Test in a routine neuropsychological test battery, but not with the clear aim of specifically exploring executive function. Paradigms that are employed in functional neuroimaging to explore the integrity of motor inhibitory systems, e.g. go–no-go (Vaidya et al., 1998) and Stop Task (Rubia et al., 1999) appear to have little place in clinical evaluation.

The WAIS has been used in only a limited way to characterize patient cohorts entering drug trials. Two small, early studies (Wood et al., 1976; Wender et al., 1981) recorded above-average scores. In a larger study (Mattes et al., 1984) patients did not differ from controls. The WRAT, a brief measure of word reading, spelling and arithmetical computation is employed, particularly in the USA, to identify the presence of learning deficits. Wood et al. (1976) noted an unexpectedly poor arithmetical ability. These findings were confirmed in a later drug study by the same group (Wender et al., 1981): male subjects fell below the 23rd percentile in spelling and arithmetic. Conversely, Roy-Byrne et al. (1997), comparing possible, probable and non-ADHD groups and using the revised version of the WRAT (Naglieri and McCarthy, 1980), found the ADHD group to have lower standard reading scores, but not to differ from the other groups on spelling or arithmetic. These limited data offer only a tentative guide to general intelligence and educational levels in adult ADHD, but it is worth noting that subjects with learning and specific educational difficulties were not excluded from any of the studies. They do not support the prediction (Silver, 2000) that between 30% and 50% of adults with ADHD would have learning difficulties, but subgroups may well have specific educational disabilities against a background of average or above-average general intelligence.

The CPT, in its various formats, is widely used as a measure of sustained attention. In two drug studies the active drug, though effective, did not improve CPT performance (Spencer et al., 1998; Willens et al., 1999). In a further drug trial (Gualtieri et al., 1985) ADD subjects tested at baseline made significantly fewer correct responses and more commissioned errors than a matched normal control group. One hour after the administration of the first dose of methylphenidate, correct responding improved significantly compared with placebo. The decline in commissioned errors did not reach significance. A study that used the computerized CPT reported complex but essentially negative findings. The MFFT was also used by Gualtieri et al. (1985) for baseline psychometric characteristics, but did not discriminate. Hechtman et al. (1984) compared treated and untreated hyperactive subjects and normal controls, but found no difference between the three groups.

Tests that are thought to reflect executive function include the Stroop Test, the Wisconsin Card Sorting Test and the Trail-making Test. Performance on the Stroop Test did not discriminate between treated hyperactive, untreated hyperactive and normal control groups (Hechtman et al., 1984). Patients treated with tomoxetine, a noradrenergic reuptake inhibitor, performed better on the Stroop when compared with placebo, but the extent to which the improvement was related to treatment response was not explored (Spencer et al., 1998). Pemoline did not improve pretreatment scores (Willens et al., 1999). Likewise, Wisconsin Card Sorting Test scores (Spencer et al., 1998; Willens et al., 1999) did not change to reflect response to treatment. The Trail-making Test did distinguish ADDH patients from patients with similar symptoms but without a childhood history of ADDH (Mattes et al., 1984). Few attempts have been made to develop a measure of hyperactivity for use in adults. Based on direct observation, 44% of adults, previously diagnosed as hyperactive children, were judged to be physically restless (Weiss et al., 1985). Gualtieri et al. (1985), in a trial of methylphenidate, employed a wrist actometer to record activity during the performance of a CPT. The ADD subjects were considerably more restless during baseline recordings, but though their scores fell 1 h after the first methylphenidate treatment, these did not reach significance.

Although widely employed in the assessment of childhood ADHD, the role of psychometric testing as an aid to diagnosis has yet to be established (Solanto, 2000). The position with adults is even less secure. Few studies have reported findings and these have been inconsistent. Most clinical tests are selected because they are in widespread use, standardized, available and because the psychometrist is familiar with their use. They often explore a range of cognitive functions and their findings may be difficult to interpret. But even the more carefully chosen tests lacked diagnostic specificity and are unable to discriminate between, say, inattention as a feature of ADHD and inattentiveness arising in the context of affective disorders. Psychometric testing must be regarded for the moment as an adjunctive rather than a critical component of the diagnostic process. It is probably at its most useful as a means of monitoring individual treatment response.

The requirement to obtain a reliable account of childhood ADHD symptomatology and behaviour is probably the most challenging aspect of adult assessment. The patients who first present as adults will usually not have undergone psychiatric assessment during childhood and, even if they have that assessment, it may not be as informative as it might have been due to a lack of familiarity with the concept of childhood ADHD. Even so, contemporaneous reports and documentation written by education and health care professionals are likely to constitute the most reliable and objective source of information. In their absence a detailed history, preferably from a parent or from another senior member of the family close to the patient as a child, should be obtained. The use of a childhood rating scale ensures that all of the salient symptoms and behaviours are canvassed and provides a quantified summary for purposes of comparison and diagnostic threshold. Ward et al. (1993) have published the Parents' Rating Scale, a modification of the Conners' Abbreviated Rating Scale (Conners, 1973; Sprague et al., 1974). The latest restandardization of the Conners' scale (Conners, 1997) includes DSM-IV subscales for hyperactivity-impulsivity and inattention, enabling the ADHD subtypes to be measured separately. Parental recall, whether in the form of a structured historical account or a completed rating scale, will extend across a considerable time interval and must inevitably lack the accuracy of immediate observation.

The patient may provide his or her own testimony. Several scales have been devised to tabulate and quantify their recall, of which the most widely used is the Wender Utah Rating Scale (WURS: Ward et al., 1993). Twenty-five of the 61 WURS items discriminate between patients with ADHD and two control groups – patients with unipolar depression and normal subjects. However, the items were drawn from Wender's 1971 monograph *Minimal Brain Dysfunction in Children* (Wender, 1971) and the ADHD diagnosis was based on the Utah criteria (Ward et al., 1993). Neither corresponds with current concepts of ADHD. The size and method of selection of the normal control group have been criticized (Conners and Barkley, 1985). Other diagnostic groups (borderline personality disorder; atypical major depression) may also achieve elevated scores (Ward et al., 1993). The WURS identified 33 of 46 (71.7%) ADHD patients but also identified 40% of normal subjects and 60% of patients with adult ADHD symptoms but who lacked a childhood history (Roy-Byrne et al., 1997). The scale thus demonstrates only moderate sensitivity and poor specificity. Other scales have been devised – the Brown Attention Deficit Disorder Scale (Brown, 1995); the University of Massachusetts Medical Center Protocol (Barkley, 1998) – but these do not have such wide currency. Patient recall may be less reliable than that of the parents: in one instance of disagreement (Wender et al., 1981) the parents proved a better predictor of treatment response. One-fifth of a cohort of ADDH adults followed up since childhood (Mannuzza et al., 1993) were unable to recall childhood symptoms of hyperactivity. A desire to acquire the diagnosis may introduce rater bias (Shaffer, 1994; van der Linden et al., 2000). It has been suggested that information from parents may be hard to come by due either to a lack of availability or to an unwillingness to cooperate (Ward et al., 1993; Shaffer, 1994). This has not been our experience. Most adults who present with persistent ADHD will be in their third decade; one or both parents will usually be alive, and the great majority will be prepared to assist in the assessment process. Every attempt should be made to obtain a parental testimony before reaching a diagnostic conclusion.

Treatment and management

Adult ADHD represents a persistence of the childhood disorder into adult years; it is essentially the same condition and, when due allowance has been made for maturational changes, the approach to treatment and management differs only in detail. Indeed, in those cases in which diagnosis was first made in childhood or adolescence, treatment may be continued unchanged into adulthood. Others will present for the first time as adults. Those that meet full DSM-IV criteria for ADHD will usually be offered treatment; those who fail to meet full criteria while providing convincing evidence of childhood ADHD – some of the symptoms of which have persisted and proved troublesome – may still be offered a therapeutic trial. Pharmacological treatment is central to the management of adult ADHD. The cerebral stimulants, a class of drugs that has as its central action an increase in intrasynaptic dopamine and noradrenaline (norepinephrine), are in the great majority of cases the treatment of first choice. Other drugs, most notably some of the tricyclic antidepressants, may have an adjunctive role, particularly in the management of comorbidity and of un-wanted side-effects. The role of psychological treatment, while of considerable potential interest, remains very largely unexplored.

Stimulants: efficacy

Cerebral stimulants remain the mainstay of pharmacological treatment of adult ADHD. Pemoline, a phenylethylamine that structurally closely resembles methylphenidate and amfetamine, has a longer half-life (11–13 h in adults), thus permitting a single daily dosage regime. Against this advantage must be set reports of serious hepatotoxicity in children (Shevell and Schreiber, 1996) and this risk may limit its usefulness as a first-choice stimulant. Methylphenidate and dextramfetamine are now the most widely prescribed stimulants for adult ADHD in the UK. Adderall, a combination of *d-l*-amfetamine, and sustained-release preparations of methylphenidate and dexamfetamine are also widely prescribed in the USA but are less readily available elsewhere.

The efficacy of the cerebral stimulants in adult ADHD has received far less attention than in children. Nine controlled studies, comprising a total of 292 subjects, have been carried out to date, seven assessing methylphenidate, three pemoline and one amfetamine compounds. Overall responsiveness is lower in adults than in children and ranges (based on controlled studies) from 25% to 73% (mean 60%) compared with a response rate in children of 6–12 years of age of 60–70% and in adolescence of 75% (Willens and Spencer, 2000). The relatively lower level of responding may be attributed in particular to unsatis-factory diagnostic criteria and inadequate doses, and perhaps also to comorbid-ity, noncompliance and poorly developed criteria for measuring responsive-ness. The evaluation of the presence of childhood ADHD symptoms in adults presenting for the first time remains contentious and may explain some of the variability in treatment outcomes. There is a lack of significant correlation between dose, serum level, symptom response and side-effects (Spencer et al., 1995): serum levels corresponding to the same dose may vary four- to fivefold between individuals. Consequently drug dosage is to a considerable extent empirical. There are however grounds for considering whether the relatively poor outcome of some earlier studies could have been due to inadequate dosage (Sachdev and Trollor, 2000). In the first four controlled studies of methylphenidate the average drug dose was 0.6 mg/kg and the average response rate was 50%. In the fifth study (Spencer et al., 1995) a dose of 1 mg/kg was used and a response rate of 78% was reported. Given the biphasic character of the behavioural response to cerebral stimulants, increasing dosage will eventually give rise to restlessness, insomnia, anorexia and other features of increased monoaminergic stimulation, but the point at which this occurs will vary greatly from individual to individual and will be difficult to predict. When due account is taken of variations in dosage there is little reason to suspect any significant difference in therapeutic potency between the three most commonly used cerebral stimulants. The sustained-release preparations have yet to be subjected to controlled trials. The cerebral stimulants would seem therefore to be effective in adult ADHD, possibly as effective as in the childhood disorder, but this must, for the moment, remain a qualified judgement given the limited database and the observation that more than half of the published controlled studies were conducted in two major centres in the USA.

Contraindications

There are few absolute contraindications to the use of cerebral stimulants in adult ADHD, although there are many situations in which they should be introduced and monitored with more than usual caution. The presence of significant comorbidity may suggest that treatment of ADHD be deferred until the comorbid state has been addressed. Indeed, until this has been done it may not be possible to evaluate the significance of ADHD symptomatology. Minor degrees of affective comorbidity may not detract from the effectiveness of treatment (Spencer et al., 1995) but in another study (Willens et al., 1999) subjects with comorbid anxiety showed a poorer response to pemoline. There is increased comorbidity due to substance abuse in adult ADHD, but although such patients overall show little response to cerebral stimulants, treatment does not appear to exacerbate abuse or cause craving (Willens and Spencer, 2000).

Side-effects

Cerebral stimulants are usually well tolerated in adults. The commonest side-effects in order of frequency of occurrence are: insomnia, edginess, diminished appetite, dysphoria and headaches (Willens and Spencer, 2000). They are most prominent shortly after the introduction of treatment or after an increase in dosage. They usually remit over time or, failing this, following a reduction in dosage. Cerebral stimulant-induced psychosis has been reported anecdotally in 20 cases in children, but not in adults. The potential for iatrogenic substance abuse clearly exists, but likewise has not been reported. The effects of cerebral stimulants on heart rate and blood pressure are, in adults, minimal. Behavioural rebound and cognitive construction phenomena have been observed in children, but have received little attention in adults.

Clinical management

The pharmacokinetics of cerebral stimulants do not differ greatly in adults from older children and adolescents, though the half-life of pemoline is longer (11–13 h in adults; 7–8 h in children). Behavioural effects for both methylphenidate and dexamfetamine peak at 1–2 h postingestion and dissipate at 4–6 h and a divided-dose regime is unavoidable. The first dose is best taken shortly after waking, the second at midday and the third (if needed) during late afternoon, but the precise timing will vary from subject to subject and should coincide with wearing-off effects. It is advisable to start at a low dose (e.g. a total daily dose of 15–30 mg in divided doses) increasing incrementally at 2–3-weekly intervals towards a dose that should reflect an optimal balance between benefit and side-effects. Some patients will respond to methylphenidate but not to dexamfetamine and vice versa. The drug, whichever one is first chosen, should be increased incrementally for as long as it is well tolerated. If it is poorly tolerated or ineffectual, even at a high dose, then the alternative drug should be substituted.

Childhood cohort follow-up studies suggest that, over a 5–10-year period, many – perhaps most late adolescents and young adults will cease to require treatment. However, it may be difficult to predict the needs of individuals. Some subjects will, deliberately or inadvertently, withdraw from medication and their response to withdrawal, if sustained, may provide a guide as to whether continued medication is necessary. In any event a judiciously timed 'drug holiday' is advisable every 1–2 years to test the need for therapy.

Other drug treatment

Although in the majority of cases the first-line treatment will be the cerebral stimulants, a definite role exists for other categories of drugs, particularly the tricyclic antidepressants. Other drug groups, such as the α-antagonists, the β-blockers, and the monoamine oxidase inhibitors (MAOIs) have been used alone or in combination with the cerebral stimulants, but though often reported on favourably in open trial, none has been subjected to the rigor of controlled studies. The tricyclic antidepressants may be used alone, in the event of failure to respond to both methylphenidate and dexamfetamine, or in conjunction with a cerebral stimulant in the presence of comorbid depression or to manage refractory cerebral stimulant side-effects such as weight loss or insomnia. In children tricyclic antidepressants compare with cerebral stimulants in their effect on hyperactivity and impulsiveness, but not on attentional symptoms. Tricyclic antidepressants and cerebral stimulants have not been directly compared in adults, but in a 6-week double-blind placebo-controlled study of desipramine (Willens et al., 1996), all three symptom groups responded. Symptoms declined steadily over the 6-week period. The same group (Spencer et al., 1998) reported that tomoxetine, a highly selective noradrenergic reuptake inhibitor, achieved a comparable reduction in symptomatology over a 3-week period.

The MAOIs have been used in both children and adults, but usage is limited to those who are able to adhere to dietary constraints. Selegeline, a partial but relatively selective MAOI B inhibitor, does not have dietary implications and was reported to have a 60% success rate in adults in a small controlled study (Wood et al., 1983).

The value of other drug treatments remains to be established. The α_{2A}-agonists such as clonidine may prove effective against impulsiveness, hyperactivity and aggression, but not against inattention. They may cause hypotension and drowsiness, but in combined therapy may offset cerebral stimulant-induced insomnia. Clomipramine may also act against aggressive behaviour, but causes seizures in 1.5% of adults. The more sedative neuroleptics may have some effect, but any consideration of their immediate or delayed side-effects should preclude any role in the management of ADHD. The selective serotonin reuptake inhibitors have received little attention by way of controlled trials, but clinical experience suggests that they are at best ineffectual and may even aggravate some ADHD symptoms.

Further research

The recognition that ADHD symptoms may persist into adulthood is a recent development and the principal parameters of the condition have yet to be adequately charted. The very existence of adult ADHD is still questioned; with more reason, the prevalence of the disorder and the indications for pharmacological treatment are keenly debated. These issues may be addressed both through population-based studies designed to estimate age-related prevalence and through the development of more uniform and standardized diagnostic procedures. Such are the vagaries of retrospective diagnosis that any attempt to determine adult prevalence must take as its starting point the longitudinal studies of childhood cohorts: only in this way can the diagnosis of adult ADHD be achieved with any reliability. The more advanced longitudinal studies (Weiss et al., 1985; Mannuzza et al., 1991a, 1993) provide valuable information about the attritional decline in ADHD symptomatology, the development of adult comorbidity and the relation of adult comorbidity to symptom persistence; based on clinical referrals they cannot offer any indication of prevalence. This can only be accomplished through large-scale unbiased community-based surveys; such programmes exist (Taylor et al., 1996) but have yet to undergo adult assessment. It is important that samples should not be restricted to pure ADHD but should include comorbid conditions, particularly conduct disorder. Longitudinal studies could also shed light on factors predicting symptom persistence, a surprisingly neglected area. In the meantime it is noteworthy that patients participating in the more advanced studies such as the New York cohorts, last reported at the age of 25 (Mannuzza et al., 1991a, 1993) would now be into their fourth decade. Further observations should confirm or refute conjectural extrapolations based on earlier sampling points.

Diagnostic assessment procedures vary between centres. The existence of dual classificatory systems may be an inconvenience, but there is no reason why data should not be collected that satisfy both sets of criteria. There must be concern that the salient features, e.g. age, gender distribution, comorbidity, that characterize the longitudinal cohorts and some of the patient groups diagnosed for the first time in adult life differ so markedly, to the extent that the possibility that the samples are drawn from quite separate populations cannot be dismissed. A direct comparison of these two broad categories of referrals, using the same assessment protocols and rating scales, might provide some clarification.

Understandably, longitudinal studies have been primarily concerned with monitoring the persistence of ADHD symptoms; the consequence of the remitted syndrome for subsequent personality and cognitive development and for social and occupational adjustment has received less attention. But there is some suggestion that ADHD in remission may also predict the emergence of similar patterns of comorbidity and socioeconomic maladjustment. Whether this is a delayed consequence of an earlier period of social and educational disadvantage or an age-related expression of a still-unfolding neurodevelopmental syndrome merits further study.

REFERENCES

American Psychiatric Association. (1968). *Diagnostic and Statistical Manual of Mental Disorders*, 2nd edn. Washington, DC: American Psychiatric Association.

American Psychiatric Association. (1980). *Diagnostic and Statistical Manual of Mental Disorders*, 3rd edn. Washington, DC: American Psychiatric Association.

American Psychiatric Association. (1987). *Diagnostic and Statistical Manual of Mental Disorders*, 3rd edn, revised. Washington, DC: American Psychiatric Association.

American Psychiatric Association. (1994). *Diagnostic and Statistical Manual of Mental Disorders*, 4th edn. Washington, DC: American Psychiatric Association.

Babinski, L.M., Hartsough, C.S. and Lambert, N.M. (1999). Childhood conduct problems, hyperactivity-impulsivity, and inattention as predictors of adult criminal activity. *Journal of Child Psychology and Psychiatry*, **40**, 347–55.

Barkley, R.A. (1990). *Attention Deficit Hyperactivity Disorder: A Handbook for Diagnosis and Treatment*. New York: Guilford Press.

Barkley, R.A. (1998). *Attention-Deficit Hyperactivity Disorder: A Handbook for Diagnosis and Treatment*, 2nd edn. New York: Guilford Press.

Beck, A.T., Ward, C.E., Mendelson, M., Mock, J. and Erbaugh, J. (1961). An inventory for measuring depression. *Archives of General Psychiatry*, **4**, 561–71.

Biederman, J., Faraone, S.V., Spencer, T. et al. (1993). Patterns of psychiatric comorbidity, cognition, and psychosocial functioning in adults with attention deficit hyperactivity disorder. *American Journal of Psychiatry*, **150**, 1792–8.

Biederman, J., Faraone, S.V., Mick, E. et al. (1995). High risk for attention deficit hyperactivity disorder among children of parents with childhood onset of the disorder: a pilot study. *American Journal of Psychiatry*, **152**, 431–5.

Bird, H.R., Canino, G., Rubio-Stipec, M. et al. (1988). Estimates of the prevalence of childhood maladjustment in a community survey in Puerto Rico. *Archives of General Psychiatry*, **45**, 1120–6.

Brown, T. (1995). *Brown Attention Deficit Disorder Scales*. San Antonio: Psychological Corporation.

Cairnes, E. and Cammock, T. (1978). Development of a more reliable version of the matching familiar figures test. *Developmental Psychology*, **14**, 555–60.

Cantwell, D.B. and Baker, L. (1992). Attention deficit disorder with and without hyperactivity: a review and comparison of matched groups. *Journal of the American Academy of Child and Adolescent Psychiatry*, **31**, 432–8.

Clements, S.D. (1966). *Minimal Brain Dysfunction in Children: Terminology and Identification*. Public Health Service publication no. 1415. Washington, DC: Department of Health, Education, and Welfare.

Conners, C.K. (1973). Rating scales for use in drug studies with children: special issue on children. *Psychopharmacological Bulletin*, 24–42.

Conners, C.K. (1997). *The Conners Rating Scales, Revised: Technical Manual*. Toronto, Canada.

Conners, C.K. and Barkley, R.A. (1985). Rating scales and checklists for child psychopharmacology. *Psychopharmacology Bulletin*, **21**, 809–38.

Erllenmeyer-Kimling, L. and Cornblatt, B. (1978). Attentional measures in a study of children at high-risk for schizophrenia. *Journal of Psychiatric Research*, **14**, 93–8.

Gittelman, R., Mannuzza, S., Shenker, R. and Bonagura, N. (1985). Hyperactive boys almost grown up. *Archives of General Psychiatry*, **42**, 937–47.

Gualtieri, C.T., Ondrusek, G. and Finley, C. (1985). Attention deficit disorders in adults. *Clinical Neuropharmacology*, **8**, 343–56.

Hart, E., Lahey, B., Loeber, R., Applegate, B. and Frick, P.J. (1995). Developmental change in attention-deficit hyperactivity disorder in boys: a four year longitudinal study. *Journal of Abnormal Child Psychology*, **23**, 729–49.

Hechtman, L. and Weiss, G. (1986). Controlled prospective fifteen year follow-up of hyperactives as adults: non-medical drug and alcohol use and anti-social behaviour. *Canadian Journal of Psychiatry*, **31**, 557–67.

Hechtman, L., Weiss, G., Perlman, T. and Amsel, R. (1984). Hyperactives as young adults: initial predictors of adult outcome. *Journal of the American Academy of Child Psychiatry*, **23**, 250–60.

Hill, J.C. and Schoener, E.P. (1996). Age-dependent decline of attention deficit hyperactivity disorder. *American Journal of Psychiatry*, **153**, 1143–6.

Jastak, J. and Jastak, S. (1978). *A Wide-range Achievement Test Manual.* Wilmington, Delaware: Jastak Associates.

Mann, A.H., Jenkins, R., Cutting, J.C. and Cowen, J.C. and Cowen, P.J. (1981). The development and use of a standardised assessment of abnormal personality. *Psychological Medicine*, **11**, 839–47.

Mannuzza, S., Klein, R.G., Bonagura, N. et al. (1991a). Hyperactive boys almost grown up, V: replication of psychiatric status. *Archives of General Psychiatry*, **48**, 77–83.

Mannuzza, S., Gittelman Klein, R. and Addalli, K.A. (1991b). Young adult mental status of hyperactive boys and their brothers: a prospective follow up study. *Journal of the American Academy of Child and Adolescent Psychiatry*, **13**, 743–51.

Mannuzza, S., Klein, R.G., Besslea, A., Malloy, P. and LaPadula, M. (1993). Adult outcome of hyperactive boys: educational achievement occupational work, and psychiatric status. *Archives of General Psychiatry*, **50**, 565–77.

Mattes, J.A., Boswell, L. and Oliver, H. (1984). Methyl phenidate effects on symptoms of attention deficit disorder in adults. *Archives of General Psychiatry*, **41**, 1059–63.

Milberger, S. Biederman, J., Faraone, S.V., Murphy, J. and Tsuang, M.T. (1995). Attention deficit hyperactivity disorder and comorbid disorders: issues of overlapping symptoms. *American Journal of Psychiatry*, **152**, 1793–9.

Murphy, K.R. and Barkley, R.A. (1996). Attention deficit hyperactivity disorder in adults. *Comprehensive Psychiatry*, **37**, 393–401.

Naglieri, J.A. and McCarthy, A. (1980). WISC-R correlations with WRAT achievement scores. *Perception and Motor Skills*, **51**, 392–7.

Pilgrim, J. and Mann, A.H. (1990). Use of the ICD-10 version of standardised assessment of personality to determine the prevalence of personality disorder in psychiatric inpatients. *Psychological Medicine*, **20**, 985–92.

Roy-Byrne, P., Scheele, L., Brinkley, J. et al. (1997). Adult attention-deficit hyperactivity disorder: assessment guidelines based on clinical presentation to a speciality clinic. *Comprehensive Psychiatry*, **38**, 133–40.

Rubia, K., Overmeyer, S., Taylor, E. et al. (1999). Hypofrontality in attention deficit hyperactivity disorder during higher order motor control: a study using fMRI. *American Journal of Psychiatry*, **156**, 891–6.

Sachdev, P.F. and Trollor, J.N. (2000). How high a dose of stimulant medication in attention deficit hyperactivity disorder? *Australian and New Zealand Journal of Psychiatry*, **34**, 645–50.

Safer, D.J. and Krager, J.N. (1988). A survey of medication treatment for hyperactive/inattentive students. *Journal of the American Medical Association*, **260**, 2256–8.

Sandberg, S. (1996). Hyperkinetic or attention deficit disorder. *British Journal of Psychiatry*, **169**, 10–17.

Shaffer, D. (1994). Attention deficit hyperactivity disorder in adults. *American Journal of Psychiatry*, **151**, 633–8.

Shevell, M. and Schreiber, M. (1996). Pemoline-associated hepatic failure: a critical analysis of the literature. *Paediatric Neurology*, **16**, 14–16.

Silver, L.B. (2000). Attention-deficit/hyperactivity disorder in adult life. *Child and Adolescent Psychiatric Clinics of North America*, **9**, 511–23.

Solanto, M.B. (2000). The predominantly inattentive sub-type of attention-deficit/hyperactivity disorder. *CNS Spectrums*, **5**, 45–51.

Spencer, T., Wilens, D. Biederman, J. et al. (1995). A double-blind, crossover comparison of methyl phenidate and placebo in adults of childhood-onset attention-deficit hyperactivity disorder. *Archives of General Psychiatry*, **52**, 434–43.

Spencer, T., Biederman, J., Wilens, T. et al. (1996). Pharmacotherapy of attention deficit disorder across the life cycle. *Journal of the American Academy of Child and Adolescent Psychiatry*, **35**, 409–32.

Spencer, T., Biederman, J., Wilens, T. et al. (1998). Affectiveness and tolerability of tomoxetine in adults with attention deficit hyperactivity disorder. *American Journal of Psychiatry*, **155**, 693–5.

Sprague, R.L., Cohen, M. and Werry, J.S. (1974). *Normative Data on the Conners Teachers' Rating Scale and Abbreviated Scale*. Technical report. Urbana-Champaign: Children's Research Centre, University of Illinois.

Taylor, E., Chadwick, O., Heptinstall, U. and Danckaerts, M. (1996). Hyperactivity and conduct problems as risk factors for adolescent development. *Journal of the American Academy of Child and Adolescent Psychiatry*, **35**, 1213–26.

Vaidya, C.J., Austin, G., Kirkorian, G. et al. (1998). Selective effects of methylphenidate in attention deficit hyperactivity disorder: a functional magnetic resonance imaging study. *Proceedings of the National Academy of Sciences of the United States of America*, **95**, 14494–9.

van der Linden, G., Young, S., Ryan, P. and Toone, B. (2000). Attention deficit hyperactivity disorder in adults – experience of the first National Health Service clinic in the United Kingdom. *Journal of Mental Health*, **9**, 527–35.

Ward, M.F., Wender, P.H. and Reimherr, F.W. (1993). The Wender Utah rating scale: an aid in the retrospective diagnosis of childhood attention deficit hyperactivity disorder. *American Journal of Psychiatry*, **150**, 885–9.

Wechsler, D. (1981). *Manual for the Wechsler Adult Intelligence Scale – Revised*. San Antonio: Psychological Corporation.

Weiss, G., Hechtman, L., Milroy, T. and Perlman, T. (1985). Psychiatric status of hyperactives as adults: a controlled prospective 15-year follow-up of 63 hyperactive children. *Journal of the American Academy of Child Psychiatry*, **24**, 211–20.

Wender, P.H. (1971). *Minimal Brain Dysfunction in Children*. New York, NY: John Wiley.

Wender, P.H., Reimherr, F.W. and Wood, D.R. (1981). Attention deficit disorder ('minimal brain dysfunction') in adults. A replication study of diagnosis and drug treatment. *Archives of General Psychiatry*, **38**, 449–56.

Wender, P.H., Reimherr, F.W., Wood, D.R. and Ward, M. (1985). A controlled study of methylphenidate in the treatment of attention deficit disorder, residual type, in adults. *American Journal of Psychiatry*, **142**, 547–52.

Willens, T.E. and Spencer, T.J. (2000). The stimulants revisited. *Child and Adolescent Psychiatric Clinics of North America*, **9**, 573–603.

Willens, T.E., Biederman, J., Prince, J. et al. (1996). Six-week, double-blind, placebo controlled study of desipramine for adult attention deficit hyperactivity disorder. *American Journal of Psychiatry*, **153**, 1147–53.

Willens, T.E., Biederman, J., Spencer, T.J. et al. (1998). Controlled trial of high doses of pemoline for adults with attention-deficit/hyperactivity disorder. *Journal of Clinical Psychopharmacology*, **19**, 257–64.

Willens, D.E., Biederman, J., Spencer, T. et al. (1999). Controlled trial of high doses of pemoline for adults with attention deficit/hyperactivity disorder. *Journal of Clinical Psychopharmacology*, **19**, 257–64.

Wood, D.R., Reimherr, F.W., Wender, P.H. and Johnson, G.E. (1976). Diagnosis and treatment of minimal brain dysfunction in adults. *Archives of General Psychiatry*, **3**, 1453–60.

Wood, D.R., Reimherr, F.W., and Wender, P.H. (1983). The use of L-deprenyl in the treatment of attention deficit disorder, residual type (ADD, RT). *Psychopharmacological Bulletin*, **19**, 627–9.

World Health Organization. (1992). *ICD-10 Classification of Mental and Behavioural Disorders: Clinical Descriptions and Diagnostic Guidelines*. Geneva: World Health Organization.

Index